FOOD, NUTRITION AND HEALTH

FOOD, NUTRITION AND HEALTH

SECOND EDITION

EDITED BY LINDA TAPSELL

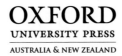

OXFORD
UNIVERSITY PRESS
AUSTRALIA & NEW ZEALAND

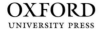

OXFORD
UNIVERSITY PRESS

Oxford University Press is a department of the University of Oxford.
It furthers the University's objective of excellence in research,
scholarship, and education by publishing worldwide. Oxford is a registered
trademark of Oxford University Press in the UK and in certain other
countries.

Published in Australia by
Oxford University Press
Level 8, 737 Bourke Street, Docklands, Victoria 3008, Australia.

A catalogue record for this
book is available from the
National Library of Australia

NATIONAL
LIBRARY
OF AUSTRALIA

ISBN 9780190304867

Reproduction and communication for educational purposes

Edited by Anne Mulvaney
Cover design by OUPANZ
Cover Image: Shutterstock
Text design by Sardine Design
Typeset by Newgen KnowledgeWorks Pvt. Ltd., Chennai, India
Proofread by Pete Cruttenden
Indexed by Jenny Browne
Printed in China by Golden Cup Printing Co. Ltd.

CONTENTS

OXFORD UNIVERSITY PRESS

EXTENDED CONTENTS

PART 1: FOOD AND NUTRITION BASICS

CHAPTER 1: FOOD AND HEALTH: WORKING WITH NUTRITION
Linda Tapsell

CHAPTER 2: DIETARY GUIDELINES: PLANNING A HEALTHY DIET
Linda Tapsell and Elizabeth Neale

CHAPTER 3: CONSUMING FOOD: DIGESTION, ABSORPTION AND METABOLISM
Linda Tapsell

CHAPTER 8: WATER, ALCOHOL AND BEVERAGES
Vinodkumar Gopaldasani and Rebecca Thorne

CHAPTER 9: FAT-SOLUBLE VITAMINS: A, D, E AND K
Olivia Wright, Vicki Flood and Linda Tapsell

CHAPTER 10: WATER-SOLUBLE VITAMINS: B AND C
Linda Tapsell

CHAPTER 11: MAJOR MINERALS: SODIUM, POTASSIUM, CALCIUM, MAGNESIUM AND PHOSPHORUS
Linda Tapsell

OXFORD UNIVERSITY PRESS

CHAPTER 15: NUTRITION DURING INFANCY AND CHILDHOOD
Sara Grafenauer, Kanita Kunaratnam and Vicki Flood

CHAPTER 16: NUTRITION DURING ADOLESCENCE
Clare Collins, Rebecca Haslam, Annette Murphy, Kristine Pezdirc and Lee Ashton

CHAPTER 17: NUTRITION DURING ADULTHOOD AND THE PREVENTION OF CHRONIC DISEASE
Linda Tapsell

LIST OF FIGURES AND TABLES

FIGURES

TABLES

LIST OF CASE STUDIES

OXFORD UNIVERSITY PRESS

LIST OF ABBREVIATIONS

AA	arachidonic acid
ABS	Australian Bureau of Statistics
ADH	anti-diuretic hormone
AEE	activity energy expenditure
AGHE	Australian Guide to Healthy Eating
AI	adequate intake
AIHW	Australian Institute of Health and Welfare
AMD	age-related macular degeneration
AMDR	acceptable macronutrient distribution range
AOAC	Association of Official Analytical Chemists
APD	accredited practising dietitian
AUSNUT	Australian Food and Nutrient Database
BGL	blood glucose level
BMI	body mass index
BMR	basal metabolic rate
CDC	Centers for Disease Control and Prevention
CHO	carbohydrate
CHS	Cardiovascular Health Study
CKD	chronic kidney disease
CMRF	cardiometabolic risk factors
CSIRO	Commonwealth Scientific and Industrial Research Organisation
CVD	cardiovascular disease
DASH	Dietary Approaches to Stop Hypertension
DIT	diet-induced thermogenesis
DNA	deoxyribonucleic acid
DPA	docosahexaenoic acid
EAR	estimated average requirement
EER	estimated energy requirement
EPA	eicosapentaenoic acid
FAO	Food and Agriculture Organization (United Nations)

FDA	Food and Drug Administration (USA)
FFQ	food frequency questionnaire
FOS	fructo oligosaccharides
FSANZ	Food Standards Australia New Zealand
GDM	gestational diabetes mellitus
GI	glycaemic index
GOS	galacto oligosaccharides
GRAS	generally recognised as safe
HACCP	Hazard Analysis Critical Control Point
HDL	high-density lipoprotein
HFAB	Healthy Food Access Basket
IDA	iron deficiency anaemia
IDD	iodine deficiency disorders
IDL	intermediate-density lipoprotein
LA	linoleic acid
LBM	lean body mass
LCN	low-calorie sweetener
LCPUFA	long chain polyunsaturated fatty acids
LDL	low-density lipoprotein
LOAEL	lowest observed adverse effect level
LOS	length of stay
MAMP	microbe associated molecular patterns
MCT	medium chain triglyceride
ME	metabolisable energy
MET	metabolic equivalent
MNA	Mini Nutritional Assessment
MUFA	monounsaturated fatty acid
NHMRC	National Health and Medical Research Council
NIP	nutrition information panel
NOAEL	no adverse effect level
NRV	Nutrient Reference Values
NUTTAB	Nutrient Tables for Australian Foods
PAL	physical activity level
PCA	principal component analysis

OXFORD UNIVERSITY PRESS

PHF	potentially hazardous food
PMSEIC	Prime Minister's Science, Engineering and Innovation Council
PTN	protein
PUFA	polyunsaturated fatty acids
RCT	randomised controlled trial
RDI	recommended dietary intake
REE	resting energy expenditure
ROS	reactive oxygen species
SCFA	short chain fatty acids
SDT	suggested dietary target
SES	socioeconomic status
SFA	saturated fatty acids
SSB	sugar-sweetened beverage
TEF	thermic effect of food
TFA	trans fatty acids
UIC	urinary iodine concentration
UL	upper level of intake
UPF	ultra-processed food
USI	universal salt iodisation
VDR	vitamin D receptor
VLDL	very-low-density lipoprotein
WHAS	Women's Health and Aging Studies
WHO	World Health Organization

ABOUT THE EDITOR

LINDA TAPSELL AM PHD FDAA

Linda Tapsell is a Senior Professor, Nutrition and Dietetics in the School of Medicine at the University of Wollongong, and the Illawarra Health and Medical Research Institute, New South Wales. She holds a Bachelor of Science (Biochemistry and Pharmacology) and Post Graduate Diploma in Nutrition and Dietetics from the University of Sydney, a Masters of Health Personnel Education from the University of New South Wales and a PhD in Nutrition and Public Health from the University of Wollongong. Professor Tapsell began her career in healthcare working in large teaching hospitals and community health. She has been an academic for 28 years, teaching multitudes of nutrition and dietetic students and supervising more than 20 PhD graduates. She has had a stellar research career, having led two major food research centres and been the chief investigator of dietary trials conducted over a 25-year period examining the effects of food consumption on health. Professor Tapsell has had over 200 articles published in scientific journals and has served on a number of national and international nutrition science advisory committees, including those relating to grant reviews, dietary guidelines and nutrient reference values. She is a Fellow of both the Dietitians Association of Australia (DAA) and the Nutrition Society of Australia, and a long-standing member of the American Society of Nutrition. In 2015, Professor Tapsell was named a member of the Order of Australia (AM) for 'significant service to health science as an academic and clinician specialising in diet and nutrition'.

OXFORD UNIVERSITY PRESS

CONTRIBUTORS

ANNE MCMAHON

Dr Anne-Therese McMahon is a Senior Lecturer at the University of Wollongong whose research focuses on understanding food behaviour and health outcomes. Her work primarily draws upon qualitative health research methodologies to understand complex human behaviour from the perspectives of the participants themselves. Dr McMahon is now also broadening her work to include planetary health imperatives and intersections with human health, focusing her attention on food sustainability practices. This includes identifying, implementing and evaluating local and international food initiatives involving students, community partners and researchers in public health and nutrition disciplines with a view to supporting healthy communities overall.

ANNETTE MURPHY

Annette Murphy is a Senior Clinical Dietitian working at the John Hunter Hospital in Newcastle. She has nearly 20 years of experience working in research fields and as a clinical dietitian. She has held positions as a Lecturer at the University of Newcastle in the areas of Paediatric Dietetics and Community and Clinical Dietetics. She has co-authored numerous book chapters and assisted in the writing of a number of academic papers.

CLARE COLLINS

Professor Clare Collins is a National Health and Medical Research Council (NHMRC) Senior Research Fellow, Professor of Nutrition and Dietetics and Director of Research for the School of Health Sciences, Faculty of Health and Medicine, and Deputy Director, Priority Research Centre in Physical Activity and Nutrition at the University of Newcastle. In 2017, Professor Collins was awarded the Hunter Medical Research Institute's Researcher of the Year. Her research areas include dietary intake assessment and evaluating the impact of food and nutrition across key life stages and chronic disease conditions. Professor Collins is a Fellow of the DAA, has published over 300 manuscripts, supervised 25 higher degree research candidates, has been a DAA media spokesperson for 18 years and is a sought-after nutrition media commentator.

ELIZABETH NEALE

Dr Elizabeth Neale is an Accredited Practising Dietitian whose current role is as a Career Development Fellow (Lecturer) in the School of Medicine at the University of Wollongong. Dr Neale's research focuses on the evidence-based framework in nutrition, with a particular focus on the methodologies of systematic reviews and meta-analyses in nutrition. She also has research expertise in exploring the impact of whole foods and dietary patterns on risk factors for chronic diseases.

GARY DYKES

Professor Gary Dykes is currently the Acting Head, School of Public Health at Curtin University. He holds a PhD in microbiology from the University of the Witwatersrand in South Africa.

Professor Dykes is an experienced researcher who has pursued a diverse international career spanning a number of research organisations and universities in South Africa, New Zealand, Canada and Malaysia, as well as in Australia. He is an active researcher in the area of public health microbiology with a focus on enteric bacterial foodborne pathogens and has published widely in this area.

JOANNA RUSSELL

Dr Joanna Russell is a public health nutritionist, lecturer and early career researcher based in the Faculty of Social Sciences at the University of Wollongong. She was awarded her PhD in 2014 and her research focuses on the methodological challenges of measuring population level food security and diet quality. Building on her PhD research, Dr Russell is involved in developing appropriate measurement tools to assess food security in Australian older adults.

KANITA KUNARATNAM

Kanita Kunaratnam is currently pursuing her PhD at the University of Sydney, looking into child and maternal dietary patterns. She has a background in nutrition and dietetics and has over 10 years of experience working as a dietitian in many different settings including hospitals, public health and community health. Her research interests are in child and maternal nutrition, nutrition policy and public health, and childhood obesity. As a mother of three young children, she thoroughly enjoys combining the experience of motherhood and parenting with evidence-based research to positively influence the growth and development of children.

KAREN CHARLTON

Dr Karen Charlton, PhD AdvAPD RPHNutr, is an Associate Professor who teaches public health nutrition at the University of Wollongong. She researches the role of diet in the prevention and management of chronic diseases, particularly hypertension and cognitive decline. She advocates for improved models of nutritional care across the lifespan, from pregnancy to nutrition in old age. Her work has been translated into policy, in the context of salt reduction strategies and iodine deficiency.

KAREN WALTON

Dr Karen Walton is an Advanced Accredited Practising Dietitian and an Associate Professor at the University of Wollongong. Her research interests include nutrition support for older adults in the community, hospitals and residential aged care; particularly regarding access to food and beverage packaging and food service interventions to enhance dietary intakes among older adults.

KRISTINE PEZDIRC

Dr Kristine Pezdirc works as a clinical trial project officer in the School of Medicine and Public Health at the University of Newcastle. She was awarded her PhD from the University of Newcastle in February 2016. She also completed a Bachelor of Nutrition and Dietetics (Hons I) at the University of Newcastle in 2010. Dr Pezdirc's research areas of interest include young adults, fruit and vegetable intake, biomarkers (carotenoids) and skin colour.

LAUREN WILLIAMS

Professor Lauren Williams is Head of Discipline of Nutrition and Dietetics at Griffith University, and has honorary professorial appointments at the University of Newcastle and the University of Canberra.

Her undergraduate degree was in science (Honours) and she also holds tertiary qualifications in social science, health promotion and dietetics, and a PhD in public health nutrition. Professor Williams has been an academic for over 25 years, primarily in dietetic education, and previously worked as a public health nutritionist. Lauren has published books, book chapters and journal articles in her research areas of weight control, gendered dieting, the rural and allied health workforce, and the sociological aspects of food and eating. She has co-edited four editions of the OUP academic text and reader *A Sociology of Food and Nutrition: The Social Appetite* with John Germov. She is a Fellow of the DAA.

LEE ASHTON

Dr Lee Ashton is a Postdoctoral researcher in the Priority Research Centre for Physical Activity and Nutrition at the University of Newcastle. He was awarded his PhD from the University of Newcastle in March 2017. He also completed a Master of Science in Nutrition, Obesity & Health at the University of Leeds in 2011 and a Bachelor of Science (Hons) in Sport and Exercise Science at Leeds Beckett University in 2010, both in the United Kingdom. His research investigates physical activity and nutrition for population health, with particular emphasis on health promotion strategies for chronic disease prevention and well-being.

MICHAEL LEVERITT

Dr Michael Leveritt is a Senior Lecturer in Nutrition and Dietetics at the University of Queensland. His research and teaching activities focus on developing a better understanding of how nutrition can positively enhance athlete participation, well-being and performance in a variety of sport and exercise contexts. He is a passionate educator, practitioner and researcher with over 100 peer-reviewed research publications and his career to date has included positions with the Australian Institute of Sport as well as academic positions in New Zealand and the United Kingdom.

OLIVIA WRIGHT

Dr Olivia Wright is a Lecturer in Nutrition and Dietetics at the University of Queensland. She is passionate about helping people to remain healthy as they age, enjoys assisting the food and nutraceutical industry to design and trial innovative products to assist people's well-being, and is driven to provide high-quality education through novel teaching and assessment strategies. She has published over 30 research papers and has mentored numerous postgraduate students to achieve their nutrition practice and/or research goals. Dr Wright has a strong focus on research collaboration across disciplines and has achieved continued success in multidisciplinary research.

RANIL COOREY

Dr Ranil Coorey he is a Senior Lecturer at Curtin University. He has developed commercial food safety management systems and worked in the food industry in research and development and product innovation. His research includes a variety of industry-funded projects on chicken and red meat safety. These projects have included active packaging for microbial inactivation, modelling storage temperature and spoilage-related changes to the microbial flora and biochemistry of meat. Dr Coorey also holds an international collaborative research project on safe chicken processing. He teachers food safety and food processing and has published in these areas.

REBECCA THORNE

Rebecca Thorne has been an Accredited Practising Dietitian since 2008 and has primarily worked within the areas of research and private practice. Her qualifications include a Bachelor of Science (Exercise Science and Nutrition) and Masters of Science (with Distinction) in Nutrition and Dietetics from the University of Wollongong. As part of her experience as a clinical trials dietitian, Ms Thorne has worked across a number of NHMRC and industry-funded projects including randomised control trials, feeding studies, consultancies and qualitative studies. Her trial experience includes investigating whole diets, individual foods or nutrients, appetite and health outcomes.

REBECCA HASLAM

Dr Rebecca Haslam is an Accredited Practising Dietitian, sports dietitian and postdoctoral researcher within the Priority Research Centre for Physical Activity and Nutrition at the University of Newcastle. She completed her undergraduate degree in Nutrition and Dietetics in 2011 through the University of Newcastle and was awarded her PhD in Human Physiology in February 2017. Her areas of expertise include assessment of dietary and clinical biomarkers and how they change with certain health conditions. Other research areas include nutrition therapy for improving cancer risk and outcomes.

SARA GRAFENAUER

Dr Sara Grafenauer is an Advanced Accredited Practising Dietitian with experience in community nutrition, clinical dietetics and nutrition communications including social media. She began her career instructing parents and, more recently, tertiary students in maternal, infant and child health nutrition. She has served as a breastfeeding adviser to the Australian Multiple Birth Association and maintains her skills through a private practice focused on women's health, family and childhood nutrition and nutrition consultations for dance students.

SCOTT WINCH

Dr Scott Winch is an Aboriginal man with Gundungurra/Ngunnawal and Wiradjuri heritage. Dr Winch has 20 years' experience in Aboriginal health including key positions in various levels of government, universities and Aboriginal community-controlled organisations. He has contributed to establishing and delivering many Aboriginal health programs including programs addressing Aboriginal food security. Dr Winch also has significant research experience. He holds a PhD, a Masters of Applied Epidemiology and a Graduate Diploma in Health Service Management.

STUART JOHNSON

Dr Stuart Johnson is an Associate Professor (Food Technology) in the School of Molecular and Life Sciences at Curtin University. His work has been based in academia, industry and government around the theme of sustainable grains for health: functional foods, nutraceuticals and biomaterials. It focuses on value-addition to grains (primarily sorghum) and legumes (e.g. lupin, chickpea) through food product and process development; extraction and purification of grain protein and dietary fibre fractions for food ingredients, nutraceuticals and biomaterials; and *in vitro* and human studies to understand the health benefits of new grain foods.

VICKI FLOOD

Professor Vicki Flood is Professor of Allied Health, Western Sydney Local Health District and Faculty of Health Sciences and Charles Perkins Centre, University of Sydney. She has a background in nutrition and dietetics, epidemiology and public health, including population-based cohort studies and intervention studies to reduce chronic disease. Her main areas of research include nutrition and eye disease, food security of vulnerable population groups and micronutrient research. Professor Flood is a member of national expert advisory groups and has represented Australia at international meetings. She has received numerous research grants, been published in 150 peer-reviewed publications and supervises several research students.

VINODKUMAR GOPALDASANI

Dr Vinodkumar Gopaldasani is an experienced physician, lecturer and researcher with broad work health and safety skills and experience in epidemiology, toxicology, chemical and physical hazards, risk management and workplace health promotion. He has received grants, in partnership with collaborators, building on his strengths in public health promotion, epidemiology and work health and safety. Dr Gopaldasani is part of a multidisciplinary team of public health academics, work health and safety professionals and academics who excel in teaching and conducting research combining public health with workplace health and safety that can be translated into national policy and good practice.

YASMINE PROBST

Dr Yasmine Probst is a Senior Lecturer with the School of Medicine at the University of Wollongong and Research Fellow at the Illawarra Health and Medical Research Institute. She holds dual Masters degrees in Dietetics and Health Informatics and is recognised as an Advanced Accredited Practising Dietitian with the DAA and a Fellow of the Australasian College of Health Informatics. Her research focuses on nutrition informatics targeting food composition and its application to nutrition practice with a specific focus on dietary methodology and dietary modelling. Dr Probst has published widely and presented her work at a number of national and international conferences.

PREFACE

Understanding how food affects health is not just an area of learning—it is part of life. As the primary source of nutrients, food is fundamental to existence, yet it can easily be taken for granted. Nutrition is a fascinating area of science, and enabling better nutrition for individuals and communities is a noble endeavour for practitioners in the field.

Food, Nutrition and Health is an introductory text for all students of food and nutrition. It covers a knowledge matrix that reflects recognised principles and practices, from the basic chemistry of nutrients in foods to the nature of the food supply and the impact of food consumption on health. This second edition includes more on nutrients and metabolism and introduces important areas in Indigenous food security, social connections with food, and aspects of food science.

The text begins with the basic principles of nutrition and the contexts in which nutrition knowledge is applied. Each chapter includes a section on pathways to practice. This helps to establish the relevance of the knowledge covered to broader policy and work environments. Improving nutritional health in the community requires input from a number of angles, so there is a range of opportunities for graduates to apply the knowledge and critical appraisal skills encouraged through the text.

An appreciation of dietary guidelines and discovering ways to plan a healthy diet provides a good start. Students can consider the implications for their own dietary habits and those around them. The details of food digestion, absorption and metabolism then follow, as we explore the breakdown of food and subsequent events at the cellular and molecular level. It is here the concept of 'Food as Medicine' may begin to be appreciated. At all times we are reminded of food as the source of nutrients.

After studying the nutrients that provide fuel (protein, fat and carbohydrate) we consider the implications of energy balance and the challenges of weight management. The issue of fad diets is considered and critically appraised, building discriminative skills through the application of nutrition principles. This is then followed with more detail on micronutrients, the hidden gems in food that make a big difference to food quality. Connections are made with contemporary food and nutrition issues. This may include interesting media coverage that raises debate, implications for public health policy and healthcare practice or the need for more or different types of research to untangle the problem.

The second part of the text considers the application of nutrition knowledge under various conditions. Beginning with the nutritional implications of exercise and sport in healthy individuals, the need to meet nutritional requirements during the human lifecycle is addressed, from conception to older age. Students are able to see how requirements for food and nutrients vary depending on physiological conditions. Links with many areas of practice are exposed, from sports science to early childhood services and aged care. Students can develop an appreciation of the different contributions that can be made in support of nutritional health, as well as opportunities for specialisation and research.

An important perspective to consider here is that of Indigenous Australian food security. The underpinning problems associated with poor nutrition in Indigenous communities is a public health priority. Gaining insight into this topic reminds us that knowledge of nutrients in food is not enough, even though it is fundamental in the practice of nutrition. Introducing a cultural, social and behavioural side to nutrition broadens the reference framework. It also enables students from a range of disciplines to appreciate the significance of nutrition and the need to work collaboratively in addressing nutrition-related problems.

This brings us to the food environment, including how food is developed, how food safety is assured, and how we identify problems with food consumption and health. The final chapter of the text ties in all the perspectives, looking to the future and describing some of the current initiatives that throw light on this path.

The fundamental aspects of food, nutrition and health remain, but concepts are continually built upon with ongoing research. Not only is new knowledge generated, but new methodologies and related technologies are also implemented. This means understanding nutrition, and ways of addressing nutrition-related problems are always evolving. This is reflected in the text, as readers are taken through historical developments and challenged to think about how issues are exposed and debated. Reference materials include useful weblinks, which readers should check to keep up to date on the latest work in that area. This is particularly the case for policy- and practice-related areas that are continually under review. Food, nutrition and health is a dynamic and exciting area of study, whether built into a career or managing your own health across the lifespan.

ACKNOWLEDGMENTS

This second edition of *Food, Nutrition and Health* has been substantially developed in size and shape, following publisher consultation with academic users. There is a new pedagogical structure and new content. We acknowledge the work of all authors in the first edition, welcome the inputs of new contributors, and thank Ms Vivian Guan for her research assistance, in particular searching reference materials and updating tables and figures.

Again it has been enjoyable and satisfying working with Oxford University Press, in particular Debra James (Publishing Manager), Melpo Christofi (Content Development Specialist) and Jordan Irving (Editorial Coordinator), and our very helpful copy editor, Anne Mulvaney.

Linda Tapsell

The author and the publisher wish to thank the following copyright holders for reproduction of their material.

AIHW Australian Institute of Health and Welfare material reproduced under Creative Commons BY 3.0 (CC-BY 3.0) licence, https://creativecommons.org/licenses/by/3.0/au/, **Alamy**, pp. 96 right, 192; **Alamy/Horst Mahr**, Figure 23.1A; **Alexmax/Dreamstime**, p. 79; **Australian Bureau of Statistics**. (2006). National Aboriginal and Torres Strait Islander Health Survey, 2004-05. Canberra: ABS, Creative Commons Attribution 4.0 International licence (ABS), https://creativecommons.org/licenses/by/4.0/, Table 19.2; **Brent Parker Jones Food Photographer**, pp. 30 top, 131 top, 153 bottom left & right; **Coperion GmbH**, Figure 23.6; **Dennis Kitchen Studio**, Figure 6.5 (tuna); **Department of Health and Ageing** (2011). *Australian Health Survey: Rationale for expanding the National Health Survey series.* Canberra: DoHA. Creative Commons Attribution 4.0 International licence (ABS) Content of table from Australian Bureau of Stats, Table 22.7; **Dreamstime**, p. 80 top left & centre; **Food Standards Australia and New Zealand** material © Food Standards Australia and New Zealand, reproduced under Creative Commons BY 3.0 (CC-BY 3.0) licence, https://creativecommons.org/licenses/by/3.0/au/, **Food Standards Australia New Zealand**. (2012). AUSNUT 2007. Canberra: FSANZ, Creative Commons Attribution 3.0 Australia (CC BY 3.0) licence, https://creativecommons.org/licenses/by/3.0/au/, Table 9.7; **Getty Images/Andy Crawford**, p. 240 left; **Getty Images/DAJ**, p. 289; **Getty Images/Dorling Kindersley**, pp. 240 right, 241 left; **Getty Images/istock**, Figure 23.5; **Getty/Robin Smith**, Figure 23.9A; **Getty Images/Stockbyte**, part openers; **National Health and Medical Research Council** (NHMRC), Tables 1.1, 2.7, 3.3, 5.2, 10.2, 14.4, 14.6, p.41; A. Lee, C. N. Mhurchu, G. Sacks, B. Swinburn, W. Snowdon, S. Vandevijvere, … C. Walker. (2013). Monitoring the price and affordability of foods and diets globally, *Obesity Reviews*, 14(S1), 82-95. doi:10.1111/obr.12078, Table 21.1; **Oxford University Press** UK for material from *Essentials of Human Nutrition* by Mann & Truswell (eds), 4th edition, Oxford University Press, reproduced with permission, Figures 3.3, 3.4, 3.5, 3.6, 3.8, 3.9, 4.2, 4.4, 5.2, 5.3, 5.4, 6.4, 7.1, 7.3, 9.1, 9.2, 10.3; G. Pocock, & C. D. Richards. (2006). Human Physiology - The basis of medicine, 3rd Edition: **Oxford University Press**, Figure 7.2; **rethinksugarydrink.org.au**, p. 193; Shutterstock, Figures 2.1, 4.1 (photos only), 6.5 (except tuna), 14.3, 23.1B, 23.8 (flour & concentrate), pp. 3, 7, 8 (scales), 10, 11, 18, 19, 21, 22, 23, 30 bottom, 30 centre, 61 top, 80 top right and bottom, 91 bottom, 91 top, 96 left, 131 bottom, 133 bottom, 133 top, 191,

207, 220, 241 bottom, 241 right, 242, 246, 294, 414,502; © **State of Western Australia** (Department of Primary Industries and Regional Development, WA), Figures 23.8 (whole seed & dehulled kernals) 23.9B & C; **World Map of Food Guides**: (Canada) Eating Well with Canada's Food Guide, Health Canada, 2011, reproduced with permission from the Minister of Health, 2013/ (Great Britian) The Eatwell Plate, Department of Health, NHS UK/ (Latvia) Ministry of Health of the Republic of Latvia/ (Germany) German Nutrition Society/ (Spain) SEDCA/ (China) Chinese Nutrition Society/ (Japan) Ministry of Health Labour and Welfare/ (Australia) National Health and Medical Research Council (2013)/ (Singapore) Health Promotion Board 2012/ (Guatemala) Institute of Nutrition of Central America and Panamar (INCAP)/ (Oman) Department of Nutrition and Ministry for Health, Oman/ (USA) U.S Department of Agriculture, Figure 1.4.

Every effort has been made to trace the original source of copyright material contained in this book. The publisher will be pleased to hear from copyright holders to rectify any errors or omissions.

NUTRITION SUBJECT KNOWLEDGE MATRIX

The Nutrition Society of Australia (NSA) has developed a range of competencies for qualified individuals while recognising the diversity amongst practising nutrition scientists and nutritionists. The competencies reflect professional expectations for those entering the field, and a framework for benchmarking courses in nutrition science. They also provide a reference for those seeking registration with NSA.

Details are published in the open access publication:

Lawlis T, Torres SJ, Coates AM, Clark K, Charlton KE, Sinclair AJ, Wood LG, Devine A. Development of nutrition science competencies for undergraduate degrees in Australia. Asia Pacific Journal of Clinical Nutrition. 2018, and is available on the society website [www.nsa.asn.au]

There are five core competency standards, underpinned by knowledge, skills, attitudes and values:

1 Nutrition Science,
2 Food and the Food System,
3 Nutrition Governance, Sociocultural and Behavioural Factors,
4 Nutrition Research and Critical Analysis,
5 Communication and Professional Conduct.

There are also three specialist competency areas: Public Health Nutrition, Food Science and Animal Nutrition. *Food, Nutrition and Health* aligns more with Public Health Nutrition although there are multiple references to food science throughout and a chapter specifically focused on this topic (Chapter 23).

While undergraduate course coordinators will map the development of competency in these areas across a number of subjects across the years, this text touches on all competency areas, with substantial components relating to nutrition science, food, nutrition governance and nutrition research. Basic nutrition science topics are covered in depth alongside food sources and dietary issues. Each chapter reviews the research in that topic and includes call-out sections covering specific areas of research under the title 'Research in Practice'. There are specific sections on evidence based review. Each chapter also contains a section entitled 'Pathways to Practice' which could form the basis for discussing communication and professional conduct, a competency largely assessed under workplace conditions.

Competency area (number of statements)	Relevant Chapter
Nutrition Science (11)	1–18, 24
Food and the Food System (15)	All chapters and specifically 21-23.
Nutrition Governance, Sociocultural and Behavioural Factors (8)	1–3; 14-21 and specifically 19–21
Nutrition Research and Critical Analysis (7)	All chapters, and specifically 2,3,22–24
Communication and Professional Conduct (8)	All chapters, and specifically 1 and 24.

GUIDED TOUR

CHAPTER OBJECTIVES

This chapter will enable the reader to:

- broadly define the relationship between food consumption and health
- recognise the ways in which nutrition knowledge can be applied throughout the life stages
- appreciate the influences of the broader social environment on nutrition and health.

CHAPTER OBJECTIVES

Each chapter opens with clearly defined and achievable objectives that will help focus your learning.

KEY TERMS

Biochemistry	Nutrients
Dietary guidelines	Physiology
Food	Social environment
Life stages	

KEY TERMS, MARGIN NOTES AND GLOSSARY

To aid your understanding of important concepts, **Key terms** are listed at the beginning of the chapter, defined in **Margin notes** where they first appear and collated in the **Glossary** at the end of the book.

INTRODUCTION

It is common knowledge that **food** is essential for health. Everyone eats food and most people have an opinion on which foods are better for them. So why do we need nutritionists? What's more, why does advice on nutrition always seem to change? The chapters in this book will address these questions from several perspectives.

One short answer to the quandary is that nutrition is both a science and a practice. The World Health Organization (WHO) defines nutrition as 'the intake of food, considered in relation to the body's dietary needs' [1]. As a science, nutrition builds a very broad knowledge base from a range of disciplines that practitioners are then able to apply in practice. A great deal of nutrition knowledge comes from the basic sciences such as chemistry, **biochemistry**, biology and **physiology**. Other knowledge comes from

Food
substance consumed as part of a meal or snack to provide energy and nutrients for sustaining health; originating from plants or animals and consumed as whole or components thereof with or without processing and blending with other ingredients.

GLOSSARY

Absorption
The process of transfer of food components across the gut barrier and into the transport systems of the body.

Acceptable macronutrient distribution range (AMDR)
'An estimate of the range of intake for each macronutrient for individuals (expressed as a contribution to energy), which would allow for an adequate intake of all other nutrients while maximizing general health outcomes' (www.nrv.gov.au).

Activities of daily living (ADL)
Activities such as walking, sitting, eating, washing and dressing.

KEY POINTS

- Nutrition is about understanding how food and nutrient consumption influences health.
- Nutrition concepts can be applied to support human health throughout the lifecycle.
- Working with nutrition involves an appreciation of the broader social environment, including the roles of a wide range of stakeholders.

KEY POINTS:

Highlight the main points covered throughout the chapter.

» RESEARCH AT WORK

THE FRAMINGHAM HEART STUDY

The Framingham Heart Study is an observational study that began in Framingham, Massachusetts. Starting in 1948, it is the longest-running cohort study in the United States aimed at understanding obesity and related disorders such as type 2 diabetes [10]. Originally, 5209 men and women were enrolled in the study and since then have returned for detailed medical examinations every two years. In 1971 a second cohort of 5124 children and spouses of the original cohort were enrolled. In 2002 the third generation (i.e. grandchildren of the original participants) were signed up to join the study. This study has led to the identification of risk factors and other related medical and psychosocial issues associated

RESEARCH AT WORK
Real-life research and study examples that draw on themes explored in the chapter.

» CASE 1.1

SHOULD WE RELY ON FOOD OR VITAMIN SUPPLEMENTS FOR ADEQUATE NUTRITION?

The debate between the relative value of foods versus vitamin supplements can be seen in many forms of media. For example, the headline 'Vitamins can harm cancer patients: scientist' appeared in the *Sydney Morning Herald* on 10 January 2013 [13]. This article reported Professor James Watson—co-discoverer of deoxyribonucleic acid (DNA)—debating in the Royal Society's journal *Open Biology* whether antioxidant use was much more likely to cause than prevent cancer. Supplementing with vitamins A, C and E was discussed. On the other hand, foods such as blueberries tend to be considered for their taste, even though they deliver vitamins. So how do we know what is better for consuming vitamins: food or supplements?

CASE
Interesting person-centred case studies that seek to reinforce chapter content and broaden your thinking on important topics.

TRY IT YOURSELF

Consider the foods in your shopping trolley at your next supermarket visit. How many of them are fresh and how many are in packages? Of those in packages, what do the labels tell you about their nutritional quality? How would you use the information on nutrient content and/or Health Star Rating to judge the contribution of this food to the quality of your overall diet?

TRY IT YOURSELF
Thought-provoking practical exercises that encourage you to draw upon the chapter material and consolidate the knowledge you have gained.

STOP AND THINK

- How do we know that food consumption affects health?
- What is the relationship between nutrients, foods and diets?
- How can we achieve nutritional balance?

STOP AND THINK
Questions that prompt you to reflect on what you're reading and think critically about the issues addressed.

serve functions that enable the organism to survive. To fully appreciate this effect (and the sciences that underpin this knowledge), there is a need to understand the structures and functions of the various components of the body (physiology), how these are affected in disease states (pathophysiology), the chemical structure of food molecules (chemistry) and how these play a role in pathways that underlie body function (biochemistry). Part of this may include understanding how the molecules in food influence genetic expression. This is just the start of a biological perspective on nutrition.

See Chapter 3 on digestion, absorption and metabolism.

TOPIC LINK
Margin notes that direct you to further material on key topics in other parts of the text.

FIGURE 1.3   RELATIONSHIP BETWEEN FOOD, NUTRIENTS AND WHOLE DIETS

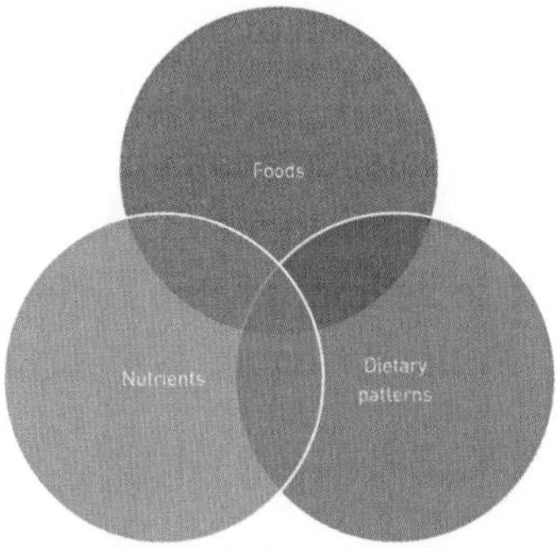

FIGURES AND TABLES
To help illustrate important concepts and invite analysis and consideration from the information presented.

TABLE 2.1   METHODS FOR ANALYSING DIETARY PATTERNS

Testing a known healthy pattern	Identifying patterns from usual intakes
Diet quality scores	Principal component analysis
Healthy eating index	Factor analysis
Mediterranean diet scores Healthy Nordic Food Index	Cluster analysis Reduced rank regression

SUMMARY

- Food delivers essential components that support the structure and function of the human body, but the concept of food synergy recognises that the effects of food may be greater than the sum of its parts.
- The stages of life provide a useful framework for applying scientific knowledge of nutrition to health-related practice.
- The applications of nutrition science in practice can occur at a number of levels, from individualised self-care through to managing individuals in healthcare institutions.

SUMMARY

At the end of each chapter the **Summary** provides an excellent starting point for revision with key points that will help consolidate your knowledge and understanding of the content.

PATHWAYS TO PRACTICE

- There are many areas of practice that relate to working with nutrition. This occurs at the individual level with consumer food choice and healthcare dietary advice, and at the population level through guidelines, standards and community programs.
- Healthcare delivery and the development and governance of policy are high-order activities, but involvement in nutrition occurs at all levels of society.
- The important issue is that contributions are appropriately located, and recognition is given for the area of expertise that is required.

PATHWAYS TO PRACTICE

Strategies, examples and key messages that allow you to gain a practical understanding of the theoretical concepts within each chapter.

DISCUSSION QUESTIONS

1 How is food defined and how is it different from vitamin supplements?
2 How does nutrition science provide evidence for the effects of food consumption on health?
3 What are some of the problems associated with communications in nutrition and the health benefits of foods and nutrients?
4 How does the concept of life stages provide a useful framework for defining nutritional needs?
5 How do we know if there are nutrition problems in the community?
6 What is a food value chain and where do stakeholders fit into this concept?

DISCUSSION QUESTIONS

Challenging summary questions designed to assist your chapter revision and recall for exam preparation.

USEFUL WEBLINKS

American Institute of Cancer Research:
www.aicr.org

Australian Bureau of Agricultural and Resource Economics and Sciences:
www.agriculture.gov.au/abares

Australian Dietary Guidelines:
www.eatforhealth.gov.au

USEFUL WEBLINKS

A list of relevant key websites that point the way to extending knowledge of the main topics covered.

FURTHER READING

Mahmood, S. S., Levy, D., Vasan, R. S. & Wang, T. J. (2014). The Framingham Heart Study and the epidemiology of cardiovascular disease: a historical perspective. *The Lancet*, 383(9921), 999–1008. doi:10.1016/S0140-6736(13)61752-3.

Mozaffarian, D. (2016). Dietary and policy priorities for cardiovascular disease, diabetes, and obesity: a comprehensive review. *Circulation*. doi:10.1161/circulationaha.115.018585.

Simpson, S. & Raubenheimer, D. (2012). *The Nature of Nutrition: A unifying framework from animal adaptation to human obesity.* Princeton, NJ: Princeton University Press.

FURTHER READING

Recommendations that allow you to access additional information relating to the themes explored in each chapter.

RESOURCES GUIDE

Food, Nutrition and Health 2e is accompanied by lecturer and student resources that reinforce and extend learning.

LECTURERS

The following resources are available for lecturers who prescribe the text for their course:
- **Instructor's Resource Manual**
- **PowerPoints**
- **Test bank**
- **Image bank**

STUDENTS

Oxford Ascend online resources can be used by students to test their knowledge, practice and discover more material. Keep an eye out for the Oxford Ascend logo throughout the text which will flag resources available that are relevant to the material you are reading. To access, visit www.oxfordascend. com, create an account and activate the code within the text. Codes can be activated once.

- **Additional Oxford resources:** Supplementary reading material that will further support your understanding of key concepts in food, health and nutrition.
- **Multiple choice questions:** Quizzes that allow you to recall and reflect upon the information they have read and understood in the chapter.
- **Weblinks:** A chapter-by-chapter catalogue of the weblinks mentioned in the text for you to easily access videos and other useful online resources.

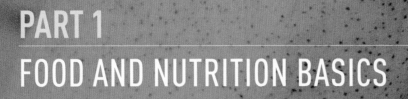

PART 1
FOOD AND NUTRITION BASICS

1

CHAPTER 1

FOOD AND HEALTH: WORKING WITH NUTRITION

LINDA TAPSELL

CHAPTER OBJECTIVES

This chapter will enable the reader to:

- broadly define the relationship between food consumption and health
- recognise the ways in which nutrition knowledge can be applied throughout the life stages
- appreciate the influences of the broader social environment on nutrition and health.

KEY TERMS

Biochemistry	Nutrients
Dietary guidelines	Physiology
Food	Social environment
Life stages	

KEY POINTS

- Nutrition is about understanding how food and nutrient consumption influences health.
- Nutrition concepts can be applied to support human health throughout the lifecycle.
- Working with nutrition involves an appreciation of the broader social environment, including the roles of a wide range of stakeholders.

INTRODUCTION

It is common knowledge that **food** is essential for health. Everyone eats food and most people have an opinion on which foods are better for them. So why do we need nutritionists? What's more, why does advice on nutrition always seem to change? The chapters in this book will address these questions from several perspectives.

One short answer to the quandary is that nutrition is both a science and a practice. The World Health Organization (WHO) defines nutrition as 'the intake of food, considered in relation to the body's dietary needs' [1]. As a science, nutrition builds a very broad knowledge base from a range of disciplines that practitioners are then able to apply in practice. A great deal of nutrition knowledge comes from the basic sciences such as chemistry, **biochemistry**, biology and **physiology**. Other knowledge comes from health disciplines such as epidemiology, dietetics and medicine, and then from humanities disciplines such as sociology and anthropology, and the study of economics.

The unifying factor is the need to better understand the relationship between food and health. Because this is a complex relationship, it needs to be considered from a number of different angles, but they can all come together to represent the science of nutrition.

It is difficult to locate the exact origins of modern nutrition science, but it can be seen in a number of settings: from the chemistry laboratories of Wilbur Atwater [2], determining the energy value of foods, to the observations of scurvy prevention with citrus fruits consumption by long-haul mariners [3]. The subsequent isolation and description of the nutrient, vitamin C, through the science of chemistry heralded the discovery of vitamins in foods and the recognition that **Nutrient Reference Values (NRVs)** [4] were required to protect the health of populations. Today the exploration of food composition continues to expand rapidly, particularly with an interest in phytochemicals found in plants that have very intriguing properties [5]. This research has also triggered food innovation, driving the development of foods with improved nutritional qualities that may be linked to better health outcomes.

From the perspective of Western populations, nutrition science also developed strongly during the world wars when food rationing became a major issue [6]. Methods for measuring population eating patterns and observing their relationships with health outcomes were developed and led to observations of the relationship between diet and the development of cardiovascular disease. This has now expanded to diet and chronic disease generally, and the identification of food components and food patterns that may prove deleterious to health when consumed in excess. Food and nutrient-based trials have tested a number of hypotheses related to food consumption and health. This research has led to a reconsideration of the emphasis on nutrients and other food components rather than whole foods and whole diets [7].

The emerging concept of **food synergy** suggests that the sum of the parts may be more effective than the component parts themselves, driving researchers to first consider food and dietary patterns in addressing the effects of food on health [8]. This has implications for how research may be evaluated, for example, in developing dietary guidelines [9].

Food
substance consumed as part of a meal or snack to provide energy and nutrients for sustaining health; originating from plants or animals and consumed as whole or components thereof with or without processing and blending with other ingredients.

Biochemistry
study of the chemistry of living organisms.

Physiology
study of the vital biological functions of plants and animals.

See Chapter 4 on phytochemicals.

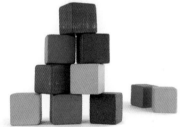

Nutrient Reference Values (NRVs)
a set of standards based on scientific evidence of nutrient requirements, used for assessing nutritional quality of dietary intakes.

Food synergy
a concept that acknowledges the sum of the parts is greater than the components of foods.

LINDA TAPSELL

>> RESEARCH AT WORK

THE FRAMINGHAM HEART STUDY

The Framingham Heart Study is an observational study that began in Framingham, Massachusetts. Starting in 1948, it is the longest-running cohort study in the United States aimed at understanding obesity and related disorders such as type 2 diabetes [10]. Originally, 5209 men and women were enrolled in the study and since then have returned for detailed medical examinations every two years. In 1971 a second cohort of 5124 children and spouses of the original cohort were enrolled. In 2002 the third generation (i.e. grandchildren of the original participants) were signed up to join the study. This study has led to the identification of risk factors and other related medical and psychosocial issues associated with cardiovascular disease. The study continues today, with research expanding into other areas such as the role genetics has in the development of cardiovascular disease. From 1950 to 2016 over 3300 articles have been published using data collected from the Framingham Heart Study.

In addition to these developments, the discovery of the human genome in the 1950s has produced significant implications for nutrition. Nutritional genomics and nutritional genetics are just some of the emerging scientific disciplines that contribute to our understanding of food and health (Figure 1.1). Research in this area shows how the components of foods can act as agents of the environment when we study the effect of environment on genetic expression. This understanding has implications for how much of a nutrient a person may need and how diet may influence when a person develops a disease state [11].

FIGURE 1.1   NUTRIGENETICS AND NUTRIGENOMICS

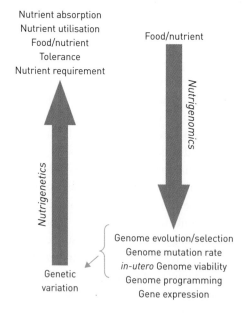

Source: P. J. Stover & M. A. Caudill (2008). Genetic and epigenetic contributions to human nutrition and health: managing genome–diet interactions. *Journal of the Academy of Nutrition and Dietetics*, 108(9), 1480–7. doi:10.1016/j.jada.2008.06.430

FIGURE 1.2   RELATIONSHIP BETWEEN BASIC BIOLOGICAL CONCEPTS IN NUTRITION,
APPLICATIONS OF THIS KNOWLEDGE TO HUMAN HEALTH, AND PRACTICE DOMAINS

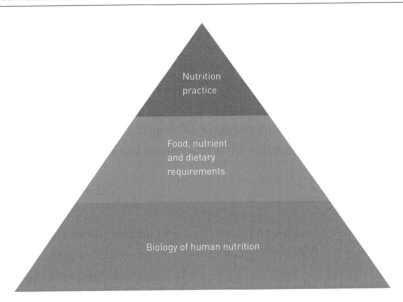

A useful framework for studying nutrition is to consider the building blocks of knowledge in a sequential manner (Figure 1.2). First we may consider the nature of food as a source of nutrients and other biological substances that serve particular functions within the body. This extends to the concept of food synergy, where the sum of the parts is greater than the individual components. We can then consider the largely observational evidence that dietary patterns are associated with the emergence of lifestyle-related disease. The knowledge derived from research in human nutrition can then be applied to examine the specific needs for nutrients and foods throughout the human lifecycle. We can also study the characteristics of dietary patterns that appear to protect against the development of lifestyle-related disease. Integrating this knowledge helps to develop guidelines and policies for practice.

Nutrition practice occurs in various contexts, from an individual making their personal food choices through to the activities of communities, healthcare systems, industry and governments. Thus there are different levels of practice and different pathways for practice. At the most basic level, nutrition practice equates to an individual looking after their health, applying nutrition knowledge to personal food choices. Practices that have an impact on the broader community require specific levels of expertise depending on the context (e.g. in healthcare, industry, research and development or public policy) and require higher levels of learning.

Regardless of the context, nutrition practice will always be dependent on quality research. This research occurs at many levels, from the basic biological underpinnings of nutrition through to clinical trials on foods, and social and environmental research on food systems. By its nature, research will introduce new knowledge.

Frameworks for evaluating research will also be applied, but in the end there may be shifts in recommendations and applications. Students of nutrition need to have this 'big picture' view of their discipline. As well as having a good grasp of basic concepts, they will also need to appreciate the need to keep up with the scientific literature and maintain strong critical evaluation skills.

STOP AND THINK

- How has knowledge about nutrition evolved within modern science?
- How has this knowledge been applied, and how might this relate to practice?
- What might the study of nutrition look like in the future?

HOW DOES FOOD CONSUMPTION AFFECT HEALTH?

The old adage 'you are what you eat' provides one of the simplest summaries of the relationship between food and health. When food is eaten, it is broken down in the digestive system and most is absorbed as small molecules into the bloodstream. From here it is transported to various parts of the body to serve functions that enable the organism to survive. To fully appreciate this effect (and the sciences that underpin this knowledge), there is a need to understand the structures and functions of the various components of the body (physiology), how these are affected in disease states (pathophysiology), the chemical structure of food molecules (chemistry) and how these play a role in pathways that underlie

See Chapter 3 on digestion, absorption and metabolism.

body function (biochemistry). Part of this may include understanding how the molecules in food influence genetic expression. This is just the start of a biological perspective on nutrition.

≫ RESEARCH AT WORK

NUTRITIONAL ECOLOGY

Before we eat food, it is worthwhile taking a moment to think about food itself. Food can be described as a variety of substances consumed to build and maintain the body's structure and function, but food also has its own biological origins as plants and animals. The composition of food reflects its genetic potential [8], nutritional environment and the way in which the food is modified for human consumption. There are parallels to understanding human health and understanding decisions behind the production of food (plants and animals) for human consumption. In reality, food is not only 'produced'; it also grows across the planet in its own right, but there is a strong human influence on the overall supply of food.

Nutritional ecology
interactions of the animal with its environment from a nutritional perspective.

Nutritional ecologists have looked closely at the dynamic interface between humans and their food environment to develop new theoretical positions on how obesity and cardiovascular disease may have emerged with our current food environment. Raubenheimer and Simpson [12], for example, have developed an approach known as 'nutritional geometry' to present a 'protein leverage hypothesis'. Through analytical means, they argue that the current state of overconsumption of food may be due to varying access to protein in a food environment that has vast amounts of food with a very wide range of nutritional quality. Raubenheimer and Simpson integrate knowledge of environment and evolution with analyses of data on food and nutrient consumption patterns to add a useful dimension to the study of nutrition science. This has implications for future developments in obesity management and the development of the food supply.

>> CASE 1.1

SHOULD WE RELY ON FOOD OR VITAMIN SUPPLEMENTS FOR ADEQUATE NUTRITION?

The debate between the relative value of foods versus vitamin supplements can be seen in many forms of media. For example, the headline 'Vitamins can harm cancer patients: scientist' appeared in the *Sydney Morning Herald* on 10 January 2013 [13]. This article reported Professor James Watson—co-discoverer of deoxyribonucleic acid (DNA)—debating in the Royal Society's journal *Open Biology* whether antioxidant use was much more likely to cause than prevent cancer. Supplementing with vitamins A, C and E was discussed. On the other hand, foods such as blueberries tend to be considered for their taste, even though they deliver vitamins. So how do we know what is better for consuming vitamins: food or supplements?

In a review of the food versus nutrient debate, Jacobs and colleagues [8] observed that vitamin supplemental trials often drew their logic from observational studies of relationships between food consumption patterns and health. Identifying the vitamins in those foods, and considering the known mechanisms of action of the vitamins, may have led to the hypothesis that vitamin supplementation may produce desired health benefits. When put to the test, however, some studies that used vitamin supplements produced unexpected negative health effects.

More recently, a group of European researchers conducted a systematic review and meta-analysis of trials involving dietary supplements and the prevention of heart disease and cancer. They examined data from 49 trials and 287,304 participants to conclude there was insufficient evidence to support the use of dietary supplementation in primary prevention. They found some small beneficial effects with some, no effects with others and a link between vitamin A supplementation and increased cancer risk [14].

- What does the research discussed above suggest about the nature of food versus vitamin supplements?
- What does it mean for the promotion of health?
- When might it be necessary to take vitamin supplements?

Given its fundamental role in human health, the nutritional value of food has a direct impact on the health of the population. The relationship between food and health goes beyond simple digestion and absorption of food at the individual level, but it is a good starting point for studying nutrition.

In the last 100 years or so, scientists have identified the chemical composition of critical food components that have proved essential for life. These are referred to as **nutrients**: macronutrients (protein, fat and carbohydrate) and micronutrients (vitamins and minerals). While it is now possible to consume nutrients in isolated and supplemental form, it is important to remember that their origins lie in food. Indeed, scientists are continuing to expand their knowledge of nutrients themselves, as well as identifying other components in food that are also proving to be significant. Breaking down food into its component parts is informative, but in the end we need to put it all back together again to understand the effect of food on health.

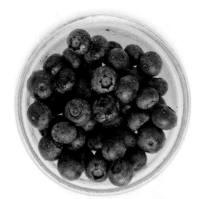

Nutrients
substances required for the nourishment of the organism, generally provided as components of foods.

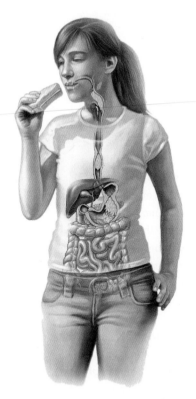

The knowledge of nutrients and other components in food does enable us to categorise foods in terms of their common composition. Thus, for example, we associate fruit with vitamin C and milk with protein and calcium. However, in classifying foods we should not be limited by our knowledge of single nutrients. By 'thinking foods first' [7], we are able to integrate new knowledge on food components as it emerges and build an understanding of why (and how) a particular food contributes to health. Of course, we do not eat one food alone, so effects are exposed in the context of a total diet.

In other words, there is interdependence between foods in promoting health (Figure 1.3). Specific foods may be associated with a total diet (e.g. extra virgin olive oil in a Mediterranean diet), but health outcomes result from all the foods consumed in the diet. Foods can be categorised in terms of their relative position in healthy diets and are likely to have that position because of their nutrient composition relative to the energy value they also contribute. Overall nutrient content is one attribute of a healthy diet, but achieving balance in total energy content and other dietary factors such as sodium and saturated fat also appears important in managing the diet–health relationship. At the same time, these dietary attributes will reflect the types of food chosen for consumption.

The concept of balance is critical in nutrition. This relates to the delivery of multiple nutrients as well as the construction of whole diets from different foods. It is consistent with the medical concept of homeostasis—the physiological process by which the internal systems of the body are maintained at equilibrium, despite variations in external conditions [15]. The ensuing chapters in this book expand on the issue of food and nutritional balance from science and practice perspectives.

Nutritional balance
meeting the required amounts of all nutrients while at the same time meeting requirements for energy intakes.

FIGURE 1.3 RELATIONSHIP BETWEEN FOOD, NUTRIENTS AND WHOLE DIETS

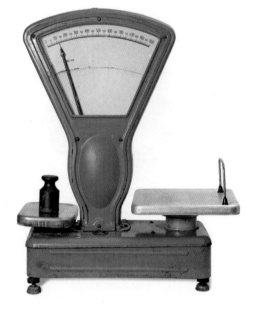

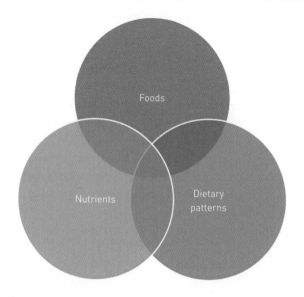

>> CASE 1.2

NUTRITION INFORMATION ON FOOD LABELS

Food labels

Food Standards Australia New Zealand (FSANZ) provides useful information for consumers on details contained on food labels. Components include:

1 nutrition information panel (including nutrients per serve)
2 percentage labelling concerning the amount of ingredients
3 name and description of the food, which must be accurate
4 food recall information (including Australian or New Zealand name and business address of manufacturer or importer)
5 information for allergy sufferers
6 date marking (best before if shelf life less than two years, or 'use by' date for safety requirements)
7 ingredient list.

For more information, see www.foodstandards.gov.au/consumer/labelling/Pages/interactive-labelling-poster.aspx.

Health Star Rating System

A Health Star Rating can be seen on many manufactured food products in Australia. The Health Star Rating System was developed by Australian state and territory governments in partnership with industry and public health and consumer groups. The ratings are based on the overall nutrient composition of the food, with reference to overall energy value alongside 'positive nutrients' (e.g. fibre, protein, vitamins and minerals) and 'risk nutrients' (e.g. saturated fat, sodium and sugar). Not all foods will have ratings.

For more information, see http://healthstarrating.gov.au/internet/healthstarrating/publishing.nsf/content/home.

• How do food labels and Health Star Ratings on food packages expose the consumer to the relationship between foods and nutrients?
• What are the challenges for consumers in using these features to make food choices?

From a biological perspective, food consumption affects health in the first instance by delivering key nutrients to support and maintain vital systems in the body. Scientific knowledge has provided a great deal of information for understanding why this is so, but there is always more to know, which means that some of our assumptions may change with time. We do not know everything that is in food and there is more to understand about the functions of the human body, but with ongoing research the picture is becoming clearer, providing stronger evidence for practice.

TRY IT YOURSELF

Consider the foods in your shopping trolley at your next supermarket visit. How many of them are fresh and how many are in packages? Of those in packages, what do the labels tell you about their nutritional quality? How would you use the information on nutrient content and/or Health Star Rating to judge the contribution of this food to the quality of your overall diet?

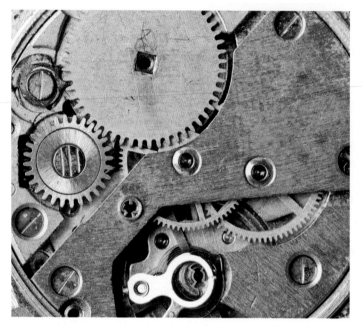

There are many ways to establish a position on how food consumption affects health. From the perspective of modern Western science, there is a strong commitment to the scientific method, and this is applied by a range of scientific disciplines. Evidence frameworks [16] apply a system by which information is appropriately assessed to produce a position that is scientifically defensible.

Identifying the different chemical compounds in food has been one of the most significant steps in understanding how food affects health. The next step has been to characterise their mode of action in the biological context [17]. This can involve highly controlled experiments that use cell cultures or animal models where a great deal is already known and the pathways under study can be isolated and observed. This form of research can explain how the isolated compounds in food might act on physiological and biochemical

Mechanistic research
research that explains natural processes in physical or deterministic terms.

processes, and is often referred to as **mechanistic research**. Given the nature of this research, it is not taken as direct evidence of effects but rather helps to explain observations that suggest this may be happening. Studying the basic sciences of chemistry, biochemistry and physiology helps the nutritionist to understand what underpins mechanistic research and to apply this knowledge appropriately in practice.

Observational research
research that examines relationships between environmental exposures and health outcomes.

Observational research looks for relationships between dietary factors and health. Observational studies emerge from the science of epidemiology and help to build knowledge for practice. Population health research can provide important observations of relationships between dietary practices and health outcomes. Findings from observational studies still provide indirect evidence, but these studies are stronger than mechanistic research because they are more directly related to the consumption of food and measurements of human health. The study context is less controlled than in a laboratory setting, but the discipline of epidemiology exerts its own controls on how the population is sampled, what is measured and the forms of statistical analyses that are conducted. Understanding these processes enables the nutritionist to evaluate the quality of the research in applying it to practice.

Randomised controlled trial (RCT)
an experimental study design that tests effects of treatments on health outcomes.

Randomised controlled trials (RCTs) are considered to provide the best evidence where people consume foods and health outcomes are measured. Such studies provide direct evidence of effects of food consumption on health. The research is conducted in a more controlled human context, although this creates limitations as people normally eat food in a more flexible environment, and so the results may not be very generalisable. Nevertheless, evidence-based methodologies tend to accept that the results from RCTs provide the highest level of evidence for effects of food on health. The practising nutritionist needs to keep up to date with food-related RCTs, bearing in mind that in most cases there will be studies showing positive effects and others that will not.

OXFORD UNIVERSITY PRESS

» RESEARCH AT WORK

PREDIMED STUDY OF THE MEDITERRANEAN DIET

The most robust method of determining a cause-and-effect relationship between an intervention (such as a diet) and outcome (such as heart disease) is the RCT. An RCT is defined by:

- randomly allocating participants into different intervention groups
- including a 'control' or 'comparison' group in order to judge the effects of the intervention.

Participants in an RCT should be unaware of the group into which they have been placed and, ideally, staff working on the trial should also be blinded to the intervention (although this is not always possible) [18].

In the PREDIMED trial, around 7500 adults aged 55–80 years with either type 2 diabetes or three risk factors for cardiovascular disease were randomly allocated to receive control (low fat) dietary advice in one of two groups advised on the Mediterranean diet, one supplemented with nuts and the other with extra virgin olive oil. The researchers found around a 30% reduced incidence of cardiovascular events (heart attack, stroke) in the Mediterranean diet groups [19].

See Chapters 1, 2, 5 and 7 on the PREDIMED trial and Mediterranean diet.

There are problems in conducting RCTs with food but, in reality, positions on the relationship between food and health are based on a body of evidence that is produced from many studies, often of different forms. The end result of all this science may appear to be that nutritionists are constantly changing their minds. This, however, is a simplistic response to a complex, evolving field.

As the science of nutrition evolves, it is expected that new knowledge will emerge and this may result in a changed recommendation. With the development of a broad framework for understanding nutrition in its own right, however, this is

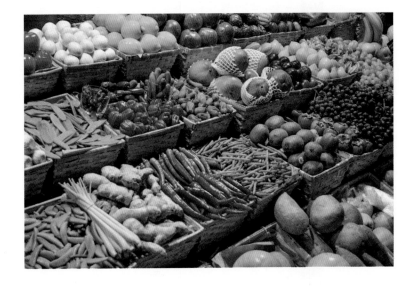

less likely to be problematic. Quality review systems for evidence-based practice in nutrition are now widespread (Table 1.1) and are used in the development of dietary guidelines (Figure 1.4)—for example, in Australia (www.eatforhealth.gov.au), the United States (http://health.gov/dietaryguidelines) and other areas of food and nutrition policy around the globe (e.g. American Institute for Cancer Research at www.aicr.org). These systems provide methods for searching the scientific literature through to analysing the content of studies, evaluating their quality and arriving at a conclusion on the body of evidence as provided. The practice of evidence-based review is another form of science that is now being taken up and developed substantively in the nutrition domain.

TABLE 1.1   LEVELS OF EVIDENCE IN HEALTH

Level	Intervention	Diagnostic accuracy	Prognosis	Aetiology	Screening intervention
I	A systematic review of level II studies	A systematic review of level II studies	A systematic review of level II studies	A systematic review of level II studies	A systematic review of level II studies
II	A randomised controlled trial	A study of test accuracy with an independent, blinded comparison with a valid reference standard, among consecutive persons with a defined clinical presentation	A prospective cohort study	A prospective cohort study	A randomised controlled trial
III-1	A pseudorandomised controlled trial (i.e. alternate allocation or some other method)	A study of test accuracy with an independent, blinded comparison with a valid reference standard, among non-consecutive persons with a defined clinical presentation	All or none	All or none	A pseudorandomised controlled trial (i.e. alternate allocation or some other method)
III-2	A comparative study with concurrent controls: • Non-randomised, experimental trial • Cohort study • Case-control study • Interrupted time series with a control group	A comparison with reference standard that does not meet the criteria required for Level II and III-1 evidence	Analysis of prognostic factors among persons in a single arm of a randomised controlled trial	A retrospective cohort study	A comparative study with concurrent controls: • Non-randomised, experimental trial • Cohort study • Case-control study
III-3	A comparative study without concurrent controls: • Historical control study • Two or more single arm study • Interrupted time series without a parallel control group	Diagnostic case-control study	A retrospective cohort study	A case-control study	A comparative study without concurrent controls: • Historical control study • Two or more single arm study
IV	Case series with either post-test or pre-test/post-test outcomes	Study of diagnostic yield (no reference standard)	Case series, or cohort study of persons at different stages of disease	A cross-sectional study or case series	Case series

Source: NHMRC Guideline Assessment Register Consultants (2009). *NHMRC Levels of Evidence and Grades for Recommendations for Developers of Guidelines.* Canberra: NHMRC. © Commonwealth of Australia

FIGURE 1.4   WORLD MAP OF FOOD GUIDES

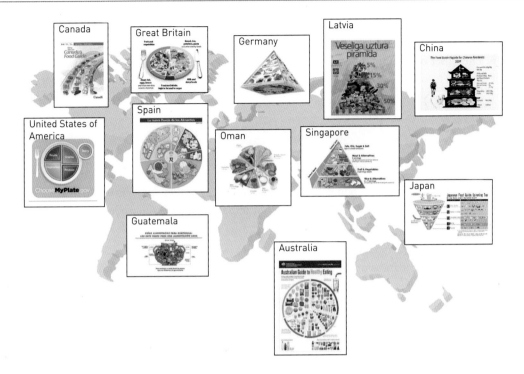

STOP AND THINK

- How do we know that food consumption affects health?
- What is the relationship between nutrients, foods and diets?
- How can we achieve nutritional balance?

HOW IS KNOWLEDGE OF NUTRITION APPLIED THROUGHOUT THE LIFECYCLE?

Translating nutrition knowledge to practice involves identifying the problem and working out how it can be changed. In the first instance, it is important to know what people are eating, the nutritional value of their diet, how it measures up to standards of nutritional requirements [4] and how it fits with **dietary guidelines**. Dietary guidelines provide recommendations for achieving a healthy diet; food standards regulate the composition of food and the statements that can be made about food products.

A consideration of **life stages** provides a useful platform for organising the application of nutrition knowledge to the healthcare of individuals and communities. Eating food is part of survival (recall that 'you are what you eat'), so understanding the needs of the body throughout the stages of life provides some insight into determining which foods might be best to consume. Not surprisingly, the resource needs of the first stages of life

Dietary guidelines

statements on strategies for choosing a healthy diet based on scientific evidence on the effects of food intake and dietary patterns on health.

Life stages

defined periods throughout the lifespan, such as infancy, childhood, adulthood and old age.

are critical, with subsequent growth and development affected by how the nutritional stage is set. For example, pregnancy and lactation are changed physiological conditions with specific requirements for nutrition resources. With maturation of the adult person and possible declines in physical activity, body composition may change, as will body chemistry and function, altering the need for energy and nutrients. The onset of chronic disease and the loss of functionality demand particular consideration in terms of changes to eating habits.

» CASE 1.3

OBESITY AND DIETARY HABITS OF AUSTRALIANS

The Australian Institute of Health and Welfare (AIHW) produces regular reports on Australia's food and nutrition. In *Australia's Health 2016* [20], it was noted in data from the Australian Bureau of Statistics (ABS) that:

- in 2014–15 around 11.2 million Australian adults were overweight or obese
- the rate of obesity is increasing, with an average weight gain of 4.4 kg between 1995 and 2014–15
- overweight and obesity is more common among Indigenous adults
- in 2014–15 most adults (93%) did not eat the recommended five serves of vegetables
- in the same period, 50% did not eat the recommended two serves of fruit
- about 35% of energy intake was consumed as discretionary foods.

See more at www.aihw.gov.au/WorkArea/DownloadAsset.aspx?id=60129556760.

- How do the obesity statistics above reflect food and nutrition problems in the Australian community?
- How are discretionary foods defined from a nutrient and food perspective?

Most people are healthy when they are born, so the focus is on meeting nutritional requirements and maintaining energy balance. In the absence of chronic disease, applying nutrition principles from the perspective of managing physiological changes and functionality is the primary concern. For example, matching physiological changes and meeting specific nutrient requirements are key focal points for pregnancy and lactation. Meeting requirements is also important for infants and children, but there are particular considerations such as the development of healthy eating patterns and the prevention of childhood obesity. The main focus in adulthood is the prevention of chronic lifestyle diseases, such as obesity, hypertension, diabetes and cardiovascular disease, with a special emphasis on dietary patterns that are proving to be protective. Nutritional requirements for older ages are different again, particularly when older people are institutionalised and may suffer from malnutrition. In each case, however, being able to assess nutrition and dietary aspects are entry points to practice, as is the reference to standards and guidelines from which to judge the extent of potential problems (Figure 1.5).

FIGURE 1.5   NUTRITION REQUIREMENTS THROUGHOUT THE LIFECYCLE

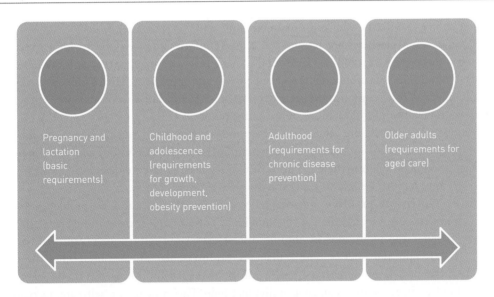

Pregnancy and lactation (basic requirements)

Childhood and adolescence (requirements for growth, development, obesity prevention)

Adulthood (requirements for chronic disease prevention)

Older adults (requirements for aged care)

≫ RESEARCH AT WORK

IDENTIFYING NUTRITION TARGETS IN OLDER AGE

Nutrition scientists are aware that the global population aged over 60 years is predicted to double by 2050. A review of nutritional considerations for healthy ageing noted that where older adults are unable to meet their nutritional requirements, 'nutritional frailty' can become a major concern. Chronic conditions likely to affect this are:

- cognitive decline
- dementia
- sarcopaenia (loss of muscle mass)
- reduced immunity to infectious disease.

There is evidence that all of these conditions may benefit from careful attention to a healthy diet, as has been shown, for example, with the Mediterranean diet in the PREDIMED study. Arguments have been made for research that examines biomarkers of these conditions, tests effects of nutritional interventions and re-evaluates current body mass index (BMI) standards for older adults. Health services may also consider how older adults can undergo a 'nutrition physical' as part of their routine healthcare [21].

In order to apply nutrition principles to individuals and populations we need valid dietary assessment methods, databases of food composition, population NRVs, and food and dietary policies and guidelines. **Dietary assessment methods** are necessary to be able to gauge the extent of nutritional problems. There are many forms of dietary assessment, ranging from surveys (questionnaires) to food records and observations of

Dietary assessment methods

surveys, interviews and records that provide an account of a person's usual eating habits.

eating behaviour. The best method for assessing intake will very much depend on the purposes of the practice, the information required and the resources available to undertake the assessment. Decisions on methods of choice also need a well-informed nutrition base.

Food composition databases are required to convert information on food to information about nutrients. It is this process that tells us, for example, that a diet with many takeaway foods has a certain level of fat. From this information judgments can be made and appropriate advice given or action taken. The development of food composition databases is another significant area of nutrition science, and it also carries considerations for limitations of use and application.

Population NRVs provide the values for nutrient intakes that would best support the health of most people in the population. As such, they enable practitioners to compare values with those reported in their dietary assessment. Because there is a great deal of science behind the derivation of these values, it is important to be able to apply this knowledge appropriately.

Nutrition practice
the application of nutrition knowledge to address an identified problem.

Nutrition practice broadly relies on the identification of problems. Nutrition problems can be identified at the individual, community or institutional level. In Western societies, the prevalence of chronic disease associated with poor nutritional habits (e.g. overweight and obesity, type 2 diabetes, cardiovascular disease) underlines the problem [22]. At the individual level, nutritional health can be managed by the person themselves through their own food choices, or they can seek individual help. The concept of 'self-care' recognises the autonomy of individuals in conducting the personal aspects of their lives, bearing in mind the responsibilities that go with them [23]. A starting point is the person's ability to assess dietary intake using valid methods and to make judgments on the quality of their diet with reference to dietary guidelines and food standards. At the individual level, people choose different foods because they have come to know they are better than others for health. They may use information on food labels in making those choices. They may look for advice, such as national dietary guidelines formulated by government health authorities [24].

Primary healthcare services provide medical, nursing and allied health support for individuals in the community and associated groups. The nutrition knowledge applied will also depend on individual circumstances, but in the first instance will reference the dietary guidelines as they relate to specific groups. For specific problems, such as the need to address the risk of cardiovascular disease, resources from related authoritative groups such as the Heart Foundation may provide more specific information. It all comes down to the level of translation required, which draws on the degree of specialised training in nutrition undertaken by the healthcare professional. If an individual becomes ill and this has implications for the food they eat, they may need to consult a health practitioner, and for specific nutrition expertise may consult a dietitian.

When disease takes hold and food intake can influence outcomes, the degree of knowledge integration, translation and application is much more demanding. It requires an understanding of where and how the condition deviates from the normal (pathophysiology) and how the components of food may influence this process. Combining this with an understanding of a person's usual eating habits and a knowledge of food composition then enables a specific dietary prescription to be drawn up that would help support the condition. The information provided in each case is usually different and therefore the application of generalised tools such as the dietary guidelines is inappropriate. The extent of nutrition knowledge required for this category of care is quite substantial, drawing on the basic sciences through to the evidence frameworks for the effects of diet on health. Medicare payments for dietetic services and employment of dietitians in hospitals reflect this required level of expertise.

At a broader community level, there is a need to protect against the development of nutrition-related illnesses in the population and ensure the food supply is supportive. Governments will also be involved at this level, developing public health-related policies, guidelines and standards aimed at protecting the health of the population (www.foodstandards.gov.au; www.nhmrc.gov.au; www.eatforhealth.gov.au). The food and agricultural industries are also important because of the role they play in the food supply to the population at large (www.agriculture.gov.au; www.agriculture.gov.au/abares). In addition, there are various forms of nutrition promotion. Groups and societies can form to disseminate nutrition information and undertake activities that support nutrition in their communities. For example, schools provide basic nutrition education (based on the dietary guidelines) to children and can engage in activities to promote healthy food choices such as through school canteen policies and fresh food gardens (www.kitchengardenfoundation.org.au). Healthcare workers within community and public health programs can provide these community groups with resources and further guidance in developing nutrition promotion activities. These services may work across all age groups, including maternal, child, home and aged care facilities. The goal of nutrition in supporting health is the same throughout, but the particular knowledge and applications will depend on the needs and circumstances of the specific group.

≫ CASE 1.4

THE OTTAWA CHARTER FOR HEALTH PROMOTION

Translating knowledge of nutrition into practice requires a comprehensive approach to health and health promotion. Growing expectations regarding health promotion in developed nations around the world led to the development of a charter for health promotion. On 21 November 1986, an International Conference on Health Promotion was held in Canada to respond to the view that public health systems were too medically and disease-focused, too oriented to the individual, and not in keeping with the environmental, social and economic challenges facing health systems into the future.

The Ottawa Charter for Health Promotion [25] continues to represent consensus agreement on health promotion today. Essentially, the Charter vowed to build healthy public policy, create supportive environments, strengthen community action, develop personal skills and reorient health services.

- How might the Ottawa Charter for Health Promotion be applied in the Australian context?
- What are the implications of the Charter for the delivery of health services in nutrition?

At the community and institutional level, food service systems play a major role in decisions about food choice. These include services such as Meals on Wheels [26] and food-service systems in childcare centres, nursing homes, hospitals and worksite canteens. The nutrition knowledge applied in food-service systems includes and goes beyond the dietary guidelines. It references a range of standards and policies that have been developed through the fundamentals of nutrition science to ensure that the food delivered to recipients meets nutritional requirements, is safe to eat and is likely to be consumed. This includes policy relating to recommended dietary intakes of nutrients for different age groups, food safety standards and knowledge of culinary preferences and needs of the recipients. Most, if not all, people working in this area would benefit from an understanding of the fundamental principles of nutrition and food safety. At higher levels of responsibility, as in the case of a food-service dietitian [27], they would also need to apply standards for determining and monitoring food and nutrition quality, while translating and integrating a number of areas of nutrition knowledge.

» CASE 1.5

MEALS ON WHEELS: MORE THAN JUST A MEAL

The concept of Meals on Wheels—delivering meals to frail elderly people who wish to remain in their own homes and maintain a degree of independence, but who require a little extra help—began in Britain during the Second World War. The service came to Australia in 1952; it was started in Melbourne by an individual, taken over by the Red Cross and then spread to other states. Millions of meals are delivered each year to many older Australians by around 70,000 volunteers. The work carried out by the service also includes food safety and labelling for Meals on Wheels, research and resource development, advocacy in regard to national policy issues, and membership support [26; 28]. See also: http://mealsonwheels. org.au.

- What are some of the critical nutritional issues that Meals on Wheels services may have to deal with in meeting the nutritional needs of older Australians?

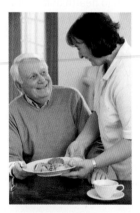

Research contributes to the generation of new knowledge, which helps to drive the practice, and practice creates new questions for research to address. Research agencies play an important role in expanding the understanding of all aspects of nutrition, from the details of how food supports health, to how better to implement strategies that have an effect on health (www.arc. gov.au; www.nhmrc.gov.au). There is a large number of locations for practice in nutrition with different pathways and requirements for applications of knowledge.

STOP AND THINK

- Why do nutritional needs vary across the lifecycle?
- How are nutritional problems identified at the individual and community level?
- What are some of the locations of nutrition practice where nutritional problems may be addressed?

HOW DOES THE BROADER SOCIAL ENVIRONMENT INFLUENCE NUTRITION AND HEALTH?

Applications of nutrition science to human health occur in a broader social and environmental context. One way to consider this is to view the systems that influence the supply of food and the way it is regulated. Key stakeholders include governments and agencies, the food industry, the health and agricultural sectors, and other groups with interests in food (Figure 1.6).

See Chapter 2 on dietary guidelines.

FIGURE 1.6   KEY SECTORS IN THE COMMUNITY RELATED TO FOOD AND NUTRITION

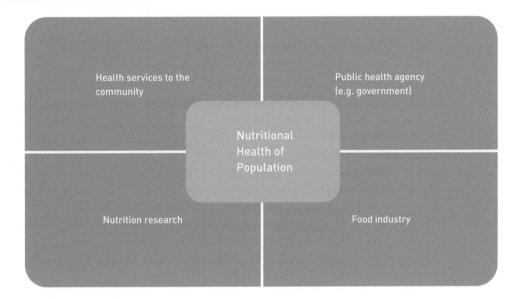

Health services to the community

Public health agency (e.g. government)

Nutritional Health of Population

Nutrition research

Food industry

Food and nutrition policy concerns plans for actions to be taken to deal with nutrition problems. Knowledge of nutrition is fundamental to ensure these policies are grounded in sound science and strong evidence. Nutrition research is an important underpinning factor in the development of policies and their related actions. Nutrition policy and related activities involve a principled approach. This approach concerns many sectors of government and the community at large, and requires agencies for implementation and standards that inform implementation. For example, food standards are set to protect public health. They govern the types of ingredients that can go into foods and the information that can be provided on labels. FSANZ [29] develops the standards and they are enforced at state government level. These standards also relate to health claims that can be made on foods, based on scientific evidence.

Food and nutrition policy

principles of action relating to the way in which food is dealt with by organisations and individuals.

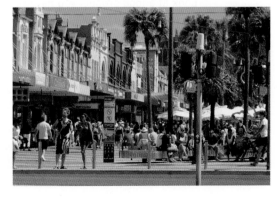

LINDA TAPSELL

>> **CASE 1.6**

MARKETING OF FOODS AND BEVERAGES

The marketing of individual foods and beverages to targeted groups within the community is standard practice for the food industry and is integral to managing a business. However, controversies often arise in food and beverage marketing. These might relate to the way in which health-related messages are constructed, or when a risk to the community is perceived from the type of products being marketed to specific groups.

There are many issues surrounding the marketing of healthy food. These include the definition of a food or defining characteristics (e.g. wholegrain versus 'brown' versus wholemeal), the ingredients used in a food, and fresh single food versus foods processed with multiple ingredients. There are also many issues concerning the marketing of beverages, particularly where there may be health risks [30].

- What are the health risks of energy drinks mixed with alcohol?
- How much do we know about the effects of caffeine and alcohol mixed together?
- What are the particular risks to the target market of young adults?

Stakeholders

people or groups with a vested interest in an area under consideration.

Food value chain

the added value that occurs in relation to events that begin with agriculture or primary food production through to food processing, manufacturing, distribution, retail and food service to consumers.

The way in which policy is developed generally involves drawing together a high level of expertise and some degree of consultation. The simple listing of stakeholder groups in food and nutrition policy demonstrates the very broad and complex social and cultural contexts in which it occurs. It also reflects the extent to which nutrition practice operates, and the levels at which this may relate to policy development.

Food is dealt with by society in a number of ways, so there are **stakeholders** at many points. Some stakeholders have a major influence on food choice behaviour. Others are important to the food value or supply chain. The **food value chain** is a concept that deals with the way food makes its way from where it is grown to where it is eaten (sometimes referred to as 'paddock to plate'). Because there are so many dimensions to food in society, linking food policy with nutrition requires a working relationship across a number of sectors. This has implications for nutrition practice, because it means the knowledge of nutrition has to be effectively applied in several settings.

TRY IT YOURSELF

Look at a food product you have recently purchased from a supermarket. Using the information on the packet, identify as many groups as possible that may be related to the production of this food and the reasons behind your purchasing it.

Health services are clearly a major stakeholder group in nutrition practice. This is because nutrition is important in the prevention of chronic disease (such as obesity, type 2 diabetes and cardiovascular disease), dietary change is required in managing disease once it is established (such as for weight loss, supporting cholesterol-lowering and hypertension management), and dietary intervention is required for certain disease conditions (e.g. malnutrition is a particular condition that has emerged in the elderly hospitalised population). As outlined previously, health services provide a key location for various forms of nutrition practice.

Government departments and agencies have many roles that have implications for food and nutrition. They need to protect public health, build an educated community, foster the creation of employment, encourage innovation and manage the economy. Food is associated with all of these components. The development of a national food and nutrition policy can be seen as one step towards integrating the functions of government to improve the nutritional health of the population.

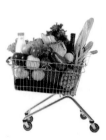

>> CASE 1.7

THE HEALTHY FOOD PARTNERSHIP

Making healthy food choices is dependent on being able to discriminate between foods, understanding how much food is appropriate (serve size), and the availability and accessibility of foods.

Under the auspices of the Australian Government's Department of Health, the Healthy Food Partnership aims to 'improve the dietary habits of Australians by making healthier food choices easier and more accessible and by raising awareness of better food choices and portion sizes' [31]. Aims include to:

- support industry to reformulate foods supported by the Health Star Rating System
- support consumers to eat more core foods—for example, fruits and vegetables
- educate consumers on portion and serve sizes
- improving consumers' knowledge and awareness of healthy food choices.

More detail can be found at: www.health.gov.au/internet/main/publishing.nsf/content/healthy-food-partnership.

- How would knowledge of food and nutrition be applied in the work of the Healthy Food Partnership?
- What do consumers need to know about food and nutrition to be able to make healthy food choices?

>> RESEARCH AT WORK

FOOD SECURITY IN A CHANGING WORLD

Climate change has significant implications for food production, with subsequent implications for nutrition. In 2010, the Prime Minister's Science, Engineering and Innovation Council (PMSEIC) formed an Expert Working Group to develop a report titled *Australia and Food Security in a Changing World* [32]. The working group members included scientists with backgrounds in plant functional genomics, agribusiness, animal studies, environmental and rural sciences, climate adaptation, rural affairs and nutrition, who produced a set of recommendations on many aspects of food production, human health and environmental management. The awareness of the importance of nutrition was a key element, as was the need to reference nutrition standards and guidelines in broader overall activities. This example shows how nutrition science can contribute to multidisciplinary teams addressing important global health and economic problems.

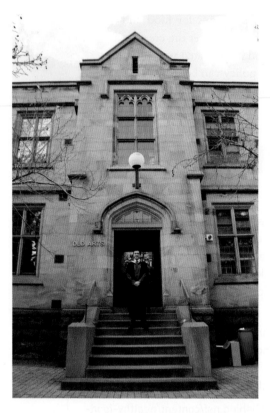

Non-government organisations and many community organisations also have an interest in nutrition. Examples in Australia include the Heart Foundation (www.heartfoundation.org.au) and the Cancer Council (www.cancercouncil.com.au). Groups such as these take a particular interest in how nutrition relates to their specific concerns, such as the links between nutrition and the prevalence of heart disease and cancer, and how community education may assist in prevention. More general consumer advocacy groups (e.g. www.choice.com.au) may address concerns supporting consumer decisions that affect food and nutrition for the population.

Professional societies and organisations link individuals in a particular area of nutrition practice. They provide a form of peer support and tend to do so by setting standards (recognised through membership), providing continuing education and interacting with governments and the general community. Examples of professional nutrition-related societies in Australia include the Dietitians Association of Australia (www.daa.asn.au), Nutrition Society of Australia (www.nsa.asn.au), Australian Institute of Food Science and Technology (www.aifst.asn.au) and Public Health Association of Australia (www.phaa.net.au).

Schools provide a basic education for life and this includes knowledge of human nutrition, often covered in health areas of the curriculum. The activities of schools can also influence nutritional behaviours, such as through policies regarding the types of foods sold in school canteens (see, for example, www.health.gov.au). *Universities and higher education institutions* provide a deeper level of knowledge and enquiry, giving students pathways to many areas of practice, including nutrition communications and policy such as in public health, media and the food industry, education in schools and elsewhere, healthcare practice such as in dietetics, and ongoing formal research, to name just a few.

Researchers from a range of disciplines contribute to working with nutrition via many paths. Researchers in basic science bring cutting-edge knowledge of mechanisms by which components in food may be affecting the function of the human body. Food scientists build knowledge on food composition and how this is affected by food production and manufacturing processes. Epidemiologists and public health practitioners expose the links between dietary patterns and health, and the surrounding circumstances influencing these relationships. Dietitians and other health practitioners evaluate the consequences for individual and population health of any action or advice given in relation to food and nutrition. Food and agriculture groups advise on the opportunities, risks and feasibility of food supply positions. Consumer groups provide another critical set of perspectives.

Research and development agencies are integral to building nutrition knowledge. Research produces new knowledge that is taken up into the various forms of nutrition practice. In Australia, the research sector includes funding agencies such as the Australian Research Council (www.arc.gov.au) and the National Health and Medical Research Council (NHMRC), which serve as primary sources of research funds for universities (www.nhmrc.gov.au) and the Commonwealth Scientific and Industrial Research Organisation (CSIRO) (www.csiro.au). The research and development (R&D) sector also considers the links between research and commercialisation.

Research and development

activities that address key questions and use valid methods to collect and analyse data or information that is evaluated and acted upon in developing new products or processes.

Agricultural and livestock industries provide primary products to the food value chain in many countries (www.agriculture.gov.au). Australia produces most of its own fruit and vegetables, grains, meat and dairy products. Each of these sectors has associated research and development arms aimed at sustaining and enhancing their productivity with food innovation. Primary food products are significant contributors to the nutritional quality of diets, and primary food production therefore is an important stakeholder group for nutrition practice.

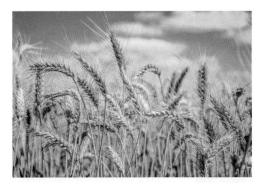

Food companies (food manufacturing industries and firms) are an important part of the food value chain. Much of the food sold in large urbanised societies is manufactured to some extent. Food companies are able to compete on the market with their products through brands that are known for particular qualities. Some of this information is given on food labels and in marketing strategies. Innovation in food manufacturing includes the development of new products and this draws on R&D. This may relate to improving nutritional quality or establishing evidence of likely nutritional effects from consumption of those products. Nutrition research and marketing are important forms of nutrition practice with this stakeholder group.

Retail outlets such as supermarkets provide the main interface between consumers and food in large urbanised societies. They provide all forms of food, and represent a significant component of the food value chain from the paddock to the plate. Other food outlets such as restaurants, cafés, fast-food chains, institutional food-service/catering systems and vending machines are also significant contributors to the food supply. These constitute key elements of exposure to the food environment in which individuals make food choices that ultimately influence their health.

From this introductory chapter it becomes apparent that we need to know more to better understand and apply nutrition knowledge more effectively. Knowledge of food and nutrition expands into a network that takes us to different areas and poses more and more questions as we go. You will soon realise why nutrition is constantly debated and why you need to keep abreast of new knowledge to get the most out of your study of nutrition. Enjoy the journey!

STOP AND THINK

- Who are the main stakeholder groups in food and nutrition in Australia?
- What is the relevance of the food value chain to the nutritional health of the population?
- How do policies and guidelines protect the nutritional health of the population?

SUMMARY

- Food delivers essential components that support the structure and function of the human body, but the concept of food synergy recognises that the effects of food may be greater than the sum of its parts.
- The stages of life provide a useful framework for applying scientific knowledge of nutrition to health-related practice.
- The applications of nutrition science in practice can occur at a number of levels, from individualised self-care through to managing individuals in healthcare institutions.

PATHWAYS TO PRACTICE

- There are many areas of practice that relate to working with nutrition. This occurs at the individual level with consumer food choice and healthcare dietary advice, and at the population level through guidelines, standards and community programs.
- Healthcare delivery and the development and governance of policy are high-order activities, but involvement in nutrition occurs at all levels of society.
- The important issue is that contributions are appropriately located, and recognition is given for the area of expertise that is required.

DISCUSSION QUESTIONS

1 How is food defined and how is it different from vitamin supplements?
2 How does nutrition science provide evidence for the effects of food consumption on health?
3 What are some of the problems associated with communications in nutrition and the health benefits of foods and nutrients?
4 How does the concept of life stages provide a useful framework for defining nutritional needs?
5 How do we know if there are nutrition problems in the community?
6 What is a food value chain and where do stakeholders fit into this concept?

USEFUL WEBLINKS

American Institute of Cancer Research:
www.aicr.org

Australian Bureau of Agricultural and Resource Economics and Sciences:
www.agriculture.gov.au/abares

Australian Dietary Guidelines:
www.eatforhealth.gov.au

Australian Government, Department of Health Healthy Food Partnership:
www.health.gov.au/internet/main/publishing.nsf/content/healthy-food-partnership

Australian Government, Department of Health. Health Star Rating System:
http://healthstarrating.gov.au/internet/healthstarrating/publishing.nsf/content/home

Australian Health Survey 2011–13:
www.abs.gov.au/australianhealthsurvey

Australian Institute of Food Science and Technology:
www.aifst.asn.au

Australian Institute of Health and Welfare—*Australia's Health 2016*:
www.aihw.gov.au/WorkArea/DownloadAsset.aspx?id=60129556760

Australian Meals on Wheels Association:
http://mealsonwheels.org.au

Australian Research Council:
www.arc.gov.au

Cancer Council:
www.cancercouncil.com.au

Choice:
www.choice.com.au

Commonwealth Scientific and Industrial Research Organisation:
www.csiro.au

Department of Agriculture and Water Resources:
www.agriculture.gov.au

Dietary Guidelines for Americans:
http://health.gov/dietaryguidelines

Dietitians Association of Australia:
https://daa.asn.au

Food Standards Australia New Zealand:
www.foodstandards.gov.au

Heart Foundation:
https://heartfoundation.org.au

National Health and Medical Research Council:
www.nhmrc.gov.au

Nutrition Society of Australia:
http://nsa.asn.au

Public Health Association of Australia:
www.phaa.net.au

Stephanie Alexander Kitchen Garden Foundation:
www.kitchengardenfoundation.org.au

FURTHER READING

Mahmood, S. S., Levy, D., Vasan, R. S. & Wang, T. J. (2014). The Framingham Heart Study and the epidemiology of cardiovascular disease: a historical perspective. *The Lancet*, 383(9921), 999–1008. doi:10.1016/S0140-6736(13)61752-3.

Mozaffarian, D. (2016). Dietary and policy priorities for cardiovascular disease, diabetes, and obesity: a comprehensive review. *Circulation*. doi:10.1161/circulationaha.115.018585.

Simpson, S. & Raubenheimer, D. (2012). *The Nature of Nutrition: A unifying framework from animal adaptation to human obesity*. Princeton, NJ: Princeton University Press.

Willett, W. (2012). *Nutritional Epidemiology*, 3rd edn. Oxford: Oxford University Press.

REFERENCES

1   World Health Organization (2017). Health Topics: Nutrition. Retrieved from: www.who.int/topics/nutrition/en.

2   W. O. Atwater (1887). The chemistry of foods and nutrition. I. The composition of our bodies and our food. *Century Magazine*, 34, 59–74.

3   K. J. Carpenter (1986). *The History of Scurvy and Vitamin C*. Cambridge: Cambridge University Press.

4   National Health and Medical Research Council (2006). *Nutrient Reference Values for Australia and New Zealand, Including Recommended Dietary Intakes*. Canberra: NHMRC.

5   M. M. Murphy, L. M. Barraj, D. Herman, X. Bi, R. Cheatham & R. K. Randolph (2012). Phytonutrient intake by adults in the United States in relation to fruit and vegetable consumption. *Journal of the Academy of Nutrition and Dietetics*, 112(2), 222–9. doi:https://doi.org/10.1016/j.jada.2011.08.044.

6   A. Keys (1990). Recollections of pioneers in nutrition: from starvation to cholesterol. *Journal of the American College of Nutrition*, 9(4), 288–91. doi:10.1080/07315724.1990.10720382.

7   D. R. Jacobs & L. C. Tapsell (2007). Food, not nutrients, is the fundamental unit in nutrition. *Nutrition Reviews*, 65(10), 439–50. doi:10.1111/j.1753-4887.2007.tb00269.x.

8   D. R. Jacobs, M. D. Gross & L. C. Tapsell (2009). Food synergy: an operational concept for understanding nutrition. *American Journal of Clinical Nutrition*, 89(5), 1543S–1548S. doi:10.3945/ajcn.2009.26736B.

9   L. C. Tapsell, E. P. Neale, A. Satija & F. B. Hu (2016). Foods, nutrients, and dietary patterns: interconnections and implications for dietary guidelines. *Advances in Nutrition: An International Review Journal*, 7(3), 445–54. doi:10.3945/an.115.011718.

10 M. T. Long & C. S. Fox (2016). The Framingham Heart Study—67 years of discovery in metabolic disease. *Nature Reviews Endocrinology*, 12, 177. doi:10.1038/nrendo.2015.226.

11 K. M. Camp & E. Trujillo (2014). Position of the academy of nutrition and dietetics: nutritional genomics. *Journal of the Academy of Nutrition and Dietetics*, 114(2), 299–312. doi:10.1016/j.jand.2013.12.001.

12 D. Raubenheimer & S. J. Simpson (2016). Nutritional ecology and human health. *Vol. 36. Annual Review of Nutrition*, 603–26.

13 M. Heffernan & J. Medew (2013). Vitamins can harm cancer patients: scientist. *Sydney Morning Herald*, 10 January. Retrieved from: www.smh.com.au/healthcare/vitamins-can-harm-cancer-patients-scientist-20130109-2cgrc.html.

14 L. Schwingshackl, H. Boeing, M. Stelmach-Mardas, M. Gottschald, S. Dietrich, G. Hoffmann & A. Chaimani (2017). Dietary supplements and risk of cause-specific death, cardiovascular disease, and cancer: a systematic review and meta-analysis of primary prevention trials. *Advances in Nutrition*, 8(1), 27–39. doi:10.3945/an.116.013516.

15 *Oxford Concise Medical Dictionary* (2010). Homeostasis. *Oxford Concise Medical Dictionary*, 8th edn. Oxford: Oxford University Press.

16 National Health and Medical Research Council (2000). *How to Use the Evidence: Assessment and application of scientific evidence. Handbook series on preparing clinical practice guidelines*. Canberra: NHMRC.

17 P. J. H. Jones, N.-G. Asp & P. Silva (2008). Evidence for health claims on foods: how much is enough? Introduction and general remarks. *Journal of Nutrition*, 138(6), 1189S–1191S. doi:10.1093/jn/138.6.1189S.

18 B. Sibbald & M. Roland (1998). Understanding controlled trials. Why are randomised controlled trials important? *British Medical Journal*, 316(7126), 201.

OXFORD UNIVERSITY PRESS

19 R. Estruch, E. Ros, J. Salas-Salvadó, M.-I. Covas, D. Corella, F. Arós, ... M. A. Martínez-González (2018). Primary prevention of cardiovascular disease with a Mediterranean diet supplemented with extra-virgin olive oil or nuts. *New England Journal of Medicine*, 378(25), e34. doi:10.1056/NEJMoa1800389.

20 Australian Institute of Health and Welfare (2016). *Australia's Health 2016*. Canberra: AIHW. Retrieved from: www.aihw.gov.au/reports/australias-health/australias-health-2016/contents/summary.

21 J. Shlisky, D. E. Bloom, A. R. Beaudreault, K. L. Tucker, H. H. Keller, Y. Freund-Levi, ... S. N. Meydani (2017). Nutritional considerations for healthy aging and reduction in age-related chronic disease. *Advances in Nutrition*, 8(1), 17–26. doi:10.3945/an.116.013474.

22 Australian Institute of Health and Welfare (2016). *Australia's Health 2016*. In brief. Canberra: AIHW. Retrieved from: www.aihw.gov.au/australias-health.

23 J. Epp (1986). Achieving health for all: a framework for health promotion. *Health Promotion International*, 1(4), 419–28. doi:10.1093/heapro/1.4.419.

24 National Health and Medical Research Council (2013). *Australian Dietary Guidelines*. Canberra: NHMRC.

25 World Health Organization (2012). *The Ottawa Charter for Health Promotion 1986*. Retrieved from: www.who.int.en.index.html.

26 K. Walton, S. Maclure, K. Sitwane & P. Williams (2009). A nutritional analysis of Meals on Wheels (MOW) meals. *Nutrition & Dietetics*, 66(S1), 33.

27 K. Walton (2012). Improving opportunities for food service and dietetics practice in hospitals and residential aged care facilities. *Nutrition & Dietetics*, 69(3), 222–5. doi:10.1111/j.1747-0080.2012.01620.x.

28 Australian Meals on Wheels Association (2012). Meals on Wheels, Australia. Retrieved from: www.mealsonwheels.org.au/Home.aspx.

29 Food Standards Australia New Zealand (2012). Food Standards Australia New Zealand. Retrieved from: www.foodstandards.gov.au.

30 J. Howland & D. J. Rohsenow (2013). Risks of energy drinks mixed with alcohol. *JAMA—Journal of the American Medical Association*, 309(3), 245–6. doi:10.1001/jama.2012.187978.

31 Department of Health (2016). Healthy Food Partnership. Retrieved from: www.health.gov.au/internet/main/publishing.nsf/Content/healthy-food-partnership.

32 Prime Minister's Science, Engineering and Innovation Council (2010). *Australia and Food Security in a Changing World*. Canberra: PMSEIC.

CHAPTER 2

DIETARY GUIDELINES: PLANNING A HEALTHY DIET

LINDA TAPSELL AND ELIZABETH NEALE

CHAPTER OBJECTIVES

This chapter will enable the reader to:

- discuss the benefit of various dietary patterns for health
- appreciate the role of dietary guidelines in planning a healthy diet
- describe how scientific evidence is evaluated for dietary guidelines and other areas concerning food and nutrition.

KEY TERMS

Diet quality

Dietary guidelines

Dietary patterns

Evidence-based review

KEY POINTS

- Cuisines are cultural ways in which foods are combined to form recipes, meals and dietary patterns. They can be described in terms of characteristic foods, flavours, ways of cooking and geographical regions from which the cuisine is identified. Some cuisines have been associated with better health outcomes in populations.
- Dietary guidelines support the planning of a healthy diet. This diet would comprise plenty of vegetables and legumes, fruits and wholegrains, and moderate amounts of milk/cheese/ yoghurt, fish, eggs, lean meats and nuts, with healthy oils for culinary use.
- The evidence base for examining the relationship between diet and health is complex. It is developed using standardised processes that evaluate a wide range of studies.

OXFORD UNIVERSITY PRESS

INTRODUCTION

A diet is characterised by the types and amounts of foods to be consumed on a regular basis. A healthy diet is one in which foods of a high nutritional quality predominate. Food patterns can develop from following diets and are formed by making regular choices of particular foods. A healthy food pattern means most of the foods chosen provide the essential nutrients required by the body, and the total amount of food supports an ideal body weight. It can also be a pattern where the particular combinations of foods protect against, for example, cardiovascular disease (CVD). A diet that is designed to contain less energy (kilojoules/calories) than the body requires is a weight-loss diet. Diets can also be characterised by food avoidance (e.g. gluten free) or specific selectivity of foods (e.g. vegetarian). Given the potential health risks with food avoidance and low energy intakes, there should be some level of clinical oversight (with doctors and dietitians), but for the population at large dietary guidelines provide general direction for the normal healthy population. Across the globe, many national guidelines now refer to 'plant-based diets', and this means that most of the food should come from plant sources (vegetables, fruit, grains).

The only food that serves as a complete food for humans is breast milk in infancy. Indeed, it is the recognised best food for infants in the first six months of life [1]. The production of breast milk is also the consequence of a human physiological process that comes after the feeding of the foetus *in utero*. The nutrient composition of human breast milk naturally follows suit in meeting nutritional needs for the early stages of life of the infant. With growth and development, nutritional needs are met through a combination of foods, but for best results this combination also has a nutritional code, just as breast milk does for the newborn. This code represents an ideal combination of foods that deliver requirements for health. There is always individual variation in requirements [2], but from a population health perspective, guidelines can be set based on best available knowledge at the time.

The fact that humans have evolved to live longer and healthier lives means better access to foods that are good to eat. It also reflects a cultural knowledge of food, and of healthy **cuisines**, where staple foods provide substantial amounts of nutrients known to be required for growth and development. Some cultures have more formally defined the relationships between food and health to the extent that foods can become somewhat medicalised (e.g. in Ayurvedic and Chinese medicines). Today, both Mediterranean and Asian cuisines have been recognised as being associated with healthier outcomes than cuisines based on other food choices [3–5]. Bridges are being built between modern nutritional science and traditional cultural knowledge of food. As the latter provides an indication of safety and potential benefits, it serves as a reasonable starting point for examining hypotheses that use scientific methods. One study exploring the relationship with nutritional composition and the Chinese concepts of 'hot' and cold' foods shows how cultural knowledge can align with concepts in nutrition science [6]. Extensive research on Mediterranean and Nordic diets, both with high **diet quality**, has linked these diets to health benefits [7–10].

Cuisine means more than a list of foods consumed in a diet—it also refers to the way foods are cooked. The concept of cuisine does recognise the use of foods available in a regional area, such as olive oil in the Mediterranean diet. The associated cuisine also includes a combination of foods combined in recipes that contain many vegetables found in countries around the Mediterranean Sea [11] (Figure 2.1). Because the foods in the Mediterranean diet are nutrient rich and the overall dietary pattern has a fatty acid profile, which is congruent with reduced CVD risk, it is recognised as healthy. On the other hand, **dietary patterns** that have too many nutrient-poor foods and have a fatty acid profile

Cuisine
the combination of foods selected on a particular basis with some reference to culinary traditions and regional foods.

Diet quality
the nutritional value of a particular combination of foods normally consumed consistently over a period of time.

Dietary patterns
the consistent choice of particular sets of foods over extended periods of time.

LINDA TAPSELL AND ELIZABETH NEALE

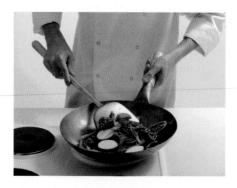

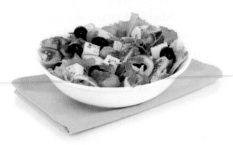

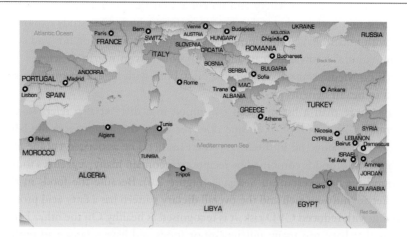

FIGURE 2.1   COUNTRIES BORDERING THE MEDITERRANEAN SEA

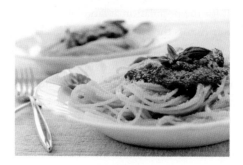

OXFORD UNIVERSITY PRESS

associated with disease risk are recognised as unhealthy. The cuisines associated with this include many 'fast' or highly processed foods characterised by high saturated fat, sugar and salt contents. As this pattern is common in Westernised communities, where food is a significant economic commodity, the cuisine is often referred to in terms of a Western diet [12]. Comparing health outcomes in populations that consume different cuisines helps to expose the diet–disease relationship in humans.

» RESEARCH AT WORK

SHIFTING CUISINE WITH MIGRATION

When people migrate they bring their food cultures and also adopt those of their new environment: the adaptation is bidirectional. For example, Asian migration into Australia has influenced the range of fresh food outlets and broadened the range of healthy food choices such as grains (rice), legumes (soy) and different types of vegetables and fruits. The influence of the new local cuisine for these migrants, however, may not always be advantageous [13]. To illustrate this point, a study of Western-style food intakes in a cohort of Chinese living in Singapore (Singapore Chinese Health Study of men and women aged 45–74) found that those who consumed Western-style fast-food items at least twice a week had an increased risk of developing type 2 diabetes and of dying from coronary heart disease compared with those who rarely ate those foods [14]. On the other hand, another study found that Anglo-Celts and Greek-Australians following a traditional Mediterranean diet in Australia had a 17% reduction in overall mortality [15]. Thus, choice of food pattern remains an important parameter for health and there is ample opportunity to learn from this across cultures, particularly in a society with a broad food supply such as Australia.

TRY IT YOURSELF

How would you describe your eating pattern? How many cuisines would be present in the meals you choose over any given week?

Establishing the evidence on what constitutes a healthy diet, however, requires a substantial amount of research. Trying to capture the nature of healthy dietary patterns and cuisines requires research and practice to work closely together. As previously stated, cultural eating patterns may reflect a common knowledge of healthy food. This can provide a starting point for modern science to understand why this may be so. Ensuing research can also correct misconceptions and consolidate the knowledge base on food overall. A good example of this kind of research is the PREDIMED study, which will be discussed in more detail later in the chapter [16]. This chapter gives an overview of the relationship between cuisines and food patterns and health. It examines research on the relationships between dietary patterns and disease risk and then outlines the science behind the Australian Dietary Guidelines, which support the planning of a healthy diet. There are particular challenges for developing dietary guidelines in the context of the globalisation of food choice and the consequent exposure to a wide range of cuisines. In addition, the evidence underpinning dietary guidelines comes from a wide range of studies using different scientific methods that need to be critiqued in a systematic and transparent way. These issues are addressed in the last part of the chapter.

STOP AND THINK

- What are the subtle differences between the terms 'dietary pattern', 'cuisine' and 'diet'?
- Why is it important to research these concepts in nutritional science?
- What kind of changes in food choices are needed for a healthier diet?

WHICH DIETARY PATTERNS ARE BEST FOR HEALTH?

Because 'you are what you eat', the effects of consuming food are likely to be seen over long periods of time [17]. Relationships between diet and disease are exposed by studying food intake patterns and comparing them to disease end points (such as diagnosis of the disease or sudden death attributed to the disease) or disease biomarkers (such as blood cholesterol levels, blood glucose levels, blood pressure and body fat). As understanding of the pathophysiology of a disease grows, so too does understanding of how diet works. New biomarkers begin to emerge that may better predict the course of the disease, or show stronger relationships with diet. It takes some time before these measures become standard clinical practice for disease assessment and management, but the scientific literature contains many new ideas and new developments that students of nutrition would find interesting to follow.

Food delivers relatively small doses of multiple small molecules over extended periods. The balance of this delivery is the result of patterns of food choices. The general effects of diet are to maintain the functions of the body, but poor diet can also lead to chronic disease. The regular selection of types of food (creating a food pattern), its preparation (referring to a cuisine) and the total combination of foods (forming a diet) all make important contributions to health. Food delivers nutrients, but the diet is not a simple nutrient delivery system. Synergies between nutrients exist within foods and can be further affected by food preparation and the combination of foods consumed within a diet [17]. It has been argued that to establish the evidence for the effects of diet on health it is best to examine relationships in the context of the whole diet rather than simply focusing on the nutrients that are delivered by the diet [17].

A schema for understanding these relationships is seen in Figure 2.2. Effects and associations can be related to diseases (such as CVD), disease risk factors (such as levels of cholesterol) and even behaviours (such as improved dietary quality). The construct of health and disease also needs to be considered. For example, while much research to date has focused on chronic diseases (e.g. coronary heart disease, type 2 diabetes, obesity and hypertension), there is emerging evidence for relationships with healthy ageing, along the lines of maintaining functionality such as eyesight.

The extent of research in this area is very broad, so only examples of key areas are given here. The framework provided by these examples and the principles discussed thus far, however, enable a wide range of potential areas to be explored in taking a more complete view of the relationship between food consumption and health.

Assessing the diet–disease relationship using a whole-of-diet approach is useful from a number of perspectives. Importantly, it avoids the limitations of studies involving single nutrients or foods [18]. Through analyses of the eating patterns of large populations, dietary patterns have been identified to be associated with the development of obesity, metabolic syndrome, type 2 diabetes and CVD.

FIGURE 2.2   RELATIONSHIPS BETWEEN NUTRIENTS, FOODS AND DIET PATTERNS

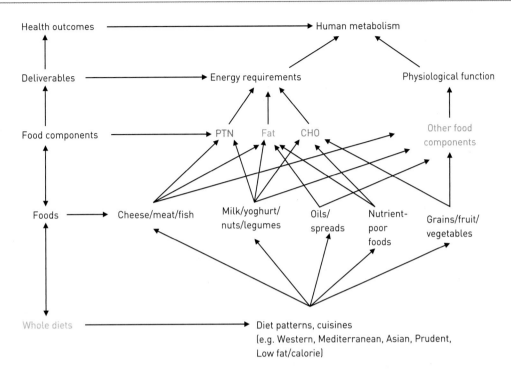

» RESEARCH AT WORK

ANALYSING DIETARY PATTERNS

There is a number of ways in which scientists expose dietary patterns by analysing records or surveys of reported food intakes among populations (see also Table 2.1). The two most common methods of analysis are *a priori* methods, which hypothesise that a given pattern will be superior (this is the basis of diet quality scores, such as a **healthy eating index**) or *posterior* methods that simply explore the data and look for relationships between foods. Examples of the latter are principal component analysis (PCA), exploratory factor analysis and cluster analysis [19].

Applying PCA, a study of baseline food records from participants attending a weight-loss trial [20] found that a dietary pattern rich in nuts, seeds, fruit and fish was inversely associated with blood pressure. It was similarly associated with the sodium:potassium ratio measured by 24-hour urine samples, a biomarker of dietary intakes.

Healthy eating index
a score obtained for an overall dietary pattern based on predetermined scores for individual foods consumed in the diet.

See Chapter 22 on dietary assessment and methods of analysis.

LINDA TAPSELL AND ELIZABETH NEALE

TABLE 2.1   METHODS FOR ANALYSING DIETARY PATTERNS

Testing a known healthy pattern	Identifying patterns from usual intakes
Diet quality scores	Principal component analysis
Healthy eating index	Factor analysis
Mediterranean diet scores Healthy Nordic Food Index	Cluster analysis Reduced rank regression

In a comparison of scores obtained from 38,428 women aged about 60 years in the Swedish Mammography Cohort study, both the modified Mediterranean diet score and the Healthy Nordic Food Index were associated with lower mortality, but the association was stronger with the modified Mediterranean diet score [21]. Thus, even though it may be assumed Swedish women consume more of a Nordic diet, the pattern captured in the modified Mediterranean diet score appeared to be more related to reduced mortality. This is both a reflection of the measurement tool and a food consumed, and leaves space for further research on the relative importance of foods that make up dietary patterns versus cuisines.

The health benefits of the Mediterranean diet have been researched for some time. This research lies at the base of the ongoing observations and interventions addressing the diet–heart disease relationship. One of the earliest investigators, Ancel Keys, examined epidemiological data on death rates from CVD from seven countries. He observed reduced mortality in peoples consuming diets rich in olives, olive oil and nuts with less meat, which was expressed as a higher ratio of dietary monounsaturated to saturated fat (MUFA:SFA) [22]. Thus, while the observation was made of the Mediterranean diet, it was often presented in terms of a nutrient profile, notably dietary fat. Keys' observations provided the impetus for many trials based on dietary fat that would test the observed relationship with actual dietary interventions. Trials that were also based on a Mediterranean-style diet showed effects on risk factors such as reduced blood pressure, reduced low-density lipoprotein (LDL) cholesterol, increased high-density lipoprotein HDL cholesterol, reduced inflammatory markers, and improved insulin sensitivity as well as reduced overall CVD risk [23–27]. The observations were confirmed in the seminal PREDIMED study. Conducted over five years in around 7500 older adults at risk of CVD, the dietary intervention demonstrated around 30% reduction in CVD events [16]. The challenge remains to translate the principles of the Mediterranean diet, some of which may relate to dietary fat, but the picture is more complicated, and there is a strong call for evidence-based research to focus more on dietary patterns than on individual nutrients [28]. This creates a particular challenge for dietary research across the globe.

During intervention trials, participants are advised on a particular diet. This usually takes the form of lists of foods to consume in varying amounts (vegetables, fruits, grains, nuts, fish etc.). This information may be translated from a food list to menus for meals, whole days or whole weeks. Advice can be further supported by providing recipes in which the foods are combined to constitute dishes. Large studies, such as the PREDIMED study, provide a great deal of this information for participants on websites (e.g. see www.predimed.es). Thus, the food list can define the diet; the menus reflect the dietary pattern and the recipes encase the cuisine. See also Table 2.2.

Given the interdependence between nutrients, foods and diets, cuisines other than those from the Mediterranean could also support health, but the principles underpinned by key nutrients, foods and

See Chapter 1 on nutrients, foods and diets.

diets are likely to be similar. Dietary fat may remain an important consideration, but the amount and type of food delivering the fat may be significant [29].

TABLE 2.2   RANGE OF FACTORS RESEARCHED IN HEALTHY DIETARY PATTERNS

Health outcome	Nutrients	Foods	Diets
LDL cholesterol	Type of fatty acids	Olive oil	Mediterranean
Hypertension	Plant phytochemicals (polyphenols, flavonoids)	Fish	Dietary Approaches to Stop Hypertension (DASH)
CVD	Fibre	Vegetables and fruits	Dietary guidelines
Cancer		Wholegrains	Nordic
All-cause mortality		Nuts	
		Yoghurt	

>> RESEARCH AT WORK

IDENTIFYING FOOD COMBINATIONS ASSOCIATED WITH HEALTH

Studies from across the globe indicate that a predominance of plant-based foods and the nature of food processing may underlie the characteristics of healthy cuisines.

A study of 12,000 men and women in the United States observed that consuming higher intakes of potatoes (including chips), sugary drinks and red meats was associated with weight increase, where the opposite was found for consuming wholegrains, vegetables, nuts, yoghurt and fruits [30]. The Swedish INTERGENE study of around 3500 men and women identified a 'healthy' eating pattern as comprising foods high in fibre and low in fat, and fewer foods rich in fat and sugar. Those who tended to be overweight ate little fruit and vegetables while consuming a lot of white bread and sugary drinks [31].

The same patterns also appear linked with disease progression. An observational study of 10,000 adults in the Korean National Health and Nutrition Examination Survey showed a lower risk of high triglyceride levels was associated with consuming mainly vegetables, grains and fish (high blood triglycerides, a type of fat, is associated with CVD. It was also inversely associated with risk of metabolic syndrome (a combination of CVD risk factors) [32]. Again from the United States, where the diet patterns was dominated by highly processed foods (potato chips, refined grains, sweets, desserts), high-fat dairy foods and red/processed meats, there was an increased risk of type 2 diabetes. The risk was higher in the presence of obesity or if there was also a low level of physical activity [33]. In another analysis of the diets of these men, breakfast emerged as significant, showing an increased risk of type 2 diabetes when breakfast was omitted. This association remained after adjustments were made for body mass index (BMI) [34]. In the Multi-Ethnic Study of Atherosclerosis (MESA) involving over 5000 men and women [35], a dietary pattern in which fats and processed meat were dominant was associated with a greater risk of CVD, but the pattern in which wholegrain cereals and fruit emerged as dominant was associated with a lower risk. This association remained after adjusting for lifestyle and demographic factors. This research shows that it is possible to expose 'healthy' and 'unhealthy' dietary patterns in terms of their relationship to the incidence of CVD.

Invariably, research shows healthy food patterns comprise foods known to be nutrient-rich, whereas foods associated with negative outcomes are either nutrient poor or may be over-consumed within the diet. Isolating individual foods is helpful, but more needs to be known about how these foods are combined and prepared (cuisine), and the impact of the broader lifestyle context, including meal settings and physical activity.

LINDA TAPSELL AND ELIZABETH NEALE

>> CASE 2.1

THE MEDITERRANEAN DIET [36], [37], [38].

The Mediterranean cuisine is characterised by a number of foods such as olive oil and vegetables. Olives are well recognised as central to the Mediterranean cuisine and the environment of the Mediterranean is ideal for their growth. Tomatoes are a main vegetable that form part of the cuisine base. Given the significance of the Mediterranean region in the history of human migration and trade, it is likely that more fruits and vegetables were added to the cuisine over time. Depending on the conditions, different fruits and vegetables may have grown better in different regions, but fish would have been available by the sea. Thus, while different combinations of foods and creations of recipes may have occurred, the common features of generous amounts of vegetables (including legumes) and fruits, the culinary use of olive oil and the inclusion of fish would characterise the Mediterranean diet. The PREDIMED study assessed compliance to the Mediterranean diet with a 14-point score (Table 2.3) based on the relative inclusion or limitation of certain categories of foods [39].

- Apply the PREDIMED diet score to your usual eating patterns. How much did you score out of 14?
- What do you think would be the average Australian's score?
- How adaptable would the Mediterranean diet in PREDIMED be in Australia?

TABLE 2.3   MEDITERRANEAN DIET SCORE USED IN PREDIMED STUDY

Preferred items	Criteria for 1 point	Limited items	Criteria for 1 point
Foods consumed			
Olive oil	>4 tbsp/day	Butter, margarine, cream	<1/day
Vegetables (200 g)	>2 serves/day	Red meat and products	<1/day
Fruit serves	>3 serves/day	Commercial sweets, pastries	<3/week
Legumes (150 g serve)	>3 serves/week		
Fish/shellfish (100–150 g serve)	>3 serves/week		
Nuts (30 g)	>3 serves/week		
Culinary behaviours			
Olive oil as culinary use	Yes	Preferring chicken, turkey to pork, sausage	Yes
Wine	>7 glasses/week	Sweetened carbonated beverages	<1/day
Dishes seasoned with sofrita (tomato, onion, olive oil)	>12/week		

Source: M. A. Martínez-González, A. García-Arellano, E. Toledo, J. Salas-Salvadó, P. Buil-Cosiales, D. Corella, ... for the PREDIMED Study Investigators (2012). A 14-Item Mediterranean diet assessment tool and obesity indexes among high-risk subjects: the PREDIMED trial. *PLOS ONE*, 7(8), e43134. doi:10.1371/journal.pone.0043134

Countries associated with Western civilisation, including Australia, have higher rates of heart disease, and the typical high saturated fat diet is associated with higher rates of CVD [40]. This dietary fat profile reflects the types of foods that are chosen and the cuisine in which they are consumed. As stated earlier, the food sources of saturated fat may need more consideration [29] and in this context, they should also be considered from a cuisine perspective. A comparison of Western dietary patterns with other regions of the world, their characteristic foods and key nutrients may be informative.

A lower risk of CVD is found in countries like Japan where traditional dietary patterns are characterised by a wide variety of foods. (The Japanese dietary guidelines emphasise the consumption of a wide variety of different foods per day [41].) Japanese people consume large amounts of fish and seafood so the traditional Japanese diet contains at least 1 g per day of the long-chain omega-3 PUFA [42]. When a cohort of Japanese people moved to Hawaii and adopted a Western diet, their rates of heart disease increased. It was also noted their omega-3 intakes dropped by more than 50% [42], but more needs to be known of the overall cuisine effect of this apparent loss of fish to the diet.

French cuisine is well known for its commitment to flavoursome, elegant meals. From a nutrient perspective, traditional French cuisine has a relatively high level of saturated fat, which in the past has created a paradox with a 30% lower mortality rate from CVD [43–45]. However, the relative amounts of foods in French cuisine suggested a more balanced diet, with more fruit and vegetables and less potatoes, biscuits and cakes than in Western diets [46]. At the food level, the diet may contain more butter, more cheese and more meat than Western diets [43–45]. There is also a notable cuisine difference, and differences in choices of foods containing fat. The traditional French diet gains most of its saturated fat from cheese and meat. Much of the saturated fat in the diet of Australians comes from foods that are baked and fried such as desserts and potato chips/crisps, but this has not been the case in France [47; 48]. There are other differences in these foods besides their saturated fat content, including the delivery of other nutrients, the form and consequences of food processing, the relative energy contribution to the diet and the meal context in which the foods are consumed.

As with other areas of the Mediterranean, the diet of France also includes wine with meals. While the negative effects of alcohol consumption are well documented, the context in which wine is consumed in the Mediterranean diet is an important differentiating factor. From a food component perspective, grapes and red wine contain compounds that research has shown reduces oxidative stress and inflammation. A range of potential mechanisms have been shown, mainly in animal and *in vitro* studies [49], but there is a need for more clinical studies in humans to untangle the evidence for benefits of consuming wine.

In contrast to the situation in France, Finland used to have the highest recorded death rates from heart dietary patterns, but this has reduced dramatically following intervention campaigns that saw reductions in smoking, blood pressure and plasma total cholesterol levels [50], and dietary changes including reduced saturated fat intakes and increased consumption of fruit and vegetables [50]. A deeper analysis of cuisine changes aligned with changes in dietary fat would help to explain how these specific modifications had an impact.

See Chapter 19 on Indigenous Australian food security.

See Chapter 8 on water, alcohol and beverages.

In contrast to European traditional cuisines, Australian cuisine has taken many turns. The cuisine of Indigenous Australians has proven to be both environmentally friendly and healthful [51].

The influence of immigrant cuisines underpins today's Australian cuisine, which is not so much a single entity but a fusion of different foods, both fresh and manufactured, with multicultural influences. The impact of the early British settlers was still apparent up to the 1950s. The menu for a typical day may contain soup but would have a main meal of meat and vegetables (usually potatoes plus two other vegetables) and dessert (often containing fruit). As Australia is a meat-producing country, meat was affordable and regularly consumed. Cooking meals was common, as were family mealtimes. Eating out of the home changed with the emergence of eat-in or takeaway restaurants set up by migrants from southern Europe and Asia [52]. Food culture has also changed, from not being discussed in polite company in the early 1800s to media shows that have won top audience-viewing ratings [53]. While there is ample opportunity for utilising cuisine development to build healthy eating patterns in the community, this has not always been the case. Analyses of dietary patterns and cuisine elements in known healthy diets need to form part of this effort.

» CASE 2.2

THE BEST DIETS

Cuisines (culinary uses of food), dietary patterns (regular choices of foods) and diets (defined foods consumed regularly) form part of everyday life. 'Dieting' (eating according to rigid rules from food lists) can be a national pastime and there is a constant barrage of information in the media on different types of diets.

'Fad diets' are diets with a questionable scientific basis. They can omit at least one entire healthy food group (e.g. grains) and promise results that are not sustainable even though results can be achieved quickly. Thus, fad diets have the potential to be harmful to health and are not recommended by health authorities. The news media often pick up on fad diets and report the latest reviews. Accredited practising dietitian Catherine Saxelby [54] provides guidance on identifying fad diets (Table 2.4).

TABLE 2.4   ISSUES WITH FAD DIETS

Characteristics	Types of fad diet	Methods	Examples
Enticing claims on quick, effortless weight loss	Single foods	Boredom from eating the same thing may lead to eating less	Soup diet
'Eat as much as you like'	Semi fasting	Fasting can produce rapid weight loss but only in short term	Grapefruit diet
Contains 'miracle foods'	Liquid diets	Meal replacements can control intake but may not be satisfying or help develop food skills	Israeli Army Diet
Requires special supplements or pills	Meal replacements		Detox diets
			Flat belly diet
'Revolutionary'	Minimal carbohydrate	Water loss	Cellulite diet
Focuses only on food			Fasting supplements
			Scarsdale diet

Source: C. Saxelby (2018). *Complete Food and Nutrition Companion*. Melbourne: Hardie Grant Books

Each year, the US News and World Report (http://health.usnews.com/best-diet) pulls together a number of experts in the scientific literature (see http://health.usnews.com/best-diet/experts) to rate the best diet for health and fitness according a scale (5 = extremely effective, to 1 = ineffective) (Table 2.5).

In 2017, the top two were the Dietary Approaches to Stop Hypertension (DASH) diet and the Mediterranean diet. One of the experts in the 2017 review, Dr David Katz MD, commented on the value of this particular media approach in informing consumers on best diets (see www.verywell.com/the-best-and-worst-of-the-best-diets-report-4122171). While recognising the benefits of this type of review, Katz cautioned against a potential emphasis on 'dieting', and stressed the need to consider the broader social context in which food is consumed and to work on sustained behavioural change.

TABLE 2.5 EVALUATING DIETS FOR HEALTH AND FITNESS

Criteria	Best diets	Benefits of review
Short-term weight loss	Dietary Approaches to Stop Hypertension (DASH)	Quality of reviewers
Long-term weight loss		Presentation of information
Preventing or managing diabetes and heart disease	Mediterranean diet	Scope of review
Ease of compliance		Public health merit
Nutritional completeness		
Health risks (including malnourishment)		

Source: US News and World Report (2018). Health—best diets. Retrieved from: http://health.usnews.com/best-diet

- Why would the best diets score highly?
- What is the relevance of the criteria applied to assess these diets?
- How can these diets help sustained dietary change?

See Chapters 11 and 17 for a discussion of the DASH diet.

Food and nutrition are central to health, and diet provides the pathway. The examination of best diets underlines the value of studying nutrition in depth to appreciate the complexities involved in building knowledge from nutrition science and translating it to effective practice.

STOP AND THINK

- Which foods emerge consistently as part of healthy dietary patterns around the globe?
- Why do excess amounts of certain nutrients appear implicated in deleterious dietary patterns?
- How does cuisine influence the healthfulness of dietary patterns?

HOW CAN A HEALTHY DIET BE PLANNED WITH DIETARY GUIDELINES?

Following a **healthy diet** can simply mean following a set of principles on which food choices are made. Behind those principles may stand 'a diet', because the consistent applications of those principles will result in an eating pattern that can be summarised down to a diet. Dietary guidelines provide those principles. In general, dietary guidelines provide advice on food choices to populations. The governments of many countries produce dietary guidelines that reflect the types of foods consumed in those regions and government priorities. Many other groups also produce guidelines and nutrition statements (some may relate to specific diseases), but this chapter focuses on dietary guidelines developed by the National Health and Medical Research Council (NHMRC) and Department of Health for the general population.

Healthy diet
the regular consumption of foods that provide the energy and nutrient requirements of an individual and at the same time protect against disease.

Generally, dietary guidelines statements are worded in a way that reflects general food choice behaviour. For planning a healthy diet, words like 'choose', 'avoid', 'limit' and 'encourage' are used. They relate to food groups (e.g. vegetables), food components (e.g. saturated fat) and cuisine issues (e.g. use of salt). As important components of evidence-based practice, however, these statements reflect the

 LINDA TAPSELL AND ELIZABETH NEALE

expertise of authoritative organisations in distilling and translating a comprehensive and complex base of scientific evidence into relatively simple messages.

≫ RESEARCH AT WORK

DIETARY GUIDELINES STATEMENTS FOR AUSTRALIANS 2013

The Australian Dietary Guidelines statements were developed with the support of evidence-based systematic literature reviews underpinned by key questions (see www.eatforhealth.gov.au). The statements that emerged are outlined below.

1   To achieve and maintain a healthy weight you should be physically active and choose amounts of nutritious foods and drinks that meet your energy needs.

- Children and adolescents should eat enough nutritious foods to grow and develop normally. They should be physically active every day and their growth should be checked regularly.
- Older people should eat nutritious foods and keep physically active to help maintain muscle strength and a healthy weight.

2   Eat a wide variety of nutritious foods from these five groups every day:

- Plenty of vegetables, including different types and colours, and legumes/beans
- Fruit
- Grain (cereal) foods, mostly wholegrain and/or high cereal fibre varieties, such as breads, cereals, rice, pasta, noodles, polenta, couscous, oats, quinoa and barley
- Lean meat and poultry, fish, eggs, nuts and seeds, legumes/beans
- Milk, yoghurt, cheese and/or their alternatives, mostly reduced fat (reduced fat milks are not suitable for children under the age of two years).
- And drink water.

3   Limit intake of food and drinks containing saturated fat, added salt, added sugars and alcohol.

- Limit intake of foods high in saturated fat such as biscuits, cakes, pastries, pies, processed meats, commercial burgers, pizza, fried foods, potato chips, crisps and other savoury snacks.
- Replace high-fat foods that contain predominantly saturated fats such as butter, cream, cooking margarine, coconut and palm oil with foods which contain predominantly polyunsaturated and monounsaturated fats such as oils, spreads, nut butters/pastes and avocado.
- Low-fat diets are not suitable for children under the age of two years.
- Limit intake of food and drink containing added salt.
- Read labels to choose lower sodium options among similar foods.
- Do not add salt to foods in cooking or at the table.
- Limit intake of foods and drinks containing added sugars such as confectionary, sugar-sweetened soft drinks and cordials, fruit drinks, vitamin waters, and energy and sports drinks.
- If you choose to drink alcohol, limit your intake. For women who are pregnant, planning a pregnancy or breastfeeding, not drinking alcohol is the safest option.

4   Encourage and support breastfeeding.

5   Care for your food; prepare and store it safely.

    OXFORD UNIVERSITY PRESS

AUSTRALIAN GUIDE TO HEALTHY EATING

Source: National Health and Medical Research Council (2013). *Australian Guide to Healthy Eating*.
Canberra: NHMRC. © Commonwealth of Australia

Essentially, dietary guidelines focus on five main food groups: vegetables, fruit, grains, protein-rich foods (fish, lean meats, eggs, legumes, nuts) and milk/cheese/yoghurt. One of the biggest problems in translating this guidance to practice is that each of these food groups can be prepared or manufactured in such a way, with or without other ingredients, that they lose nutritional value [55]. They then become the foods to limit (potato chips, cakes, processed meats). The ability to differentiate between 'core foods' and 'discretionary foods' remains one of the challenges in using dietary guidelines to develop a healthy diet. Instead of a minimal amount, Australians consume about 35% of their energy from discretionary foods, the major contribution coming from cereal products and dishes [56].

See Case 7.3 on Chapter 7 on the relationship between serving sizes and weight.

See Chapter 1 for information about food labels and Health Star Ratings.

TRY IT YOURSELF

Record all the foods you consumed in the past 24 hours. Categorise them according to the foods listed to include and those to limit in the ADG. Which category of foods formed most of your intake? Which foods could you exchange so that your eating pattern fits the guidelines better?

Identifying the best type of food to consume is an important first step. Food labels and Health Star Ratings help with this process. The next question is: how much food is in a healthy diet? Large serving sizes can be a problem in an obesogenic environment. The companion document to the dietary guidelines, the

                                              LINDA TAPSELL AND ELIZABETH NEALE

Australian Guide to Healthy Eating (AGHE)

a companion document to the Australian Dietary Guidelines that serves as a food selection tool outlining healthy dietary patterns using core food groups.

See Chapter 3 for a discussion of dietary modelling and the ADG.

Australian Guide to Healthy Eating (AGHE) [57] outlines the numbers of serves of each food group that would meet the requirements of individuals bearing in mind that this would vary for different ages, body sizes and levels of activity (Table 2.6).

The AGHE is based on dietary modelling that inputs the energy and nutrient needs of groups in the population with information on food consumption patterns from national surveys, and considers the evidence of the potential impact of food consumption on health [58]. Like all forms of modelling, dietary modelling constructs theoretical examples of food combinations. Decisions are made on how many food groups to work with, and to allow for flexibility in the models. Not everyone has the same requirement for food, but everyone requires adequate amounts of nutrients, so the choice of foods remains important. It is possible to build in various forms of any food group—for example, full-fat and low-fat milk or yoghurt and different types of vegetables or grains—and to accommodate cuisine differences defined by different foods—for example, vegetable foods or meat. Outputs of the modelling process include sets of food combinations that theoretically constitute a healthy diet. Nutritional requirements are addressed with reference to the required intakes given by Nutrient Reference Values (NRVs). In the dietary modelling carried out for the ADG, the recommended dietary intake (RDI) value was used because the advice was targeted to individuals within the population [58]. Dietary modelling underpinned the foundation and total diets reflected in the types and amounts of foods described in the AGHE.

TABLE 2.6   SERVING SIZES OF RECOMMENDED FOODS (AGHE)

Food group	Recommended serves/day*	Examples	Single serve size
Vegetables	5	Green/orange vegetables	½ cup
		Canned beans, lentils	½ cup
		Green leafy/salad	1 cup
Fruit	2	Apples	1 medium
		Plums	2
		Fruit salad	1 cup
Cereals/grains	6	Bread	1 slice
		Cereal/porridge	½ cup
		Rice/pasta	½ cup
Meats/eggs/legumes/ nuts	2½	Beef, lamb, pork	65 g
		Chicken, turkey	80 g
		Fish	100 g
		Eggs	2 large
		Legumes	1 cup
		Nuts	30 g
Milk/cheese/yoghurt	2½	Milk	250 mL
		Cheese	30 g
		Yoghurt	200 g

*Based on recommendations for women 19–50 years.

Source: National Health and Medical Research Council (2013). *Australian Dietary Guidelines*. Canberra: NHMRC. © Commonwealth of Australia

TRY IT YOURSELF

Go to the 'Average Recommended Number of Serves Calculator' on the Australian Dietary Guidelines website: www.eatforhealth.gov.au/node/add/calculator-servings. Enter your details and see whether your diet matches a healthy diet.

National dietary guidelines are a very public example of how nutrition science interfaces with practice at the level of population health. Commentary on dietary guidelines can be found in the media [59], in the scientific literature [60] and in social networks. This reflects the broad range of stakeholders in the development and applications of the guidelines. In Australia, guidance on healthy dietary patterns has occurred for over 75 years, primarily through the NHMRC and government departments (e.g. www.eatforhealth.gov.au). Expert working committees are formed to undertake the considerable process of evidence review and translation. Because the guidelines are underpinned by nutrition science, the development of dietary guidelines over the decades has been evolutionary, producing different types of guidelines and food guides. For example, the most recent Australian Dietary Guidelines (2013) follow on from the 2003 Dietary Guidelines for Australian Adults [61] and incorporate previously separate Dietary Guidelines of Older Australians (1999), and for Children and Adolescents (2003) [62]. The most recent review of the ADG (2012) incorporated the concurrent review of the AGHE, which, as discussed earlier, was built around the concept of five core food groups. The important thing for practitioners is that they keep up to date and use the most current version. The statements outlined in dietary guidelines represent a culmination of evidence and translation to meaningful messages for the public (Table 2.7). These processes are outlined in the main body of the ADG report [1].

TABLE 2.7   DOCUMENTS ASSOCIATED WITH THE AUSTRALIAN DIETARY GUIDELINES (2013) AND INFANT FEEDING GUIDELINES (2012)

Evidence reports	Health professional resources	Consumer resources
A Review of the Evidence to Address Targeted Questions to Inform the Revision of the Australian Dietary Guidelines (2011)	Australian Dietary Guidelines	Australian Guide to Healthy Eating (Food Modelling Tool)
A Modelling System to Inform the Revision of the Australian Guide to Healthy Eating (2011)	Infant Feeding Guidelines	Summary booklet for the Australian Dietary Guidelines
Review: Nutritional Requirements and Dietary Advice Targeted for Pregnant and Breastfeeding Women (2013)	Australian Guide to Healthy Eating (Food Modelling Tool)	Brochures for infants, children, pregnant women and adults
Infant Feeding Guidelines Literature Review (2012)	Educator Guide	Posters
	Summary booklet for the Australian Dietary Guidelines	Interactive web tools
	Summary booklet for the Infant Feeding Guidelines	Healthy eating information such as fact pages and tips

Source: National Health and Medical Research Council (2013). *Australian Dietary Guidelines.* Canberra: NHMRC, p. 4. © Commonwealth of Australia

>> CASE 2.3

TRANSLATING DIETARY GUIDELINES IN VARYING CULTURAL CONTEXTS

The translation of dietary guidelines to different cultural contexts requires further understanding of the significance of food in everyday life. For example, kosher regulations in the Jewish faith and halal dietary laws in the Islamic faith have defined specifications for dietary practices. While different people keep kosher rules in different ways because of the many levels of religious observance in Judaism [63], essentially following a traditional kosher regime would mean the need to follow certain rules extending beyond the avoidance of certain foods. For example, certain animals may not be eaten, slaughtering of the permitted animals must be conducted in a certain way, and even then certain parts of the animals may not be allowed to be consumed. Two sets of cooking utensils would be needed, as one may not come into contact with dairy and the other should not touch meat. This may extend to the necessity for two areas for refrigeration [64]. People following the Islamic religion also have dietary laws and these are known as halal. The foods that are avoided include certain meats such as pork, alcohol and other stimulating beverages. There are certain rules around the way in which animals are slaughtered for their meat. Observance of the Muslim faith includes observance of Ramadan, a month-long fast where neither food nor drink is consumed from sunrise to sunset [65].

- What are the implications of these specifications of dietary practices for the application of Australian Dietary Guidelines?
- How do these examples throw light on the significance of cuisine in developing healthy diets?

While developed with population health in mind, dietary guidelines can serve as first points of reference for individuals and organisations. Guideline materials serve as useful reference standards for a number of settings—for example, the design of the Kids Nutrition and Physical Activity Survey [66] and the Illawarra Healthy Food Basket survey [67]. Evidence supporting dietary guidelines continues to mount. Compliance with the dietary guidelines has been shown to be one of seven health behaviours that are associated with greater longevity against coronary heart disease in the United States (others included not smoking and being physically active) [68]. Methodological advances in the development of dietary guidelines will naturally occur [55; 69], and the science underpinning dietary guidelines will continue to be produced. It remains important to appreciate the science underpinning the evidence-based review that delivers on the guidelines.

STOP AND THINK

- How do dietary guidelines assist individuals develop a healthy diet?
- How is scientific evidence integrated into the development of dietary guidelines?
- What are some of the challenges in translating dietary guidelines to practice at the population level?

HOW ARE EVIDENCE-BASED REVIEWS APPLIED IN DIETARY GUIDELINES AND OTHER AREAS OF FOOD AND NUTRITION?

The development of dietary guidelines has evolved over many years. From originally relying on the deliberations of expert scientists, critical methods have been formally defined and applied to demonstrate the planning, analysis and interpretation of evidence from which the guidelines are constructed. Today, the analysis of the relevant available scientific research has come to be known as **systematic review**.

Systematic reviews contain a number of key elements, designed to ensure the risk of **bias** is minimised.

A starting point for the systematic review is the research question. Because guidelines aim to improve the health of populations, these questions need to relate to the target population and specify the health effects (or outcomes) of interest. Thus, the components of research questions for systematic reviews follow a formula summarised as PICO: population (P), intervention (I), comparator (C) and outcome (O). The next stage involves the development of a search strategy, which involves identifying search terms based on PICO components, and deciding which scientific databases to search—for example, MEDLINE or the Cochrane Central Register of Controlled Trials (CENTRAL). As part of developing the search strategy, review authors must also define criteria for deciding which papers to include and which to leave out (inclusion and exclusion criteria).

It is also at this point that the types of study designs to be included in the review (e.g. randomised controlled trials and cohort studies) would also be decided. The process of developing the search strategy and inclusion/exclusion criteria is guided by the research question, and is consistently applied throughout the review.

After the search has been conducted and the inclusion/exclusion criteria applied, key components of eligible studies are extracted into summary tables. Components included in summary tables will vary depending on the type of study and research question, but could include: study citation, study design, weight of the study population, study duration, sample size, details of the intervention and study results.

Systematic review
a method of combining and appraising all evidence on a topic.

Bias
a systematic error in results or inferences, which can lead to either underestimating or overestimating effects.

≫ RESEARCH AT WORK

SYSTEMATIC REVIEWS

In 2016, Neale and colleagues [70] conducted a systematic review to explore the effect of healthy dietary patterns (such as the Mediterranean diet) on biomarkers associated with inflammation, insulin resistance and adiposity. The design for this review is summarised in Table 2.8.

The systematic search initially found 1597 articles, and after applying the inclusion and exclusion criteria, 17 studies were found to be eligible for the review. Data from these studies was pooled in a meta-analysis.

The systematic review found that consumption of a healthy dietary pattern was associated with significant reductions in C-reactive protein, suggesting a reduction in inflammation. Limited evidence was available for other biomarkers, highlighting how systematic reviews can also be used to guide future research directions.

LINDA TAPSELL AND ELIZABETH NEALE

TABLE 2.8   DESIGN OF A SYSTEMATIC REVIEW

Question: What is the effect of consumption of healthy dietary patterns (I) on biomarkers of adiposity, insulin resistance and inflammation (O) in adults (P), compared with unhealthy dietary patterns (C)?

Databases	Keywords	Inclusion criteria	Exclusion criteria
Scopus, PubMed, Web of Science Cochrane Central Register of Controlled Trials	('diet* pattern*' OR 'food pattern*' OR 'Mediterranean diet' OR 'prudent diet' OR 'western diet' OR 'diet* score*' OR 'diet* index*), in combination with (biomarker* AND ('metabolic syndrome' OR 'metabolic health')) OR ('tumour necrosis factor' OR 'tumor necrosis factor' OR 'TNF*') OR ('retinol binding protein 4' OR 'RBP4') OR ('leptin' OR 'leptin:adiponectin' OR 'leptin/adiponectin') OR ('CRP' OR 'hsCRP' OR 'high sensitivity C-reactive protein') OR ('resistin') OR ('adiponectin' OR 'high molecular weight adiponectin')	Randomised controlled trials conducted in humans 18 years or over, which assessed the effect of a specific cuisine-based dietary pattern on biomarkers (e.g. C-reactive protein).	Studies were not included in the review if they were conducted in pregnant or breastfeeding women; were published as conference abstracts only; or reported only post-prandial effects of dietary patterns.

Source: E. P. Neale, M. J. Batterham & L. C. Tapsell (2016). Consumption of a healthy dietary pattern results in significant reductions in C-reactive protein levels in adults: a meta-analysis. *Nutrition Research*, 36(5), 391–401. doi:https://doi.org/10.1016/j.nutres.2016.02.009

An important key feature of systematic reviews is the appraisal of the risk of bias in studies included in the review. Risk of bias can vary substantially between studies due to reasons such as blinding of participants and personnel, and reporting all study outcomes, and it important that this is taken into account when drawing conclusions.

There are a number of methods for appraising risk of bias in studies. For example, the Cochrane Risk of Bias tool [71] considers components such as:

- random allocation sequence (how participants are allocated to different groups in a trial)
- allocation concealment (who knows about the allocation to groups)
- blinding of participants (not knowing which groups they have been allocated to), personnel and outcome assessors (whether researchers know which groups participants have been allocated to)
- incomplete outcome data (were reasons for missing data explained, and was missing data dealt with appropriately?)
- selective reporting (whether all study results have been reported).

This system provides a clear and transparent means for classifying each study as being at low, unclear or high risk of bias. During reviews of the evidence for the 2013 Australian Dietary Guidelines, for example, each included study was critiqued to determine how likely it was that bias, confounding or chance could have influenced study results [72]. This added to the scientific rigour under which the guidelines were developed.

In addition to considering individual studies, a strength of systematic reviews is their ability to consider the evidence base as a whole. This can be done qualitatively, by summarising and discussing the main features and findings of the body of evidence in a narrative style, or quantitatively, via a **meta-analysis.**

The final step in a systematic review involves making a judgment regarding the body of evidence. As with quality appraisal of individual studies, there are a number tools available to appraise the body of evidence on a topic. In 2013, the Australian Dietary Guidelines used the method designed by the NHMRC, which included the following components:

Meta-analysis
a statistical method used in some systematic reviews that involves combining the results of individual studies.

- attributes of the body of evidence (the number of studies, level of evidence and risk of bias in individual studies)
- consistency of results within the body of evidence
- clinical impact from application of the guideline to the population
- generalisability to the target population
- applicability to various settings and contexts within the population.

>> CASE 2.4

STANDARDS FOR EVIDENCE-BASED REVIEWS

With the development of systematic review methods as a global effort, it was soon recognised that any differences between tools and rating systems could limit the ability of guidelines to be compared between organisations and countries [73]. As a result, a new method, known as GRADE, was developed by a working group with expertise in guideline development. GRADE was designed to be a consistent global method for systematic review. It is now used by a broad range of international organisations, including the Cochrane Collaboration, World Health Organization (WHO), American College of Physicians, and National Institute of Health and Clinical Excellence (NICE).

In recent years, there have been other improvements to systematic review methodology to ensure reduced risk of bias. One such strategy is the Preferred Reporting Items for Systematic Reviews and Meta-Analyses (PRISMA) [74], which sets out required items to be reported in the review. Another improvement has been the pre-registration of research questions and methods for systematic reviews, which minimises the risk of bias by ensuring authors' decisions on review questions and inclusion criteria are not dependent on the findings of the review. Pre-registration of review protocols also decreases the risk of duplication of research questions. PROSPERO is a website where review authors can pre-register their reviews (see: www.crd.york.ac.uk/PROSPERO).

- What is the value of international agreement on how evidence in food and health is assessed?
- Where does discussion on systematic review come into debates on best diets and super foods?

Systematic reviews are used widely in nutrition. In addition to evaluating the evidence base for dietary guidelines, systematic reviews form part of the update of NRVs [75] and guidelines for clinical practice [76]. They also underpin the evidence for general level health claims on the effects of foods on health for display on food labels and advertisements. These must be self-substantiated by a process involving a systematic review of the literature [77].

STOP AND THINK

- Why is it important to have systematic review systems to assess the scientific evidence on food consumption and health?
- What might be more general perceptions of bias in statements on health effects of foods and diets? How do this compare with how scientific methods describe bias?
- How does the practice of evidence-based review in nutrition compare with general discussion on food and nutrition issues in the media?

SUMMARY

- A healthy diet is characterised by a combination of foods that deliver essential nutrients and has an energy value that supports an ideal body weight. This diet could be achieved through cuisines that traditionally combine foods with known health benefits in attractive and modest proportions, such as Mediterranean cuisines.
- Healthy dietary patterns are based on the regular consumption of foods such as vegetables, fruits, wholegrains, lean meats, fish, eggs, legumes and nuts, and dairy products such as milk, yoghurt and cheese.
- Evidence for the effects of dietary patterns on health is established by systematic review methodology that accounts for the populations of interest, the type of health outcomes assessed, the quality of each study and totality of evidence from scientific research.

PATHWAYS TO PRACTICE

- Working with nutrition means being able to identify the difference between dietary patterns that are examined in the scientific literature via observational studies or clinical trials, and 'fad diets' that are promoted commercially, often with very little scientific evidence.

- A good place to start when providing nutrition education is to focus attention on the food categories defined in the Australian Guide to Healthy Eating, and in particular emphasising the importance of vegetables, legumes, nuts, fruits and wholegrains forming the base of the diet.

- Appreciating the value of, and possibly developing skills in, systematic review methodology enables a deeper understanding of the scientific processes that underpin quality nutrition and dietary advice.

DISCUSSION QUESTIONS

1 Why do new 'diets' appear to gain more attention in the general media than research on the effects of healthy dietary patterns?
2 How well do the dietary guidelines statements relate to the food choices that are available for the general public?
3 Why do we need evidence-based review methodology for establishing guidelines and reference standards in relation to food and nutrition?

USEFUL WEBLINKS

Australian Dietary Guidelines:
www.eatforhealth.gov.au

Australian Health Survey 2011–13:
www.abs.gov.au/australianhealthsurvey

Best Diets US News and World Report:
http://health.usnews.com/best-diet

Cochrane Handbook for Systematic Reviews of Interventions:
http://handbook.cochrane.org

Diets on Parade: The Best and Worst of the 2017 Best Diets Report:
www.verywell.com/the-best-and-worst-of-the-best-diets-report-4122171

GRADE:
https://gradepro.org

NHMRC levels of evidence and grades:
www.nhmrc.gov.au/_files_nhmrc/file/guidelines/developers/nhmrc_levels_grades_evidence_
120423.pdf

PREDIMED study:
www.predimed.es

Preferred Reporting Items for Systematic Reviews and Meta-Analyses (PRISMA):
www.prisma-statement.org

PROSPERO (International prospective register of systematic reviews):
www.crd.york.ac.uk/PROSPERO

Public Workshop #3: Review of the process to update the Dietary Guidelines for Americans:
http://nationalacademies.org/hmd/Activities/Nutrition/DietaryGuidelinesforAmericans/2017-
JAN-10/Videos/Session%203%20Videos/12-Garza-Video.aspx

FURTHER READING

Adriouch, S., Julia, C., Kesse-Guyot, E., Méjean, C., Ducrot, P., Péneau, S., ... Fezeu, L. K. (2016). Prospective association between a dietary quality index based on a nutrient profiling system and cardiovascular disease risk. *European Journal of Preventive Cardiology*, 23(15), 1669–76. doi:10.1177/2047487316640659

Astrup, A., Brand-Miller, J., Jenkins, D. J. A., Livesey, G. & Willett, W. C. (2016). Weighing up dietary patterns. *The Lancet*, 388(10046), 758–9. doi:10.1016/S0140-6736(16)31337-X

Baldermann, S., Blagojević, L., Frede, K., Klopsch, R., Neugart, S., Neumann, A., ... Schreiner, M. (2016). Are neglected plants the food for the future? *Critical Reviews in Plant Sciences*, 35(2), 106–19. doi:10.1080/07352689.2016.1201399

Brown, K. A., Timotijevic, L., Barnett, J., Shepherd, R., Lähteenmäki, L. & Raats, M. M. (2011). A review of consumer awareness, understanding and use of food-based dietary guidelines. *British Journal of Nutrition*, 106(1), 15–26.

Christie, C., Worel, J. N. & Hayman, L. L. (2016). Implementation of the 2015 Dietary Guidelines: who, what, why, where, and when. *Journal of Cardiovascular Nursing*, 31(1), 5–8. doi:10.1097/JCN.0000000000000316

Delgado-Lista, J., Perez-Martinez, P., Garcia-Rios, A., Perez-Caballero, A. I., Perez-Jimenez, F. & Lopez-Miranda, J. (2016). Mediterranean diet and cardiovascular risk: beyond traditional risk factors. *Critical Reviews in Food Science and Nutrition*, 56(5), 788–801. doi:10.1080/10408398.2012.726660

DeSalvo, K. B., Olson, R. & Casavale, K. O. (2016). Dietary Guidelines for Americans. *JAMA—Journal of the American Medical Association*, 315(5), 457–8. doi:10.1001/jama.2015.18396

Dwyer, J. T., Rubin, K. H., Fritsche, K. L., Psota, T. L., Liska, D. J., Harris, W. S., ... Lyle, B. J. (2016). Creating the future of evidence-based nutrition recommendations: case studies from lipid research. *Advances in Nutrition*, 7(4), 747–55. doi:10.3945/an.115.010926

Fayet, F., Mortensen, A. & Baghurst, K. (2012). Energy distribution patterns in Australia and its relationship to age, gender and body mass index among children and adults. *Nutrition & Dietetics*, 69(2), 102–10.

Frank, A. P. & Clegg, D. J. (2016). Dietary Guidelines for Americans—eat less salt. *JAMA—Journal of the American Medical Association*, 316(7), 782. doi:10.1001/jama.2015.14433

Frank, A. P. & Clegg, D. J. (2016). Dietary Guidelines for Americans—eat less saturated fat. *JAMA—Journal of the American Medical Association*, 315(17), 1919.

Frank, A. P. & Clegg, D. J. (2016). Dietary Guidelines for Americans—eat less sugar. *JAMA—Journal of the American Medical Association*, 315(11), 1196.

Fung, T. T., Pan, A., Hou, T., Mozaffarian, D., Rexrode, K. M., Willett, W. C. & Hu, F. B. (2016). Food quality score and the risk of coronary artery disease: a prospective analysis in 3 cohorts. *American Journal of Clinical Nutrition*, 104(1), 65–72. doi:10.3945/ajcn.116.130393

Galli, A., Iha, K., Halle, M., El Bilali, H., Grunewald, N., Eaton, D., ... Bottalico, F. (2017). Mediterranean countries' food consumption and sourcing patterns: an ecological footprint viewpoint. *Science of the Total Environment*, 578, 383–91. doi:10.1016/j.scitotenv.2016.10.191

Guyatt, G. H., Oxman, A. D., Vist, G. E., et al. (2008). GRADE: an emerging consensus on rating quality of evidence and strength of recommendations. *British Medical Journal*, 336(7650), 924–6.

Henderson, G., Zinn, C. & Schofield, G. (2017). Dietary guidelines are not beyond criticism. *The Lancet*, 389(10069), 598. doi:10.1016/S0140-6736(17)30278-7

Hendrie, G. A., Baird, D., Golley, R. K. & Noakes, M. (2017). The CSIRO healthy diet score: an online survey to estimate compliance with the Australian dietary guidelines. *Nutrients*, 9(1). doi:10.3390/nu9010047

Henriksen, H. B., Ræder, H., Bøhn, S. K., Paur, I., Kværner, A. S., Billington, S., … Blomhoff, R. (2017). The Norwegian dietary guidelines and colorectal cancer survival (CRC-NORDIET) study: a food-based multicentre randomized controlled trial. *BMC Cancer*, 17(1). doi:10.1186/s12885-017-3072-4

Jin, J. (2016). Dietary Guidelines for Americans. *JAMA—Journal of the American Medical Association*, 315(5), 528. doi:10.1001/jama.2016.0077

Jones, A. D., Hoey, L., Blesh, J., Miller, L., Green, A. & Shapiro, L. F. (2016). A systematic review of the measurement of sustainable diets. *Advances in Nutrition*, 7(4), 641–64. doi:10.3945/an.115.011015

Kennedy, E. (2004). Dietary diversity, diet quality, and body weight regulation. *Nutrition Reviews*, 62, S78–S81.

Khanna, S. K. (ed. in chief) (2016). Understanding the impact of globalization on food preferences, dietary patterns, and health. *Ecology of Food and Nutrition*, 55(4), 339–40. doi:10.1080/03670244.2016.1213557

Kothe, E. J. & Mullan, B. A. (2011). Perceptions of fruit and vegetable dietary guidelines among Australian young adults. *Nutrition & Dietetics*, 68(4), 262–6.

Kromhout, D., Spaaij, C. J. K., De Goede, J., Weggemans, R. M., Brug, J., Geleijnse, J. M., … Zwietering, M. H. (2016). The 2015 Dutch food-based dietary guidelines. *European Journal of Clinical Nutrition*, 70(8), 869–78. doi:10.1038/ejcn.2016.52

Mann, J., Morenga, L. T., McLean, R., Swinburn, B., Mhurchu, C. N., Jackson, R., … Beaglehole, R. (2016). Dietary guidelines on trial: the charges are not evidence based. *The Lancet*, 388(10047), 851–3. doi:10.1016/S0140-6736(16)31278-8

Martínez-González, M. A. (2016). Benefits of the Mediterranean diet beyond the Mediterranean Sea and beyond food patterns. *BMC Medicine*, 14(1). doi:10.1186/s12916-016-0714-3

Martínez-González, M. A. & Martin-Calvo, N. (2016). Mediterranean diet and life expectancy: beyond olive oil, fruits, and vegetables. *Current Opinion in Clinical Nutrition and Metabolic Care*, 19(6), 401–7. doi:10.1097/MCO.0000000000000316

McNaughton, S. A., Ball, K., Crawford, D. & Mishra, G. D. (2008). An index of diet and eating patterns is a valid measure of diet quality in an Australian population. *Journal of Nutrition*, 138(1), 86–93.

Mitka, M. (2016). New dietary guidelines place added sugars in the crosshairs. *JAMA—Journal of the American Medical Association*, 315(14), 1440–1. doi:10.1001/jama.2016.1321

Mozaffarian, D. & Ludwig, D. S. (2015). The 2015 US dietary guidelines: lifting the ban on total dietary fat. *JAMA—Journal of the American Medical Association*, 313(24), 2421–2. doi:10.1001/jama.2015.5941

Murray, E. K., Baker, S. & Auld, G. (2017). Nutrition recommendations from the US Dietary Guidelines critical to teach low-income adults: expert panel opinion. *Journal of the Academy of Nutrition and Dietetics*, 118(20), 201–10. doi:10.1016/j.jand.2016.11.007

Ndanuko, R. N., Tapsell, L. C., Charlton, K. E., Neale, E. P. & Batterham, M. J. (2016). Dietary patterns and blood pressure in adults: a systematic review and meta-analysis of randomized controlled trials. *Advances in Nutrition: An International Review Journal*, 7(1), 76–89. doi:10.3945/an.115.009753

Nelson, M. E., Hamm, M. W., Hu, F. B., Abrams, S. A. & Griffin, T. S. (2016). Alignment of healthy dietary patterns and environmental sustainability: a systematic review. *Advances in Nutrition*, 7(6), 1005–25. doi:10.3945/an.116.012567

Opie, L. (2014). Dietary patterns need emphasising. *The Lancet*, 384(9958), 1925. doi:10.1016/S0140-6736(14)62275-3

Raber, M., Chandra, J., Upadhyaya, M., Schick, V., Strong, L. L., Durand, C. & Sharma, S. (2016). An evidence-based conceptual framework of healthy cooking. *Preventive Medicine Reports*, 4, 23–8. doi:10.1016/j.pmedr.2016.05.004

Rautiainen, S., Manson, J. E., Lichtenstein, A. H. & Sesso, H. D. (2016). Dietary supplements and disease prevention: a global overview. *Nature Reviews Endocrinology*, 12(7), 407–20. doi:10.1038/nrendo.2016.54

Rooney, C., McKinley, M. C., Appleton, K. M., Young, I. S., McGrath, A. J., Draffin, C. R., … Woodside, J. V. (2017). How much is '5-a-day'? A qualitative investigation into consumer understanding of fruit and vegetable intake guidelines. *Journal of Human Nutrition and Dietetics*, 30(1), 105–13. doi:10.1111/jhn.12393

Sherzai, A., Heim, L. T., Boothby, C. & Sherzai, A. D. (2012). Stroke, food groups, and dietary patterns: a systematic review. *Nutrition Reviews*, 70(8), 423–35.

Verger, E. O., Dop, M. C. & Martin-Prével, Y. (2016). Not all dietary diversity scores can legitimately be interpreted as proxies of diet quality. *Public Health Nutrition*, 1–2. doi:10.1017/S1368980016003402

REFERENCES

1 National Health and Medical Research Council (2011). *A Review of the Evidence to Address Targeted Questions to Inform the Revision of the Australian Dietary Guidelines: Evidence statements*. Canberra: NHMRC.

2 P. J. Stover (2006). Influence of human genetic variation on nutritional requirements. *American Journal of Clinical Nutrition*, 83(2), 436S–442S. doi:10.1093/ajcn/83.2.436S

3 F. Sofi, R. Abbate, G. F. Gensini & A. Casini (2010). Accruing evidence on benefits of adherence to the Mediterranean diet on health: an updated systematic review and meta-analysis. *American Journal of Clinical Nutrition*, 92(5), 1189–96. doi:10.3945/ajcn.2010.29673

4 A. Drewnowski & B. M. Popkin (1997). The nutrition transition: new trends in the global diet. *Nutrition Reviews*, 55(2), 31–43.

5 P. A. Gilbert & S. Khokhar (2008). Changing dietary habits of ethnic groups in Europe and implications for health. *Nutrition Reviews*, 66(4), 203–15. doi:10.1111/j.1753-4887.2008.00025.x

6 C. Liu, Y. Sun, Y. Li, W. Yang, M. Zhang, C. Xiong & Y. Yang (2012). The relationship between cold–hot nature and nutrient contents of foods. *Nutrition and Dietetics*, 69(1), 64–8. doi:10.1111/j.1747-0080.2011.01565.x

7 C. M. Kastorini, H. J. Milionis, K. Esposito, D. Giugliano, J. A. Goudevenos & D. B. Panagiotakos (2011). The effect of Mediterranean diet on metabolic syndrome and its components: a meta-analysis of 50 studies and 534,906 individuals. *Journal of the American College of Cardiology*, 57(11), 1299–313. doi:10.1016/j.jacc.2010.09.073

8 S. K. Poulsen, A. Due, A. B. Jordy, B. Kiens, K. D. Stark, S. Stender, … T. M. Larsen (2014). Health effect of the New Nordic Diet in adults with increased waist circumference: a 6-mo randomized controlled trial. *American Journal of Clinical Nutrition*, 99(1), 35–45. doi:10.3945/ajcn.113.069393

9 T. Liyanage, T. Ninomiya, A. Wang, B. Neal, M. Jun, M. G. Wong, … V. Perkovic (2016). Effects of the Mediterranean diet on cardiovascular outcomes: a systematic review and meta-analysis. *PLOS ONE*, 11(8), e0159252. doi:10.1371/journal.pone.0159252

10 V. B. Gunge, I. Andersen, C. Kyrø, C. P. Hansen, C. C. Dahm, J. Christensen, … A. Olsen (2017). Adherence to a healthy Nordic food index and risk of myocardial infarction in middle-aged Danes: the diet, cancer and health cohort study. *European Journal of Clinical Nutrition*, 71, 652. doi:10.1038/ejcn.2017.1

11 W. C. Willett, F. Sacks, A. Trichopoulou, G. Drescher, A. Ferro-Luzzi, E. Helsing & D. Trichopoulos (1995). Mediterranean diet pyramid: a cultural model for healthy eating. *American Journal of Clinical Nutrition*, 61(suppl. 6), 1402s–1406s. doi:10.1093/ajcn/61.6.1402S

12 L. Cordain, S. B. Eaton, A. Sebastian, N. Mann, S. Lindeberg, B. A. Watkins, … J. Brand-Miller (2005). Origins and evolution of the Western diet: health implications for the 21st century. *American Journal of Clinical Nutrition*, 81(2), 341–54. doi:10.1093/ajcn.81.2.341

13 M. L. Wahlqvist (2002). Asian migration to Australia: food and health consequences. *Asia Pacific Journal of Clinical Nutrition*, 11(s3), S562–S568. doi:10.1046/j.1440-6047.11.supp3.13.x

14 A. O. Odegaard, W. P. Koh, J.-M. Yuan, M. D. Gross & M. A. Pereira (2012). Western-style fast food intake and cardiometabolic risk in an eastern country: clinical perspective. *Circulation*, 126(2), 182–8. doi:10.1161/circulationaha.111.084004

15 A. Kouris-Blazos, C. Gnardellis, M. L. Wahlqvist, D. Trichopoulos, W. Lukito & A. Trichopoulou (1999). Are the advantages of the Mediterranean diet transferable to other populations? A cohort study in Melbourne, Australia. *British Journal of Nutrition*, 82(1), 57–61. doi:10.1017/S0007114599001129

16 R. Estruch, E. Ros, J. Salas-Salvadó, M.-I. Covas, D. Corella, F. Arós, … M. A. Martínez-González (2018). Primary prevention of cardiovascular disease with a Mediterranean diet supplemented with extra-virgin olive oil or nuts. *New England Journal of Medicine*, 378(25), e34. doi:10.1056/NEJMoa1800389

17 D. R. Jacobs, M. D. Gross & L. C. Tapsell (2009). Food synergy: an operational concept for understanding nutrition. *American Journal of Clinical Nutrition*, 89(5), 1543S–1548S. doi:10.3945/ajcn.2009.26736B

18 R. W. Kimokoti & B. E. Millen (2011). Diet, the global obesity epidemic, and prevention. *Journal of the American Dietetic Association*, 111(8), 1137–40. doi:https://doi.org/10.1016/j.jada.2011.05.016

19 H. P. Fransen, A. M. May, M. D. Stricker, J. M. A. Boer, C. Hennig, Y. Rosseel, … J. W. J. Beulens (2014). *A posteriori* dietary patterns: how many patterns to retain? *Journal of Nutrition*, 144(8), 1274–82. doi:10.3945/jn.113.188680

20 R. N. Ndanuko, L. C. Tapsell, K. E. Charlton, E. P. Neale, K. M. O'Donnell & M. J. Batterham (2017). Relationship between sodium and potassium intake and blood pressure in a sample of overweight adults. *Nutrition*, 33, 285–90. doi:http://dx.doi.org/10.1016/j.nut.2016.07.011

21 E. Warensjö Lemming, L. Byberg, A. Wolk & K. Michaëlsson (2018). A comparison between two healthy diet scores, the modified Mediterranean diet score and the Healthy Nordic Food Index, in relation to all-cause and cause-specific mortality. *British Journal of Nutrition*, 119(7), 836–46. doi:10.1017/S0007114518000387

22 A. Keys, A. Menott, M. J. Karvonen, C. Aravanis, H. Blackburn, R. Buzina, … H. Toshima (2017). The diet and 15-year death rate in the seven countries study. *American Journal of Epidemiology*, 185(11), 1130–42. doi:10.1093/aje/kwx101

23 R. Estruch, M. A. Martínez-González, D. Corella, J. Salas-Salvadó, V. Ruiz-Gutiérrez, M. I. Covas, … E. Ros (2006). Effects of a Mediterranean-style diet on cardiovascular risk factors a randomized trial. *Annals of Internal Medicine*, 145(1), 1–11. doi:10.7326/0003-4819-145-1-200607040-00004

24 R. Solá, M. Fitó, R. Estruch, J. Salas-Salvadó, D. Corella, R. de La Torre, … M.-I. Covas (2011). Effect of a traditional Mediterranean diet on apolipoproteins B, A-I, and their ratio: a randomized, controlled trial. *Atherosclerosis*, 218(1), 174–80. doi:https://doi.org/10.1016/j.atherosclerosis.2011.04.026

25 M. de Lorgeril, P. Salen, J.-L. Martin, N. Mamelle, I. Monjaud, P. Touboul & J. Delaye (1996). Effect of a Mediterranean type of diet on the rate of cardiovascular complications in patients with coronary artery disease insights into the cardioprotective effect of certain nutriments. *Journal of the American College of Cardiology*, 28(5), 1103–8. doi:https://doi.org/10.1016/S0735-1097(96)00280-X

26 S. Vincent-Baudry, C. Defoort, M. Gerber, M.-C. Bernard, P. Verger, O. Helal, … D. Lairon (2005). The Medi-RIVAGE study: reduction of cardiovascular disease risk factors after a 3-mo intervention with a Mediterranean-type diet or a low-fat diet. *American Journal of Clinical Nutrition*, 82(5), 964–71. doi:10.1093/ajcn/82.5.964

27 K. Esposito, R. Marfella, M. Ciotola, C. Di Palo, F. Giugliano, G. Giugliano, … D. Giugliano (2004). Effect of a Mediterranean-style diet on endothelial dysfunction and markers of vascular inflammation in the metabolic syndrome: a randomized trial. *JAMA—Journal of the American Medical Association*, 292(12), 1440–6. doi:10.1001/jama.292.12.1440

28 R. J. de Souza & S. S. Anand (2016). Saturated fat and heart disease. *British Medical Journal*, 355. doi:10.1136/bmj.i6257

29 D. I. Givens & S. S. Soedamah-Muthu (2016). Dairy fat: does it increase or reduce the risk of cardiovascular disease? *American Journal of Clinical Nutrition*, 104(5), 1191–2. doi:10.3945/ajcn.116.144766

30 D. Mozaffarian, T. Hao, E. B. Rimm, W. C. Willett & F. B. Hu (2011). Changes in diet and lifestyle and long-term weight gain in women and men. *New England Journal of Medicine*, 364(25), 2392–404. doi:10.1056/NEJMoa1014296

31 C. M. Berg, G. Lappas, E. Strandhagen, A. Wolk, K. Torén, A. Rosengren, … L. Lissner (2008). Food patterns and cardiovascular disease risk factors: the Swedish INTERGENE research program. *American Journal of Clinical Nutrition*, 88(2), 289–97. doi:10.1093/ajcn/88.2.289

32 J. Kim & I. Jo (2011). Grains, vegetables, and fish dietary pattern is inversely associated with the risk of metabolic syndrome in South Korean adults. *Journal of the American Dietetic Association*, 111(8), 1141–9. doi:https://doi.org/10.1016/j.jada.2011.05.001

33 R. M. van Dam, E. B. Rimm, W. C. Willett, M. J. Stampfer & F. B. Hu (2002). Dietary patterns and risk for type 2 diabetes mellitus in US men. *Annals of Internal Medicine*, 136(3), 201–9. doi:10.7326/0003-4819-136-3-200202050-00008

34 R. A. Mekary, E. Giovannucci, W. C. Willett, R. M. van Dam & F. B. Hu (2012). Eating patterns and type 2 diabetes risk in men: breakfast omission, eating frequency, and snacking. *American Journal of Clinical Nutrition*, 95(5), 1182–9. doi:10.3945/ajcn.111.028209

35 J. A. Nettleton, J. F. Polak, R. Tracy, G. L. Burke & J. D. R. Jacobs (2009). Dietary patterns and incident cardiovascular disease in the Multi-Ethnic Study of Atherosclerosis. *American Journal of Clinical Nutrition*, 90(3), 647–54. doi:10.3945/ajcn.2009.27597

36 T. Antonia & L. Pagona (1997). Healthy traditional Mediterranean diet: an expression of culture, history, and lifestyle. *Nutrition Reviews*, 55(11), 383–9. doi:10.1111/j.1753-4887.1997.tb01578.x

37 I. Paran & E. van der Knaap (2007). Genetic and molecular regulation of fruit and plant domestication traits in tomato and pepper. *Journal of Experimental Botany*, 58(14), 3841–52. doi:10.1093/jxb/erm257

38 A. Blum, M. Monir, I. Wirsansky & S. Ben-Arzi (2005). The beneficial effects of tomatoes. *European Journal of Internal Medicine*, 16(6), 402–4. doi:https://doi.org/10.1016/j.ejim.2005.02.017

39 M. A. Martínez-González, A. García-Arellano, E. Toledo, J. Salas-Salvadó, P. Buil-Cosiales, D. Corella, … for the PREDIMED Study Investigators (2012). A 14-Item Mediterranean Diet Assessment Tool and obesity

indexes among high-risk subjects: the PREDIMED Trial. *PLOS ONE*, 7(8), e43134. doi:10.1371/journal.pone.0043134

40 D. Mozaffarian & D. S. Ludwig (2010). Dietary guidelines in the 21st century—a time for food. *JAMA—Journal of the American Medical Association*, 304(6), 681–2. doi:10.1001/jama.2010.1116

41 N. Yoshiike, F. Hayashi, Y. Takemi, K. Mizoguchi & F. Seino (2007). A new food guide in Japan: the Japanese food guide spinning top. *Nutrition Reviews*, 65(4), 149–54. doi:10.1111/j.1753-4887.2007.tb00294.x

42 Y. Nakamura, H. Ueshima, N. Okuda, K. Miura, Y. Kita, T. Okamura, … J. Stamler (2012). Relation of dietary and lifestyle traits to difference in serum leptin of Japanese in Japan and Hawaii: the INTERLIPID study. *Nutrition, Metabolism and Cardiovascular Diseases*, 22(1), 14–22. doi:https://doi.org/10.1016/j.numecd.2010.03.004

43 J. Ferrières (2004). The French paradox: lessons for other countries. *Heart*, 90(1), 107–11.

44 A. Schmid (2010). The role of meat fat in the human diet. *Critical Reviews in Food Science and Nutrition*, 51(1), 50–66. doi:10.1080/10408390903044636

45 S. M. Artaud-Wild, S. L. Connor, G. Sexton & W. E. Connor (1993). Differences in coronary mortality can be explained by differences in cholesterol and saturated fat intakes in 40 countries but not in France and Finland. A paradox. *Circulation*, 88(6), 2771–9. doi:10.1161/01.cir.88.6.2771

46 A. E. Evans, E. E. McCrum, R. McClean, Z. M. Mathewson, C. C. Patterson, J. B. Ruidavets, … F. Cambien (1995). Autres pays, autres coeurs? Dietary patterns, risk factors and ischaemic heart disease in Belfast and Toulouse. *QJM: An International Journal of Medicine*, 88(7), 469–77. doi:10.1093/oxfordjournals.qjmed.a069090

47 J.-L. Volatier & P. Verger (1999). Recent national French food and nutrient intake data. *British Journal of Nutrition*, 81(S1), S57–S59. doi:10.1017/S0007114599000902

48 T. A. O'Sullivan, G. Ambrosini, L. J. Beilin, T. A. Mori & W. H. Oddy (2011). Dietary intake and food sources of fatty acids in Australian adolescents. *Nutrition*, 27(2), 153–9. doi:https://doi.org/10.1016/j.nut.2009.11.019

49 R. Nakata, S. Takahashi & H. Inoue (2012). Recent advances in the study on resveratrol. *Biological and Pharmaceutical Bulletin*, 35(3), 273–9. doi:10.1248/bpb.35.273

50 T. Laatikainen, J. Critchley, E. Vartiainen, V. Salomaa, M. Ketonen & S. Capewell (2005). Explaining the decline in coronary heart disease mortality in Finland between 1982 and 1997. *American Journal of Epidemiology*, 162(8), 764–73. doi:10.1093/aje/kwi274

51 C. Bannerman (2006). Indigenous food and cookery books: redefining Aboriginal cuisine. *Journal of Australian Studies*, 30(87), 19–36. doi:10.1080/14443050609388048

52 L. Deborah (2000). The heart of the meal: food preferences and habits among rural Australian couples. *Sociology of Health & Illness*, 22(1), 94–109. doi:10.1111/1467-9566.00193

53 TV Tonight (2010). The top 100. Retrieved from: www.tvtonight.com.au/2010/12/2010-the-top-100.html.

54 C. Saxelby (2018). *Complete Food and Nutrition Companion*. Melbourne: Hardie Grant Books.

55 L. C. Tapsell, E. P. Neale, A. Satija & F. B. Hu (2016). Foods, nutrients, and dietary patterns: interconnections and implications for dietary guidelines. *Advances in Nutrition: An International Review Journal*, 7(3), 445–54. doi:10.3945/an.115.011718

56 Australian Bureau of Statistics (2015). *Australian Health Survey: First results, 2011–12*. Canberra: ABS.

57 National Health and Medical Research Council (2013). *Australian Dietary Guidelines*. Canberra: NHMRC.

58 National Health and Medical Research Council (2011). *A Modelling System to Inform the Revision of the Australian Guide to Healthy Eating*. Canberra: NHMRC.

59 M. Metherell & J. Swan (2011). Easy on the spuds, but chow down the carrots to meet new dietary guidelines. *Sydney Morning Herald*, 13 December.

60 R. Hughes (2009). Public health nutrition. Dietary guidelines. We have traction in Australia. *Public Health Nutrition*, 12(2), 290–1. doi:10.1017/s136898000800445x

61 National Health and Medical Research Council (2003). *Dietary Guidelines for Australian Adults*. Canberra: Commonwealth of Australia.

62 National Health and Medical Research Council (2003). *Dietary Guidelines for Children and Adolescents in Australia Incorporating the Infant Feeding Guidelines for Health Workers*. Canberra: Commonwealth of Australia.

63 S. Fishkoff (2010). Keeping kosher—but just on holidays. *Washington Jewish Week*, 19 August, pp. 16–18.

64 S. M. Barbieri (2001). Keeping kosher. *Minnesota Monthly*, 9(5), 38–40.

65 H. Skanchy (2009). A cultural look at the diet and health issues of the Middle East. Retrieved from: http://citeseerx.ist.psu.edu/viewdoc/download?doi=10.1.1.513.9699&rep=rep1&type=pdf.

66 CSIRO Preventative Health National Research Flagship and the University of South Australia (2008). *Australian National Children's Nutrition and Physical Activity Survey: Main findings*. Canberra: Commonwealth of Australia.

67 P. Williams, M. Reid & K. Shaw (2004). The Illawarra Healthy Food Price Index. 1. Development of the food basket. *Nutrition and Dietetics*, 61(4), 200–7.

68 Q. Yang, M. E. Cogswell, W. Flanders, et al. (2012). Trends in cardiovascular health metrics and associations with all-cause and CVD mortality among US adults. *JAMA—Journal of the American Medical Association*, 307(12), 1273–83. doi:10.1001/jama.2012.339

69 The National Academies of Sciences, Engineering, Medicine (2017). *Public Workshop #3: Review of the Process to Update the Dietary Guidelines for Americans*. Retrieved from: http://nationalacademies.org/hmd/Activities/Nutrition/DietaryGuidelinesforAmericans/2017-JAN-10/Videos/Session%203%20Videos/12-Garza-Video.aspx

70 E. P. Neale, M. J. Batterham & L. C. Tapsell (2016). Consumption of a healthy dietary pattern results in significant reductions in C-reactive protein levels in adults: a meta-analysis. *Nutrition Research*, 36(5), 391–401. doi:https://doi.org/10.1016/j.nutres.2016.02.009

71 J. P. T. Higgins & S. Green (2011). *Cochrane Handbook for Systematic Reviews of Interventions Version 5.1.0 [updated March 2011]*. The Cochrane Collaboration.

72 National Health and Medical Research Council (2009). *NHMRC Additional Levels of Evidence and Grades for Recommendations for Developers of Guidelines*. Canberra: NHMRC.

73 G. H. Guyatt, A. D. Oxman, G. E. Vist, R. Kunz, Y. Falck-Ytter, P. Alonso-Coello & H. J. Schünemann (2008). GRADE: an emerging consensus on rating quality of evidence and strength of recommendations. *British Medical Journal*, 336(7650), 924–6. doi:10.1136/bmj.39489.470347.AD

74 D. Moher, A. Liberati, J. Tetzlaff, D. G. Altman & the PRISMA Group (2009). Preferred reporting items for systematic reviews and meta-analyses: the PRISMA Statement. *PLOS Medicine*, 6(7), e1000097. doi:10.1371/journal.pmed.1000097

75 Department of Health (2015–17). *Methodological Framework for the Review of Nutrient Reference Values*. Canberra: Department of Health. Retrieved from: www.nrv.gov.au/file/methodological-framework-pdf-705kb.

76 National Health and Medical Research Council (2013). *Clinical Practice Guidelines for the Management of Overweight and Obesity in Adults, Adolescents and Children in Australia*. Canberra: NHMRC.

77 Food Standards Australia New Zealand (2013). *Guidance on Establishing Food–Health Relationships for General Level Health Claims (Version 1.1)*. Canberra: FSANZ.

LINDA TAPSELL AND ELIZABETH NEALE

CHAPTER 3

CONSUMING FOOD: DIGESTION, ABSORPTION AND METABOLISM

LINDA TAPSELL

CHAPTER OBJECTIVES

This chapter will enable the reader to:

- describe the processes involved in the digestion of food and the absorption of nutrients
- outline the main metabolic processes influenced by food consumption
- describe Nutrient Reference Values and identify dietary patterns designed to meet them.

KEY TERMS

Absorption

Digestion

Metabolism

Nutrient Reference
Values (NRVs)

KEY POINTS

- When food is consumed it is broken down into its component parts. Nutrients are absorbed through the gut in various forms and transported throughout the body by a range of mechanisms.
- Macronutrients are the major nutritional components of foods and serve as fuel sources; carbohydrate is the main source, and the components of digested protein and fat also serve important structural and functional roles.
- Micronutrients (vitamins and minerals) are delivered and absorbed in smaller quantities by a range of mechanisms, often to maintain a balance in physiological levels.
- Nutrient Reference Values (NRVs) are sets of science-referenced standards for macro and micronutrient consumption that address requirements for age and sex, and target prevention of diet-related chronic disease.
- Choosing a healthy diet implies a combination of foods that deliver essential nutrients in the forms that adequately meet requirements and in a dietary pattern that is protective against chronic disease.

INTRODUCTION

The science of nutrition concerns itself with the study of food and the way in which food consumption affects health. Understanding what happens to food when it is consumed is part of understanding nutrition. Examining the process of food digestion and nutrient absorption and metabolism takes us into the realm of the chemical composition of food and the actions of food components on biological pathways within the human body. From the moment food is placed in the mouth through to the excretion of waste through faeces and urine, most of the components of foods are variously released, modified, transported and generally made available for the systems of the body.

The term 'nutrient' describes components in food that we have known about for some time as more or less essential for survival. Scientists are continually discovering new components in food, and there is some discussion on how the definition of nutrients might be extended [1]. Nevertheless, this chapter will focus on the main nutrients required for the human lifecycle, which involves stages of early development and growth through to maturation and senescence. Nutritional needs vary throughout these stages and are dependent on a number of conditions including sex, physical activity, functional capacities and genetics. New research on the **human microbiome** has added a layer of complexity to our understanding of how the body utilises and produces or needs nutrients (Figure 3.1). From a population perspective, individual variation in requirements

Human microbiome
profile of the bacteria in the large bowel (gut).

FIGURE 3.1　LOCATION OF GUT MICROBIOME

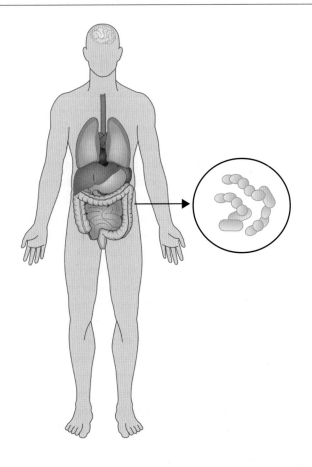

for nutrients must be considered. Setting standards (or NRVs) is a complex task that needs to address this variation and consider the risks involved. The application of these standards is also important in supporting the nutritional quality of the food supply.

Appreciating the processes involved in the digestion, absorption and metabolism of food may help in translating requirements for nutrients into food choices for a healthy diet. All foods are combinations of nutrients, but some foods are better sources of nutrients than others. This relates to the natural composition of the food as well as the form of food from which nutrients may become available. In the end, however, foods themselves tend to be eaten in combinations, in meals comprising a number of individual foods and/or mixed dishes in which the foods are ingredients that have been prepared together. Cooking processes can change the context further. In this chapter we examine the sequelae of the breakdown of food into nutrients, consider how a balance is achieved in the body, and relate this to actual foods consumed in a healthy diet.

Visit Oxford Ascend to watch a video and read more on the digestive system.

STOP AND THINK

- What kind of system does the gut resemble in breaking down food for eventual release and use in the body?
- Why are indigestible food components relevant to health?
- Why would different transport systems be useful in absorbing nutrients?
- How does a new understanding of the human microbiome change our perspective on how food choices may influence health?

WHAT HAPPENS TO FOOD WHEN IT IS EATEN?

Digestion

the process of breaking down food into its components when it is consumed.

Absorption

the process of transfer of food components across the gut barrier and into the transport systems of the body.

Macronutrients

components of food that deliver energy and comprise the main nutrient part of food by weight: protein, fat and carbohydrate—all carbon-containing molecules but with different chemical structures.

The process of digestion begins when food enters the mouth. Chewing and grinding breaks it down into smaller parts. Mixing with saliva allows chemical breakdown to begin, but the main part of **digestion** and **absorption** occurs in the small and large intestines. The component parts of foods, and in particular the **macronutrients**, are dealt with in different ways, but generally they are broken down to smaller molecules and prepared for action. Further details of the significance of these actions are provided in the ensuing chapters on specific nutrients.

Remember that foods are combinations of nutrients, and this combination varies depending on the food. Bread, for example, has a large component of carbohydrate, but it also contains protein and some fat, as well as vitamins and minerals (Table 3.1). On the other hand, cooking oil is nearly all fat, and milk contains roughly equal amounts of protein, fat and carbohydrate. In reality, foods themselves tend to be eaten in combinations, such as in meals, so digestion and absorption occurs in the context of multiple foods and multiple nutrients. Nevertheless, we have come to understand these processes in terms of the individual nutrients concerned.

The function of the human gastrointestinal tract is to break down food and then its component parts and control the entry and distribution of those components into systems that package and deliver the key molecules to do the work of the body. Enzymes are the agents of this breakdown. There are many classes of enzymes with specific duties depending on the types of compounds they break down. Absorption of nutrients into the human system may be active or passive, depending on the chemical structure of the nutrient. Once through

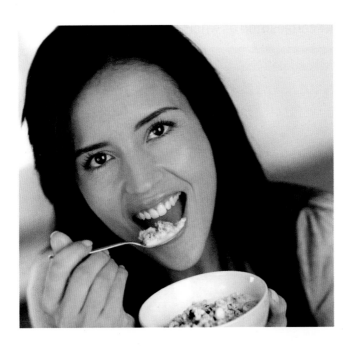

the gut wall, the transport systems also befits the class of compounds and the organs or tissues to which they are delivered. Not all food components make it through, but the system picks up again with the microbiome, or bacterial colony in the large bowel, which makes further use of potential energy sources, utilising molecules for its own benefit or making other forms further available to the body. End products are produced and excreted. Meanwhile, the molecules working their way through the system are further transported, modified, repackaged and metabolised as part of the functioning of the human system. The whole process adds meaning to the saying 'you are what you eat'.

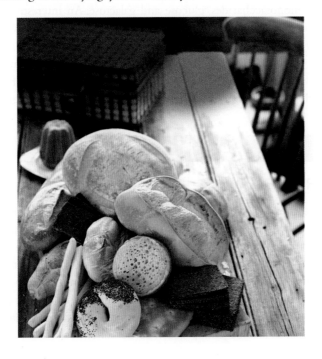

TABLE 3.1   NUTRIENT COMPOSITION OF WHOLEMEAL BREAD

Nutrient components of wholemeal bread	Amount per 100 g*
Protein	9 g
Fat	2.9 g
Dietary fibre	6.3 g
Carbohydrates	39.7 g
Niacin (vitamin B3)	3.18 mg
Biotin (vitamin B7)	7.8 µg
Folic acid	118 µg
Iodine	48 µg
Potassium	183 mg
Zinc	1.06 mg

*Values shown are taken from the *NUTTAB 2010* food composition database [2].

Carbohydrate

In the first instance, the grinding of food by teeth and mixing with saliva helps to create a softer texture that can be swallowed. One of the first enzymes along the tract, salivary amylase, starts the process for the carbohydrate component of the food, but it is soon inactivated as food passes into the acidic stomach region. Pancreatic amylase carries on that work in the small intestine, with three more carbohydrate digesting enzymes emerging at the brush border (microvilli): α glucosidase, sucrose isomaltase and α galactosidase (also known as lactase). Lactase is responsible for breaking down the sugar in milk (lactose), producing the monosaccharides, glucose and galactose. An interesting point to note here is that enzymes are proteins, and proteins are synthesised from genetic material. Only a small proportion of the global population retain the lactase enzyme into maturity, making them lactose tolerant. If lactose

See Chapter 4 on carbohydrates for more details on terms.

cannot be digested it is passed through the gut and, in association with water, can create gastrointestinal disturbance. The same is true of large amounts of sugar alcohols, such as sorbitol, which are not well absorbed (although some is absorbed through passive diffusion).

>> CASE 3.1

LACTOSE INTOLERANCE

Lactose intolerance is a condition when the intestinal cells are unable to secrete enough lactase to digest lactose in the food ingested (e.g. from milk or other dairy foods) [3; 4]. The undigested lactose, unable to be absorbed into the blood, will reach the large intestine, where the microbiota ferment the lactose, creating irritating acids and gas (Figure 3.2). Lactose itself will also draw water into the large intestinal lumen and cause bloating and diarrhoea. Lactose intolerance is more common among Asians and native North Americans whose traditional post-weaning diets do not include dairy products. It is also more common after gastrointestinal illnesses as the layers of the gut may be damaged, decreasing the production of enzymes such as lactase (called 'brush border' enzymes).

FIGURE 3.2   SCHEMA FOR LACTOSE INTOLERANCE

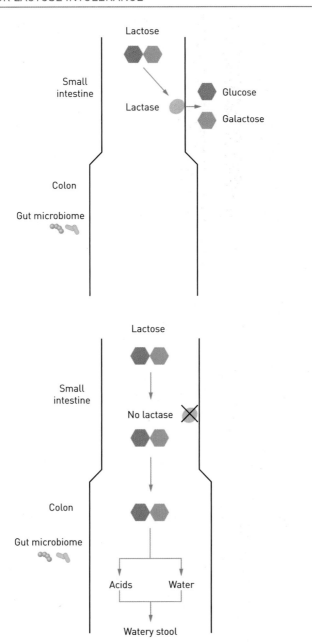

- Which foods and beverages should you avoid if you are lactose intolerant?
- Which nutrients may be at risk of inadequate consumption without these foods and beverages in the diet?

On the other hand, the sugars glucose and galactose are absorbed into the gut cells (enterocytes) via an active transport system involving sodium-glucose co-transporters. They are then pumped into the intracellular space with the help of glucose transporters. Because glucose is such a critical fuel source, the levels in the blood are controlled by a complex system of responses and counterbalances. As glucose emerges in the blood, it stimulates further hormonal secretion by the pancreas (Figure 3.3). In contrast, other forms of carbohydrate, including categories of fibre, are not digested and absorbed at this point and do not directly contribute to blood glucose levels, but their physical presence may otherwise influence the availability of glucose from the gut. Thus the type and amount of carbohydrate in a food or a meal will have different effects on blood glucose responses. While this is a highly controlled system, glucose, fructose and galactose are also sent to the liver and muscle for storage.

See Chapter 4 on carbohydrates for details on fibre.

FIGURE 3.3   PRINCIPAL PATHWAYS OF CARBOHYDRATE DIGESTION AND ABSORPTION

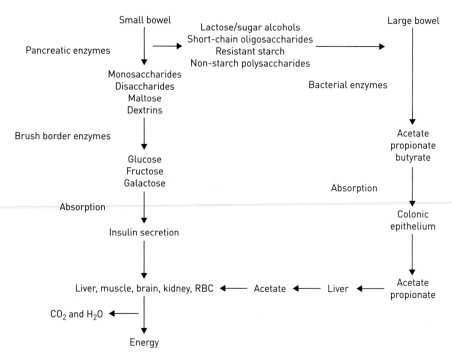

Source: J. Cummings & J. Mann (2012). Chapter 3: Carbohydrates. In J. Mann & S. Truswell (eds), *Essentials of Human Nutrition*, 4th edn. Oxford University Press, Incorporated

Fat

At the same time, the fat in the meal, which is mostly triglyceride, forms an emulsion in the stomach. This passes to the intestine where it binds with bile salts to create droplets. Lipase enzymes work on these droplets to release fatty acids. Other dietary lipids are also present, such as phospholipids (digested by phospholipases), cholesterol esters (digested by cholesterol ester hydrolases) and fat soluble vitamins. Smaller products of triglyceride digestion, namely glycerol and short-chain fatty acids (<12 carbon lengths), enter the portal system by diffusion across the enterocytes. Others form micelles and enter the enterocytes for resynthesis to ultimately form chylomicrons, which are then absorbed into the portal and lymph systems. These lipid transport units comprise an internal lipophilic combination of cholesterol esters and reformed triglycerides surrounded by a polar lipid layer of cholesterol and lipoproteins, wrapped in apolipoproteins (Figures 3.4 and 3.5). Chylomicrons, which first appear in the blood after a meal, provide transport to the liver for lipids and fat soluble vitamins. The enzyme lipoprotein lipase acts on chylomicrons to release fatty acids from triglycerides to the tissues. (Cholesterol remains in the chylomicron remnants and is taken up by the liver. The liver also synthesises cholesterol, which is a part of cell membranes and is also used to make bile acids and steroid hormones.)

See Chapter 5 on fats and lipids for details on triglyceride.

Portal system
vascular system that delivers nutrients from the gut to the liver.

The processes of packaging and repackaging lipids reflect the chemical nature of the lipid molecules and the watery environment in which transport takes place (Figure 3.6). Disruptions to these systems or lack of enzymes can result in fat malabsorption.

Transport lipoproteins vary in size and the amount of triglyceride transported (Figure 3.7). Chylomicrons (CM) carry the most triglyceride, followed by very-low-density lipoproteins (VLDL).

FIGURE 3.4   STRUCTURE OF CHOLESTEROL AND CHOLESTEROL ESTER

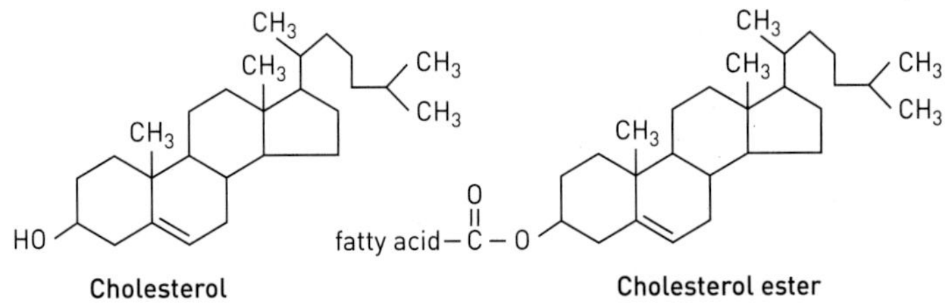

Cholesterol

Cholesterol ester

Source: C. M. Skeaff & J. Mann (2012). Chapter 4: Lipids. In J. Mann & S. Truswell (eds), *Essentials of Human Nutrition*, 4th edn. Oxford University Press, Incorporated

FIGURE 3.5   FORMATION OF A TRIACYLGLYCEROL MOLECULE

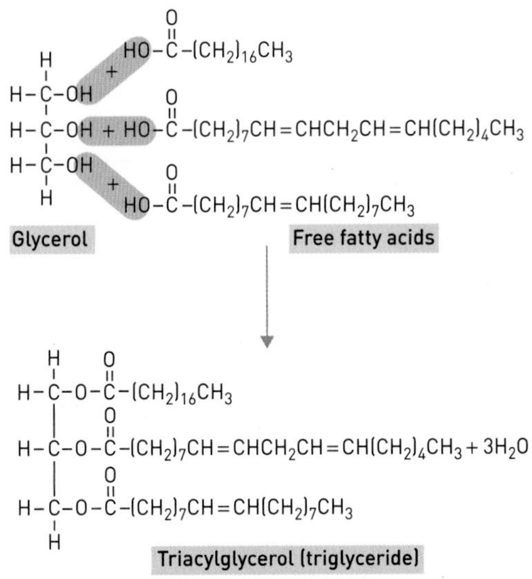

Glycerol   Free fatty acids

Triacylglycerol (triglyceride)

Source: C. M. Skeaff & J. Mann (2012). Chapter 4: Lipids. In J. Mann & S. Truswell (eds), *Essentials of Human Nutrition*, 4th edn. Oxford University Press, Incorporated (Figure 4.1, p. 50)

FIGURE 3.6   DIGESTION AND ABSORPTION OF DIETARY LIPIDS

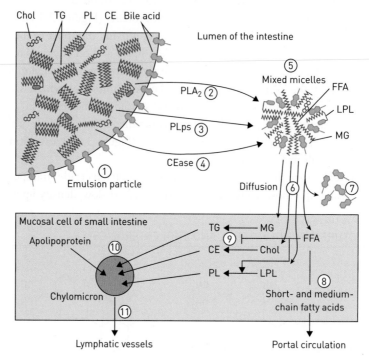

Source: C. M. Skeaff & J. Mann (2012). Chapter 4: Lipids. In J. Mann & S. Truswell (eds),
Essentials of Human Nutrition, 4th edn. Oxford University Press, Incorporated. (Figure 4.6, p. 58)

FIGURE 3.7   PERCENTAGE OF TRIGLYCERIDE IN LIPOPROTEINS

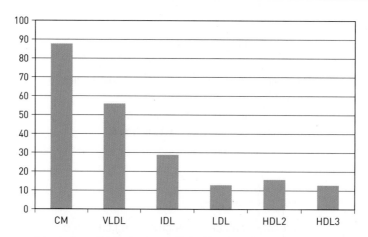

Abbreviations: CM: Chylomicrons; VLDL: Very-low-density lipoprotein from high-density lipoprotein;
IDL: Intermediate-density lipoprotein; LDL: low-density lipoprotein; HDL: High-density lipoprotein

Source: Adapted from C. M. Skeaff & J. Mann (2012). Chapter 4: Lipids. In J. Mann & S. Truswell (eds),
Essentials of Human Nutrition, 4th edn. Oxford University Press, Incorporated

Protein

The protein in the meal or food is also first prepared in the mouth, but then partially broken | See Chapter 6 on protein.
down by the acidic environment of the stomach. This serves to untangle (or denature) the chemical
strands of the protein. The hydrochloric acid from the stomach also activates the protein-splitting enzyme,
pepsin, from its inactive form, pepsinogen. Smaller polypeptides are then formed. In turn, the pancreas
and the small intestine secrete protease enzymes to break down the polypeptides further into amino
acids and peptides. The di and tri peptides are further hydrolysed at the gut wall, and mostly amino acids
are absorbed with the assistance of transporter molecules. The amino acids may be used by the cells
themselves or transported into the surrounding fluid and capillaries, eventually going to the liver. About
half of protein synthesis occurs in the visceral tissues (mostly liver) and the other half in the carcass (mostly
muscle), but the daily rate of protein turnover (synthesis and degradation) is much higher in the liver, the
'engine room' of metabolism. Table 3.2 shows the process of protein digestion.

TABLE 3.2   PROTEIN DIGESTION IN HUMANS

Organ	Activation	Enzyme	Substrate	Product
Stomach	pH <4	Pepsin	Whole protein	Very large polypeptides with C-terminal Tyr, Phe, Trp, also Leu, Glu, Gln
Pancreas	pH 7.5 Enterokinase secreted by small intestinal mucosa	Endopeptidases	Bonds with peptide chain	Peptide with basic amino acid at C terminus (Arg, Lys)
		Trypsin	Peptides	Peptide with neutral amino acid at C terminus
		Chymotrypsin	Peptides	Amino acids
		Exopeptidases	C-terminal bonds	Amino acids
		Carboxypeptidase	Successive amino acids at C terminus	
		Aminopeptidase	Successive amino acids at N terminus	

Source: A. A. Jackson & S. Truswell (2012). Chapter 5: Protein. In J. Mann & S. Truswell (eds), *Essentials of Human Nutrition*, 4th edn. Oxford University Press, Incorporated (Table 5.1, p. 76)

Amino acids can go on to produce the protein elements of genetic expression (such as deoxyribonucleic
acid; DNA), neurotransmitters (such as adrenaline), hormones (such as thyroid hormone) and fat digestion
(such as bile acids). They form important components of membrane structure (as in phospholipids) and
blood components (e.g. albumin). If utilised for energy, the excretory product urea is produced, and this is
passed through the kidneys (Figure 3.8).

Visit Oxford Ascend for more on the excretory system.

In summary, while enzymes are involved in the digestion of food, and the macronutrients therein, there
are differences in the subsequent treatment of nutrients, and the absorption mechanisms vary, reflecting to
some extent differences in chemical properties. Functional properties also vary: amino acids
may be utilised immediately in the cells of the gut, the maintenance of blood glucose levels
is directly influenced by glucose absorption, and fatty acid transport reflects a dynamic state

See Chapters 7–12 on energy, water, fats, vitamins and minerals.

LINDA TAPSELL

FIGURE 3.8   PROCESSES OF PROTEIN SYNTHESIS AND DEGRADATION

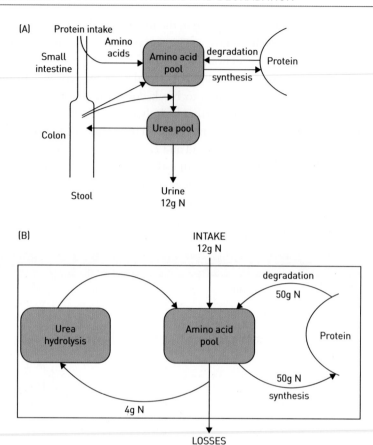

Source: A. A. Jackson & S. Truswell (2012). Chapter 5: Protein. In J. Mann & S. Truswell (eds), *Essentials of Human Nutrition*, 4th edn. Oxford University Press, Incorporated

FIGURE 3.9   FERMENTATION OF CARBOHYDRATE IN THE LARGE BOWEL

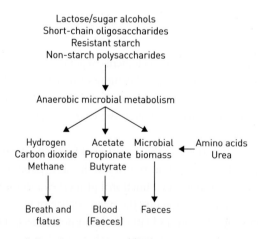

Source: J. Cummings & J. Mann (2012). Chapter 3: Carbohydrates. In J. Mann & S. Truswell (eds), *Essentials of Human Nutrition*, 4th edn. Oxford University Press, Incorporated (Figure 3.5, p. 33)

of flux within the cardiovascular system, in particular. Micronutrient (vitamin and mineral) digestion and absorption also occurs in this environment and is subject to various degrees of control depending on how balance is maintained in the body. Some micronutrients are also synthesised in the large bowel (colon), which is also the site of a second wave of fuel delivery via the action of resident bacteria (microbes) on 'resistant' carbohydrates (Figure 3.9) and proteins that have made their way to the colon.

Microbiome

The **microbiome** refers to the population of microbes (and their genetic material) that represent a distinctive ecological environment within the human body. A balance between two main classes of microbes, the bacteroidetes and firmicutes, is implicated in metabolic health, including susceptibility to obesity [5]. Ongoing research has explored how the microbiome changes with weight loss, including that resulting from surgical procedures [6]. There is much to be learnt about the lifelong association between the microbiome and the food we eat [7], with further implications for confirming the evidence on foods that promote health.

> **Microbiome**
> ecological system of the
> intestinal flora.

» RESEARCH AT WORK

THE GUT MICROBIOME AND METABOLIC HEALTH

In the past 10 years science has exposed the role of the gut microbiota on human metabolism. While we have been aware that food components such as fibre make it through to the large bowel, this research has exposed how microbes themselves utilise these components, producing new molecules or 'microbe associated molecular patterns' (MAMP), which affect human metabolism. A recent review summarised these effects in the areas of gut function, communication with other organs and tissues, and a range of physiological processes [8]. These relate to feedback systems associated with energy metabolism and food consumption as well as the functioning of the immune system, which has its base in the human gut.

The gut microbiome is also responsible for the production of secondary bile acids that enable recycling of bile salts present in the colon via the enterohepatic circulation. More recent interest has looked at the gut–brain axis, with a focus on the secretion of neurohormones and neurotransmitters, with implications for regulating food intake. The central role of basal inflammation in the pathogenesis of obesity and related metabolic disease has also drawn attention to how the gut microbiome may be implicated. A link has been suggested between gut inflammation and/or permeability and dysfunction of visceral fat leading to inflammation in the liver with associated insulin resistance [9]. Interest then follows on foods that deliver components that may improve gut integrity and function.

STOP AND THINK

- What methods of research might expose what happens to food when it is consumed?
- How do we know about individual nutrients when they are consumed as combinations in foods?
- How would the form of a food, or the combination of foods in a meal, influence the availability of macronutrients for an individual?

WHAT ARE THE MAJOR METABOLIC PROCESSES INFLUENCED BY FOOD CONSUMPTION?

Metabolism

the utilisation of food components in the chemical processes within the body.

While it is easy to see that food consumption must affect all **metabolism** because it provides the raw materials, science has exposed substantial detail on the intricacies of this relationship in certain domains, to the extent that dietary modification can be tested and utilised for positive effects. In many cases, this has occurred where malfunction is apparent, resulting in diseases such as diabetes and cardiovascular disease. Given the nature of these diseases, these insights were related to carbohydrate and fat metabolism, but it must be remembered that the human biological system works as a whole (i.e. there is an interdependence between these nutrients), and everything comes back to food eventually. In addition, as the metabolic complexities associated these diseases are better understood, the connections between them also become apparent, such that today they are grouped together as cardiometabolic disorders [10; 11], with the precursor state known as 'metabolic syndrome' [12].

The utilisation of food to produce energy is biochemical in nature (Figure 3.10). An important end point is the production of the molecule adenosine triphosphate (ATP), which harnesses chemical energy via electron transport. The metabolic pathway begins with the breakdown of food into macronutrients (carbohydrate, protein and fat), then into subunits (glucose, amino acids, fatty acids and glycerol). These subunits are further broken down by specific pathways, delivering fragments to co-enzyme A producing the molecule acetyl CoA which is taken up into the Krebs cycle (also known as the tricarboxylic acid or citric acid cycle). In the presence of oxygen, cell mitochondria utilise two molecules produced by the

FIGURE 3.10 METABOLISM OF MACRONUTRIENTS FROM FOOD TO PRODUCE ENERGY

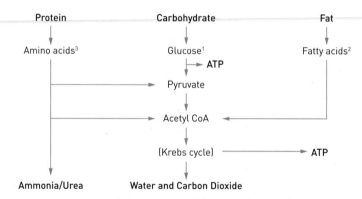

[1] The breakdown of glucose to pyruvate also produces energy in the form of ATP. This process, known as glycolysis, occurs outside the cell mitochondria (the engine room of energy metabolism) and does not require oxygen. It is therefore referred to as anaerobic metabolism. When there is insufficient oxygen to progress through the Krebs cycle, lactate can be produced, and this process enables further energy (ATP) production, relevant to heavy exercise (see Chapter 13).

[2] Fatty acids combined with CoA are broken down in the mitochondria to produce acetyl CoA through a process known as β oxidation. Fatty acids cannot be converted to glucose, so when glucose energy reserves are low, more acetyl CoA is produced from fatty acids in the liver. When this cannot all be taken up in the Krebs cycle, other compounds, known as ketone bodies, are produced. These can be utilised by the heart and kidney for ATP production, but acetone can be produced which is clinically noticeable in some cases.

[3] The amino acids in muscle proteins (i.e. all except leucine and lysine) can be converted to glucose via the process of gluconeogenesis. They can enter the energy metabolism pathway via conversion to pyruvate (glucogenic amino acids) or follow the pathway of fatty acids, producing acetyl CoA through β oxidation (ketogenic amino acids). Amino acids not required for protein synthesis lose their nitrogen-containing amino group, which is excreted in the ammonia–urea pathway.

Krebs cycle—reduced nicotinamide adenine dinucleotide (NADH) and flavine adeninedinucleotide (FADH2)—to generate ATP via an electron transport chain. This is known as aerobic metabolism. The waste products of energy metabolism are carbon dioxide (CO_2) and water (H_2O), reflecting the chemical building blocks of the macronutrients. As amino acids contain nitrogen as well as carbon, hydrogen and oxygen, their breakdown produces ammonia (NH_3), which is metabolised to urea in the liver and excreted in the kidneys.

Glucose homeostasis

To begin to understand the relationships between nutrients and the various metabolic cascades, it is helpful to return to the processing of nutrients. Despite the varying pathways for absorption, the three macronutrients are delivered to the liver, a very significant processing organ of the body. Glucose is the major fuel source of the brain and other tissues, and the body will do what it can to maintain **glucose homeostasis**. This is achieved by two main processes (Figure 3.11).

Gluconeogenesis is the formation of new glucose from amino acids and from glycerol, which becomes available after free fatty acids are delivered to adipose tissue. Thus high protein diets can also influence blood glucose (and fat storage). The situation exposed so far for dietary fat is very complex. Fat is implicated not only as a fuel source but also in cascades of metabolic events; for example, in cell signalling related to the action of insulin [13].

Glucose homeostasis
the maintenance of blood glucose levels within a range that best supports health; occurs when all stimulus and response mechanisms are in balance.

Gluconeogenesis
formation of new glucose from amino acids and glycerol.

FIGURE 3.11 HORMONAL REGULATION OF GLUCOSE

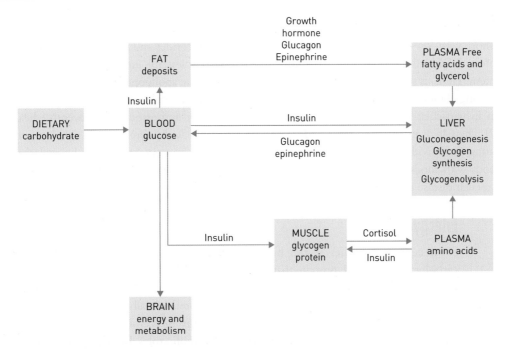

Source: Adapted from G. Pocock & C.D. Richards (2006). *Human Physiology. The basis of medicine.* Oxford University Press (Figure 27.5, p. 541)

Glycogenolysis
the breakdown of glycogen
to deliver free glucose.

Glycogenolysis occurs with the breakdown of stored carbohydrate (glycogen) in the liver for distribution or in the muscle for its own purposes. In all this, hormonal control systems are at play: low blood sugar stimulates the release of glucagon, which sets off gluconeogenesis, whereas high blood sugar stimulates the release of insulin, which promotes the formation of glycogen. Disorders of insulin action, insufficiency or depletion of insulin, result in the disease state known as diabetes mellitus.

Glucose serves as a fuel through a process known as glycolysis, where further enzyme-assisted reactions lead to the production of energy and related metabolites in the cell mitochondria. This is the end point of a complex pathway, which began with eating a food such as a piece of bread. Glucose metabolism is a fundamental biological process linked to food consumption. Obviously, diet plays an important role, not only in the management of disorders of carbohydrate (and possibly fat) metabolism such as diabetes, but also in supporting the system, which seeks to maintain homeostatic conditions and thereby functionality throughout life.

Lipid transport

The study of diet and heart disease has helped to also expose the significance of diet in relation to fat metabolism. Cholesterol has been implicated in cardiovascular disease and myocardial infarction (heart attack) for some time, through the identification of cholesterol build-up in diseased vessels, and epidemiological observations of the association between high blood cholesterol levels and the prevalence of cardiovascular disease in populations [14; 15]. The transport of lipids in packaged forms underpins a great deal of research on cardiovascular health, particularly in relation to lipoproteins of varying density and the major apolipoprotein subclasses. While there is a genetic basis to these profiles

See Chapter 5 on fats and lipids for details about SFA content.

(noting that proteins are part of both lipoproteins and enzymes), a degree of generalisation can be applied, particularly for Western societies and in the context of Western food and activity environments.

In short, very-low-density lipoprotein (VLDL) releases triglycerides and free fatty acids. Low-density lipoprotein (LDL) connects to LDL receptors and releases cholesterol into the tissues. High-density lipoprotein (HDL) is secreted by the liver and intestine, transferring apolipoprotein, and is also responsible for returning cholesterol from the tissues to the liver (reverse cholesterol transport). The LDL cholesterol fraction in particular is implicated in cardiovascular disease risk and assessed in preventive healthcare [16; 17]. Diets high in saturated fatty acids (SFA) are associated with increased LDL cholesterol levels, implicating foods with a high SFA content. Reducing the SFA content of the diet, by replacing high SFA foods with foods that are high in polyunsaturated fatty acids (PUFA), is associated with reduced cardiovascular disease risk [18].

Energy balance

See Chapters 4–7 on carbohydrates, fats and lipids, protein and energy intake.

Energy balance
a state that occurs when the energy consumed is equal to the energy expended.

Food consumption lies at the heart of **energy balance** because food provides the carbohydrate, fat and protein that replenishes the body stores and provides new fuel. Humans belong to the animal kingdom and they store very little carbohydrate (as glycogen in liver and muscle), and dietary carbohydrate is preferentially metabolised for energy or stored as fat. Fatty acids are also utilised for energy (glycerol is eventually converted to glucose), but they have additional important metabolic roles. Because protein forms large structural and functional parts of the body, stores are protected, but protein is also used as a fuel source and excess stored ultimately as fat. Amino acids and the products of protein degradation are absorbed (and reabsorbed) into the system to form what is known as the 'amino acid pool'. This pool is drawn on to form specific structures and serve specific functions, or is utilised for energy.

Manipulating the macronutrient proportions of the diet with different food patterns may have some advantages in some individuals, but adherence to these patterns is often difficult to achieve, and if weight loss is the target, dietary energy is the most effective nutritional factor [19].

Gut integrity and immune health

It has been known for some time that short chain fatty acids (SCFA), in particular butyrate, acetate and propionate, are produced by bacterial fermentation of fibres. Non-digestible polysaccharides are broken down by enzymes that are produced by bacteria. Butyrate is used as fuel by cells in the gut (colonocytes), while acetate and propionate are absorbed into the bloodstream and transported to the liver (from there, acetate is further transported as fuel), and the remaining SCFA are eventually excreted in faeces. Further research has added to this knowledge, exposing extensive roles for SCFA in maintaining gut integrity and supporting immune function. More broadly, microbe associated molecular patterns (MAMPs) are related to a range of signalling cascades that influence the immune system and play a role in the delicate balance of pro- and anti-inflammatory responses.

See Chapter 4 for details on polysaccharides.

Visit Oxford Ascend for more on the immune system.

STOP AND THINK

* Which foods would be important in supporting glucose homeostasis in people with impaired insulin action?
* Which lipoprotein entities are routinely measured to assess risk of cardiovascular disease, and why?
* What types of foods appear to support a healthy gut microbiome?

WHAT ARE NUTRIENT REFERENCE VALUES AND HOW ARE THEY MET IN THE DIET?

Food delivers nutrients which have multiple functions within human biology that support health. Nutrients engage in a complex set of chemical pathways that serve a purpose. This creates a form of interdependence (or synergy) between nutrients, defined by the physiological and biochemical blueprint of the body. Problems with nutrient intakes are observed with clinical signs of deficiency or toxicity implicating the relevant chemical pathways. Balance is a central concept in nutrition (Figure 3.12), as it is in health. Problems can also arise where there is a strong relationship between a nutrient and a dietary pattern associated with chronic disease, or biomarkers of that disease. In all cases, the integral relationship between nutrients, foods and whole diets remains pivotal in working with nutrition and health.

With this in mind, Australian and New Zealand health authorities develop and work with a set of scientifically defined standards known as Nutrient Reference Values (NRVs) (see www.nrv.gov.au). These are known as Dietary Reference Intakes in the United States and Canada [20] and Dietary Reference Values in the United Kingdom [21]. The primary functions of these standards are to assess the nutritional quality of dietary intakes of individuals, groups and populations.

Behind this assessment is the need to protect public health and the increasing evidence from scientific research exposing the health effects of food consumption. The suite of NRVs available today reflects the

FIGURE 3.12 REPRESENTATIONAL IMAGE OF THE CONCEPT OF BALANCE IN NUTRIENT REQUIREMENTS

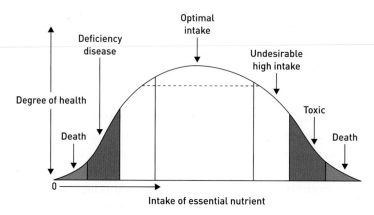

Source: Adapted from Department of Health (2017). *General Principles for Establishing Safe Upper Levels of Intake for Micronutrients—Issues for consideration.* Canberra: Department of Health

extent of this evidence and the range of purposes that NRVs must now serve. The applications of these standards have wide-reaching potential for public health, including use in dietary modelling for dietary guidelines documents (such as the Australian Guide to Healthy Eating) [22; 23], referencing in food labelling practices, and the formulation of food products. They can also be used in menu assessments for institutions such as childcare, boarding schools, workplaces and aged care facilities.

≫ CASE 3.2

SCIENTIFIC RESEARCH AND THE NRVs

As the NRVs are based on the best available science at the time, and scientific investigation is ongoing, a great deal of methodological work has been undertaken in maintaining the NRVs.

In Europe, an evidence-based methodology for deriving micronutrient requirements was published in 2013 [24], introducing new concepts such as risk analysis and risk management in standards development. In the United States, scientific literature, editorial debates [25] and commentary [26] on the evidence framework have emerged. Others have commented on the funding for relevant research [27], drawing attention to the operational networks of science.

In Australia, a new methodological framework was developed and utilised in the round of NRV reviews published in 2017 [28; 29]. This new framework clarified the conceptual basis and applications of the NRVs, provided a process for review of the NRVs and outlined methods for deriving NRV recommendations.

* Why is there a need for methodological development in reviewing NRVs?
* When are international considerations relevant, and when should the focus be on national concerns?
* What would be the spectrum of nutrition science specialties required to support this activity in practice?

The methods for deriving NRVs in Australia involve a number of stages based on evidence review [28]. The first stage begins with defining the question. This includes identifying the details of the population of interest (e.g. children, adults, males, females) and clarifying the health outcomes of concern (e.g. goitre, scurvy, hypertension, cardiovascular disease). Today, NRVs are not only concerned with deficiency states, but also relationships with the prevention of chronic disease risk. The exploration of food components is also extending these boundaries [1]. For the purposes of the current Australian NRVs, a nutrient is defined as 'a substance that provides nourishment essential for the maintenance of health and for growth' [28], and the list of nutrients has remained fairly constant.

Addressing both concerns for deficiency and chronic disease means separating the research that addresses nutrient adequacy and clinical deficiency states from the research that examines the relationship between diet and chronic disease. There are also other considerations, such as the bioavailability profile of nutrients, the different forms (chemical structures) of a nutrient class, the balance between dietary and endogenous production of nutrients (e.g. some are also produced in the gut or skin) and the interactions between nutrients. Without doubt, this is a complex scientific endeavour requiring a breadth of expertise.

The different NRVs reflect their utility in practice. They are also linked to other aspects of nutrition practice. In particular, they provide a base for dietary modelling in the dietary guidelines, ensuring the food-based guidance meets requirements for nutrients (www.eatforhealth.gov.au). Both the dietary guidelines and NRVs reference dietary data from national nutrition surveys [22; 30]. This embeds the processes in the available food supply and the realities of dietary consumption patterns. Again, the interdependence between nutrients, foods and dietary patterns is played out, this time in policy and standards development.

The NRVs that are used to assess **nutritional adequacy** are the **estimated average requirement (EAR)**, **adequate intake (AI)** and **recommended dietary intake (RDI)** The EAR provides the best estimate of the prevalence of inadequate intakes in populations (Table 3.3). Because nutrient requirements of individuals are assumed to fall into a symmetrical distribution, where most individuals would have a requirement close to the midpoint and a few at the extremes, the EARs of nutrients were set at the midpoint, covering 50% of the population, as the name implies. Intake below the EAR indicates a ≥50% risk of dietary nutrient inadequacy. When data is not available to assess an EAR, an AI is set, based on the amount of a nutrient consumed by healthy individuals in the population. It is expected that the AI would normally exceed the average requirement, but the exact proportion of the population it covers is unknown. When no experimental data exists for the usual intake of healthy individuals, the population median is used as the AI. The RDI is an older version of this NRV. Also considering a population distribution of intakes (Figure 3.12), the RDI was originally set at two standard deviations above the EAR, so that it theoretically covered 97.5% of people. Since consuming small amounts above the actual requirement of a nutrient is usually not harmful, the RDI can be used as a target for daily intake, and intake above the RDI indicates a low risk of dietary nutrient inadequacy for an individual (Figure 3.13). The RDI should not be used to assess the adequacy of population dietary intakes (Table 3.3).

These reference points were set after a review of scientific literature to determine the requirement of the average healthy person within various age ranges. Because people of different age and gender may have different nutrient requirements—for example,

See Chapter 2 on dietary guidelines.

Nutritional adequacy
the amount of nutrients consumed that would reduce the probability of deficiency disease or inadequate growth.

Estimated average requirement (EAR)
'Nutrient level required meeting the needs of approximately half the healthy individuals in a sex and particular life stage group' (www.nrv.gov.au).

Adequate intake (AI)
'The average daily nutrient intake level based on observed or experimentally-determined approximations or estimates of nutrient intake by a group (or groups) of apparently healthy people that are assumed to be adequate' (www.nrv.gov.au).

Recommended dietary intake (RDI)
'The average daily intake level that is sufficient to meet the nutrient requirements of nearly all (97–98%) healthy individuals in a sex and particular life stage group' (www.nrv.gov.au).

FIGURE 3.13 RELATIONSHIP AMONG UPPER LEVEL OF INTAKE (UL), RECOMMENDED DIETARY
INTAKE (RDI) AND ESTIMATED AVERAGE REQUIREMENT (EAR)

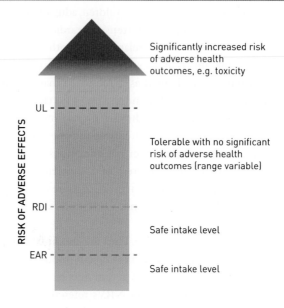

TABLE 3.3   USES OF NRVs FOR ASSESSING ADEQUACY OF INTAKE FOR INDIVIDUALS AND GROUPS

Nutrient Reference Value	For individuals	For groups
EAR	**Use to examine the probability that usual intake is inadequate** (best estimate)	**Use to estimate the prevalence of inadequate intakes within a group**
RDI	**Use to assess probability that usual intake is inadequate** (≥RDI implies a low probability of inadequacy)	*Do not use* to assess intakes of populations
AI (in absence of EAR)	**Use to examine the probability that usual intake is inadequate** (≥AI implies low probability of inadequacy. When the AI is based on median intakes of healthy populations, this assessment is made with less confidence.)	**In the absence of EAR, use to estimate the prevalence of inadequate intakes within a group** (Median intake ≥AI implies a low prevalence of inadequate intakes. When the AI is based on median intakes of healthy populations, this assessment is made with less confidence.)
Upper level of intake (UL)	Usual intake above this level may place an individual at risk of adverse effects from excessive nutrient intake	**Use to estimate the percentage of the population at potential risk of adverse effects from excessive nutrient intake**

Source: National Health and Medical Research Council (2006). *Nutrient Reference Values for Australia and New Zealand, Including Recommended Dietary Intakes*. Canberra: NHMRC. © Commonwealth of Australia

menstruating women would need more iron than men of the same age due to menstrual loss of iron—NRVs were clustered into groups based on age and gender. However, even within groups the requirement can still vary from individual to individual. Thus NRVs should not be used to diagnose nutrient deficiencies. Nutrient deficiency is confirmed by clinical means—for example, when deficiency symptoms occur, such as the presence of scurvy in vitamin C deficiency.

The NRV used to assess **negative health effects** of nutrient intakes is the **upper level of intake (UL)**. It is a general misconception that overconsumption of nutrients is harmless, particularly for fat-soluble vitamins such as vitamin A. The UL is set at a point where nutrient intakes may increase the risk of adverse health outcomes. Two estimations are involved in the determination of the UL: the LOAEL (lowest observed adverse effect level), defined as the 'lowest dose at which there is a measureable adverse effect from a test substance in a test subject or population' [28]; and the NOAEL (no adverse effect level), defined as the 'highest dose at which there is a measureable adverse effect from a test subject or population' [28]. The Australian NRV methodology allows for four descriptors for UL, based on the availability of data to undertake the necessary reviews: these include UL and three qualifiers: provisional, not determined and not required.

The NRVs used to address the risk of chronic lifestyle-related disease are the **suggested dietary target (SDT)** and the **acceptable macronutrient distribution range (AMDR)**. Evidence for the relationship with chronic disease is generally provided through clinical trials and population cohort studies, where disease outcomes are assessed. The focal point may be a single nutrient (indicating the need for an SDT) or relative amounts of macronutrients in the diet (relating to the AMDR). Meta-analysis of data from multiple studies may be possible to determine the nature and extent of this relationship. Where there is a convincing relationship between intakes of a nutrient and the health outcome, population intake patterns provide the means for setting the SDT. When the target is set at the median intake (as in the AI), most people would need to reduce their intake, so this is a reasonable level to set. It is important to note that this is a statistically derived population target, bearing in mind that 50% of the population would theoretically be consuming the nutrient above this target.

The AMDR brings to bear research on whole diets (e.g. low fat, high protein, low carbohydrate), and highlights the fact that meeting nutritional requirements often leaves an energy gap that could be met by any of the three macronutrients. However, the value of an AMDR may be questioned as it appears the evidence for defining optimum diets is better placed by addressing cuisine patterns based on key identifiable foods rather than proportions of macronutrients in which foods have not been defined (and can have varying effects). The methodological framework for the Australian NRVs [28] states that a review of this area is needed.

A number of NRVs reference the energy requirements of an individual. The AMDRs refer to the relative amounts of macronutrients as a percentage of energy. Vitamins associated with energy metabolism are naturally linked to energy expenditure and, thereby, energy requirements. The **estimated energy requirement (EER)** provides a value for groups within the population defined by age, sex, size and activity, all of which impinge on energy expenditure.

Negative health effects measurable adverse events or outcomes following consumption of a substance.

Upper level of intake (UL) 'The highest daily average intake level likely to pose no adverse health effects to almost all individuals in the general population. As intake increase above the UL, the potential risk of adverse effects increases' (www.nrv.gov.au).

Suggested dietary target (SDT) 'A daily average intake from food and beverages for certain nutrients that may help in the prevention of chronic disease' (www.nrv.gov.au).

Acceptable macronutrient distribution range (AMDR) 'An estimate of the range of intake for each macronutrient for individuals (expressed as a contribution to energy), which would allow for an adequate intake of all other nutrients while maximizing general health outcomes' (www.nrv.gov.au).

See Chapter 10 on water soluble vitamins.

Estimated energy requirement (EER) 'The average dietary energy intake that is predicted to maintain energy balance in a healthy adult of defined age, sex, weight, height and level of activity consistent with good health' (www.nrv.gov.au).

>> RESEARCH AT WORK

REVISED NRVs FOR SODIUM

Using the methodological framework for the review of NRVs [28], revised positions on the SDT and UL of intake were published in 2017 [28; 29].

The SDT was noted as a target for average population intake levels to help in the prevention of chronic disease. The revised level was 2000 mg/day, which is about half that of the current intake in Australia and New Zealand of about 3600 mg/day. To achieve a population median of 2000 mg/day, most people would need to reduce their sodium intake. This level would also allow for a total diet to meet requirements for all other nutrients, given the current food supply.

The UL was noted as the average intake likely to pose no risk in the general population. Following analysis of currently available data, which clearly showed increasing blood pressure with increasing sodium intakes, a point at which this relationship did not occur could not be identified. In keeping with the definitions outlined in the methodological framework, the UL was set at 'not determined'. This was because a point of low risk could not be determined and a safe upper limit was not identifiable in the available data (which addressed intakes of between 1200 and 3300 mg sodium) [31]. A full review of the supporting documents for this analysis and the processes undertaken can be found at www.nrv.gov.au.

TRY IT YOURSELF

Refer to the NRVs for calcium to identify the amount of calcium you require for your age and sex. Note the amount of dairy-based foods you consume on a regular daily basis (the following provide roughly 300 mg calcium per serve: one cup of milk, 200 g tub of yoghurt or one slice of cheese). Evaluate your calcium intake using this information and the nutrition information panels on other products that may contain calcium.

See Chapter 2 dietary guidelines and planning a healthy diet.

Addressing the recommendations for NRVs in the diet requires an understanding of food sources of nutrients and the intake levels that can be achieved with the current food supply. This has all been factored into the dietary guidance provided in the Australian Guide to Healthy Eating (www.eatforhealth.gov.au) and its related online resources. The recommended combination of foods and the suggested serving sizes can be determined for individuals given their age, sex and level of activity.

There may be little concern for meeting requirements of some nutrients, as they may be plentifully supplied across a broad range of commonly consumed foods. In others cases, the nutrient may be limited in concentration to a few main food sources, while yet other nutrients may be appearing in excess because of an overemphasis in the foods supplied and consumed (e.g. sodium, saturated fat and sugars). Just as the biological processes of the human body work to maintain balance, so too does the delivery of nutrients to serve those processes. Given the characteristics of the Australian food environment and the prevalence of hypertension, cardiovascular disease and obesity, it is imperative that most Australians achieve their required intake of nutrients while constraining sodium, saturated fat and energy intakes, and that changes are made in the food system to support those actions.

The concepts of **nutrient density** and **energy density** may assist in discriminating between foods for this purpose [32]. As the names of these terms imply, nutrient density refers to the concentration of a micronutrient within a food, while energy density refers to its kilojoule content. Foods with a high nutrient density provide a significant amount of nutrients, whereas those with a high energy density are also referred to as high calorie foods. Because food is made up of multiple components, energy and nutrient density are affected by components that can dilute the density, such as water and fibre. Thus foods with a high water and fibre content may be less energy-dense [33]. Foods with a high fat content may be more energy-dense because fat is an energy-dense nutrient (37 kJ/g) compared with protein (17 kJ/g) and carbohydrate (16 kJ/g). Thus some energy-dense foods, such as nuts and cheese, may also be nutrient-dense, so it is important to include them in the diet. To enable the delivery of nutrients in the diet with this extra energy cost, smaller serving sizes of foods tend to be recommended, in contrast to large serving sizes for nutrient-dense foods with low energy density (such as green leafy vegetables).

On the other hand, the energy density of a food may be highly influenced by its method of preparation (Table 3.4). The influence of food preparation often results in foods such as vegetables or cereals being classified as 'core' (including vegetables and grains) or 'discretionary'. The Australian Dietary Guidelines define discretionary foods as those with high levels of added saturated fat, sodium or sugar [23]. In the Nutrition First analysis of the Australian Health Survey data, discretionary foods appeared to contribute to 35% energy, with major sources including cereal and vegetable-based foods [34].

Nutrient density
Amount of nutrients/ Energy value (kJ).

Energy density
Energy value (kJ)/Weight of food (g).

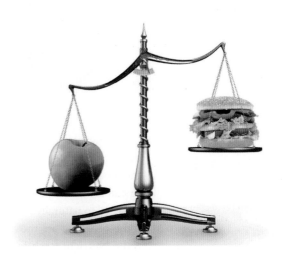

TABLE 3.4   ENERGY DENSITY OF POTATO DISHES PREPARED BY DIFFERENT MEANS

Potato (100 g)	Energy (kJ)*	Total fat (g)*	Energy density (kJ/g)*
Sebago potato (unpeeled) boiled	261	0	2.61
Sebago potato (unpeeled) baked	318	0.4	3.18
Sebago potato (peeled) mashed	279	0.4	2.79
Potato crisps (plain) salted	2160	33.9	21.6
Hot potato chips (takeaway outlet)	968	10.8	9.68
Potato hash brown (takeaway)	934	13.2	9.34

*Calculated from *NUTTAB 2010* [2].

TRY IT YOURSELF

Cottage cheese contains 529 kJ/100 g and 89 mg calcium/100 g. Natural plain yoghurt contains 367 kJ/ 100 g and 193 mg calcium/100 g. Estimate the amount of calcium that would be delivered in the amount of food that would deliver 100 kJ at the same time. If you were both limiting energy intakes and needing to meet calcium requirements, which food might be the better choice, and why?

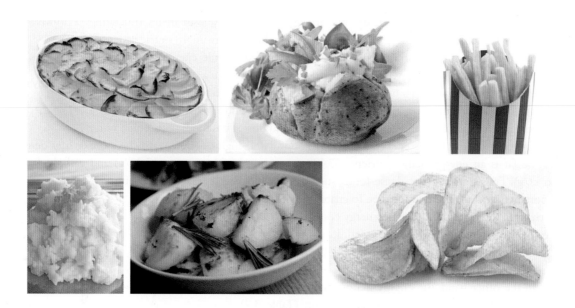

Nutrient profiling

a system of ranking and categorising foods based on nutritional value with respect to a predetermined set of nutrients.

In the past decade, **nutrient profiling** has emerged as a process for distinguishing between foods by addressing nutrient density (Figure 3.14). As an artificial construction, the process is limited by its inputs, reflecting what we know about food and its components to date. In principle, however, the application could be useful for manufactured foods (as opposed to naturally occurring foods), which are constructed from a number of ingredients, some of which are proving to be problematic. An example of a nutrient profiling system is the Nutrient Rich Food Index, which is based on nine nutrients to be encouraged and

FIGURE 3.14 CATEGORISING FOODS IN TERMS OF ENERGY AND NUTRIENT VALUE COMBINED

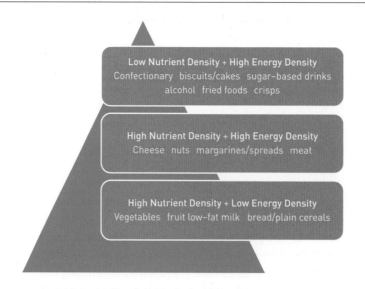

Low Nutrient Density + High Energy Density
Confectionary biscuits/cakes sugar–based drinks
alcohol fried foods crisps

High Nutrient Density + High Energy Density
Cheese nuts margarines/spreads meat

High Nutrient Density + Low Energy Density
Vegetables fruit low–fat milk bread/plain cereals

OXFORD UNIVERSITY PRESS

three nutrients to be limited. This system has been used to rank individual foods, meals and menus by their nutritional value [35; 36]. Recently, it has been used to rank different snack foods for children, demonstrating that yoghurt, milk and fruit have emerged as the most nutrient rich (scoring >30 points), while carbonated soft drinks, pies, cakes and ice-cream have emerged as the most nutrient poor (with negative scores) [37].

The concept of nutrient profiling is applied in the voluntary Australian Health Star Rating System (www.healthstarrating.gov.au), which helps consumers discern the nutritional profile of packaged foods. As products receive from a ½ star to 5 stars, it provides a simple score on ranking within food categories. This information complements the additional nutrition information panels (NIP) provided on packaged foods, which outline the amount of energy, protein, fat, saturated fat, carbohydrate, sugars and sodium in the food (per 100 g and per serve) [38]. Additional information on nutrients is also required when claims are made—for example, if a food claims to be a source of fibre then the amount of fibre must be listed.

STOP AND THINK

- Why do we need NRVs?
- How does scientific research underpin the setting of NRVs?
- How is nutrient profiling useful in discriminating between foods?

SUMMARY

- Foods have their origins in plants and animals, so the nutrient composition is interrelated.
- Foods can be categorised as principal sources of protein, fat and carbohydrate. Macronutrients are the major nutritional components of foods and serve as fuel sources. Carbohydrate is the main source, whereas the components of digested protein and fat also serve important structural and functional roles.
- Foods also deliver significant amounts of essential vitamins and minerals. When food is consumed, it is broken down into its component parts. Nutrients are absorbed through the gut in various forms and transported throughout the body by a range of mechanisms. Micronutrients (vitamins and minerals) are delivered and absorbed in smaller quantities by a range of mechanisms, often to maintain a balance in physiological levels.
- Nutrient Reference Values are a set of science-referenced standards for macro and micronutrient consumption that address requirements for age and sex, and target prevention of diet-related chronic disease. Requirements for nutrients are derived from the principle of balance, with the 'upside down U' reference. Not enough of a particular nutrient is likely to cause problems, with increasing amounts leading to improvements but only to a certain point. After that any further increase may result in negative effects and toxicity is a real consideration.
- Choosing a healthy diet implies a combination of foods that deliver essential nutrients in the forms that adequately meet requirements and in a dietary pattern that is protective against chronic disease.
- Evaluating which foods are best requires an understanding of the relative nutritional value of foods, the amount of dietary energy available and the need to allocate some of this energy to foods that deliver the required nutrients.

PATHWAYS TO PRACTICE

- In all forms of practice, understanding the mechanisms of food digestion and nutrient absorption and transport is fundamental in appreciating the role of nutrients and their significant relationship with food.

- Applications of nutrition knowledge covered in this chapter occur in a range of settings—for example, food regulations and food-based nutrition communications and promotions. This has relevance to those working in government and industry.

- Establishing the significance of research on individual nutrients can be achieved with an understanding of how they are delivered through food and made available to the body.

DISCUSSION QUESTIONS

1   Why are foods sometimes referred to as 'carbohydrates' when carbohydrates are actually only a food component?
2   Which foods are major sources of protein and how is this related to the original plant or animal from which the food came?
3   Why do higher levels of protein and fat often occur in the same foods?
4   What are some of the meanings of the word 'fat' in food and nutrition?
5   How are foods that contain mostly fat used in the diet?
6   What are some of the ways for remembering which foods contain fat-soluble or water-soluble vitamins? Give some examples.
7   Together, which food groups would provide all the essential nutrients in the diet?
8   How useful are the terms 'nutrient-dense' and 'energy-dense' in differentiating between foods on nutritional terms?

USEFUL WEBLINKS

Dietary Reference Intakes in the United Kingdom:
www.nutrition.org.uk/nutritionscience/nutrients-food-and-ingredients/nutrient-requirements.html

Dietary Reference Intakes in the United States and Canada:
https://ods.od.nih.gov/Health_Information/Dietary_Reference_Intakes.aspx

Eat for Health:
www.eatforhealth.gov.au

Health Star Rating System:
www.healthstarrating.gov.au

Nutrient Reference Values in Australia:
www.nrv.gov.au

Nutrition Information Panels:
www.foodstandards.gov.au/consumer/labelling/panels/Pages/default.aspx

Resources—2017 Revisions of the Nutrient Reference Values:
www.nrv.gov.au/resources

The Human Microbiome:
http://learn.genetics.utah.edu/content/microbiome

FURTHER READING

Bach Knudsen, K. E., Nørskov, N. P., Bolvig, A. K., Hedemann, M. S. & Lærke, H. N. (2017). Dietary fibers and associated phytochemicals in cereals. *Molecular Nutrition and Food Research*, 61(7). doi:10.1002/mnfr.201600518

Bondonno, N. P., Bondonno, C. P., Ward, N. C., Hodgson, J. M. & Croft, K. D. (2017). The cardiovascular health benefits of apples: whole fruit vs. isolated compounds. *Trends in Food Science & Technology*. doi:https://doi.org/10.1016/j.tifs.2017.04.012

de Clercq, N. C., Groen, A. K., Romijn, J. A. & Nieuwdorp, M. (2016). Gut microbiota in obesity and undernutrition. *Advances in Nutrition: An International Review Journal*, 7(6), 1080–9. doi:10.3945/an.116.012914

Desmarchelier, C. & Borel, P. (2017). Overview of carotenoid bioavailability determinants: from dietary factors to host genetic variations. *Trends in Food Science & Technology*. doi:https://doi.org/10.1016/j.tifs.2017.03.002

Drewnowski, A., Rehm, C. D., Maillot, M., Mendoza, A. & Monsivais, P. (2015). The feasibility of meeting the WHO guidelines for sodium and potassium: a cross-national comparison study. *BMJ Open*, 5(3). doi:10.1136/bmjopen-2014-006625

Giacco, R., Costabile, G. & Riccardi, G. (2016). Metabolic effects of dietary carbohydrates: the importance of food digestion. *Food Research International*, 88, 336–41. doi:10.1016/j.foodres.2015.10.026

Gleeson, J. P. (2017). Diet, food components and the intestinal barrier. *Nutrition Bulletin*, 42(2), 123–31. doi:10.1111/nbu.12260

Grundy, M. M. L., Edwards, C. H., Mackie, A. R., Gidley, M. J., Butterworth, P. J. & Ellis, P. R. (2016). Re-evaluation of the mechanisms of dietary fibre and implications for macronutrient bioaccessibility, digestion and postprandial metabolism. *British Journal of Nutrition*, 116(5), 816–33. doi:10.1017/S0007114516002610

Jacome-Sosa, M., Parks, E. J., Bruno, R. S., Tasali, E., Lewis, G. F., Schneeman B. O. & Rains, T. M. (2016). Postprandial metabolism of macronutrients and cardiometabolic risk: recent developments, emerging concepts, and future directions. *Advances in Nutrition: An International Review Journal*, 7(2), 364–74. doi:10.3945/an.115.010397

Karaś, M., Jakubczyk, A., Szymanowska, U., Złotek, U. & Zielińska, E. (2017). Digestion and bioavailability of bioactive phytochemicals. *International Journal of Food Science and Technology*, 52(2), 291–305. doi:10.1111/ijfs.13323

Link, J. C. & Reue, K. (2017). Genetic basis for sex differences in obesity and lipid metabolism. *Annual Review of Nutrition*, 37(1), 225–45. doi:10.1146/annurev-nutr-071816-064827

Martinez, K. B., Pierre, J. F. & Chang, E. B. (2016). The gut microbiota: the gateway to improved metabolism. *Gastroenterology Clinics of North America*, 45(4), 601–14. doi:10.1016/j.gtc.2016.07.001

Martínez-Huélamo, M., Vallverdú-Queralt, A., Di Lecce, G., Valderas-Martínez, P., Tulipani, S., Jáuregui, O., … Lamuela-Raventós, R. M. (2016). Bioavailability of tomato polyphenols is enhanced by processing and fat addition: evidence from a randomized feeding trial. *Molecular Nutrition and Food Research*, 60(7), 1578–89. doi:10.1002/mnfr.201500820

Maukonen, J. & Saarela, M. (2015). Human gut microbiota: does diet matter? *Proceedings of the Nutrition Society*, 74(1), 23–36. doi:10.1017/S0029665114000688

Murphy, S. P., Yates, A. A., Atkinson, S. A., Barr, S. I. & Dwyer, J. (2016). History of nutrition: the long road leading to the dietary reference intakes for the United States and Canada. *Advances in Nutrition: An International Review Journal*, 7(1), 157–68. doi:10.3945/an.115.010322

Pocock, G. & Richards, C. D. (2006). *Human Physiology: The basis of medicine*, 3rd edn. Oxford: Oxford University Press.

Prentice, A. M., Mendoza, Y. A., Pereira, D., Cerami, C., Wegmuller, R., Constable, A. & Spieldenner, J. (2017). Dietary strategies for improving iron status: balancing safety and efficacy. *Nutrition Reviews*, 75(1), 49–60. doi:10.1093/nutrit/nuw055

Sommer, F., Anderson, J. M., Bharti, R., Raes, J. & Rosenstiel, P. (2017). The resilience of the intestinal microbiota influences health and disease. *Nature Reviews Microbiology*, 15(10), 630–8. doi:10.1038/nrmicro.2017.58

Sonnenburg, J. L. & Bäckhed, F. (2016). Diet-microbiota interactions as moderators of human metabolism. *Nature*, 535(7610), 56–64. doi:10.1038/nature18846

Thorning, T. K., Bertram, H. C., Bonjour, J. P., De Groot, L., Dupont, D., Feeney, E., … Givens, I. (2017). Whole dairy matrix or single nutrients in assessment of health effects: current evidence and knowledge gaps. *American Journal of Clinical Nutrition*, 105(5), 1033–45. doi:10.3945/ajcn.116.151548

Wolfe, R. R., Cifelli, A. M., Kostas, G. & Kim, I.-Y. (2017). Optimizing protein intake in adults: interpretation and application of the recommended dietary allowance compared with the acceptable macronutrient distribution range. *Advances in Nutrition: An International Review Journal*, 8(2), 266–75. doi:10.3945/an.116.013821

Woting, A. & Blaut, M. (2016). The intestinal microbiota in metabolic disease. *Nutrients*, 8(4). doi:10.3390/nu8040202

Yates, A. A., Erdman. Jr, J. W., Shao, A., Dolan, L. C. & Griffiths, J. C. (2017). Bioactive nutrients—time for tolerable upper intake levels to address safety. *Regulatory Toxicology and Pharmacology*, 84, 94–101. doi:10.1016/j.yrtph.2017.01.002

REFERENCES

1   S. Jew, J.-M. Antoine, P. Bourlioux, J. Milner, L. C. Tapsell, Y. Yang & P. J. H. Jones (2015). Nutrient essentiality revisited. *Journal of Functional Foods*, 14, 203–9. doi:http://dx.doi.org/10.1016/j.jff.2015.01.024

2   Food Standards Australia New Zealand (2012). *NUTTAB 2010*. Canberra: FSANZ.

3   T. H. Vesa, R. Korpela & P. Marteau (2000). Lactose intolerance. *Journal of the American College of Nutrition*, 19, 165S–175S. doi:10.1080/07315724.2000.10718086

4   Y. Deng, B. Misselwitz, N. Dai & M. Fox (2015). Lactose intolerance in adults: biological mechanism and dietary management. *Nutrients*, 7(9), 5380.

5   P. J. Turnbaugh, M. Hamady, T. Yatsunenko, B. L. Cantarel, A. Duncan, R. E. Ley, … J. I. Gordon (2009). A core gut microbiome in obese and lean twins. *Nature*, 457(7228), 480–4. doi:http://www.nature.com/nature/journal/v457/n7228/suppinfo/nature07540_S1.html

6   Z. E. Ilhan, J. K. DiBaise, N. G. Isern, D. W. Hoyt, A. K. Marcus, D.-W. Kang, … R. Krajmalnik-Brown (2017). Distinctive microbiomes and metabolites linked with weight loss after gastric bypass, but not gastric banding. *ISME Journal*, 11(9), 2047–58. doi:10.1038/ismej.2017.71

7   L. J. Brandt (2013). American Journal of Gastroenterology lecture: intestinal microbiota and the role of fecal microbiota transplant (FMT) in treatment of *C. difficile* infection. *American Journal of Gastroenterology*, 108(2), 177–85.

8   M. P. Francino (2017). The gut microbiome and metabolic health. *Current Nutrition Reports*, 6(1), 16–23. doi:10.1007/s13668-017-0190-1

9   Y.Y. Lam, A. J. Mitchell, A. J. Holmes, G. S. Denyer, A. Gummesson, I. D. Caterson, … L. H. Storlien (2011). Role of the gut in visceral fat inflammation and metabolic disorders. *Obesity*, 19(11), 2113–20. doi:10.1038/oby.2011.68

10 D. S. Siscovick (2017). Scientific discovery, contextual factors, and cardiometabolic health research: back to the future. *Circulation Research*, 120(10), 1555–7. doi:10.1161/circresaha.116.310254

11 A. F. G. Cicero & A. Colletti (2017). Food and plant bioactives for reducing cardiometabolic disease: how does the evidence stack up? *Trends in Food Science & Technology*. doi:https://doi.org/10.1016/j.tifs.2017.04.001

12 M. Laakso, J. Kuusisto, A. Stančáková, T. Kuulasmaa, P. Pajukanta, A. J. Lusis, … M. Boehnke (2017). The Metabolic Syndrome in Men study: a resource for studies of metabolic and cardiovascular diseases. *Journal of Lipid Research*, 58(3), 481–93. doi:10.1194/jlr.O072629

13 L. H. Storlien, Y. Y. Lam, B. J. Wu, L. C. Tapsell & A. B. Jenkins (2016). Effects of dietary fat subtypes on glucose homeostasis during pregnancy in rats. *Nutrition & Metabolism*, 13(1), 58. doi:10.1186/s12986-016-0117-7

14 E. J. Benjamin, M. J. Blaha, S. E. Chiuve, M. Cushman, S. R. Das, R. Deo, … P. Muntner (2017). Heart disease and stroke statistics—2017 update: a report from the American Heart Association. *Circulation*, 135(10), e146–e603. doi:10.1161/cir.0000000000000485

15 Australian Institute of Health and Welfare (2015). *Cardiovascular Disease, Diabetes And Chronic Kidney Disease—Australian facts: Risk factors. Cardiovascular, diabetes and chronic kidney disease series no. 4. Cat. no. CDK 4.* Canberra: AIHW.

16 K. N. Karmali, S. D. Persell, P. Perel, D. M. Lloyd-Jones, M. A. Berendsen & M. D. Huffman (2017). Risk scoring for the primary prevention of cardiovascular disease. *Cochrane Database of Systematic Reviews*, 3. doi:10.1002/14651858.CD006887.pub4

17 M. F. Piepoli, A. W. Hoes, S. Agewall, C. Albus, C. Brotons, A. L. Catapano, … W. M. M. Verschuren (2016). 2016 European Guidelines on cardiovascular disease prevention in clinical practice: the Sixth Joint Task Force of the European Society of Cardiology and Other Societies on Cardiovascular Disease Prevention in Clinical Practice (constituted by representatives of 10 societies and by invited experts). Developed with the special contribution of the European Association for Cardiovascular Prevention & Rehabilitation (EACPR). *Atherosclerosis*, 252(suppl. C), 207–74. doi:https://doi.org/10.1016/j.atherosclerosis.2016.05.037

18 F. M. Sacks, A. H. Lichtenstein, J. H. Y. Wu, L. J. Appel, M. A. Creager, P. M. Kris-Etherton, … L. V. Van Horn (2017). Dietary fats and cardiovascular disease: a presidential advisory from the American Heart Association. *Circulation*. doi:10.1161/cir.0000000000000510

19 F. M. Sacks, G. A. Bray, V. J. Carey, S. R. Smith, D. H. Ryan, S. D. Anton, … D. A. Williamson (2009). Comparison of weight-loss diets with different compositions of fat, protein, and carbohydrates. *New England Journal of Medicine*, 360(9), 859–73. doi:10.1056/NEJMoa0804748

20 Food and Nutrition Board of the Institute of Medicine National Academy of Sciences (n.d.). *Nutrient Recommendations: Dietary Reference Intakes (DRI)*. Retrieved from: https://ods.od.nih.gov/Health_Information/Dietary_Reference_Intakes.aspx.

21 British Nutrition Foundation (2016). *Nutrient Requirements*. British Nutrition Foundation. Retrieved from: www.nutrition.org.uk/attachments/article/261/Nutrition%20Requirements_Revised%20Oct%202016.pdf.

22 National Health and Medical Research Council (2011). *A Modelling System to Inform the Revision of the Australian Guide to Healthy Eating*. Canberra: NHMRC.

23 National Health and Medical Research Council (2013). *Australian Dietary Guidelines*. Canberra: NHMRC.

24 R. A. M. Dhonukshe-Rutten, J. Bouwman, K. A. Brown, A. E. J. M. Cavelaars, R. Collings, E. Grammatikaki, … P. V.T. Veer (2013). EURRECA—evidence-based methodology for deriving micronutrient recommendations. *Critical Reviews in Food Science and Nutrition*, 53(10), 999–1040. doi:10.1080/10408398.2012.749209

25 D. M. Bier & W. C. Willett (2016). Dietary Reference Intakes: resuscitate or let die? *American Journal of Clinical Nutrition*, 104(5), 1195–6. doi:10.3945/ajcn.116.144469

26 P. M. Brannon, C. M. Weaver, C. A. Anderson, S. M. Donovan, S. P. Murphy & A. L. Yaktine (2016). Scanning for new evidence to prioritize updates to the Dietary Reference Intakes: case studies for thiamin and phosphorus. *American Journal of Clinical Nutrition*, 104(5), 1366–77. doi:10.3945/ajcn.115.128256

27 J. D. Chambers, J. E. Anderson, M. N. Salem, S. G. Bügel, M. Fenech, J. B. Mason, … S. L. Booth (2017). The decline in vitamin research funding: a missed opportunity? *Current Developments in Nutrition*, 1(8). doi:10.3945/cdn.117.000430

28 Department of Health (2015–17). *Methodological Framework for the Review of Nutrient Reference Values*. Canberra: Department of Health. Retrieved from: www.nrv.gov.au/file/methodological-framework-pdf-705kb.

29 National Health and Medical Research Council (2017). *Resources—2017 Revisions of the Nutrient Reference Values*. Canberra: NHMRC. Retrieved from: www.nrv.gov.au/resources.

30 National Health and Medical Research Council (2017). *Introduction—What are Nutrient Reference Values?* Canberra: NHMRC. Retrieved from: www.nrv.gov.au/introduction.

31 Department of Health (2017). *Nutrient Reference Values for Australia and New Zealand. Revised Sodium Nutrient References Values*. Retrieved from: www.nrv.gov.au.

32 A. Drewnowski (2005). Concept of a nutritious food: toward a nutrient density score. *American Journal of Clinical Nutrition*, 82(4), 721–32.

33 N. Darmon, A. Briend & A. Drewnowski (2007). Energy-dense diets are associated with lower diet costs: a community study of French adults. *Public Health Nutrition*, 7(1), 21–7. doi:10.1079/PHN2003512

34 Australian Bureau of Statistics (2014). *Australian Health Survey: Nutrition First results—Foods and nutrients, 2011–12—Discretionary food*. Canberra: ABS.

35 A. Drewnowski & V. Fulgoni (2008). Nutrient profiling of foods: creating a nutrient-rich food index. *Nutrition Reviews*, 66(1), 23–39. doi:10.1111/j.1753-4887.2007.00003.x

36 A. Drewnowski (2009). Defining nutrient density: development and validation of the Nutrient Rich Foods Index. *Journal of the American College of Nutrition*, 28(4), 421S–426S. doi:10.1080/07315724.2009.10718106

37 J. Hess, G. Rao & J. Slavin (2017). The nutrient density of snacks: a comparison of nutrient profiles of popular snack foods using the Nutrient-Rich Foods Index. *Global Pediatric Health*, 4. doi:10.1177/2333794X17698525

38 Food Standards Australia New Zealand (2015). Nutrition information panels. Retrieved from: www.foodstandards.gov.au/consumer/labelling/panels/Pages/default.aspx.

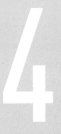

CHAPTER 4

CARBOHYDRATES AND PHYTOCHEMICALS: MAJOR COMPONENTS OF PLANT FOODS

LINDA TAPSELL

CHAPTER OBJECTIVES

This chapter will enable the reader to:

- describe the range of the chemical structures in carbohydrates, dietary fibres and phytonutrients
- outline the functions of carbohydrates, dietary fibres and phytochemicals in human health
- describe the food and beverage choices that would ensure a healthy intake of carbohydrate, dietary fibre and other plant-based nutrients.

KEY TERMS

Carbohydrate

Dietary fibre

Flavonoids

Sugars

KEY POINTS

- Carbohydrates are macronutrients in food providing the major source of fuel for the human body in the form of glucose.
- Carbohydrates are mainly delivered in plant foods, which also deliver fibre or indigestible carbohydrate. Plants also deliver phytochemicals such as flavonoids with significant anti-oxidant potential.
- In normal healthy individuals, carbohydrates are best sourced from wholegrain cereals, vegetables and fruits, legumes and, to some extent, milk and yoghurt.
- There is considerable scientific activity around the form and function of dietary carbohydrates that drives major areas of ongoing research in addressing clinical and public health issues as well as food innovation and product development.

INTRODUCTION

Carbohydrate is the major fuel source for humans. Different forms of carbohydrate are delivered by the diet and then broken down to glucose and other sugars that are delivered to cells for energy. As carbohydrates serve a fundamental component of metabolism, the rate at which carbohydrate-rich foods release sugar has been a major focus for studying the properties of these foods. This is particularly the case in the prevention and management of chronic lifestyle diseases such as diabetes mellitus. Recall that insulin, a hormone produced by the pancreas, plays a major role in controlling the release of glucose from the blood to the cells. High blood glucose levels result when this system is not functioning adequately, either through insulin resistance, which can occur with excess body fat or during pregnancy, or because of a lack of insulin, which is the case in type 1 diabetes. As high blood glucose can have damaging effects on various systems of the body, there is a need to manage glucose delivery.

With a better understanding of the processes of ageing and the development of chronic disease, other aspects of carbohydrate metabolism have been addressed in greater detail by scientific means. These include the influences of types of carbohydrate on appetite and the gut microbiome [1; 2]. In specialised clinical areas, carbohydrate metabolism is implicated in inborn errors of metabolism where certain enzymes for carbohydrate breakdown are missing [3], resulting in a form of carbohydrate intolerance.

Bearing in mind the interdependence between nutrients, foods and diets, the term 'carbohydrate' is often coined in debates on the relative value of foods and total diets, rather than the nutrient or chemical entity of carbohydrate alone. For example, bread may be referred to as a carbohydrate (or 'carb') when in fact it is a food also containing protein and fat, but it is a major source of carbohydrate in the diet. Other dietary items, such as sugar-sweetened beverages, have gained attention in public health circles as potential sources of excess energy, implicated in the problem of obesity. The issue of high carbohydrate diets is also debated in metabolic health circles [4; 5]. On the other hand, a vegetarian diet may well be a high-carbohydrate diet because of the choices of foods in the cuisine pattern (Figure 4.1).

Carbohydrates form the main component of most fully grown plant foods, such as vegetables, fruits and grains. (Note that plants grow from nuts and seeds so the relative amount of carbohydrate in these foods is different.) Plants are different from animals in many ways, so it would be expected that their chemical composition will also be distinctive. As with all living things, the chemical composition of plant foods reflects the essential biological processes that occur throughout the plant lifecycle [6; 7]. Thus, the carbohydrates in plants occur in the presence of other vitamins and minerals, reflecting the physiology of the plants and the soils in which they have grown. There are many different types of carbohydrate in plant foods, from sugars to largely indigestible forms generally referred to as fibre. In recent years, scientific interest has developed in other classes of compounds in plant foods, particularly those with a high antioxidant potential such as flavonoids [8]. These compounds have been collectively referred to as phytonutrients [9; 10]. In this chapter we describe the different types of dietary carbohydrate, examine their roles and functions, and discuss the significance of food and beverage sources when identifying the effects of carbohydrate on health.

STOP AND THINK

- How can understanding carbohydrate metabolism help you to manage your health?
- Which foods are best to consider first as overall nutritious foods, and then as major sources of carbohydrates?
- What is the difference between sugar and carbohydrate?

FIGURE 4.1   RELATIONSHIP BETWEEN NUTRIENTS, FOODS AND DIETS: THE CASE
FOR CARBOHYDRATE

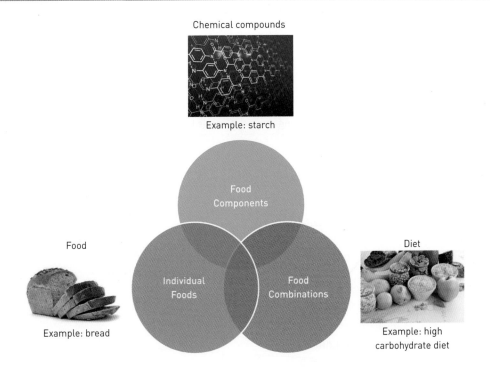

WHAT ARE THE DIFFERENT TYPES OF CARBOHYDRATE AND THEIR FUNCTIONS?

Different approaches to the classification of carbohydrate have evolved over time as the functions of carbohydrates in the body are studied (Table 4.1). Even though the body will store some carbohydrate in a number of forms and at various places, it is generally broken down to glucose for fuel. Glucose provides energy for muscle movement, and basic bodily function. Most importantly, it is an essential energy source for the brain. The human body will not function without glucose, but the basic nutrition principle of balance is important for delivering glucose through carbohydrate-rich foods.

A primary function of carbohydrates in the diet is to deliver glucose and other sugars to the cell, and early classifications focused on the structures of sugar. The term **sugar** has multiple meanings: in everyday language it is the white crystalline substance known as 'table sugar' (or in different forms as brown, raw, icing or castor sugar); in more scientific terms it refers to molecules containing saccharides—that is, specific chemical entities of a carbohydrate backbone with oxygen and hydrogen molecules attached (Figure 4.2). Glucose and fructose (the sugar in fruit) are monosaccharides, whereas sucrose (table sugar; glucose + fructose) and lactose (the sugar in milk; glucose + galactose) are disaccharides.

Glucose is a sugar with six carbon atoms. Glucose molecules exist predominantly in ring structures (Figure 4.2), forming (in the language of chemistry) α-D-glucose and β-D-glucose, which differ only

Sugars
sweet-tasting carbohydrates that dissolve in water and are chemically classified as monosaccharides and disaccharides. Sucrose is a disaccharide of a glucose molecule and a fructose molecule, which is commonly known as table sugar.

TABLE 4.1   CLASSIFICATION OF CARBOHYDRATES

Chemical term	Examples	General term	Location
Monosaccharides	Glucose Fructose	Simple Simple	Blood sugar Fruit sugar
Disaccharides	Sucrose Lactose	Simple Simple	'Table' sugar Milk sugar
Oligosaccharides	3–10 glucose chains	Complex	Food starch
Polysaccharides	>10 glucose chains	Complex	Food starch

FIGURE 4.2   THE STRUCTURE OF MONOSACCHARIDES AND DISACCHARIDES

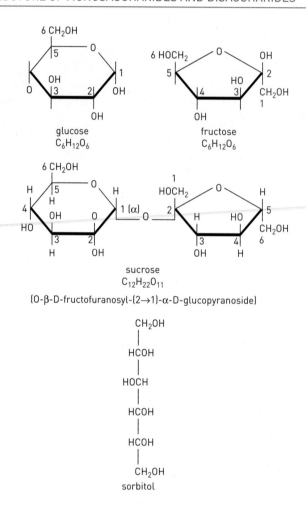

glucose
$C_6H_{12}O_6$

fructose
$C_6H_{12}O_6$

sucrose
$C_{12}H_{22}O_{11}$

(O-β-D-fructofuranosyl-(2→1)-α-D-glucopyranoside)

sorbitol

Source: J. Cummings & J. Mann (2012). Chapter 3: Carbohydrates. In J. Mann & S. Truswell (eds), *Essentials of Human Nutrition*, 4th edn. Oxford University Press, Incorporated

in the orientation of the hydroxyl group at carbon 1. In the α form, the hydroxyl group at carbon 1 is oriented in the same direction as the hydroxyl group at carbon 4. In the β form, the hydroxyl groups at carbon 1 and 4 are in opposite directions.

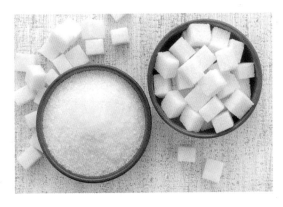

The most common monosaccharides are glucose, *fructose* and *galactose*, and these are the basic building blocks of commonly occurring carbohydrates in food, such as sugars in honey, fruit and some vegetables. Glucose syrups are often used as sweeteners in commercial foods and are commonly treated to cause partial isomerisation of the glucose to create high-fructose syrups. These syrups are at least as sweet as sucrose and are therefore used extensively in the food industry.

Sucrose and *lactose* are the most common disaccharides. Sucrose is found in many fruits but is also the common sweetener in the household pantry in the form of table sugar. Lactose is naturally occurring in milk and found in dairy products generally, although it is less commonly used as a commercial sweetener. Lactose intolerance occurs when there is a lack of the enzyme lactase, which hydrolyses the disaccharide into the monosaccharides glucose and galactose.

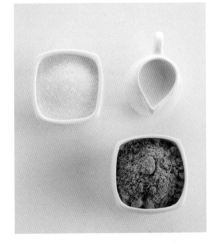

When sucrose is hydrolysed, glucose and fructose are produced and readily available for energy. Thus low-calorie alternatives to sucrose have been developed as food sweeteners. As an innovation, the emergence of this new category of food ingredient (or additive) generates debate. Food regulatory authorities, such as Food Standards Australia New Zealand (FSANZ) and the American Academy of Nutrition and Dietetics, have published positions in relation to the consumption of artificial sweeteners within a healthy diet [11–13].

Fructose was identified as an alternative to sugar more than a hundred years ago, based on the understanding that it was handled differently from a metabolic perspective. Since that time, the scientific path for arguing the risks and benefits of fructose consumption has swung around in opposite directions [14], and persists today. One perspective on the relationship between fructose-containing sugars (sucrose and high-fructose corn syrup) and obesity and diabetes argued that fructose can affect their development by influencing a 'fat switch' [15]. In addition, an analysis of National Health and Nutrition Examination Survey (NHANES) 2003–06 data showed that combinations of beverages with high excess free fructose was significantly associated with coronary heart disease in adults (45–59 years) [16]. However, two more systematic reviews and meta-analyses [17; 18] have indicated detrimental effects were not demonstrated in human studies. Aside from research design problems, such as accurately estimating fructose intake, and the need for longer-term studies, attention might be better placed on consumption patterns of foods and beverages with a high overall sugar content, particularly in at-risk groups [14]. These issues are discussed in the next section of this chapter.

Sorbitol is a naturally occurring sugar (or polyhydric) alcohol that can also be made synthetically from glucose, with 60% sweetening activity of sugar (sucrose) and about a third of the calories (see https://pubchem.ncbi.nlm.nih.gov/compound/D-Sorbitol). It has been used as a sugar substitute, but reduced absorption in the gut produces gastrointestinal symptoms such as bloating and diarrhoea, an intolerance that has been known for some time [19].

Visit Oxford Ascend for more on sugar.

TABLE 4.2   SWEETNESS SCALE FOR SUGARS AND ALTERNATIVES

Compound	Sweetness ranking
Monosaccharides[1]	
Glucose	70–80
Fructose	140
Galactose	35
Disaccharides[1]	
Sucrose	100
Lactose	20
Maltose	30–50
High fructose corn syrup	120–160
Low-calorie sweeteners[2]	
Saccharin	300X
Cyclamate	30X
Aspartame	180X
Acesulfame	200X
Sucralose	600X

[1]Sucrose = 100
[2]Sucrose = 1

Adapted from C. E. Ophardt (2003). *Elmhurst College's Virtual ChemBook*. Available at: http://chemistry.elmhurst.edu/vchembook/549sweet.html

Low-calorie sweeteners (LCNs) have been developed in response to concerns about the energy value of foods containing substantial amounts of added sugar (sucrose or fructose). LCNs can have a variety of chemical forms and sources, but their energy value is less than that of sucrose and are recognised as artificial sweeteners, non-nutritive sweeteners or high-intensity sweeteners. While individual studies provide evidence for effects and the safety on food components, strategic directions for studying LCNs are warranted given their relative novelty and, therefore, concerns for safe use. Despite many LCNs being generally recognised as safe (GRAS) in the United States under the Food and Drug Administration (FDA) food additive provisions, they do not have a history of common usage as table sugars and this may cause concern among consumers.

≫ RESEARCH AT WORK

ALTERNATIVES TO SUGAR AS A SOURCE OF SWEETNESS IN FOODS

A future research needs (FRN) process developed by the US Government's Agency for Healthcare Research and Quality was conducted to identify and prioritise future research needs on low-calorie sweeteners and health outcomes (Figure 4.3). Five outcome areas were included: brain energy sensing, gut hormones that influence energy homeostasis, taste preference and satiety, eating behaviour, and body weight and body composition. A stakeholder panel identified 18 research questions that related to five broad research areas, with the main concerns relating to body weight, appetite and dietary intake [20]. The review enabled discussions on the current state of research and the potential for public health impact. It also raised issues around how the evidence base for public health nutrition policy is developed and the challenges of knowledge translation from scientific research to policy and practice, including the significance of communicating science to the general public.

FIGURE 4.3   AREAS OF FUTURE RESEARCH ON SUGAR ALTERNATIVES

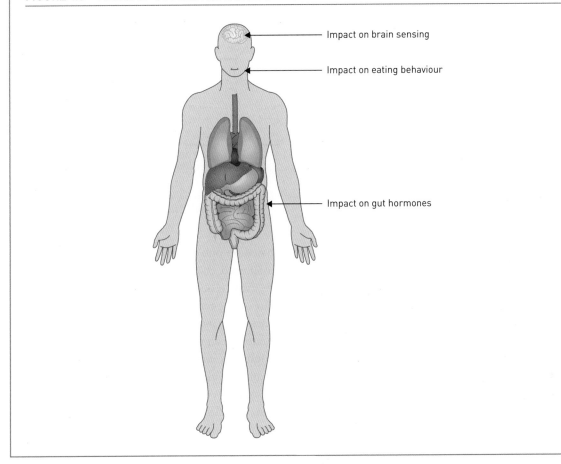

TRY IT YOURSELF

Examine the labels on food products and beverages you have recently purchased. What are the names given to the carbohydrate ingredients in these products? How many different forms of carbohydrate are present?

Carbohydrates commonly referred to as starches have multiple α-D-glucose structures. These units form the two main sub-units of which starch is comprised: amylose (linear combination of hundreds to thousands of glucose units) and amylopectin (branched combination of up to two million glucose units) (Figure 4.4).

FIGURE 4.4   STRUCTURE OF AMYLOSE AND AMYLOPECTIN

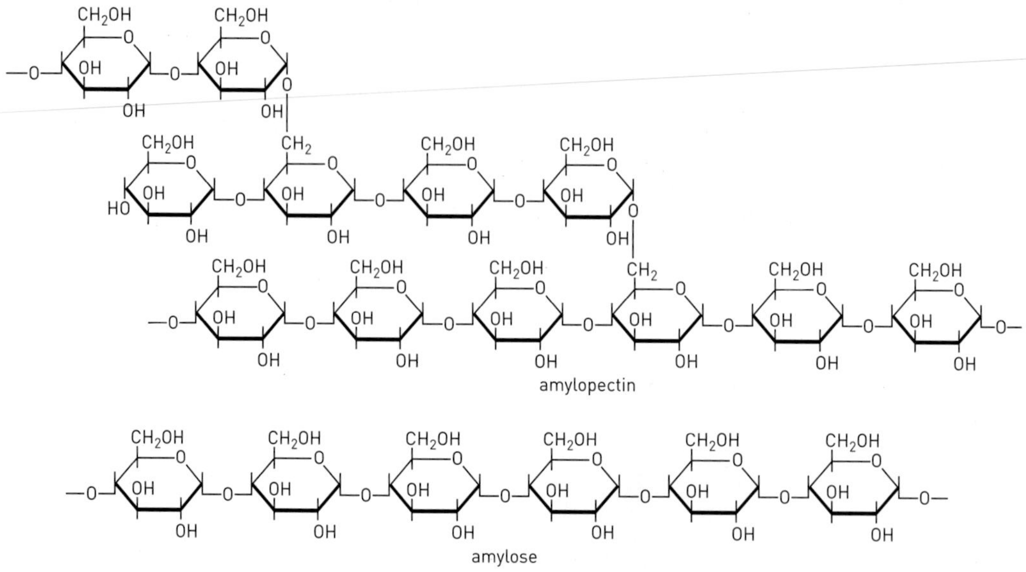

Source: J. Cummings & J. Mann (2012). Chapter 3: Carbohydrates. In J. Mann & S. Truswell (eds), *Essentials of Human Nutrition*, 4th edn. Oxford University Press, Incorporated

In the past, carbohydrates were classified as 'simple', based on one or two units of a sugar molecule (such as glucose or sucrose), or 'complex', based on a branched chain structure of sugar molecules, such as in 'starch' (Table 4.1). Today, a range of terms are used to describe dietary carbohydrates. For example, by focusing on the saccharide moiety, carbohydrate can be referred to as sugars (or saccharides), oligosaccharides (short chain combinations) or polysaccharides (many sugars) [21]. With the exception of table sugar, which could be called a food, carbohydrate is naturally delivered in more complex foods such as vegetables and bread, where other macronutrients are also present. Thus, attributes of carbohydrate-rich foods other than the simple delivery of glucose are of research interest, and the study of carbohydrate as a nutrient becomes more complex. For example, one of the most exciting new areas is the study of milk oligosaccharides in immune function, specifically in relation to its potential for reduced infectivity from human rotavirus [22].

Visit Oxford Ascend for more on carbohydrates.

Glycaemic index (GI)
a standardised measure of the glucose response to a carbohydrate load.

A more recent conceptual development has been that of the **glycaemic index (GI)** (Figure 4.5). The GI is a systematic and physiologically based measure of the effect of carbohydrate-containing foods on post-meal blood glucose levels (BGLs). Foods with minimal or no carbohydrate do not have a GI value, nor would they significantly affect post-meal BGLs. The GI is defined methodologically as the ratio of the incremental area under the curve in response to the test food versus that of the reference food, usually pure glucose or white bread, in 10 or more individuals; although the current international consensus is to report GI values on the glucose scale [23]. To convert GI values obtained on the white bread scale (GIwb) into values on the glucose scale (GIglu), a conversion factor of 0.71 is used. For example, a food with GIwb of 100 would have a GIglu of 71 when tested using glucose as the reference food, and should be reported as such. Foods with easily digested and absorbed carbohydrates, such as those with a high amylopectin (a highly branched starch molecule) and/or glucose content, would be expected to have a higher GI. Other food

FIGURE 4.5   REPRESENTATION OF THE GLYCAEMIC INDEX

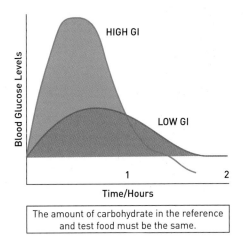

Source: Glycemic Index Foundation (2017). What is GI? Available from: www.gisymbol.com/about-glycemic-index

components such as fat and protein, as well as the acidity of the food, have been shown to affect the GI. Based on evidence from epidemiological studies, researchers have classified foods as low (GI <= 55), medium (GI between 56 and 69) and high (GI >=70) GI [24].

» CASE 4.1

CLASSIFYING CARBOHYDRATE-RICH FOODS BY FORM OR FUNCTION

From a chemical perspective, carbohydrates are now most commonly classified as oligosaccharides and polysaccharides, although in the non-scientific literature the terms 'complex carbohydrate' or 'starches' can still be found. In these cases, simple carbohydrates or sugars were assumed to be rapidly absorbed and requiring little digestion. The terms complex carbohydrates and starchy foods were sometimes used interchangeably. A slower digestion and absorption was assumed from consumption of these foods based on the length and branching of the chains of basic sugar units in the carbohydrate-rich foods.

In time, research that tested the actual properties of these foods challenged those assumptions, broadening the ways in which carbohydrate-rich foods were classified (Table 4.3). Concepts such as the GI of foods and the identification of novel fibres in foods changed these positions considerably. Today, there is wide recognition that the digestion and absorption of carbohydrate in different foods can vary considerably. The food matrix plays a large part in how sugars are released, as does the composition of the total diet. The genetic profile of individuals and the composition of the microbiome add further complexity.

- Why is it necessary to distinguish between 'carbohydrate as a nutrient' and 'carbohydrate-rich foods' in research?
- How has the concept of the GI helped to classify carbohydrate-rich foods?
- Why would the fibre content be included in classification systems for carbohydrate-rich foods?

TABLE 4.3   CARBOHYDRATE FORM, FUNCTION, FOOD AND DIETS

CHO descriptor	Characteristic
Form (nutrient)	Sugars, starches, fibres
Function (food)	Glycaemic response Digestibility
CHO-rich foods	Plant based (grain/cereal foods, vegetables, legumes, fruits)
High CHO diet	Mostly plant-based foods

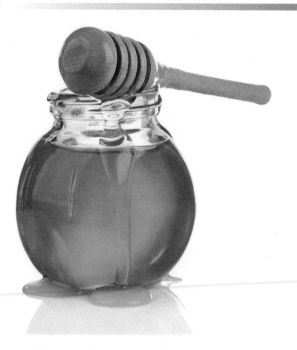

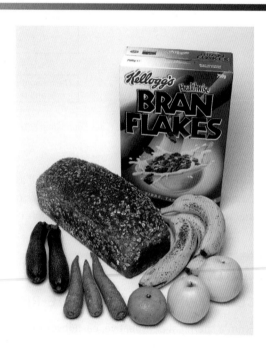

STOP AND THINK

- How does using 'simple' and 'complex' to describe carbohydrates help (or hinder) nutrition messages?
- What other effects do carbohydrate-rich foods have besides raising blood glucose?
- What does 'quitting sugar' mean in practical terms?

WHAT IS DIETARY FIBRE AND WHAT FUNCTION DOES IT SERVE?

Dietary fibre

the component of plant foods that escapes digestion and absorption in the small intestine.

Dietary fibre is the component of foods that is not digested and absorbed in the small intestine. Fibre is recognised as beneficial to health, with links to improved laxation, as well as glucose- and lipid-lowering effects in humans. Theoretically, some definitions of fibre will include a range of components of food, but it usually refers to carbohydrates from the plant cell wall such as cellulose, hemicelluloses, pectin and lignin, gums, mucilages, oligosaccharides and associated substances such as waxes.

As with carbohydrate categorisation generally, the definition and classification of dietary fibre has evolved with advances in analytical methods and other forms of research on nutrients and health. Fibre was traditionally defined according to the analytical methods that were used to measure it. To see what could be measured, scientists needed to develop a rigorous method of mimicking digestion of foods, and the process needed to be able to be repeated in multiple laboratories. In time, definitions also reflected the physiological effects of fibre (Table 4.4). The original hypotheses linking fibre intake and disease prevention have been well described [25–28], but scientists have found it much more difficult to define the precise effects of individual fibres.

Visit Oxford Ascend for more on fibre.

TABLE 4.4   DIETARY FIBRE FORM AND FUNCTION

Form	Function
Carbon chain structure	Degree of digestibility
Molecular weight	Microbial utilisation

>> CASE 4.2

MEASUREMENTS AND DEFINITIONS OF DIETARY FIBRE

Many tables of food composition describe fibre levels that are determined by the 'Prosky' method, recognised by the Association of Official Analytical Chemists (AOAC) as method 985.29 [29]. However, further research has identified that this method did not measure resistant starch or non-digestible oligosaccharides such as galacto oligosaccharides (GOS) and fructo oligosaccharides (FOS). A new method was validated (AOAC 2009.01) that includes all compounds recognised as dietary fibre, including the resistant starch, non-digestible oligosaccharides and available carbohydrates [30]. Interestingly, because the defined health benefits of fibre are based on the measures obtained with the old method, it may be that thresholds that provide physiological effects are actually higher than originally anticipated. This would be most likely in foods where there are predominantly short chain units of fibre as these are the fibres that were previously not measured. The total fibre of many common foods may not be affected by this improved method.

Definitions of dietary fibre, however, are not limited to the actual measurement of their presence in food, although the degree of polymerisation of the molecules is part of the debate. Other differences in the definitions include references to physiological effects and the allowable sources of fibre (whether naturally occurring or added).

A number of definitions of dietary fibre have emerged from various sources over time (Table 4.5). There is no universally accepted definition beyond a recognition that they are a group of carbohydrate polymers, oligomers and lignin that are not digested in the small intestine, making their way to the large intestine where they can be partially or completely fermented by gut bacteria [31]. Debate remains on the significance of degree of polymerisation, particularly those with a degree of polymerisation of 3–9. The impact of food processing is implicated in debate on whether only intrinsic fibre should be recognised rather than extrinsic (added to a food); and the breadth of recognised physiological effects beyond laxation, and effects on blood glucose and cholesterol levels [31].

- Why might fibre added in manufacturing be excluded in a definition of fibre in a food?
- If natural or added fibres had the same effects, should their different origins still be declared?
- Why would physiological effects need to be included in a definition of fibre?
- How is scientific investigation helping to clarify the definition of dietary fibre?

LINDA TAPSELL

Definitions of fibre have also differentiated between soluble and insoluble fibres. Insoluble fibre is not soluble in water, but absorbs water through the colon and therefore aids defecation. Insoluble fibre is most commonly found in wholegrain foods, wheat bran, nuts and seeds, and skins from fruits and vegetables. Soluble fibre is soluble in water and fermented in the colon. Soluble fibre is most commonly found in oats, rye, barley, fruits, vegetables, psyllium and legumes. These definitions are not rigorous, as the amount of solubility of a fibre will depend on the pH of the extraction and, therefore, the amount measured is significantly altered by food-processing techniques. Still, the general association of insoluble and soluble fibre with well-known health effects is a useful characterisation in understanding the types of benefits that are associated with fibre intake from different sources. In applying these definitions, it is important to remember that people eat whole foods, not just ingredients or nutrients, and the type of food may affect the functionality of food components such as fibre.

Resistant starch does not really fit as a soluble or insoluble fibre and was not actually measured by some of the early measurement techniques of fibre researchers. Resistant starch is, as suggested by its name, resistant to digestion in the small intestine but ferments in the large intestine. Production of end products of bacteria, such as butyrate, have been linked with positive gut health [36]. The promotion of large numbers of bacteria in the bowel, particularly through ingestion of soluble fibres and resistant starch, is an area of great interest for researchers who link the levels of microbiota with improved immune function and general gastrointestinal health. Resistant starch is found in commercial products with added fibre such as those containing Hi-maize®, some fruits, particularly unripened bananas, and pasta that is only just cooked. Cooking and cooling affects the levels of resistant starch in a food.

TABLE 4.5   DEFINITIONS OF DIETARY FIBRE

Agency	Definition
American Association of Cereal Chemists (AACC) 2001 [32], p. 112	'Dietary fibre is the edible parts of plants or analogous carbohydrates resistant to digestion and absorption in the human small intestine with complete or partial fermentation in the large intestine. Dietary fibre includes polysaccharides, oligosaccharides, lignin, and associated plants substances. Dietary fibres promote beneficial physiological effects including laxation, and/or blood cholesterol attenuation, and/or blood glucose attenuation.'
Codex Alimentarius Commission (2010) [33]	Dietary fibre means carbohydrate not hydrolysed by the endogenous enzymes in the human small intestine including: • edible carbohydrate polymers naturally occurring in food as consumed • carbohydrate polymers which have been obtained from raw materials by physical enzymatic or chemical means • synthetic carbohydrate polymers. The latter two must have been shown to have physiological effects of benefit to health. Dietary fibre will include fractions of lignin and other compounds associated with plant polysaccharides. The decision on whether to include carbohydrates from 3–9 monomeric units should be left to national authorities.
Institute of Medicine 2001 [34]	Dietary fibre consists of non-digestible carbohydrates and lignin intrinsic and intact in plants. Functional fibre consists of isolated, non-digestible carbohydrates which have beneficial physiological effects in humans. Total fibre is the sum of dietary and functional fibre.
CODEX Alimentarius Commission 2006 [35]	Dietary fibre consists of intrinsic plant cell wall polysaccharides.

TABLE 4.6   TYPES OF DIETARY FIBRE

Name	Source	Structure/function
Cellulose	Plant tissue Wheat bran	High molecular weight; large unbranched glucose units; insoluble in water but can swell
Hemicellulose (non-starch polysaccharides)	Plant tissue cereals	High molecular weight; polymers of at least three carbohydrate units; minimal solubility in water
Lignin	Woody components of cereals, some vegetables	High molecular weight; polymer of phenylpropane units, highly insoluble fibre
Pectins	Fruits mainly, vegetables, legumes	High molecular weight; water-soluble polysaccharide; forms gels at low concentration
β glucans	Cereals, mainly barley and oats	High molecular weight; generally soluble non-starch polysaccharides
Gums and mucilages	Plant, seed, seaweed exudates	High molecular weight; hydrocolloids, water-soluble fibre; form viscous solutions at low concentration
Oligosaccharides (Fructans: inulin & fructo oligosaccharides (FOS) or galacto oligosaccharides (GOS))	Fruits, vegetables Legumes, seeds Wheat (inulin)	Low molecular weight (mostly); polymers with typically 3-10 saccharide units; water soluble. FOS (inulin and oligofructose) contain short chains of fructose molecules; GOS (raffinose, stachyose, verbascose) contain short chains of galactose molecules
Synthetic analogues	Synthetic compounds	Carbohydrate compounds with properties of intrinsic dietary fibres
Resistant starch	Wholegrains, legumes, unripe bananas, pasta	Broad and diverse starches categorised from RS1-RS5

Source: Adapted from S. Fuller, E. Beck, H. Salman & L. Tapsell (2016). New horizons for the study of dietary fiber and health: a review. *Plant Foods for Human Nutrition*, 71(1), 1–12

The energy content of fibre is often not accounted for as it has been considered 'non-digestible', but in reality a reasonable percentage of fibre is fermentable and therefore contributes energy to the diet [37]. A contribution of around 50–70% of the energy from 1 g of carbohydrate (50–70% fermentation) is considered a reasonable estimation—that is, 9–11 kJ/g of fibre.

TRY IT YOURSELF

Write down everything you consumed in the past 24 hours. How many forms of dietary fibre did you likely consume?

Epidemiological research has shown that diets high in fibre can protect against obesity [38], cardiovascular disease [39; 40], diabetes [41] and all-cause mortality [42]. Specific fibres may have specific effects, but the

TABLE 4.7   POTENTIAL HEALTH EFFECTS OF DIETARY FIBRE

Potential health effects	Possible mechanisms
Laxation	Adds bulk to the stool and decreases intestinal transit time
Weight regulation and satiety	Increases food bulk with minimal increase in energy intake Soluble fibre (β glucan) has a viscous nature and may prolong cholecystokinin (CCK) release influencing appetite
Cholesterol-lowering (total and LDL)	Soluble fibre forms a viscous bolus in the gut, decreasing contact with the luminal service and increasing excretion of bile salts
Attenuation of blood glucose response	Soluble fibre forms a viscous bolus, decreasing exposure to digestive enzymes and delaying absorption of carbohydrate
Increases short chain fatty acids in colon that may be associated with decreased risk of colonic cancers	Decreased digestion allows fermentable products to enter large bowel
Alteration to gut microbiota	Shifts composition towards relative increase in desirable microflora

Source: Adapted from S. Fuller, E. Beck, H. Salman & L. Tapsell (2016). New horizons for the study of dietary fiber and health: a review. *Plant Foods for Human Nutrition*, 71(1), 1–12

generally accepted positive effects of fibre are quite broad (Table 4.7). Generally speaking, high-fibre foods are ingested more slowly due to a greater need for chewing (mastication). The higher fibre tends to mean the foods are bulkier, distending the stomach and increasing physical signals of fullness. There is slowed gastric emptying [38; 41] and decreased contact of the food with digestive enzymes. Nutrients are therefore able to reach further into the gastrointestinal tract and this tends to inhibit the hunger hormone ghrelin, while increasing release of cholecystokinin (CCK), which is a satiety hormone [43]. The nutrients are not absorbed in the further reaches of the small intestine and in the colon and so further stimulate satiety hormones such as glucagon-like-peptide-1 (GLP-1) and peptide-YY3-36 (PYY3-36).

It is this action of fibre that supports the epidemiological evidence that fibre protects against overweight and obesity [38]. An example is seen when African nations with fibre intakes of up to 80 g/day are compared with the United States, with four times the rate of overweight and obesity but only an average of 15 g/day of fibre. In the 10-year CARDIA (Coronary Artery Risk Development in Young Adults) study, researchers found that over 10 years, an individual with greater intake of dietary fibre is likely to weigh less and be leaner, and have less risk of lifestyle diseases such as heart disease, stroke and diabetes [44; 45]. There are also other positive associations of increased fibre intake, including a decreased risk of colorectal cancers [46; 47]. Considering all the evidence, there is little doubt that increasing dietary fibre intake is associated with positive health outcomes. Research in all the areas of potential benefit adds to the evidence base supporting communications on dietary fibre. For example, in two separate meta-analyses, a dose of 3 g/day of the soluble fibre $(1{\rightarrow}3)(1{\rightarrow}4)$-β-D-glucan (β-glucan) from oats and barley was been shown to significantly lower low-density lipoprotein (LDL) cholesterol, particularly if subjects had elevated cholesterol [48; 49]. Reflecting research like this, a health claim was approved in the United States: that 'a diet high in soluble fiber from whole oats (barley, oat bran, oatmeal and oat flour) and low in saturated fat and cholesterol may reduce the risk of heart disease' [50].

Evaluating the evidence base for the effects of dietary fibre is fraught due to the changes to fibre characterisation. In a recent systematic review, researchers examined the influence of fibre characteristics on appetite-related outcomes in healthy individuals [1]. Much of the literature needed to be excluded because of inadequate characterisation of the dietary fibre in the studies. Inconsistent relationships with appetite-related outcomes and dietary fibre characteristics (viscosity, fermentability, molecular weight, gel-forming capacity) were found but this reflected study designs, including elements relating to the methods of characterising the fibre, and the nature and preparation of the dietary fibre matrix. Future research is required to address these limitations in research designs to better answer the questions needed for the evidence base of dietary fibre effects.

STOP AND THINK

- What are the challenges in defining dietary fibre so that (a) research is consistent, and (b) consumers will understand a message about dietary fibre?
- What is the value in manufactured fibre that can be added to foods?
- What are the relative benefits of dietary fibre for people living in an obesogenic environment versus a food insecure environment?

WHAT ARE PHYTONUTRIENTS AND WHAT ARE THEIR FUNCTIONS?

In addition to historically recognised nutrients, an increasing number of chemical compounds have been isolated in plant foods. These phytochemical compounds can be described as secondary plant metabolites and are distinguished from the primary components (carbohydrate and fibre, protein and fat) and from micronutrients (vitamins and minerals). These **phytonutrient** compounds reflect the relationship between plants and their environment (Figure 4.6), providing defensive mechanisms, promoting growth and appearance, and their role in human health is being increasingly exposed [51; 52].

Phytonutrients
(or phytochemicals) compounds found in plants with biological activity and not otherwise classified as vitamins or minerals; include flavonoids, phytosterols and phenolic acids.

See Chapter 9 on fat soluble vitamins.

A number of main categories of phytochemicals have been reported in the literature [53], with a great deal known about phenolic acids, flavonoids, in particular carotenoids, and phytosterols. Carotenoids, for example, contain precursors of vitamin A in the form of carotene, and these compounds have been part of nutrition knowledge for some time. More recently, known compounds of this class, such as lutein and lycopene, have been the subject of exciting new developments in nutrition, particularly as they link the maintenance of functions such as eyesight to studies of food consumption patterns. The physiological effects of phytochemicals are highly varied.

As with the discovery of vitamins and minerals, the isolation of phytochemicals has come about through advances in chemistry and the associated scientific techniques utilised in this discipline. The exercise is also associated with categorisation of chemical compounds based on their structure and function (Table 4.8). For example, flavonoids include a double bond between carbon positions 2 and 3, a carboxyl group in carbon position 3, a carbonyl group in carbon position 4 and polyhydroxylation of the A and B aromatic rings. This structural feature is thought to explain the antioxidant and free-radical-scavenging functions of this class of compounds [54].

The absorption of phytochemicals following the digestion of food and their subsequent bioavailability and action varies across chemical species. Flavonoids, for example, are absorbed from the gut and then

FIGURE 4.6   PHYTOCHEMICALS

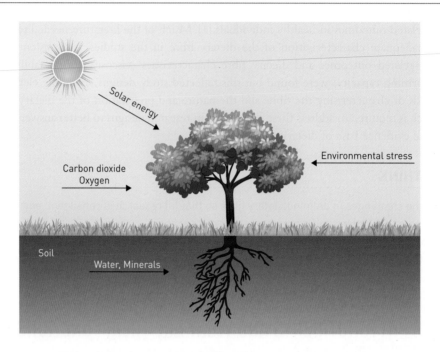

TABLE 4.8   CLASSIFICATION OF FLAVONOIDS AND FOOD SOURCES

Category	Food sources
Anthocyanins	Berries, grapes, cherries
Flavones	Herbs, leafy vegetables
Flavanols[1]	Green tea, grapes, cocoa
Flavanols[2]	Apples, onions, broccoli
Isoflavones	Soy beans
Flavanones	Citrus fruits, tomatoes

[1]Includes catechins
[2]Includes quercetin

Source: Adapted from K. R. Gildawie, R. L. Galli, B. Shukitt-Hale & A. N. Carey (2018). Protective effects of foods containing flavonoids on age-related cognitive decline. *Current Nutrition Reports*, 7(2), 39–48. doi:10.1007/s13668-018-0227-0

excreted in either the urine or faeces, either unchanged or as metabolites following modification within the body [54]. Their availability is also affected by whether or not the food is cooked. Moving from an understanding of the antioxidant activity of a class of compounds and providing a causal, mechanistic explanation for disease risk reduction, however, is a difficult task. Only limited evidence linking consumption of polyphenol-rich products with biomarkers of oxidative damage has been found, bearing in mind that extensive metabolism follows ingestion of these compounds and only low circulating levels are found in blood [55]. Thus, while understanding the chemical composition of foods is useful, it is likely that the effects we see are due to the whole diet rather than single chemical compounds within foods [56]. The path back to food, however, is made possible through the multidisciplinary nature of nutrition research and practice.

Once identified, new components of foods can be assessed and the data added to food composition tables. Once this data is available it is possible to assess the intakes of these compounds in the population, and then to associate intakes with disease risk. Additions of flavonoid values to food composition tables in the United States enabled a study comparing the flavonoid intakes of a large population sample of adults with risk of type 2 diabetes. The analysis of food frequency questionnaire data on women in the Nurses' Health Study (1984–2008; 1991–2007) and the Health Professional Follow-up Study (1986–2006) found that a higher consumption of anthocyanins and of fruit rich in anthocyanins was associated with a lower risk of developing type 2 diabetes. The study also found that no associations existed for intakes of total flavonoids and subclasses other than anthocyanins [57]. This human observational study followed mechanistic research on flavonoids, from early work on free radical scavenging to the modulation of nitrous oxide metabolism that is implicated in damage to blood vessels. The researchers noted specifically that animal model studies had shown that anthocyanin subclasses improved glucose metabolism through a particular regulatory pathway. Thus their findings were plausible from a mechanistic perspective, but the authors also noted that the fruits that delivered these anthocyanins (e.g. blueberries, apples, pears) may also contain other components that may be beneficial in preventing type 2 diabetes. Clinical trials would be required to provide more direct evidence of effects.

In another study, researchers used data from the Nurse Health Study (1995–2001) to examine the relationships between intakes of blueberries and strawberries in those aged 70 and over [58]. They assessed diet using a food frequency questionnaire and assessed cognition using six cognitive tests twice at two-year intervals. They found higher intake of flavonoids, notably from berries, to be associated with a lower rate of cognitive decline in the study sample. Noting the limitations of an observational study, the authors referred to research showing that berry-derived anthocyanidines can cross the blood–brain barrier to the hippocampus, which is associated with learning and memory. They were also able to describe various signalling pathways that may be implicated in the functionality of cognition. Thus, the research was plausible, but again clinical trials would provide more direct evidence of the potential benefits.

>> RESEARCH AT WORK

FOOD CONTAINING FLAVONOIDS AND AGE-RELATED COGNITIVE DECLINE

Two recent reviews have added to the growing knowledge that consuming foods containing flavonoids has the potential to have a positive impact on age-related cognitive decline (Figure 4.7) [59; 60]. Most of the work has been done in animal model studies underpinning the need for human clinical trials. The mechanisms are thought to be associated with a reduction in neuro-inflammation, reduced oxidative stress and improvements in neuroplasticity. The effects may occur at the level of brain regions responsible for memory where there are interactions between cellular and molecular architecture. There may be interactions with gut microbiota and interference with the accumulation of pathological proteins associated with Alzheimer's disease. Research on foods to date has focused on blueberries, grapes, citrus fruits and green tea.

As the collective science contributions for the study of phytonutrients increase, the applications for evidence-based nutrition practice grow. For example, based on research on flavanols derived from the cocoa bean, the European Food Safety Authority published a scientific substantiation on a claim stating that 'cocoa flavanols help maintain endothelium-dependent vasodilation, which contributes to normal

FIGURE 4.7   CAN PHYTOCHEMICALS REDUCE COGNITIVE DECLINE?

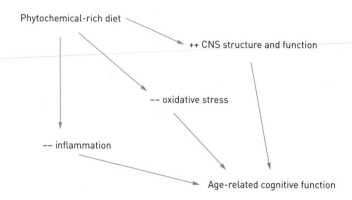

blood flow' [61]. The claim relates to 200 mg of cocoa flavanols daily which can be provided by 2.5 g of high-flavanol cocoa powder or 10 g of dark (high-flavanol) chocolate in a balanced diet. On the other hand, fruits and vegetables are major sources of phytonutrients, and this may help to explain why this food category emerges so consistently as part of dietary guidance for health. The link between the two can be seen in a study of the dietary patterns of adults in the United States, where the intakes of carotenoids and flavonoids was highest in those people who consumed levels of vegetable and fruit intake aligned with dietary guidelines [62]. Interestingly, tomatoes, carrots, oranges, orange juice and strawberries, spinach and onions accounted for most of the intakes. As is the case with food sources of vitamins, this reflected a high concentration of specific phytonutrients in some foods (e.g. carotene in carrots), but possibly also a lack of variety in fruit and vegetable consumption.

STOP AND THINK

- How does scientific research build on knowledge of carbohydrates, fibre and other plant components and their functions in the human body?
- How could food processing have an effect on the nutritional value of plant-based foods?
- Why is it useful to study the intrinsic chemical composition of plant-based foods?

WHAT ARE THE BEST FOODS AND BEVERAGE CHOICES TO ENSURE HEALTHY INTAKES OF CARBOHYDRATE, DIETARY FIBRE AND OTHER PLANT-BASED NUTRIENTS?

Plant-based foods (bread and cereals, fruit and vegetables) are the primary carbohydrate-rich food groups in the Australian diet. Although carbohydrates can be classified by various means, it is often the total carbohydrate content that is considered when grouping foods as sources of carbohydrate.

Foods containing sugars and starches

Some of the carbohydrate in plant foods is in the form of sugars. Sugars form part of the composition of fruit (fructose is the name of the sugar in fruit [63]), some vegetables (e.g. melibiose in legumes [64]) and dairy foods (lactose is the name of the sugar in milk; lactose is a disaccharide combination of glucose and galactose). It is important to note that these foods have additional important nutritional attributes, such as providing vitamin C, calcium or protein. On the other hand, food commonly referred to as sugar (including table sugar and the main ingredients in confectionery) mainly contain carbohydrate without additional significant nutrients. Thus, fruit and confectionery would not fall into the same food category even though they both contain sugars.

>> CASE 4.3

SUGAR CONSUMPTION AND PUBLIC HEALTH

With obesity a major public health problem, high-energy foods and beverages that deliver little concurrent nutritional value are of interest to public health campaigns. The challenge lies in focusing on identifiable strategies that may help reduce excess energy intake. At the same time, it is difficult to single out one food or nutrient, such as sugar, in this process [65].

While epidemiological studies enable the relationships between dietary intakes and disease risk to be exposed, methods for accurately assessing dietary intakes are crucial within that research. Apart from table sugar *per se*, sugars are contained in foods in many forms, both intrinsic and extrinsic (i.e. added). Intrinsic sugars can occur in high nutritional value foods, such as fruits and milk, which form part of dietary guidance, whereas extrinsic sugars can be oversupplied and occur in foods and beverages of little nutritional value. Research that establishes a systematic methodology for estimating added sugar content [66] is helpful in building standardised research on added sugars. For example, in an analysis of nutrient dilution in the diet of Australian children and adolescents, it was shown that intakes of added sugars gave a better indication of diet quality than assessing intakes of total sugars [67].

Sugar-sweetened beverages (SSBs) are one of the foods of interest in the added sugar debate. The previous day of reporting in the Australian Health Survey 2010–11 indicated that 39% males and 29% females consumed SSBs, which in turn contributed significantly to sugar in the Australian diet [68]. A sugar tax has been suggested in Australia [69–71]. In Mexico, the implementation of a sugar tax in January 2014 resulted in a 6.3% reduction in observed purchases that year compared with expectation s in 2008–12, mostly in lower-income urban areas and in households with children [72].

Working with added sugar in foods is more complex. In a cross-sectional analysis of the US-based National Health and Nutrition Examination Survey (NHANES) 2009–10, ultra-processed foods (UPFs) were found to contribute 57.9% of energy intake and 89.7% of energy intake from added sugars. In the highest quintile of UPF consumption, 82.1% of participants exceeded the recommended limit of 10% energy from added sugars [73]. The UPFs were identified through a food classification system that addressed the purpose and extent of industrial food processing, known as NOVA [74], but for a number of reasons, caution has been expressed in the use of this categorisation process as an alternative to linking nutrient intakes and associated foods to chronic disease outcomes [75].

Finally, food processing is a part of the modern food environment, and food technology can make a significant contribution to reducing available sugar in the food supply. For example, research on consumer sensory and hedonic perceptions of taste and texture was able to show how increasing both the vanilla and starch content of milk-based desserts helped to overcome the loss of acceptable features when the sugar content was reduced [76]. Reducing the fat content of foods can also reduce acceptability, but adding more sugar may undo any intended benefit for energy reduction and nutritional quality. Using the

US Department of Agriculture (USDA) nutrient database, a systematic analysis of data on food products for which low-fat alternatives were developed (low-calorie, light, low-fat) or non-fat versions, found the sugar content was significantly higher than the regular versions of those products [77].

- What are the benefits and challenges of focusing on dietary sugar in addressing the problems of obesity and diabetes in the community?
- How can further research on sugar intakes better inform public health strategies?
- What are some of the problems that may emerge when food categorisation systems are applied universally across the globe?

Foods also containing fibre

Apart from sugar content, carbohydrate-rich foods can be further categorised according to levels of soluble and insoluble fibre [63; 78]. Recall that dietary fibre is found in food of plant origin, namely grains, fruits and vegetables. Soluble fibre, which attracts water, forming a gelatinous mass during digestion and in turn slowing the rate at which the food is digested, is commonly found in legumes, nuts and seeds, some fruit such as plums, pears, apples and bananas, vegetables such as root vegetables and onions, and some grains such as oats and barley. On the other hand, insoluble fibre, which does not attract water during digestion but moves undigested to the large intestine to help bulk up the faecal matter and speed up the bowel movements that help to regulate gut health, is fund in wholegrains, brans and the edible skins of some fruits and vegetables. This is because insoluble fibres primarily consist of cellulose matter, though other constituents such as hemicelluloses and lignin also belong to this nutrient group.

Cereal-based foods are a major source of dietary fibre. Cereal grains have various layers, primarily the starchy endosperm, bran and germ layers. The fibre is found primarily in the outer and germ layers. The removal of fibre in the manufacture of cereal-based foods has a number of nutritional implications in terms of nutritional losses. Epidemiological studies also indicate that a lack of fibre in the diet may increase the risk of nutrition-related disease, but the link between fibre and the wholegrain needs also to be considered [79]. In cereal foods, fibre is a component of the wholegrain. Epidemiological evidence strongly suggests that consumption of wholegrain foods is associated with a reduced risk of cardiovascular disease [80], and the Australian Dietary Guidelines recommend the consumption of grain foods, mostly wholegrain [80].

Wholegrain foods

Wholegrain foods
Naturally occurring grain foods where the individual components of the wholegrain—the endosperm, germ and bran—are present in the food in the same proportions that would naturally occur in that grain.

There are many types of grains (such as wheat, barley, oats and rye). For human consumption, grains undergo various forms of processing and may be combined with other ingredients to form staple foods. For example, oats require minimal processing to be consumed as a breakfast cereal, whereas wheat and rye are common main ingredients in recipes for bread. Whether the final food can be called a wholegrain food has been the subject of much debate, but the nutritional value of grain foods defined as 'wholegrain' has been well characterised to support this position [81] (see also Figure 4.8). The question is how much of the final food product contains wholegrain, when there is such a broad range of food products in the cereal category [78]. In some cases such as oats, it is not difficult to evaluate the wholegrain content, as oats are naturally a wholegrain food. In others, such as bread or breakfast cereal, the amount of wholegrain in the product needs to be defined to enable consumers to translate the advice to choose mostly wholegrain foods.

FIGURE 4.8   HISTOLOGICAL STRUCTURE OF WHEAT GRAIN

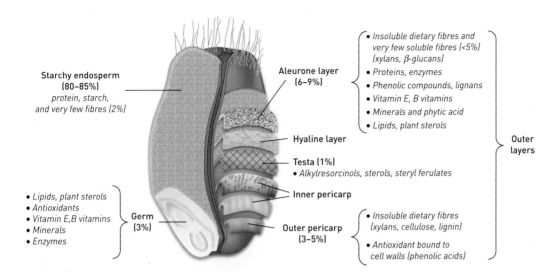

Adapted from A. Surget & C. Barron (2005). Histologie du gratin de ble. *Industrie des cereals*, 145, 3–7.

TABLE 4.9   CARBOHYDRATE CONTENT OF SELECTED FOODS

Food	Serving size*	g of carbohydrate per serve**	g of fibre per serve**
Wholemeal bread	1 slice (~40 g)	15.88	2.52
White bread	1 slice (~40 g)	18	1.12
Brown rice (boiled)	½ cup (~103 g***)	32.75	1.54
White rice (boiled)	½ cup (~95 g***)	34.2	0.95
Wholemeal pasta (boiled)	½ cup (~48 g***)	10.94	2.54
Pasta (regular, boiled)	½ cup (~74 g***)	17.61	1.48
Rolled oats	30 g/¼ cup	17.43	2.85
Wholewheat breakfast biscuit (e.g. Weetbix)	2 biscuits (~35 g***)	21.98	3.85
Pearl barley (boiled)	½ cup (~95 g***)	17.1	3.325
Chickpeas (canned, drained)	170 g/1 cup	22.61	7.99
Lentils (dried, boiled, drained)	170 g/1 cup	16.15	6.29
Desiree potato (boiled)	75 g	8.17	1.27
Orange sweet potato (boiled)	75 g	11.4	2.4
Plum (raw, with skin)	150 g (~2 plums)	10.65	3.0
Apple (red delicious, with skin)	150 g (~1 apple)	19.65	3.3
Banana (Cavendish, peeled)	150 g (~1 banana)	29.4	3.6

*Based on the Australian Dietary Guidelines [80].
**Calculated from *NUTTAB 2010* [82].
***Calculated using FoodWorks (Xyris Software Pty Ltd, Kenmore Hills, QLD, Australia, version 8, 2016).

TRY IT YOURSELF

Examine your diet and the products in your pantry for wholegrain composition. How would you describe the quantity of wholegrain you normally consume? How does this measure against a standard of 48 g/day?

Epidemiological evidence also strongly suggests that consumption of wholegrain foods is associated with a reduced risk of cardiovascular disease [83], and the Australian Dietary Guidelines recommend the consumption of grain foods, mostly wholegrain [80]. The effect of substituting wholegrains for refined grains is an ongoing area of research. Some studies have shown positive effects on gut microbiota and inflammatory markers [2] and on stool energy excretion that may have a positive influence on energy balance [84], but questions remain on potential confounding with cereal fibre (connected to micronutrients and phytochemicals), and accurate estimations of wholegrain content, bearing in mind problems with definitions and the influence of processing [85]. The type and amount of wholegrains consumed, the level of processing and the dietary context all need consideration [36].

≫ RESEARCH AT WORK

A REVIEW OF INTERNATIONAL RECOMMENDATIONS FOR DIETARY CARBOHYDRATE (CHO)

This review was published from an expert group of the European branch of the International Life Sciences Institute (ILSI) [86]. It searched the World Health Organization (WHO) and various national sources of information (including Australia) and found that dietary recommendations usually referred to a high fibre and total CHO intake with limited intake of added and free sugars. The justifications for recommendations could differ depending on classifications of CHO and of CHO-rich foods, considerations of exposure and health outcomes, and to a lesser extent the review methodology underpinning the recommendations.

The review summarises various national positions on dietary carbohydrate, foods and beverages, and reflects a number of the challenges presenting to nutrition science, particularly in the area of translation to policy and practice.

Foods delivering phytochemicals: flavonoids, phenolic acids and phytosterols

Fruits, vegetables, legumes, nuts and seeds, along with wholegrains, deliver plant phytonutrients. While the research may reflect individual foods, consuming a diet with a range of different coloured fruits and vegetables, along with nuts, seeds and wholegrains, will deliver these compounds. Foods with known high flavonoid content are citrus fruits, tea, parsley, onions, berries, as well as dark chocolate and red wine. Phenolic compounds are delivered in extra virgin olive oil along with plant sterols also found in nuts and wheat bran. The increasing knowledge of the effects of these compounds adds support to the advice to consume a minimally processed plant-based diet, rich in vegetables and fruits.

STOP AND THINK

- How are carbohydrates, dietary fibre and foods connected? Where do wholegrains fit?
- Why is sugar in food a problem in health today?
- What more needs to be known to optimise the intakes of carbohydrate-rich foods?

SUMMARY

- Carbohydrates are food components based on a glucose unit comprising six carbon atoms with attached hydroxyl groups. Glucose is the primary fuel source for the human body.
- There are a number of methods based on chemical properties and functionality in the body for measuring dietary fibre, the component in food that is not digested and absorbed in the small intestine.
- There is evidence to suggest that the presence of dietary fibre in the diet protects against disease, and that specific types of dietary fibre may have particular roles in a number of pathways that may protect health.
- Phytonutrients in plant foods are a particular category of new compounds of interest because of their powerful antioxidant activity, although much more needs to be known about their absorption, bioavailability and metabolism in the body.

PATHWAYS TO PRACTICE

- Opinions on carbohydrates and their roles regularly emerge in the media. Health workers need to have a reasonable understanding of carbohydrate forms and functions and the key principles of nutrition research that provide the evidence for practice to deal with this information in a discerning manner.
- The significance of fresh vegetables and fruits and wholegrain food products in advice on a healthy diet is underpinned by an understanding of the role of carbohydrates in human health.
- There are many opportunities to work with the food industry and in areas of food technology in which nutrition principles related to carbohydrate may be considered alongside novel food production initiatives.

DISCUSSION QUESTIONS

1   Why is chemical structure important in understanding the roles of macronutrients?
2   How does the glycaemic index principle work?
3   Why is it that not all dietary fibre has the same effect?

USEFUL WEBLINKS

Australian Guide to Healthy Eating tool:
> www.eatforhealth.gov.au/page/eat-health-calculators/calculated/1504843086

Best Plant-Based Diet:
> http://health.usnews.com/best-diet/best-plant-based-diets

Eat for Health:
> www.eatforhealth.gov.au

Food Composition Tables: see Australian Food Composition Program, Food Standards Australia New Zealand
> www.foodstandards.gov.au/science/monitoringnutrients/Pages/default.aspx

Food Standards Australia New Zealand:
www.foodstandards.gov.au

Grains & Legumes Nutrition Council:
www.glnc.org.au

Health Direct:
www.healthdirect.gov.au

Intense sweeteners—Food Standards Australia New Zealand:
www.foodstandards.gov.au/consumer/additives/intensesweetener/Pages/default.aspx

Nutrient Reference Values for Australia and New Zealand—Dietary Fibre:
www.nrv.gov.au/nutrients/dietary-fibre

Nutrient Reference Values for Australia and New Zealand—Macronutrient Balance:
www.nrv.gov.au/chronic-disease/macronutrient-balance

Nutrition and Diet—Cancer Council Australia:
www.cancercouncil.com.au/cancer-prevention/diet-exercise/nutrition-and-diet

FURTHER READING

Augustin, L. S. A., Kendall, C. W. C., Jenkins, D. J. A., Willett, W. C., Astrup, A., Barclay, A. W., ... Poli, A. (2015). Glycemic index, glycemic load and glycemic response: an international scientific consensus summit from the International Carbohydrate Quality Consortium (ICQC). *Nutrition, Metabolism and Cardiovascular Diseases*, 25(9), 795–815. doi:10.1016/j.numecd.2015.05.005

Balakumar, M., Raji, L., Prabhu, D., Sathishkumar, C., Prabu, P., Mohan, V. & Balasubramanyam, M. (2016). High-fructose diet is as detrimental as high-fat diet in the induction of insulin resistance and diabetes mediated by hepatic/pancreatic endoplasmic reticulum (ER) stress. *Molecular and Cellular Biochemistry*, 423(1–2), 93–104. doi:10.1007/s11010-016-2828-5

Carreiro, A. L., Dhillon, J., Gordon, S., Higgins, K. A., Jacobs, A. G., McArthur, B. M., ... Mattes, R. D. (2016). The macronutrients, appetite, and energy intake. *Annual Review of Nutrition*, 36(1), 73–103. doi:10.1146/annurev-nutr-121415-112624

Choudhary, A. K. & Pretorius, E. (2017). Revisiting the safety of aspartame. *Nutrition Reviews*. doi:10.1093/nutrit/nux035

Dahl, W. J. & Stewart, M. L. (2015). Position of the Academy of Nutrition and Dietetics: health implications of dietary fiber. *Journal of the Academy of Nutrition and Dietetics*, 115(11), 1861–70. doi:10.1016/j.jand.2015.09.003

Hardy, K., Brand-Miller, J., Brown, K. D., Thomas, M. G. & Copeland, L. (2015). The importance of dietary carbohydrate in human evolution. *Quarterly Review of Biology*, 90(3), 251–68.

Khan, T. A. & Sievenpiper, J. L. (2016). Controversies about sugars: results from systematic reviews and meta-analyses on obesity, cardiometabolic disease and diabetes. *European Journal of Nutrition*, 55, 25–43. doi:10.1007/s00394-016-1345-3

Kieffer, D. A., Martin, R. J. & Adams, S. H. (2016). Impact of dietary fibers on nutrient management and detoxification organs: gut, liver, and kidneys. *Advances in Nutrition: An International Review Journal*, 7(6), 1111–21. doi:10.3945/an.116.013219

Kusnadi, D. T. L., Barclay, A. W., Brand-Miller, J. C. & Louie, J. C.Y. (2017). Changes in dietary glycemic index and glycemic load in Australian adults from 1995 to 2012. *American Journal of Clinical Nutrition*, 106(1), 189–98. doi:10.3945/ajcn.116.150516

Lei, L., Rangan, A., Flood, V. M. & Louie, J. C.Y. (2016). Dietary intake and food sources of added sugar in the Australian population. *British Journal of Nutrition*, 115(5), 868–77. doi:10.1017/S0007114515005255

Lockyer, S., Spiro, A. & Stanner, S. (2016). Dietary fibre and the prevention of chronic disease—should health professionals be doing more to raise awareness? *Nutrition Bulletin*, 41(3), 214–31. doi:10.1111/nbu.12212

Lovegrove, A., Edwards, C. H., De Noni, I., Patel, H., El, S. N., Grassby, T., ... Shewry, P. R. (2017). Role of polysaccharides in food, digestion, and health. *Critical Reviews in Food Science and Nutrition*, 57(2), 237–53. doi:10.1080/10408398.2014.939263

Ma, J., Karlsen, M. C., Chung, M., Jacques, P. F., Saltzman, E., Smith, C. E., ... McKeown, N. M. (2016). Potential link between excess added sugar intake and ectopic fat: a systematic review of randomized controlled trials. *Nutrition Reviews*, 74(1), 18–32. doi:10.1093/nutrit/nuv047

Magnuson, B. A., Carakostas, M. C., Moore, N. H., Poulos, S. P. & Renwick, A. G. (2016). Biological fate of low-calorie sweeteners. *Nutrition Reviews*, 74(11), 670–89. doi:10.1093/nutrit/nuw032

Makarem, N., Nicholson, J. M., Bandera, E. V., McKeown, N. M. & Parekh, N. (2016). Consumption of whole grains and cereal fiber in relation to cancer risk: a systematic review of longitudinal studies. *Nutrition Reviews*, 74(6), 353–73. doi:10.1093/nutrit/nuw003

Malik, V. S. & Hu, F. B. (2015). Fructose and cardiometabolic health: what the evidence from sugar-sweetened beverages tells us. *Journal of the American College of Cardiology*, 66(14), 1615–24. doi:10.1016/j.jacc.2015.08.025

Montoya, C. A., Henare, S. J., Rutherfurd, S. M. & Moughan, P. J. (2016). Potential misinterpretation of the nutritional value of dietary fiber: correcting fiber digestibility values for nondietary gut-interfering material. *Nutrition Reviews*, 74(8), 517–33. doi:10.1093/nutrit/nuw014

Moshtaghian, H., Louie, J. C.Y., Charlton, K. E., Probst, Y. C., Gopinath, B., Mitchell, P. & Flood, V. M. (2016). Added sugar intake that exceeds current recommendations is associated with nutrient dilution in older Australians. *Nutrition*, 32(9), 937–42. doi:10.1016/j.nut.2016.02.004

Moynihan, P. (2016). Sugars and dental caries: evidence for setting a recommended threshold for intake. *Advances in Nutrition: An International Review Journal*, 7(1), 149–56. doi:10.3945/an.115.009365

Munsell, C. R., Harris, J. L., Sarda, V. & Schwartz, M. B. (2016). Parents' beliefs about the healthfulness of sugary drink options: opportunities to address misperceptions. *Public Health Nutrition*, 19(1), 46–54. doi:10.1017/S1368980015000397

Rebello, C. J., O'Neil, C. E. & Greenway, F. L. (2016). Dietary fiber and satiety: the effects of oats on satiety. *Nutrition Reviews*, 74(2), 131–47. doi:10.1093/nutrit/nuv063

Rippe, J. M., Sievenpiper, J. L., Lê, K.-A., White, J. S., Clemens, R. & Angelopoulos, T. J. (2017). What is the appropriate upper limit for added sugars consumption? *Nutrition Reviews*, 75(1), 18–36. doi:10.1093/nutrit/nuw046

Ross, A. B., Kristensen, M., Seal, C. J., Jacques, P. & McKeown, N. M. (2015). Recommendations for reporting whole-grain intake in observational and intervention studies. *American Journal of Clinical Nutrition*, 101(5), 903–7. doi:10.3945/ajcn.114.098046

Schaffer-Lequart, C., Lehmann, U., Ross, A. B., Roger, O., Eldridge, A. L., Ananta, E., ... Robin, F. (2017). Whole grain in manufactured foods: current use, challenges and the way forward. *Critical Reviews in Food Science and Nutrition*, 57(8), 1562–8. doi:10.1080/10408398.2013.781012

Schlesinger, S., Chan, D. S. M., Vingeliene, S., Vieira, A. R., Abar, L., Polemiti, E., ... Norat, T. (2017). Carbohydrates, glycemic index, glycemic load, and breast cancer risk: a systematic review and dose–response meta-analysis of prospective studies. *Nutrition Reviews*, 75(6), 420–41. doi:10.1093/nutrit/nux010

Seal, C. J. & Brownlee, I. A. (2015). Whole-grain foods and chronic disease: evidence from epidemiological and intervention studies. *Proceedings of the Nutrition Society*, 74(3), 313–19. doi:10.1017/S0029665115002104

Seal, C. J., Nugent, A. P., Tee, E. S. & Thielecke, F. (2016). Whole-grain dietary recommendations: the need for a unified global approach. *British Journal of Nutrition*, 115(11), 2031–8. doi:10.1017/S0007114516001161

Singh, G. M., Micha, R., Khatibzadeh, S., Shi, P., Lim, S., Andrews, K. G., ... Zajkás, G. (2015). Global, regional, and national consumption of sugar-sweetened beverages, fruit juices, and milk: a systematic assessment of beverage intake in 187 countries. *PLOS ONE*, 10(8). doi:10.1371/journal.pone.0124845

Stanhope, K. L. (2016). Sugar consumption, metabolic disease and obesity: the state of the controversy. *Critical Reviews in Clinical Laboratory Sciences*, 53(1), 52–67. doi:10.3109/10408363.2015.1084990

Sylvetsky, A. C., Edelstein, S., Delahanty, L., Walford, G., Boyko, E., Horton, E., ... Rother, K. (2016). Associations of dietary carbohydrates and carbohydrate subtypes with diabetes risk factors in the Diabetes Prevention Program. *Advances in Nutrition: An International Review Journal*, 7(1), 14A.

Thompson, H. J. & Brick, M. A. (2016). Perspective: closing the dietary fiber gap: an ancient solution for a 21st century problem. *Advances in Nutrition: An International Review Journal*, 7(4), 623–6. doi:10.3945/an.115.009696

Tryon, M. S., Stanhope, K. L., Epel, E. S., Mason, A. E., Brown, R., Medici, V., ... Laugero, K. D. (2015). Excessive sugar consumption may be a difficult habit to break: a view from the brain and body. *Journal of Clinical Endocrinology and Metabolism*, 100(6), 2239–47. doi:10.1210/jc.2014-4353

Wise, P. M., Nattress, L., Flammer, L. J. & Beauchamp, G. K. (2016). Reduced dietary intake of simple sugars alters perceived sweet taste intensity but not perceived pleasantness. *American Journal of Clinical Nutrition*, 103(1), 50–60. doi:10.3945/ajcn.115.112300

Yamini, S. & Trumbo, P. R. (2016). Qualified health claim for whole-grain intake and risk of type 2 diabetes: an evidence-based review by the US Food and Drug Administration. *Nutrition Reviews*, 74(10), 601–11. doi:10.1093/nutrit/nuw027

Yokoyama, Y., Levin, S. M. & Barnard, N. D. (2017). Association between plant-based diets and plasma lipids: a systematic review and meta-analysis. *Nutrition Reviews*.

OXFORD UNIVERSITY PRESS

Zheng, M., Allman-Farinelli, M., Heitmann, B. L. & Rangan, A. (2015). Substitution of sugar-sweetened beverages with other beverage alternatives: a review of long-term health outcomes. *Journal of the Academy of Nutrition and Dietetics*, 115(5), 767–79. doi:10.1016/j.jand.2015.01.006

REFERENCES

1   K. S. Poutanen, P. Dussort, A. Erkner, S. Fiszman, K. Karnik, M. Kristensen, ... D. J. Mela (2017). A review of the characteristics of dietary fibers relevant to appetite and energy intake outcomes in human intervention trials. *American Journal of Clinical Nutrition*, 106(3), 747–54. doi:10.3945/ajcn.117.157172

2   S. M. Vanegas, M. Meydani, J. B. Barnett, B. Goldin, A. Kane, H. Rasmussen, ... S. N. Meydani (2017). Substituting whole grains for refined grains in a 6-wk randomized trial has a modest effect on gut microbiota and immune and inflammatory markers of healthy adults. *American Journal of Clinical Nutrition*, 105(3), 635–50. doi:10.3945/ajcn.116.146928

3   E. Mayatepek, B. Hoffmann & T. Meissner (2010). Inborn errors of carbohydrate metabolism. *Best Practice & Research Clinical Gastroenterology*, 24(5), 607–18. doi:http://dx.doi.org/10.1016/j.bpg.2010.07.012

4   P. W. Siri-Tarino, S. Chiu, N. Bergeron & R. M. Krauss (2015). Saturated fats versus polyunsaturated fats versus carbohydrates for cardiovascular disease prevention and treatment. *Annual Review of Nutrition*, 35(1), 517–43. doi:10.1146/annurev-nutr-071714-034449

5   M. Dehghan, A. Mente, X. Zhang, S. Swaminathan, W. Li, V. Mohan, ... R. Mapanga (2017). Associations of fats and carbohydrate intake with cardiovascular disease and mortality in 18 countries from five continents (PURE): a prospective cohort study. *The Lancet*. doi:10.1016/S0140-6736(17)32252-3

6   D. R. Jacobs & L. C. Tapsell (2013). Food synergy: the key to a healthy diet. *Proceedings of the Nutrition Society*, 72(2), 200–6. doi:10.1017/S0029665112003011

7   D. R. Jacobs, Jr & L. C. Tapsell (2007). Food, not nutrients, is the fundamental unit in nutrition. *Nutrition Reviews*, 65(10), 439–50.

8   J. L. Clark, P. Zahradka & C. G. Taylor (2015). Efficacy of flavonoids in the management of high blood pressure. *Nutrition Reviews*, 73(12), 799–822. doi:10.1093/nutrit/nuv048

9   A. Rodriguez-Casado (2016). The health potential of fruits and vegetables phytochemicals: notable examples. *Critical Reviews in Food Science and Nutrition*, 56(7), 1097–1107. doi:10.1080/10408398.2012.755149

10 A. Scalbert, C. Andres-Lacueva, M. Arita, P. Kroon, C. Manach, M. Urpi-Sarda & D. Wishart (2011). Databases on food phytochemicals and their health-promoting effects. *Journal of Agricultural and Food Chemistry*, 59(9), 4331–48. doi:10.1021/jf200591d

11 C. Fitch & K. S. Keim (2012). Position of the Academy of Nutrition and Dietetics: use of nutritive and nonnutritive sweeteners. *Journal of the Academy of Nutrition and Dietetics*, 112(5), 739–58. doi:http://dx.doi.org/10.1016/j.jand.2012.03.009

12 Food Standards Australia New Zealand (2017). *Intense Sweeteners*. Canberra: FSANZ.

13 Food Standards Australia New Zealand (2004). *Consumption of Intense Sweeteners in Australia and New Zealand. Benchmark Survey 2003*. Canberra: FSANZ.

14 J. L. Sievenpiper (2017). Fructose: back to the future? *American Journal of Clinical Nutrition*, 106(2), 439–42. doi:10.3945/ajcn.117.161539

15 R. J. Johnson, L. G. Sánchez-Lozada, P. Andrews & M. A. Lanaspa (2017). Perspective: a historical and scientific perspective of sugar and its relation with obesity and diabetes. *Advances in Nutrition: An International Review Journal*, 8(3), 412–22. doi:10.3945/an.116.014654

16 L. R. DeChristopher, J. Uribarri & K. L. Tucker (2017). Intake of high fructose corn syrup sweetened soft drinks, fruit drinks and apple juice is associated with prevalent coronary heart disease, in U.S. adults, ages 45–59 y. *BMC Nutrition*, 3(1), 51. doi:10.1186/s40795-017-0168-9

17 R. A. Evans, M. Frese, J. Romero, J. H. Cunningham & K. E. Mills (2017). Fructose replacement of glucose or sucrose in food or beverages lowers postprandial glucose and insulin without raising triglycerides: a systematic review and meta-analysis. *American Journal of Clinical Nutrition*, 106(2), 506–18. doi:10.3945/ajcn.116.145151

18 R. A. Evans, M. Frese, J. Romero, J. H. Cunningham & K. E. Mills. (2017). Chronic fructose substitution for glucose or sucrose in food or beverages has little effect on fasting blood glucose, insulin, or triglycerides: a systematic review and meta-analysis. *American Journal of Clinical Nutrition*, 106(2), 519–29. doi:10.3945/ajcn.116.145169

19 N. K. Jain, D. B. Rosenberg, M. J. Ulahannan, M. J. Glasser & C. S. Pitchumoni (1985). Sorbitol intolerance in adults. *American Journal of Gastroenterology*, 80(9), 678–81.

20 O.-J. M. Bright, D. D. Wang, M. Shams-White, S. N. Bleich, J. Foreyt, M. Franz, … M. Chung (2017). Research priorities for studies linking intake of low-calorie sweeteners and potentially related health outcomes: research methodology and study design. *Current Developments in Nutrition*, 1(7). doi:10.3945/cdn.117.000547

21 J. H. Cummings & A. M. Stephen (2007). Carbohydrate terminology and classification. *European Journal of Clinical Nutrition*, 61(S1), S5–S18.

22 S. M. Donovan (2017). Human milk oligosaccharides: potent weapons in the battle against rotavirus infection. *Journal of Nutrition*, 147(9), 1605–6. doi:10.3945/jn.117.255836

23 J. C. Y. Louie, V. M. Flood, F. S. Atkinson, A. W. Barclay & J. C. Brand-Miller (2015). Methodology for assigning appropriate glycaemic index values to an Australian food composition database. *Journal of Food Composition and Analysis*, 38, 1–6. doi:http://dx.doi.org/10.1016/j.jfca.2014.06.002

24 J. Brand-Miller, T. M. Wolever, K. Foster-Powell & S. Colagiuri (2003). *The New Glucose Revolution*. New York: Marlowe & Company.

25 D. P. Burkitt, A. R. P. Walker & N. S. Painter (1972). Effect of dietary fibre on stools and transit-times, and its role in the causation of disease. *The Lancet*, 300(7792), 1408–11. doi:10.1016/S0140-6736(72)92974-1

26 H. Trowell (1972). Crude fibre, dietary fibre and atherosclerosis. *Atherosclerosis*, 16(1), 138–40. doi:http://dx.doi.org/10.1016/0021-9150(72)90017-2

27 H. Trowell (1972). Ischemic heart disease and dietary fiber. *American Journal of Clinical Nutrition*, 25(9), 926–32.

28 N. S. Painter (1975). *Diverticular Disease of the Colon: A deficiency disease of Western civilization*. London: Heinemann.

29 L. Prosky, N. G. Asp, I. Furda, J. W. DeVries, T. F. Schweizer & B. F. Harland (1985). Determination of total dietary fiber in foods and food products: collaborative study. *Journal—Association of Official Analytical Chemists*, 68(4), 677–9.

30 B. V. McCleary (2007). An integrated procedure for the measurement of total dietary fibre (including resistant starch), non-digestible oligosaccharides and available carbohydrates. *Analytical and Bioanalytical Chemistry*, 389(1), 291–308. doi:10.1007/s00216-007-1389-6

31 S. Fuller, E. Beck, H. Salman & L. Tapsell (2016). New horizons for the study of dietary fiber and health: a review. *Plant Foods for Human Nutrition*, 71(1), 1–12. doi:10.1007/s11130-016-0529-6

32 American Association of Cereal Chemists (2001). The definitions of dietary fibre. *Cereal Food World*, 46(3), 112–26.

33 Joint FAO/WHO Food Standards Programme (2010). *Secretariat of the CODEX Alimentarius Commission: CODEX Alimentarius (CODEX) Guidelines on Nutrition Labeling CAC/GL 2–1985 as Last Amended 2010.* Rome: FAO.

34 Institute of Medicine (2001). *Dietary Reference Intakes: Proposed definition of dietary fiber.* Washington, DC: National Academies Press.

35 Codex Alimentarius Commission (2006). *Report of the 27th Session of the Codex Committee on Nutrition and Foods for Special Dietary Uses (CCNFSDU).* Bonn: Codex Alimentarius Commission.

36 J.M. W.Wong, R. de Souza, C. W. C. Kendall, A. Emam & D. J.A. Jenkins (2006). Colonic health: fermentation and short chain fatty acids. *Journal of Clinical Gastroenterology*, 40(3), 235–43.

37 Food and Agriculture Organization of the United Nations (1998). *Physiological Effects of Dietary Fibre: Carbohydrates in human nutrition.* Geneva: FAO.

38 N. C. Howarth, E. Saltzman & S. B. Roberts (2001). Dietary fiber and weight regulation. *Nutrition Reviews*, 59(5), 129–39. doi:10.1111/j.1753-4887.2001.tb07001.x

39 D. Lairon, N. Arnault, S. Bertrais, R. Planells, E. Clero, S. Hercberg & M.-C. Boutron-Ruault (2005). Dietary fiber intake and risk factors for cardiovascular disease in French adults. *American Journal of Clinical Nutrition*, 82(6), 1185–94.

40 Y. Park, A. F. Subar, A. Hollenbeck & A. Schatzkin (2011). Dietary fiber intake and mortality in the NIH-AARP Diet and Health Study. *Archives of Internal Medicine*, 171(12), 1061–8. doi:10.1001/archinternmed.2011.18

41 C. S. Brennan (2005). Dietary fibre, glycaemic response, and diabetes. *Molecular Nutrition & Food Research*, 49(6), 560–70. doi:10.1002/mnfr.200500025

42 S.-C. Chuang, T. Norat, N. Murphy, A. Olsen, A. Tjønneland, K. Overvad, ... P. Vineis (2012). Fiber intake and total and cause-specific mortality in the European Prospective Investigation into Cancer and Nutrition cohort. *American Journal of Clinical Nutrition,* 96(1), 164–74. doi:10.3945/ajcn.111.028415

43 S. B. Roberts & M. B. Heyman (2000). Dietary composition and obesity: do we need to look beyond dietary fat? *Journal of Nutrition*, 130(2), 267S–267S.

44 D. S. Ludwig, M. A. Pereira, C. H. Kroenke, et al. (1999). Dietary fiber, weight gain, and cardiovascular disease risk factors in young adults. *JAMA—Journal of the American Medical Association*, 282(16), 1539–46. doi:10.1001/jama.282.16.1539

45 J. Montonen, P. Knekt, R. Järvinen, A. Aromaa, A. Reunanen (2003). Whole-grain and fiber intake and the incidence of type 2 diabetes. *American Journal of Clinical Nutrition*, 77(3), 622–9.

46 K.W. Heaton (1990). Dietary fibre: after 21 years of study the verdict remains one of fruition and frustration. *British Medical Journal*, 300(6738), 1479–80.

47 J. D. Leach (2007). Evolutionary perspective on dietary intake of fibre and colorectal cancer. *European Journal of Clinical Nutrition*, 61(1), 140–2. doi:http://dx.doi.org/10.1038/sj.ejcn.1602486

48 C. M. Ripsin, J. M. Keenan, D. R. Jacobs, Jr, et al. (1992). Oat products and lipid lowering: a meta-analysis. *JAMA—Journal of the American Medical Association*, 267(24), 3317–25. doi:10.1001/jama.1992.03480240079039

49 L. Brown, B. Rosner, W. W. Willett & F. M. Sacks (1999). Cholesterol-lowering effects of dietary fiber: a meta-analysis. *American Journal of Clinical Nutrition*, 69(1), 30–42.

50 Food and Drug Administration HHS (2008). Food labeling: health claims; soluble fiber from certain foods and risk of coronary heart disease. Interim final rule. *Federal Register*, 73(37), 9938–47.

51 J. W. Lampe (1999). Health effects of vegetables and fruit: assessing mechanisms of action in human experimental studies. *American Journal of Clinical Nutrition*, 70(3), 475s–490s.

52 C. J. Dillard (2000). Phytochemicals: nutraceuticals and human health. *Journal of the Science of Food and Agriculture*, 80(12), 1744–56. doi:10.1002/1097-0010(20000915)80:12<1744::AID-JSFA725>3.0.CO;2-W

53 R. H. Liu (2004). Potential synergy of phytochemicals in cancer prevention: mechanism of action. *Journal of Nutrition*, 134(12), 3479S–3485S.

54 N. C. Cook & S. Samman (1996). Flavonoids—chemistry, metabolism, cardioprotective effects, and dietary sources. *Journal of Nutritional Biochemistry*, 7(2), 66–76. doi:http://dx.doi.org/10.1016/S0955-2863(95)00168-9

55 P. C. H. Hollman, A. Cassidy, B. Comte, M. Heinonen, M. Richelle, E. Richling, ... S. Vidry (2011). The biological relevance of direct antioxidant effects of polyphenols for cardiovascular health in humans is not established. *Journal of Nutrition*, 141(5), 989S–1009S. doi:10.3945/jn.110.131490

56 D. R. Jacobs, M. D. Gross & L. C. Tapsell (2009). Food synergy: an operational concept for understanding nutrition. *American Journal of Clinical Nutrition*, 89(5), 1543S–1548S. doi:10.3945/ajcn.2009.26736B

57 N. M. Wedick, A. Pan, A. Cassidy, E. B. Rimm, L. Sampson, B. Rosner, ... R. M. van Dam (2012). Dietary flavonoid intakes and risk of type 2 diabetes in US men and women. *American Journal of Clinical Nutrition*, 95(4), 925–33. doi:10.3945/ajcn.111.028894

58 E. E. Devore, J. H. Kang, M. M. B. Breteler & F. Grodstein (2012). Dietary intakes of berries and flavonoids in relation to cognitive decline. *Annals of Neurology*, 72(1), 135–43. doi:10.1002/ana.23594

59 E. Flanagan, M. Müller, M. Hornberger & D. Vauzour (2018). Impact of flavonoids on cellular and molecular mechanisms underlying age-related cognitive decline and neurodegeneration. *Current Nutrition Reports*, 7(2), 49–57. doi:10.1007/s13668-018-0226-1

60 K. R. Gildawie, R. L. Galli, B. Shukitt-Hale & A. N. Carey (2018). Protective effects of foods containing flavonoids on age-related cognitive decline. *Current Nutrition Reports*, 7(2), 39–48. doi:10.1007/s13668-018-0227-0

61 European Food Safety Authority (2012). Scientific opinion on the substantiation of a health claim related to cocoa flavanols and the maintenance of normal endothelium-dependent vasodilation pursuant to Article 13(5) of Regulation (EC) No 1924/2006. *European Food Safety Authority Journal*, 10(7), 2809–30.

62 M. M. Murphy, L. M. Barraj, D. Herman, X. Bi, R. Cheatham & R. K. Randolph (2012). Phytonutrient intake by adults in the United States in relation to fruit and vegetable consumption. *Journal of the Academy of Nutrition and Dietetics*, 112(2), 222–9. doi:http://dx.doi.org/10.1016/j.jada.2011.08.044

63 Food and Agriculture Organization of the United Nations (1998). Dietary carbohydrate composition. In *Carbohydrates in Human Nutrition*. Rome: FAO.

64 P. Lin, X. Ye & T. B. Ng (2008). Purification of melibiose-binding lectins from two cultivars of Chinese black soybeans. *Acta Biochimica et Biophysica Sinica*, 40(12), 1029–38. doi:10.1111/j.1745-7270.2008.00488.x

65 M. D. Schorin, K. Sollid, M. S. Edge & A. Bouchoux (2012). The science of sugars, part 2: sugars and a healthful diet. *Nutrition Today*, 47(4), 175–82.

66 J. C. Y. Louie, H. Moshtaghian, S. Boylan, V. M. Flood, A. M. Rangan, A. W. Barclay, ... T. P. Gill (2015). A systematic methodology to estimate added sugar content of foods. *European Journal of Clinical Nutrition*, 69(2), 154–61. doi:10.1038/ejcn.2014.256

67 J. C. Y. Louie & L. C. Tapsell (2015). Association between intake of total vs added sugar on diet quality: a systematic review. *Nutrition Reviews*, 73(12), 837–57. doi:10.1093/nutrit/nuv044

68 Australian Bureau of Statistics (2015). *Australian Health Survey: First Results, 2011–12*. Canberra: ABS.

69 N. J. Talley (2017). National Health Summit on Obesity calls for Australia to take action to stem the pandemic. *Medical Journal of Australia*, 206(3), 106–7.

70 J. L. Veerman, G. Sacks, N. Antonopoulos & J. Martin (2016). The impact of a tax on sugar-sweetened beverages on health and health care costs: a modelling study. *PLOS ONE*, 11(4), e0151460. doi:10.1371/journal.pone.0151460

71 T. Nomaguchi, M. Cunich, B. Zapata-Diomedi & J. L. Veerman (2017). The impact on productivity of a hypothetical tax on sugar-sweetened beverages. *Health Policy*, 121(6), 715–25. doi:10.1016/j.healthpol.2017.04.001

72 M. A. Colchero, M. Molina & C. M. Guerrero-López (2017). After Mexico implemented a tax, purchases of sugar-sweetened beverages decreased and water increased: difference by place of residence, household composition, and income level. *Journal of Nutrition*, 147(8), 1552–7. doi:10.3945/jn.117.251892

73 E. Martínez Steele, L. G. Baraldi, M. L. d. C. Louzada, J.-C. Moubarac, D. Mozaffarian & C. A. Monteiro (2016). Ultra-processed foods and added sugars in the US diet: evidence from a nationally representative cross-sectional study. *BMJ Open*, 6(3). doi:10.1136/bmjopen-2015-009892

74 C. A. Monteiro, R. B. Levy, R. M. Claro, I. R. Castro & G. Cannon (2010). A new classification of foods based on the extent and purpose of their processing. *Cad Saude Publica*, 26(11), 2039–49.

75 M. J. Gibney, C. G. Forde, D. Mullally & E. R. Gibney (2017). Ultra-processed foods in human health: a critical appraisal. *American Journal of Clinical Nutrition*, 106(3), 717–24. doi:10.3945/ajcn.117.160440

76 F. Alcaire, L. Antúnez, L. Vidal, A. Giménez & G. Ares (2017). Aroma-related cross-modal interactions for sugar reduction in milk desserts: influence on consumer perception. *Food Research International*, 97, 45–50. doi:http://dx.doi.org/10.1016/j.foodres.2017.02.019

77 P. K. Nguyen, S. Lin & P. Heidenreich (2016). A systematic comparison of sugar content in low-fat vs regular versions of food. *Nutrition & Diabetes*, 6, e193. doi:10.1038/nutd.2015.43

78 Grains & Legumes Nutrition Council (2009). *Wholegrain Communication Guide*. Sydney: Grains & Legumes Nutrition Council. Retrieved from: www.glnc.org.au/wp-content/uploads/2011/04/Wholegrain-Communication-Guide-Aug-09_Final-2.pdf.

79 S. Lillioja, A. L. Neal, L. Tapsell & D. R. Jacobs (2013). Whole grains, type 2 diabetes, coronary heart disease, and hypertension: links to the aleurone preferred over indigestible fiber. *BioFactors*, 39(3), 242–58. doi:10.1002/biof.1077

80 National Health and Medical Research Council (2013). *Australian Dietary Guidelines*. Canberra: NHMRC.

81 S. M. C. Dalton, L. C. Tapsell & Y. Probst (2012). Potential health benefits of whole grain wheat components. *Nutrition Today*, 47(4), 163–74. doi:10.1097/NT.0b013e31826069d0

82 Food Standards Australia New Zealand (2012). *NUTTAB 2010*. Canberra: FSANZ.

83 National Health and Medical Research Council (2011). *A Review of the Evidence to Address Targeted Questions to Inform the Revision of the Australian Dietary Guidelines: Evidence statements*. Canberra: NHMRC.

84 J. P. Karl, M. Meydani, J. B. Barnett, S. M.Vanegas, B. Goldin, A. Kane, ...S. B. Roberts (2017). Substituting whole grains for refined grains in a 6-wk randomized trial favorably affects energy-balance metrics in healthy men and postmenopausal women. *American Journal of Clinical Nutrition*, 105(3), 589–99. doi:10.3945/ajcn.116.139683

85 I. Tetens (2017). Substituting whole grain for refined grain: what is needed to strengthen the scientific evidence for health outcomes? *American Journal of Clinical Nutrition*, 105(3), 545–6. doi:10.3945/ajcn.117.152496

86 A. E. Buyken, D. J. Mela, P. Dussort, I. T. Johnson, I. A. Macdonald, J. D. Stowell & F. J. P. H. Brouns (2018). Dietary carbohydrates: a review of international recommendations and the methods used to derive them. *European Journal of Clinical Nutrition*. doi:10.1038/s41430-017-0035-4

CHAPTER 5

FATS AND LIPIDS: MAJOR COMPONENTS OF OILS, SEEDS AND ANIMAL FOODS

LINDA TAPSELL

CHAPTER OBJECTIVES

This chapter will enable the reader to:

- describe the chemical structure and functions of fat
- describe the relationship between dietary fat and health
- describe the best food choices to ensure healthy intakes of fat.

KEY TERMS

Fatty acids

Lipids

Saturated fatty acids

Unsaturated fatty acids

KEY POINTS

- Dietary fat refers to a wide range of chemical structures that reflect many important functions in the human body.
- Some classes of polyunsaturated fatty acids cannot be synthesised by the body, making them essential in the diet, but other fatty acids can be interconverted.
- High intakes of saturated fatty acids are implicated in raised cholesterol levels and the prevalence of cardiovascular disease in the community.
- Obtaining the ideal proportions of fatty acids in the diet requires discrimination in food choices that are reflected in meals and the overall dietary pattern.

INTRODUCTION

Dietary fat is a macronutrient found in a wide range of foods, often consumed in patterns that reflect local cuisines. Since the 1950s, with the identification of lipoproteins and their observed links with dietary fat and cardiovascular disease, a healthy debate on dietary fat could be readily found in the scientific literature [1], and this is still the case today [2]. The original advice to reduce saturated fat intake appears to have stood the test of time [3], and deaths from heart disease have also declined [1].

The story of dietary fat draws on an immense amount of science in the last seven decades. Translating this to dietary intakes that promote health requires a broad understanding of scientific methods, and discipline in making sound interpretations of research.

From the perspective of chemical characterisation, fat is more correctly referred to as a class of water insoluble compounds known as **lipids**. Dietary fat comprises a number of these compounds, mostly in the form of triglycerides (or triacylglycerols), and including sterols (such as cholesterol and phytosterols) and phospholipids. Triglycerides are broken down to a glycerol chain and fatty acid components. The biochemical and cellular pathways in which fatty acids play a role continue to be a great source of intrigue and serve as an inspiration for budding scientists.

Lipids
organic oily compounds, insoluble in water.

Essential fatty acids
fatty acids that cannot be made by the body.

At a basic science level, it is known that fatty acids can be converted from carbohydrate and protein, and from other forms of each other, but this is not always the case. Thus, certain classes of fatty acids are termed **essential fatty acids**—that is, they must be consumed in the diet. Starting at the population level, research has also exposed relationships between dietary fat and cardiometabolic diseases, indicating a need to balance the intake of fatty acids delivered in foods.

Visit Oxford Ascend for more on fat.

Fat is utilised for energy, delivering around 37 kJ/g and making it the most energy-dense nutrient. Although a great deal of dietary advice has focused on this attribute, fat is much more than an energy source. It is an integral component of cell structure and function (including signalling), and a potent gene regulator [4]. In past decades, a great deal of research has addressed the metabolic functions of polyunsaturated fats and, in particular, omega-3 fatty acids, notably eicosapentaenoic acid (EPA) and docosahexaenoic acid (DHA) found in fish oils. For example, we know that DHA forms an integral part of the brain and related functions; EPA and omega-6 fatty acids compete in eicosanoid pathways, which implicate them in balancing the processes of vascular blood clotting (thrombosis) and inflammation. Other pathways relate to regulation of the immune system and insulin signalling. Research on the function of human and dietary fat is therefore not limited to energy balance and substrate utilisation; it also addresses areas such as lipid transport and inflammation (with implications for cardiovascular disease) and insulin action (with implications for diabetes).

Evidence for the health effects of dietary fat can be found in large cohort studies and randomised controlled trials, with improvements in methodologies over time. Research has also focused on individual fatty acids, not only considering the total proportion of energy from fat (as in low-fat diets), but also on manipulations of dietary fatty acid profiles. However, conducting these studies in humans requires an intricate knowledge of food composition and how different food patterns deliver particular dietary fat profiles. A major limitation of this approach is that foods deliver many other bioactive components besides fat, so ultimately dietary advice addressing optimum requirements for fat must also address other components in the diet and consider the role of food synergy in achieving health effects [5].

OXFORD UNIVERSITY PRESS

This chapter begins by outlining the basic structure of fatty acids and their fundamental pathways in human health. It then considers the evidence for effects of dietary fats on human health and how this translates to dietary guidance targeting the achievement of nutritional requirements and protection against chronic diet-related disease.

STOP AND THINK

- Which developments in scientific research helped to first expose understanding of the possible roles of dietary fat in the development of chronic disease?
- Why is it necessary to consume some dietary fat?
- How might the fat profile of different types of food vary, and how could the different types of foods be categorised?

WHAT ARE THE STRUCTURES AND FUNCTIONS OF DIETARY FAT?

'Fat' is a general term that can cover a multitude of meanings. The term 'lipid' is the more correct chemical term for these compounds distinguished by being insoluble in water. The most common lipid is called **triacylglycerol** (or triglyceride). This compound comprises a three carbon alcohol structure (glycerol) and three attached fatty acids. To a large extent, the different chemical structures of fatty acids characterise the nature of dietary fat (triglyceride). Understanding the structure of individual fatty acids (Figure 5.1) helps to explain their function in the body [6; 7].

Triacylglycerol
also known as triglyceride, a molecule with a three carbon alcohol structure (glycerol) and three attached fatty acids.

In general, fatty acids are formed by carbon chains, with hydrogen attached to carbon along the way, and carboxyl and methane groups at each end. A major difference between fatty acids occurs when there is a difference in the 'saturation' of the bonds along the carbon chain. A saturated fatty acid only has single bonds (i.e. hydrogen is attached to each carbon atom; it is 'saturated'), whereas unsaturated fatty acids include double bonds—one (mono) or more (poly)—where the bonds are not saturated with hydrogen and a methylene group is present (Figure 5.2).

FIGURE 5.1   GENERAL STRUCTURE OF FATTY ACIDS

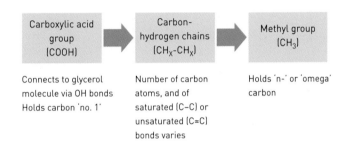

Carboxylic acid group (COOH)
Connects to glycerol molecule via OH bonds
Holds carbon 'no. 1'

Carbon-hydrogen chains (CH_x-CH_x)
Number of carbon atoms, and of saturated (C–C) or unsaturated (C=C) bonds varies

Methyl group (CH_3)
Holds 'n-' or 'omega' carbon

 LINDA TAPSELL

FIGURE 5.2 NAMES AND CHEMICAL STRUCTURES OF COMMON FATTY ACIDS

Common name: stearic acid   Chemical name: octadecanoic acid
Fatty acid notation: C18:0

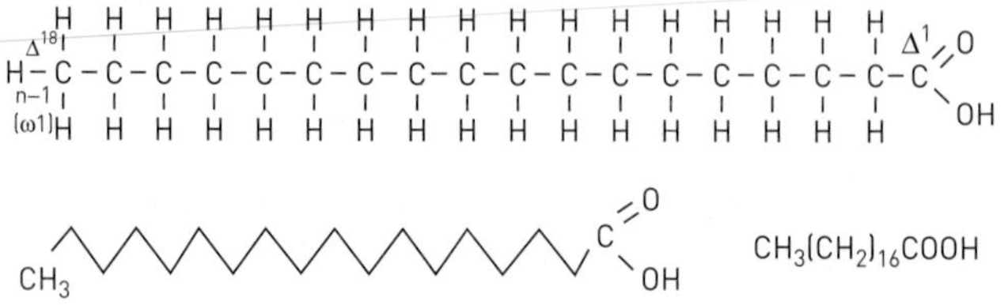

$CH_3(CH_2)_{16}COOH$

Common name: oleic acid   Chemical name: Δ^9-octadecenoic acid
Fatty acid notation: C18:1n-9, or C18:1ω-9, or C18:1Δ^9

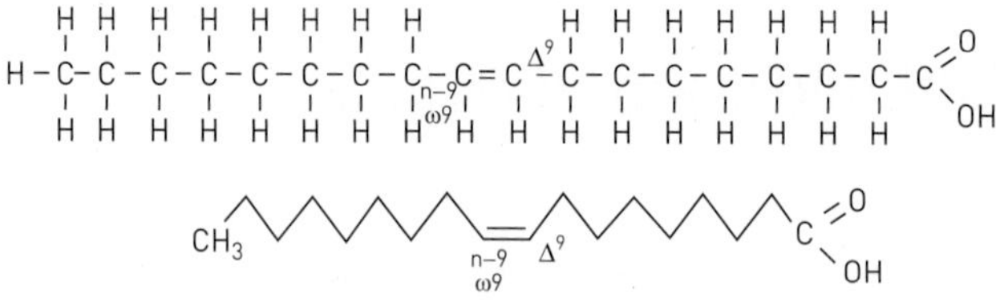

$CH_3(CH_2)_7CH=CH(CH_2)_7COOH$

Common name: linoleic acid   Chemical name: $\Delta^{9,12}$-octadecadienoic acid
Fatty acid notation: C18:2n-6, or C18:2ω-6, or C18:2$\Delta^{9,12}$

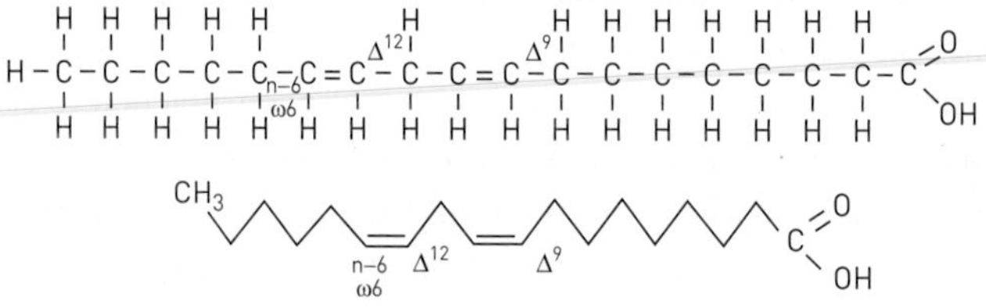

$CH_3(CH_2)_4CH=CHCH_2CH=CH(CH_2)_7COOH$

Common name: linolenic acid   Chemical name: $\Delta^{9,12,15}$-octadecatrienoic acid
Fatty acid notation: C18:3n-3, or C18:3ω-3, or C18:3$\Delta^{9,12,15}$

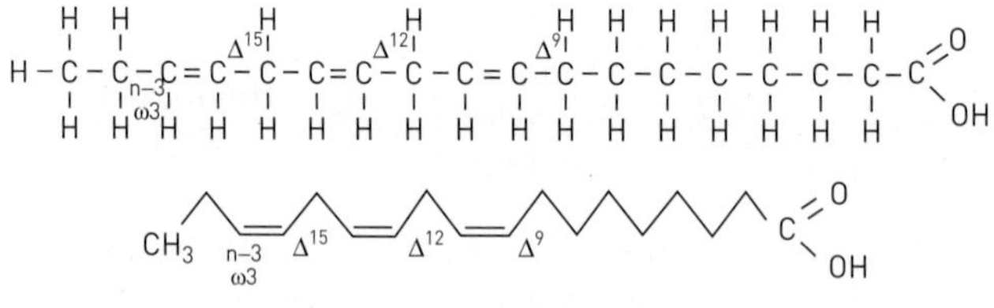

$CH_3CH_2CH=CHCH_2CH=CHCH_2CH=CH(CH_2)_7COOH$

Source: C. M. Skeaff & J. Mann (2012). Chapter 4: Lipids. In J. Mann & S. Truswell (eds), *Essentials of Human Nutrition*, 4th edn. Oxford University Press, Incorporated

TABLE 5.1   NOMENCLATURE OF SIGNIFICANT FATTY ACIDS

Common name	Class	Chemical name	Notation
Stearic acid	Saturated	Octadecanoic acid	18:0
Oleic acid	Monounsaturated	Delta 9 octadecanoic acid	18:1 n-9
Linoleic acid	Polyunsaturated	Delta 9,12 octadecadienoic acid	18:1 n-9
Linolenic acid	Polyunsaturated	Delta 9,12,15 octadecatrienoic acid	18:3 n-3

The nomenclature, or chemical naming, of fatty acids reflects these structural differences (Table 5.1). First, the carbon atoms in the fatty acid chain are numbered, starting at where the glycerol molecule joins with the fatty acid (the carboxyl end). The presence of unsaturated fats is identified by counting the number of carbon atoms from the other end of the chain (the methyl end), using the terms 'n minus (n-)' or 'omega'. Thus, the first double bond appearing in **omega-3 fatty acids** lies after the third carbon atom from the methyl end. Classes of fatty acids can also be described by their carbon chain length—for example, as seen in **medium chain triglycerides (MCTs)**.

The presence of double bonds has both structural and functional implications, including a greater susceptibility to chemical reactions such as oxidation.

In more general dietary terms, **saturated fat** refers to fat delivered by foods where the fatty acids attached to the triglyceride molecule tend to be saturated. Foods high in saturated fat, such as butter, mostly contain triglycerides with these chemical structures. A diet high in saturated fat contains a combination of foods that together deliver a large amount of saturated fatty acids relative to other types of fatty acids (and/or macronutrients) in the total diet.

Carbohydrate and protein can be converted to saturated or monounsaturated fatty acids, so in addition to dietary sources these fatty acids are readily available to the body. Polyunsaturated fatty acids (PUFA) can be interconverted in the body due to the presence of elongating and desaturating enzymes (Figure 5.3), but two PUFA with an 18 carbon chain length cannot be synthesised as the body lacks the enzymes to insert a double bond at the required points. Linoleic acid (LA, from the omega-6 class) and α–linolenic acid (ALA, from the omega-3 class) are essential in the diet. Symptoms of deficiency present as dry scaly skin, but the incidence is rare.

Omega-3 fatty acids

also known as n-3 fatty acids where the double bond occurs on the third carbon atom after the methyl end of the carbon chain. Fish oils contain the omega-3 fatty acids eicosapentaenoic acid (EPA) and docosahexaenoic acid (DHA).

Medium chain triglycerides (MCTs)

triacylglyceride compounds where the carbon chain of the fatty acids attached to the glycerol moiety comprise medium chain fatty acids.

Saturated fat

triglyceride containing fatty acids where all carbon atoms have hydrogen attached, creating single bonds along their carbon chain.

>> **CASE 5.1**

BALANCING PROPORTIONS OF ESSENTIAL FATTY ACIDS

Research on the pathways of fatty acid conversion has informed health research and supported debates on balancing the amount of essential fatty acids in the diet fat [8; 9]. As the conversion from LA to arachidonic acid (AA) uses the same enzymes as the conversion between ALA and eicosapentaenoic acid (EPA), docosapentaenoic acid (DPA) and docosahexaenoic acid (DHA) (Figure 5.3), it has been argued that the competition for enzymes could be problematic, particularly as the AA pathway is pro-thrombotic and pro-inflammatory [10].

One review on desaturase enzymes, however, argues in the first instance that the genetic transcription of the three main enzymes Δ9, Δ6 and Δ5 desaturase is regulated in a sophisticated differential manner. It is further argued that the main functions of the essential fatty acids relates to the stability of membrane phospholipids (see below). While the synthesis of EPA and DHA requires Δ6 and Δ5 desaturases, these fatty acids have a major role in maintaining cell membrane fluidity, in particular in relation to cell signalling. The functions of Δ9 desaturase relate to a more diverse group of lipids. It has a major role in the synthesis of oleic acid (a monounsaturated fatty acid, MUFA) found in adipocytes, phospholipids and cholesterol esters (a cholesterol molecule with an attached fatty acid) [11]. The genetic basis underpinning the issues raised here continues as a major challenge for research aimed at understanding the delicate balances in fatty acid metabolism [12].

In clinical research it is noted that the N-6 and N-3 PUFA do not interconvert. The n-3 PUFA contribute little energy to the diet and are delivered in limited food sources, mainly in plant foods (ALA) and fish oils (EPA/DHA/DPA). Both these factors have implications for considerations in dietary guidance [3].

- How does this case reflect the challenges in translating knowledge of cellular mechanisms to dietary advice?
- How might genetics play a role in the susceptibility of individuals to health risks implied in this case?
- What further research would help clarify issues in this debate?

FIGURE 5.3   DESATURATION AND ELONGATION OF POLYUNSATURATED FATTY ACIDS

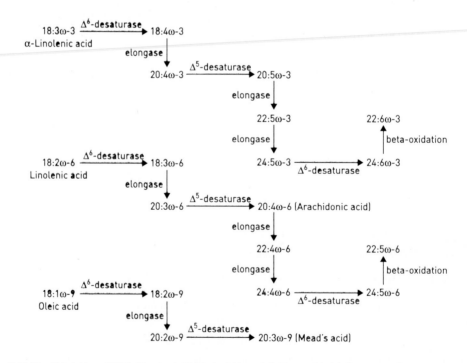

Source: C. M. Skeaff & J. Mann (2012). Chapter 4: Lipids. In J. Mann & S. Truswell (eds), *Essentials of Human Nutrition*, 4th edn. Oxford University Press, Incorporated

All fatty acids can be oxidised in cells to produce energy, with some variation in how this occurs. In the past, experimental research showed there may be differential rates of fatty acid oxidation, with the short chain saturated fatty acid (SFA), lauric acid, being highly oxidised, but for SFA generally, oxidation decreased as the chain length increased. PUFA and MUFA were fairly well oxidised [13]. In a more recent experiment, increasing the PUFA content of the diet was found to improve total fat oxidation following a meal high in saturated fat [14]. While total energy intake will always be the main dietary factor in weight loss, this and other research [15] suggests additional value with dietary PUFA. **Ketones** are a metabolic product that emerge with substantial fat oxidation, but levels are managed under normal healthy conditions (i.e. not severe cases of either starvation or diabetes). Excess dietary macronutrients are stored as fat, mainly in the form of triglycerides in adipose tissue, which contains numerous fat cells (adipocytes).

While ketones are produced by the body under certain conditions of fuel utilisation, **trans fatty acids** (TFA) are produced in foods when polyunsaturated and monounsaturated fatty acids are exposed to partial hydrogenation during manufacturing processes. There is also a small amount found in foods sourced from ruminant animals. The term 'trans' relates to the chemical structure of the fatty acid, where the hydrogen atoms are found on the opposite side of the double bond, unlike the natural 'cis' form, where they are on the same side. Cis fatty acids are bent at the double bond, whereas trans fatty acids are straight. As form follows function, these trans fatty acids (such as elaidic acid) act in similar way to saturated fatty acids [16].

Less abundant than triglycerides, **phospholipids** and sterols comprise the other major dietary lipids (Figure 5.4). Like triglycerides, the chemical structure of phospholipids also utilises a glycerol chain, but there are important differences. The inclusion of phosphorus and other attachments enables the molecule to sit between aqueous and lipid bilayers, so they have important structural functions across cell membranes. On a three carbon glycerol molecule, one end is water soluble (with a polar base group, linked with phosphate) and the other contains water insoluble lipid (non-polar fatty acids). Given this structure and function, phospholipids are ubiquitous in plant and animal food sources, delivering fatty acids as well as other compounds such as choline (in lecithin) and inositol.

Sterols have a very different structure from triglycerides and phospholipids as they contain ring-like chemical entities. This means they also have different functions that relate to a variety of processes in the body. Given the distinctive biology of plants and animals, it is not surprising that different forms of sterols are found in plant-sourced foods (phytosterols) and animal-sourced foods (cholesterol). High serum cholesterol levels are a risk factor for cardiovascular disease, but the pathophysiology is complex. Cholesterol levels reflect both dietary and endogenous sources, and the ability to balance cholesterol levels varies between individuals. Put simply, cholesterol is transported in the blood in lipoproteins—away from the tissues and back to the liver via high-density lipoprotein (HDL) or from the liver to tissues via low-density lipoprotein (LDL). Cholesterol balance is controlled in the body, but defects can occur, as seen in familial hypercholesterolaemia. Bile salts from the liver help to excrete cholesterol, with some reabsorption in the gut (and food components, such as fibres and plant sterols can affect this process). In line with its chemical structure, cholesterol has also been shown to play important roles in other areas of metabolism, including that related to sex hormones and vitamin D.

See Chapter 3 on beta oxidation.

Ketones
(or ketone bodies) metabolic by-products of fat oxidation.

Trans fatty acids
partially hydrogenated unsaturated fatty acids produced in manufacturing with similar effects as saturated fatty acids.

Phospholipids
glycerol moieties with water-soluble and water-insoluble (fatty acid) ends, such as lecithin.

See Chapter 3 on HDL and LDL.

Sterols
lipids with ring-based structures of carbon, hydrogen and oxygen. Cholesterol is found in animals and phytosterols are found in plants.

FIGURE 5.4   CHEMICAL STRUCTURES OF TRIGLYCERIDES, PHOSPHOLIPIDS AND CHOLESTEROL

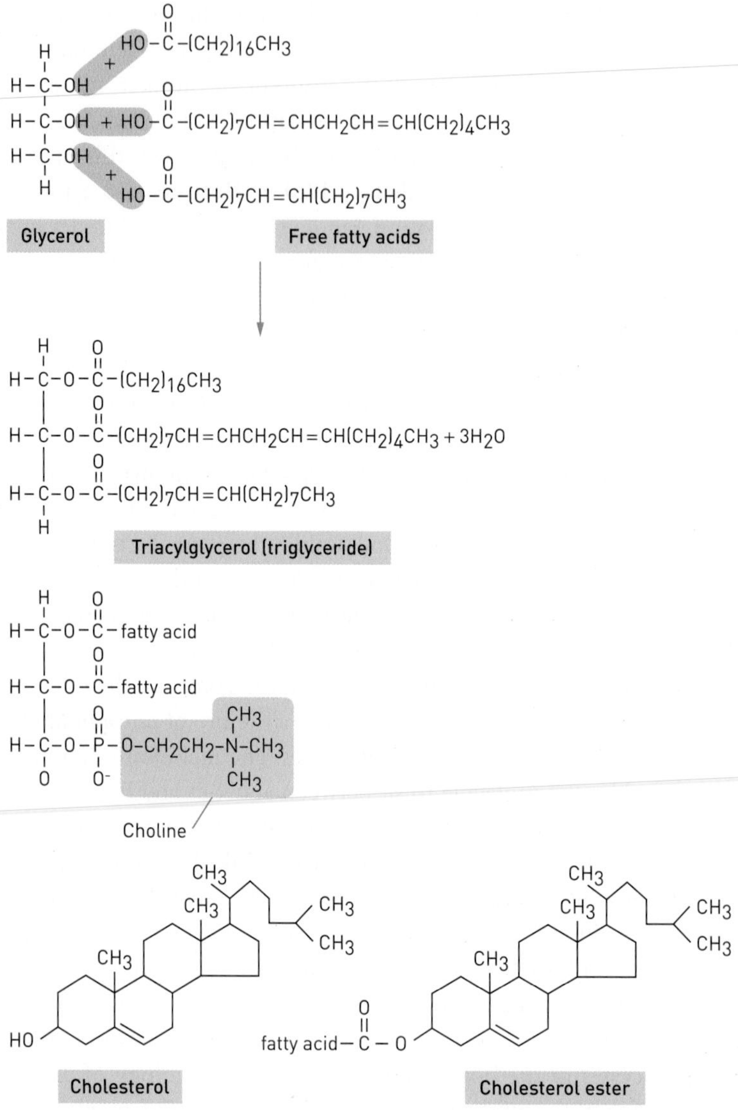

Source: C. M. Skeaff & J. Mann (2012). Chapter 4: Lipids. In J. Mann & S. Truswell (eds), *Essentials of Human Nutrition*, 4th edn. Oxford University Press, Incorporated

STOP AND THINK

- How does the chemical structure of fat relate to its function in the human body?
- What is the most common form of dietary fat, and how is it classified?
- What are the limitations of considering single fats or fatty acids in isolation from other nutrients and their food sources?

WHAT IS THE RELATIONSHIP BETWEEN DIETARY FATS AND HEALTH?

Following the early observations of the diet–cardiovascular disease relationship, guidance for optimising the relative amount and type of fat in the diet remains one of the most interesting areas of nutrition. The challenge of defining the best position for dietary fat, particularly in Western societies, becomes more complex as research contributes new knowledge from a broad platform of inquiry. This research ranges from cellular mechanisms to creating an ecological understanding of food and nutrients being delivered for a global population. From a practical perspective, however, it remains necessary to acknowledge the **nutritional interdependence** between nutrients, foods and whole diets [17]. A total diet delivers 100% of dietary energy, but this is delivered by foods with defined macronutrient composition. Changing foods can change dietary characteristics, including the relative proportion of macronutrients. For example, under iso-caloric conditions, when energy from dietary fat is reduced, the proportion of dietary carbohydrate and or protein must increase.

> **Nutritional interdependence**
> the consequence of total diets being comprised of individual foods, and foods being a source of nutrients.
>
> See Chapter 2 on critical review of study designs.

To consolidate the evidence for effects on human health, new methodological developments have helped to synthesise research conducted on all levels. This includes the critical review of study designs and their elements. In addition to the processes followed by dietary guidelines committees [18; 19] and food standards authorities [20], authoritative bodies such as the American Heart Association and the Academy of Nutrition and Dietetics have undertaken reviews and published position papers. Other groups have provided reviews addressing historical perspectives on where it all started [2], or called for extending attention to risk-related pathways beyond risk factors such as cholesterol levels [21].

The first consideration for dietary fat is meeting requirements for intakes of essential fatty acids. The National Health and Medical Research Council (NHMRC) has defined adequate intakes (AI) for LA, ALA and EPA/DHA/DPA for all age groups (Table 5.2). The values for AIs were based on median intakes within the population, as there was no apparent deficiency noted for LA and ALA, and there was a lack of studies indicating dose–response relationships for intakes of EPA/DHA and EPA [22].

The next consideration for health concerns the relationship between dietary fat and the risk of chronic lifestyle-related disease. There are a number of issues to consider here—for example, disease endpoints (such as cardiovascular disease, diabetes), biomarkers of disease (such as cholesterol levels), amount of fat, types of fatty acid and whole dietary patterns.

It is critical to note that the amount and relative proportion of fatty acids in the diet is a *total diet issue* (Figure 5.5). The total diet sets the context in which advice is made. This advice does not relate to the nutrient alone, nor even to a single food, although they are connected. For example, a low saturated fat diet means less saturated fat is consumed, and this is achieved by limiting foods that are high in saturated fat. The fundamental nutrition principle of balance must be appreciated.

The connection between nutrients, foods and diets creates challenges for evidence review. Given that reducing saturated fat means increasing another macronutrient in the diet, the position of saturated fat must be considered in light of the replacement nutrients. In practical terms, this means substantial changes in choices of foods (which deliver multiple nutrients) and shifts in dietary patterns (Figure 5.6).

TABLE 5.2   ADEQUATE INTAKE LEVELS FOR FATTY ACIDS

Age	Linoleic acid	α-linolenic acid	Total long chain n-3
Boys and girls			
1–3 years	5 g/day	0.5 g/day	40 mg/day
4–8 years	8 g/day	0.8 g/day	55 mg/day
Boys			
9–13 years	10 g/day	1.0 g/day	70 mg/day
14–18 years	12 g/day	1.2 g/day	125 mg/day
Girls			
9–13 years	8 g/day	0.8 g/day	70 mg/day
14–18 years	8 g/day	0.8 g/day	85 mg/day
Adults 19+ years			
Men	13 g/day	1.3 g/day	160 mg/day
Women	8 g/day	0.8 g/day	90 mg/day
Pregnancy			
14–18 years	10 g/day	1.0 g/day	110 mg/day
19–50 years	10 g/day	1.0 g/day	115 mg/day
Lactation			
14–18 years	12 g/day	1.2 g/day	140 mg/day
19–50 years	12 g/day	1.2 g/day	145 mg/day

Source: National Health and Medical Research Council (2006). *Nutrient Reference Values for Australia and New Zealand—Fats: total fat & fatty acids.* Canberra: NHMRC. © Commonwealth of Australia

FIGURE 5.5   MANIPULATING PROPORTIONS OF MACRONUTRIENTS PROVIDING TOTAL DIETARY ENERGY

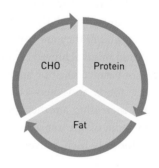

FIGURE 5.6   PROPORTIONS OF FAT IN THE DIET AND FOODS

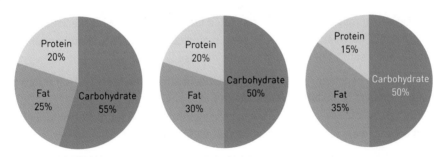

Source: Adapted and modified from (1) National Health and Medical Research Council (2015). Sample meal plans for men aged 19–50 years. Retrieved from: www.eatforhealth.gov.au/sites/default/files/content/adg_sample_meal_plan_men.pdf.
© Commonwealth of Australia

(2) National Health and Medical Research Council (2015). Sample meal plans for women aged 19–20 years. Retrieved from: www.eatforhealth.gov.au/sites/default/files/content/The%20Guidelines/adg_sample_meal_plan_women.pdf.
© Commonwealth of Australia

(3) Calculated using FoodWorks (Xyris Software Pty Ltd, Kenmore Hills, QLD, Australia, version 8, 2016)

» CASE 5.2

SATURATED FAT AND HEART DISEASE

In 2017 the Presidential Advisory of the American Heart Association addressed the question: What are the effects of dietary saturated fat (and its replacement by other nutrients) on cardiovascular disease? [3] The review addressed clinical trials and prospective cohort studies in humans using rigorous criteria for assessing causality [23]. It was noted that controversy had arisen in recent years because studies were not always in agreement on whether intakes of saturated fat increased the risk of cardiovascular disease.

However, when replacement nutrients were taken into account, the negative effects of saturated fat (SFA) were evident when SFA was replaced with polyunsaturated fat (PUFA), but not when replaced with carbohydrate (especially carbohydrate from refined grains). In trials that replaced SFA with PUFA, the risk of cardiovascular disease was reduced by about 30% [3]. The mechanism of action was a reduction in LDL-cholesterol levels, addressing a causal relationship with atherosclerosis that is recognised in clinical guidelines [24–26].

There were other important aspects of study design under consideration. Research was excluded if it was conducted over 50 years ago and the margarine contained trains fatty acids, and if there was low adherence to the dietary profiles being tested. A minimum two-year study duration was applied because it was noted that it takes about two years for tissues to equilibrate with the fatty acid levels in the diet [3]. Lifelong diet and body composition are further important considerations as they reflect the way diet has its effect in chronic disease. Results from studies where long-term diets differ from Western societies (i.e. high-energy, high saturated-fat diet) may indicate different associations with dietary factors, particularly if a single time point is taken, as in cross-sectional studies. Indeed, some heterogeneity has been noted across countries in global analyses of dietary intakes and risk of coronary heart disease. However, there is still a strong indication that non-optimal intakes of SFA, TFA and n-6PUFA contribute to estimated mortality [27].

Bearing in mind that nutrients are delivered in foods, the total diet must still be considered. Given that there are a multitude of other nutrients and dietary factors that can be implicated in the pathology of cardiovascular disease, it may be that a high saturated fat intake is also a marker of a poor-quality diet, with inadequate balance between nutrients. Research on dietary patterns will add to our understanding of the position of dietary saturated fat and in chronic disease [28; 29].

- Why is it important to consider replacement nutrients in strategies to reduce saturated fat?
- What does this mean in terms of foods and dietary patterns?
- How has the debate on saturated fat been both helpful and a source of potential confusion in determining optimal diets for prevention of cardiovascular disease?

The position taken by the Australian Dietary Guidelines is that foods containing saturated fats need to be limited, and food delivering unsaturated fats such as nuts and fish could be increased in the diet [18; 30]. Both the Lyon Heart Study [31] and the PREDIMED [32] trials demonstrated that a Mediterranean-style diet, which contained foods delivering substantial amounts of unsaturated fats, reduced the incidence of cardiovascular disease, but there were also cuisine elements in these interventions.

See Chapters 1, 2, 5 and 7 on the PREDIMED trial and Mediterranean diet.

Total diet is also important in managing diabetes, but the impact of saturated fat on the development of diabetes that may lead to cardiovascular disease has also been considered. Given the differential role of fatty acids in metabolic and signalling pathways associated with diabetes [7], saturated fat has also been implicated in the development of insulin resistance and diabetes [33]. The Finnish Diabetes Prevention Trial [34], which targeted a reduction in total fat and saturated fat in a lifestyle intervention, produced a 58% reduced risk of diabetes, an effect that was replicated in the later Diabetes Prevention Trial in the United States [35]. Finland has also conducted a population health program in which substantial dietary shifts were achieved including, but not limited to, the promotion of low saturated fat core foods (such as low saturated fat dairy products). Substantial decreases in population cholesterol levels and coronary heart disease mortality were subsequently observed [36]. Thus, while the total diet will always be central to the problem, saturated fat appears to consistently emerge as a nutrient of concern. Specific foods and the total diet still remain relevant because the observational and intervention research that informed this position involved converting total dietary intakes into nutrient characteristics.

STOP AND THINK

- Why is dietary fat implicated in the development of chronic disease in Western societies?
- How has evidence-based research advanced to better elucidate the impact of dietary fat on health?
- What other dietary aspects besides the types of fat are important for reducing cardiovascular disease risk and why?

WHAT ARE THE BEST FOOD CHOICES TO ENSURE HEALTHY INTAKES OF FAT?

There are a number of ways to address the fat composition of the diet. The first is to recognise animal- and plant-sourced foods that naturally contain a high proportion of fat, and in particular SFA or PUFA. Animal-sourced foods high in SFA include pork (lard) and beef (beef tallow and milk fat, concentrated in butter and cream), while vegetable sources are palm oil (including palm kernel oil) and coconut oil [3]. To reduce intakes from these sources requires avoidance of fat on meat, and replacing butter, palm oil and coconut oil with oils and spreads rich in PUFA or MUFA.

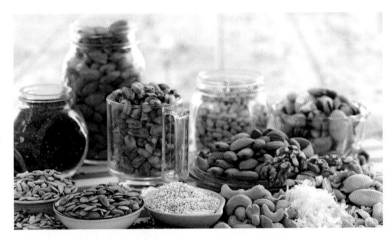

Foods with a high concentration of polyunsaturated fatty acids tend to be sourced from plants and fish. Unlike other nuts, which tend to be higher in MUFA, walnuts have a high proportion of PUFA, as LA and ALA. Note that the high PUFA content of this food also comes naturally with high levels of compounds with potent antioxidant activity, such as vitamin E and melatonin. Other foods with a high proportion of PUFA are vegetable oils (canola, corn, soybean, peanut, safflower, sunflower) and seeds. As polyunsaturated fatty acids tend to be unstable, manufacturing of safflower and sunflower oils has increased the MUFA component. Foods with a high concentration of MUFA also include olive oil, avocados and other tree nuts such as pecans, almonds, cashews, hazelnuts and pistachios [3].

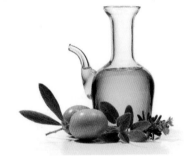

Creating shifts in the diet where SFA is replaced with PUFA will require more than simply avoiding these SFA-rich foods and including more PUFA-rich foods. This is because both types of fats are used for culinary purposes or ingredients in many food products. Evaluating the relative proportion of PUFA and SFA in the diet means assessing the contributions of a wide range of foods. Equally important is the influence of cuisine, in which fat-rich foods may be central. For example, olive oil is a key component of the Mediterranean diet, and the amount consumed would significantly influence the fatty acid profile of the diet [32]. Olive oil also delivers other important dietary components such as phenolic compounds that have a powerful antioxidant activity. Nuts are another key food in the Mediterranean diet, delivering fibre, fat-soluble vitamins and minerals and polyphenolic compounds in addition to fatty acids.

» CASE 5.3

VEGETABLES AND FAT

Understanding nutrition can be a complex task with so much detail at the food level alone. One way of making messages simple is to create categories that reduce the detail to manageable levels. In the case of food sources of saturated fat, a simple dichotomy of plant-sourced versus animal-sourced food helped to create a focus on areas where dietary saturated fat could be identified and reduced; however, translation is never so simple.

Coconut oil is a case in point. It is a vegetable oil but it has a high saturated fat content, making it less desirable as a culinary fat than, say, olive oil. Nevertheless, the plant nature of the food is worth considering further. Avocados, for example, were once considered with caution because of their fat content, but this was recognised as largely monounsaturated fat and therefore suitable within the confines of a balanced dietary intake. It also provided new culinary opportunities—for example, replacing saturated fat (e.g. butter) when spread on bread.

A systematic review of the benefits of coconut oil found eight clinical trials and 13 observational studies that examined effects on cardiovascular disease risk. The effect of coconut oil on LDL cholesterol appeared less than butter but still higher than unsaturated oils [37]. This means that the largely unsaturated plant oils currently available (olive oil, canola oil) remain superior and preferable. Translating this to practice implies a need to consider how much might be consumed in a total diet (implicating other foods) and the potential deleterious effects if use of coconut oil became widespread—for example, in creating an upsurge in the saturated fat profile of the overall dietary pattern (Table 5.3). The point is made that consumption of coconut in traditional dietary patterns does not lead to cardiovascular disease, but consumption in more complex dietary environments needs to be carefully considered [37].

- Why would the impact of the saturated fat in coconuts be different in a traditional diet (and environment) than in a Western society with an abundance of highly processed foods?
- If coconut oil were to be included in the diet, which foods would need to be removed to maintain fat balance within the diet? What are the implications for cuisine patterns?

TABLE 5.3   TOTAL FAT AND FATTY ACID CONTENT OF FOODS

Food	Serving size[1]	g of total fat per serve[3]	g of SFA per serve[3]	g of MUFA per serve[3]	g of PUFA fat per serve[3]
Almond (with skin)	30 g	16.41	1.11	10.76	3.84
Pine nuts (raw)	30 g	21.0	1.26	6.88	11.94
Walnuts (raw)	30 g	20.76	1.32	3.63	14.88
Sunflower seeds	30 g	15.3	1.29	2.95	10.35
Sunflower oil	7 g[2]	6.43	0.69	1.62	3.84
Olive oil	7 g[2]	6.43	0.99	4.58	0.56
Canola oil	7 g[2]	6.43	0.47	3.82	1.83
Polyunsaturated margarine	10 g[2]	8.05	1.6	2.45	3.66
Monounsaturated margarine	10 g[2]	6.59	1.46	3.16	1.64
Butter	10 g[2]	8.15	5.38	1.99	1.8
Coconut cream	75 mL[4]/~600 kJ[2]	14.47	13.05	0.50	0.075
Cream	40 mL[4]/~600 kJ[2]	14.36	9.2	3.49	0.56
Milk, skim	250 mL	0.25	0.25	0.075	0
Milk, reduced fat	250 mL	3.0	2.0	0.75	0
Milk, full cream	250 mL	8.75	5.75	2.3	0.25
Grilled beef rump steak (trimmed)	65–130 g	3.57–7.15	1.23–2.47	1.60–3.21	0.32–0.65
Roast leg lamb (trimmed)	65–130 g	5.72–11.44	2.27–4.55	2.24–4.47	0.52–1.04

Food	Serving size[1]	g of total fat per serve[3]	g of SFA per serve[3]	g of MUFA per serve[3]	g of PUFA fat per serve[3]
Roast leg pork	65–130 g	6.95–13.91	2.47–4.94	3.07–6.15	1.04–2.08
Grilled chicken breast (no skin)	65–130 g	1.62–3.25	0.52–1.04	0.77–1.55	0.19–0.39
Pink salmon (canned, drained)	1 small can (80 g)	5.44	1.2	1.90	1.68

[1]Based on the Australian Dietary Guidelines [18].
[2]Based on modelling of the Australian Dietary Guidelines [38].
[3]Calculated from *NUTTAB 2010* [39].
[4]Calculated using FoodWorks (Xyris Software Pty Ltd, Kenmore Hills, QLD, Australia, version 8, 2016).

A number of dietary patterns have been promoted to meet the needs for cardiovascular health. For lowering LDL cholesterol and blood pressure, the American Heart Association recommends a pattern based on vegetables and fruits, wholegrains, nuts, legumes, poultry and fish, and using low-fat dairy products and vegetable oils referred to as 'non-tropical' (not palm or coconut) [40]. As these foods contribute towards the total diet, the optimal amounts are dependent on energy (kilojoule/calorie) requirements.

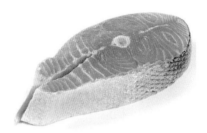

Most people do not limit their intakes to these food categories. In Australia, for example, it has been estimated that 35% of energy intake comes from 'discretionary food' [41]. These foods include cereal and vegetable products produced with saturated fats. In order to create the desired shift in dietary fat profile, a whole range of foods need to be displaced by the desired core foods (Table 5.4).

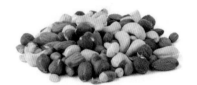

TABLE 5.4   FOOD ALTERNATIVES TO REDUCE DIETARY SATURATED FAT

Food to displace	Healthy alternative
Fried vegetables, hot chips, prepared with oils and sauces containing saturated fat	Fresh or frozen vegetables, cooked with water, herbs and spices and/or extra virgin olive oil
Fruit pies	Fresh or frozen fruit
Commercial cakes, biscuits, muffins	Wholegrain bread, fruit bread
Fried and battered fish and chicken	Grilled, baked fish, skinless chicken
Sausages, processed meats	Lean meat
Commercial snack bars, chips	Nuts, seeds, plain popcorn
Butter, coconut oil, palm oil, hard margarines	Olive oil, canola oil, soft margarines

Moving from food choices to cuisines, menus and meals is another major step in translation. This context layers in additional factors such as taste, texture, availability, traditional recipes and the social conditions for eating, to name a few. Given the variation in food combinations and meal situations, ideal macronutrient intakes may not occur in each meal, but patterns of usual choices can place the total diet in the right space (Table 5.5).

TRY IT YOURSELF

Write down all the foods you ate in the past 24 hours. What changes do you think are necessary to improve the fat quality of your diet?

TABLE 5.5   EXAMPLES OF HEALTHY FOOD COMBINATIONS

Meal suggestion	Food combinations
Breakfast	Rolled oats, mixed wholegrains, topped with nuts, seeds, fresh fruit, yoghurt
Breakfast	Green leafy vegetables, tomatoes, onions, mushrooms cooked in olive oil, topped with poached egg
Breakfast or lunch	Wholegrain seeded sourdough bread topped with tomatoes, onions and mashed sardines; or avocado, ricotta cheese and green leafy vegetables or herbs
Lunch	Herb- and nut-encrusted fish sautéed in olive oil and served with salad vegetables, dressed in citrus juice and olive oil
Lunch	Mixed vegetables sautéed in olive oil with added herbs and topped with cheese
Dinner	Beans and lean meat cooked with tomatoes, onions, capsicum and other vegetables in unsaturated vegetable oil and added herbs and spices
Dinner	Stir-fried vegetables and beans, tofu, chicken or lean meats served with rice or noodles (preferably wholegrain)
Light meal	Sandwiches, wraps, rolls, flat breads (preferably wholegrain) with avocado, nut, olive or unsaturated vegetable oil spreads, including combinations of salad or cooked vegetables, beans, fish, lean meats, egg, nuts, hard sliced fruit

>> RESEARCH AT WORK

DIETARY ALA, FISH OILS AND FISH CONSUMPTION

The requirements for ALA, EPA and DHA remain under scientific investigation, particularly as omega-3 fatty acids have apparent cardio-protective roles and the balance between plant and fish sources will be important to understand. Fish provide the main dietary source of EPA and DHA, and plant foods such as walnuts provide ALA. This study examined data from the PREDIMED trial to examine the relationship between meeting dietary requirements for these fatty acids and mortality from all causes and cardiovascular disease [42].

The PREDIMED trial was a large Mediterranean diet study targeting cardiovascular disease prevention [32]. The study was conducted in Spain, where people ate a lot of fish, and the participants who started in the trial did not have established cardiovascular disease. Also, one of the supplemented foods in the trial was walnuts (ALA intake correlated highly with walnut consumption). The analysis reported here on data from over 7000 people referred to the recommendations of the International Society for the Study of Fatty Acids and Lipids (ISSFAL) for ALA (0.7% energy) and EPA+DHA (≥500 mg/day).

When examining risk parameters for mortality, the researchers found that the group who met the recommendations for both types of fatty acid showed the greatest reduction in deaths from all causes. However, deaths from heart disease were related to meeting the requirements for EPA+DHA. The authors concluded that the two types of fatty acids are partners rather than competitors in reducing mortality.

Importantly, they noted that the sources of ALA (walnuts and extra virgin olive oil) were also sources of phytochemicals with antioxidant and anti-inflammatory properties, which may serve to address other mechanisms associated with ageing and mortality.

The main target for achieving optimal fatty acid intakes is also a dietary pattern that comprises foods with a combined nutrient intake that meets all requirements. The Australian Guide to Healthy Eating [43] was developed based on dietary modelling that took into account all the required parameters [38]. Ultimately, it is the total diet that counts, but meeting fatty acid requirements and consuming the various types in the best-known proportions is achievable once the types of foods can be adequately recognised and then translated to actual choices in everyday life.

STOP AND THINK

- How would you know if the fatty acid content of your diet was meeting recommended intakes?
- Whys does some saturated fat need to be in the diet?
- How do food combinations reflect trends in cuisines, and what drives the changes?

SUMMARY

- The main chemical structure of dietary fat is triacylglycerol or triglyceride, which delivers fatty acids on a glycerol chain. The fatty acids may be saturated, monounsaturated or polyunsaturated in nature, and this has implications for functional roles within the body.
- Fat is the most energy-dense nutrient, delivering about twice the energy of protein and carbohydrate per gram, but different types of fat (lipids) also serve important roles in cell structure, cell signalling, genetic expression and various metabolic and immunological pathways.
- Linolenic and alpha linoleic acids cannot be made by the body and must be provided in the diet. Deficiency is rare and an adequate intake (AI) level has been defined for Australians.
- A dietary pattern that has a high overall intake of saturated fatty acids is implicated in high LDL cholesterol levels and higher rates of cardiovascular disease, particularly in populations with traditional food supplies high in energy and saturated fat.
- Given the Australian food supply, dietary patterns that achieve the desired balance in fatty acid intakes are aligned with the Australian Guide to Healthy Eating.

PATHWAYS TO PRACTICE

- Understanding the relationships between dietary fat intakes and health is a central area in healthcare for the community, particularly in relation to healthy ageing and the development of cardiometabolic disorders.
- At a population level, work that involves strategies promoting food choices targeting lower intakes of saturated fat (Table 5.3) in the context of a broader intake of well-prepared meals is warranted.
- At a clinical level, manipulating dietary fat as a preventive or adjunct therapy in primary care requires skilled dietary assessment and a detailed knowledge of food composition and cuisine applied in the context of professional counselling for behaviour change. Accredited practising dietitians are trained for this purpose.

DISCUSSION QUESTIONS

1 Why is chemical structure important in understanding the various roles of dietary fat?
2 Why has saturated fat emerged as problematic in Western societies?
3 How does diet fit with cholesterol-lowering medications?
4 How difficult is it to consume a diet with a fatty acid profile that would protect health in most people?

USEFUL WEBLINKS

Australian Guide to Healthy Eating tool:
   www.eatforhealth.gov.au/page/eat-health-calculators/calculated/1504843086

Eat for Health:
   www.eatforhealth.gov.au

Food Composition Tables—Food Standards Australia New Zealand:
   www.foodstandards.gov.au/science/monitoringnutrients/Pages/default.aspx

Food Standards Australia New Zealand:
   www.foodstandards.gov.au

Health Direct:
   www.healthdirect.gov.au

Nutrient Reference Values for Australia and New Zealand—Fats: Total fat and fatty acids:
   www.nrv.gov.au/nutrients/fats-total-fat-fatty-acids

Nutrient Reference Values for Australia and New Zealand—Macronutrient Balance:
   www.nrv.gov.au/chronic-disease/macronutrient-balance

FURTHER READING

Abdullah, M. M. H., Jew, S. & Jones, P. J. H. (2017). Health benefits and evaluation of healthcare cost savings if oils rich in monounsaturated fatty acids were substituted for conventional dietary oils in the United States. *Nutrition Reviews*, 75(3), 163–74. doi:10.1093/nutrit/nuw062

Bolhuis, D. P., Costanzo, A., Newman, L. P. & Keast, R. S. (2016). Salt promotes passive overconsumption of dietary fat in humans. *Journal of Nutrition*, 146(4), 838–45. doi:10.3945/jn.115.226365

Covas, M. I., De La Torre, R. & Fitó, M. (2015). Virgin olive oil: a key food for cardiovascular risk protection. *British Journal of Nutrition*, 113(S2), S19–S28. doi:10.1017/S0007114515000136

Dias, C. B., Wood, L. G. & Garg, M. L. (2016). Effects of dietary saturated and n-6 polyunsaturated fatty acids on the incorporation of long-chain n-3 polyunsaturated fatty acids into blood lipids. *European Journal of Clinical Nutrition*, 70(7), 812–18. doi:10.1038/ejcn.2015.213

Drewnowski, A. (2015). The carbohydrate-fat problem: can we construct a healthy diet based on dietary guidelines? *Advances in Nutrition: An International Review Journal*, 6(3), 318S–325S. doi:10.3945/an.114.006973

Dwyer, J. T., Rubin, K. H., Fritsche, K. L., Psota, T. L., Liska, D. J., Harris, W. S., ... Lyle, B. J. (2016). Creating the future of evidence-based nutrition recommendations: case studies from lipid research. *Advances in Nutrition: An International Review Journal*, 7(4), 747–55. doi:10.3945/an.115.010926

Emerson, S. R., Kurti, S. P., Harms, C. A., Haub, M. D., Melgarejo, T., Logan, C. & Rosenkranz, S. K. (2017). Magnitude and timing of the postprandial inflammatory response to a high-fat meal in healthy adults: a systematic review. *Advances in Nutrition: An International Review Journal*, 8(2), 213–25. doi:10.3945/an.116.014431

Ericson, U., Hellstrand, S., Brunkwall, L., Schulz, C. A., Sonestedt, E., Wallström, P., ... Orho-Melander, M. (2015). Food sources of fat may clarify the inconsistent role of dietary fat intake for incidence of type 2 diabetes. *American Journal of Clinical Nutrition*, 101(5), 1065–80. doi:10.3945/ajcn.114.103010

Jakobsen, M. U., Madsen, L., Skjoth, F., Berentzen, T. L., Halkjær, J., Tjonneland, A., ... Overvad, K. (2017). Dietary intake and adipose tissue content of long-chain n-3 PUFAs and subsequent 5-y change in body weight and waist circumference. *American Journal of Clinical Nutrition*, 105(5), 1148–57. doi:10.3945/ajcn.116.140079

Krishnan, S., Steffen, L. M., Paton, C. M. & Cooper, J. A. (2017). Impact of dietary fat composition on prediabetes: a 12-year follow-up study. *Public Health Nutrition*, 20(9), 1617–26. doi:10.1017/S1368980016003669

Lackey, D. E., Lazaro, R. G., Li, P., Johnson, A., Hernandez-Carretero, A., Weber, N., ... Osborn, O. (2016). The role of dietary fat in obesity-induced insulin resistance. *American Journal of Physiology—Endocrinology and Metabolism*, 311(6), E989–E997. doi:10.1152/ajpendo.00323.2016

Li, K., McNulty, B. A., Tiernery, A. M., Devlin, N. F. C., Joyce, T., Leite, J. C., ... Nugent, A. P. (2016). Dietary fat intakes in Irish adults in 2011: how much has changed in 10 years? *British Journal of Nutrition*, 115(10), 1798–1809. doi:10.1017/S0007114516000787

Ludwig, D. S. (2016). Lowering the bar on the low-fat diet. *JAMA—Journal of the American Medical Association*, 316(20), 2087–8. doi:10.1001/jama.2016.15473

McClements, D. J. (2015). Reduced-fat foods: the complex science of developing diet-based strategies for tackling overweight and obesity. *Advances in Nutrition: An International Review Journal*, 6(3), 338S–52S. doi:10.3945/an.114.006999

Morio, B., Fardet, A., Legrand, P. & Lecerf, J.-M. (2016). Involvement of dietary saturated fats, from all sources or of dairy origin only, in insulin resistance and type 2 diabetes. *Nutrition Reviews*, 74(1), 33–47. doi:10.1093/nutrit/nuv043

Naughton, S. S., Mathai, M. L., Hryciw, D. H. & McAinch, A. J. (2015). Australia's nutrition transition 1961–2009: a focus on fats. *British Journal of Nutrition*, 114(3), 337–46. doi:10.1017/S0007114515001907

Navarro, S. L., Neuhouser, M. L., Cheng, T. Y. D., Tinker, L. F., Shikany, J. M., Snetselaar, L., ... Lampe, J. W. (2016). The interaction between dietary fiber and fat and risk of colorectal cancer in the Women's Health Initiative. *Nutrients*, 8(12).

Nettleton, J. A., Lovegrove, J. A., Mensink, R. P. & Schwab, U. (2016). Dietary fatty acids: is it time to change the recommendations? *Annals of Nutrition and Metabolism*, 68(4), 249–57. doi:10.1159/000446865

Olvera, F. M. R., Hernández, M. A. M., Mehta, R. & Salinas, C. A. A. (2017). Setting the lipid component of the diet: a work in process. *Advances in Nutrition: An International Review Journal*, 8(1), 165S–172S. doi:10.3945/an.116.013672

Reed, D. R. & Xia, M. B. (2015). Recent advances in fatty acid perception and genetics. *Advances in Nutrition: An International Review Journal*, 6(3), 353S–360S. doi:10.3945/an.114.007005

Sánchez-Tainta, A., Zazpe, I., Bes-Rastrollo, M., Salas-Salvadó, J., Bullo, M., Sorlí, J. V., ... Martínez-González, M. A. (2016). Nutritional adequacy according to carbohydrates and fat quality. *European Journal of Nutrition*, 55(1), 93–106. doi:10.1007/s00394-014-0828-3

Sayon-Orea, C., Carlos, S. & Martínez- González, M. A. (2015). Does cooking with vegetable oils increase the risk of chronic diseases?: a systematic review. *British Journal of Nutrition*, 113(S2), S36–S48. doi:10.1017/S0007114514002931

Simopoulos, A. (2016). An increase in the omega-6/omega-3 fatty acid ratio increases the risk for obesity. *Nutrients*, 8(3), 128.

Storlien, L. H., Lam, Y. Y., Wu, B. J., Tapsell, L. C. & Jenkins, A. B. (2016). Effects of dietary fat subtypes on glucose homeostasis during pregnancy in rats. *Nutrition & Metabolism*, 13(1), 58. doi:10.1186/s12986-016-0117-7

Storlien, L. H., Tapsell, L. C. & Calvert, G. D. (2000). Role of dietary factors: macronutrients. *Nutrition Reviews*, 58(3 Pt 2), S7–9.

Szajewska, H. & Szajewski, T. (2016). Saturated fat controversy: importance of systematic reviews and meta-analyses. *Critical Reviews in Food Science and Nutrition*, 56(12), 1947–51. doi:10.1080/10408398.2015.1018037

Tapsell, L. C. (2014). Foods and food components in the Mediterranean diet: supporting overall effects. *BMC Medicine*, 12(1), 100. doi:10.1186/1741-7015-12-100

Tapsell, L. C., Batterham, M. J., Charlton, K. E., Neale, E. P., Probst, Y. C., O'Shea, J. E., ... Louie, J. C. Y. (2013). Foods, nutrients or whole diets: effects of targeting fish and LCn3PUFA consumption in a 12mo weight loss trial. *BMC Public Health*, 13, 1231. doi:10.1186/1471-2458-13-1231

Tapsell, L., Batterham, M., Huang, X. F., Tan, S. Y., Teuss, G., Charlton, K., ... Warensjö, E. (2010). Short term effects of energy restriction and dietary fat sub-type on weight loss and disease risk factors. *Nutrition, Metabolism and Cardiovascular Diseases*, 20(5), 317–25. doi: https://doi.org/10.1016/j.numecd.2009.04.007

Tapsell, L. C., Batterham, M. J., Teuss, G., Tan, S. Y., Dalton, S., Quick, C. J., ... Charlton, K. E. (2009). Long-term effects of increased dietary polyunsaturated fat from walnuts on metabolic parameters in type II diabetes. *European Journal of Clinical Nutrition*, 63(8), 1008–15.

Vallgårda, S., Holm, L. & Jensen, J. D. (2015). The Danish tax on saturated fat: why it did not survive. *European Journal of Clinical Nutrition*, 69(2), 223–6. doi:10.1038/ejcn.2014.224

Vessby, B., Uusitupa, M., Hermansen, K., Riccardi, G., Rivellese, A. A., Tapsell, L. C., ... Storlien, L. H. (2001). Substituting dietary saturated for monounsaturated fat impairs insulin sensitivity in healthy men and women: the KANWU Study. *Diabetologia*, 44(3), 312–19.

Vieira, S. A., McClements, D. J. & Decker, E. A. (2015). Challenges of utilizing healthy fats in foods. *Advances in Nutrition: An International Review Journal*, 6(3), 309S–317S.

Wang, D. D. & Hu, F. B. (2017). Dietary fat and risk of cardiovascular disease: recent controversies and advances. *Annual Review of Nutrition*, 37(1), 423–46. doi:10.1146/annurev-nutr-071816-064614

REFERENCES

1   D. Kritchevsky (1998). History of recommendations to the public about dietary fat. *Journal of Nutrition*, 128(2), 449S–452S.

2   K. D. Pett, J. Kahn, W. C. Willett & D. L. Katz (2017). *Ancel Keys and the Seven Countries Study: An evidence based response to revisionist histories. White paper commissioned by the True Health Initiative*. The True Health Initiative. Retrieved from: www.truehealthinitiative.org/wordpress/wp-content/uploads/2017/07/SCS-White-Paper.THI_.8-1-17.pdf.

3   F. M. Sacks, A. H. Lichtenstein, J. H.Y. Wu, L. J. Appel, M. A. Creager, P. M. Kris-Etherton, ... L. V.Van Horn (2017). Dietary fats and cardiovascular disease: a presidential advisory from the American Heart Association. *Circulation*. doi:10.1161/cir.0000000000000510

4   L. H. Storlien, Y. Y. Lam, B. J. Wu, L. C. Tapsell & A. B. Jenkins (2016). Effects of dietary fat subtypes on glucose homeostasis during pregnancy in rats. *Nutrition & Metabolism*, 13(1), 58. doi:10.1186/s12986-016-0117-7

5   D. R. Jacobs, M. D. Gross & L. C. Tapsell (2009). Food synergy: an operational concept for understanding nutrition. *American Journal of Clinical Nutrition*, 89(5), 1543S–1548S. doi:10.3945/ajcn.2009.26736B

6   A. J. Hulbert, N. Turner, L. H. Storlien & P. L. Else (2005). Dietary fats and membrane function: implications for metabolism and disease. *Biological Reviews*, 80(1), 155–69. doi:10.1017/S1464793104006578

7   L. H. Storlien, A. J. Hulbert & P. L. Else (1998). Polyunsaturated fatty acids, membrane function and metabolic diseases such as diabetes and obesity. *Current Opinion in Clinical Nutrition & Metabolic Care*, 1(6), 559–63.

8   D. Mozaffarian & J. H.Y. Wu (2011). Omega-3 fatty acids and cardiovascular disease: effects on risk factors, molecular pathways, and clinical events. *Journal of the American College of Cardiology*, 58(20), 2047–67. doi:https://doi.org/10.1016/j.jacc.2011.06.063

9   A. P. Simopoulos (2002). The importance of the ratio of omega-6/omega-3 essential fatty acids. *Biomedicine & Pharmacotherapy*, 56(8), 365–79. doi:https://doi.org/10.1016/S0753-3322(02)00253-6

10 W. C. Willett (2007). The role of dietary n-6 fatty acids in the prevention of cardiovascular disease. *Journal of Cardiovascular Medicine*, 8, S42–S45. doi:10.2459/01.jcm.0000289275.72556.13

11 M.T. Nakamura & T. Y. Nara (2004). Structure, function, and dietary regulation of Δ6, Δ5, and Δ9 desaturases. *Annual Review of Nutrition*, 24(1), 345–76. doi:10.1146/annurev.nutr.24.121803.063211

12 B. S. Mühlhäusler (2017). Variability in the cardiometabolic effects of ω-3 long-chain PUFAs: background diet, timing, and genetics. *American Journal of Clinical Nutrition*, 105(5), 1029–30. doi:10.3945/ajcn.117.155739

13 J. P. DeLany, M. M. Windhauser, C. M. Champagne & G. A. Bray (2000). Differential oxidation of individual dietary fatty acids in humans. *American Journal of Clinical Nutrition*, 72(4), 905–11.

14 J. L. Stevenson, M. K. Miller, H. E. Skillman, C. M. Paton & J. A. Cooper (2017). A PUFA-rich diet improves fat oxidation following saturated fat-rich meal. *European Journal of Nutrition*, 56(5), 1845–57. doi:10.1007/s00394-016-1226-9

15 L. C. Tapsell, M. J. Batterham, G. Teuss, S. Y. Tan, S. Dalton, C. J. Quick, ... K. E. Charlton (2009). Long-term effects of increased dietary polyunsaturated fat from walnuts on metabolic parameters in type II diabetes. *European Journal of Clinical Nutrition*, 63(8), 1008–15.

16 A. H. Lichtenstein (2014). Dietary trans fatty acids and cardiovascular disease risk: past and present. *Current Atherosclerosis Reports*, 16(8), 433. doi:10.1007/s11883-014-0433-1

17 L. C. Tapsell, E. P. Neale, A. Satija & F. B. Hu (2016). Foods, nutrients, and dietary patterns: interconnections and implications for dietary guidelines. *Advances in Nutrition: An International Review Journal*, 7(3), 445–54. doi:10.3945/an.115.011718

18 National Health and Medical Research Council (2013). *Australian Dietary Guidelines*. Canberra: NHMRC.

19 US Department of Health and Human Services & US Department of Agriculture (2015). *2015–2020 Dietary Guidelines for Americans*, 8th edn. Retrieved from: https://health.gov/dietaryguidelines/2015/resources/2015-2020_Dietary_Guidelines.pdf.

20 Food Standards Australia New Zealand (2018). Our science. Retrieved from: www.foodstandards.gov.au/science/Pages/default.aspx.

21 D. Mozaffarian (2016). Dietary and policy priorities for cardiovascular disease, diabetes, and obesity: a comprehensive review. *Circulation*, 133(2), 187–225. doi:10.1161/circulationaha.115.018585

22 National Health and Medical Research Council (2014). *Nutrient Reference Values for Australia and New Zealand—Fats: Total fat and fatty acids*. Canberra: NHMRC.

23 A. B. Hill (1965). The environment and disease: association or causation? *Proceedings of the Royal Society of Medicine*, 58(5), 295–300.

24 R. H. Eckel, J. M. Jakicic, J. D. Ard, J. M. de Jesus, N. H. Miller, V. S. Hubbard, ... S. Z. Yanovski (2014). 2013 AHA/ACC guideline on lifestyle management to reduce cardiovascular risk. *A Report of the American College of Cardiology/American Heart Association Task Force on Practice Guidelines*, 129(25 suppl. 2), S76–S99. doi:10.1161/01.cir.0000437740.48606.d1

25 Department of Health and Human Services & US Department of Agriculture (2015). *Scientific Report of the 2015 Dietary Guidelines Advisory Committee*. Washington, DC: Department of Health and Human Services, US Department of Agriculture. Retrieved from: https://health.gov/dietaryguidelines/2015-scientific-report/pdfs/scientific-report-of-the-2015-dietary-guidelines-advisory-committee.pdf.

26 T. A. Jacobson, K. C. Maki, C. E. Orringer, P. H. Jones, P. Kris-Etherton, G. Sikand, ... W. V. Brown (2015). National Lipid Association recommendations for patient-centered management of dyslipidemia: part 2. *Journal of Clinical Lipidology*, 9(6), S1–S122.e121. doi:10.1016/j.jacl.2015.09.002

27 Q. Wang, A. Afshin, M. Y. Yakoob, G. M. Singh, C. D. Rehm, S. Khatibzadeh, ... D. Mozaffarian (2016). Impact of nonoptimal intakes of saturated, polyunsaturated, and trans fat on global burdens of coronary heart disease. *Journal of the American Heart Association*, 5(1). doi:10.1161/jaha.115.002891

28 R. J. de Souza, A. Mente, A. Maroleanu, A. I. Cozma, V. Ha, T. Kishibe, ... S. S. Anand (2015). Intake of saturated and trans unsaturated fatty acids and risk of all cause mortality, cardiovascular disease, and type 2 diabetes: systematic review and meta-analysis of observational studies. *British Medical Journal*, 351. doi:10.1136/bmj.h3978

29 D. I. Givens & S. S. Soedamah-Muthu (2016). Dairy fat: does it increase or reduce the risk of cardiovascular disease? *American Journal of Clinical Nutrition*, 104(5), 1191–2. doi:10.3945/ajcn.116.144766

30 National Health and Medical Research Council (2011). *A Review of the Evidence to Address Targeted Questions to Inform the Revision of the Australian Dietary Guidelines: Evidence statements*. Canberra: NHMRC.

31 M. de Lorgeril, P. Salen, J.-L. Martin, I. Monjaud, J. Delaye & N. Mamelle (1999). Mediterranean diet, traditional risk factors, and the rate of cardiovascular complications after myocardial infarction. *Final Report of the Lyon Diet Heart Study*, 99(6), 779–85. doi:10.1161/01.cir.99.6.779

32 R. Estruch, E. Ros, J. Salas-Salvadó, M.-I. Covas, D. Corella, F. Arós, … M. A. Martínez-González (2018). Primary prevention of cardiovascular disease with a Mediterranean diet supplemented with extra-virgin olive oil or nuts. *New England Journal of Medicine*, 378(25), e34. doi:10.1056/NEJMoa1800389

33 B. Vessby, M. Uusitupa, K. Hermansen, G. Riccardi, A. A. Rivellese, L. C. Tapsell, … L. H. Storlien (2001). Substituting dietary saturated for monounsaturated fat impairs insulin sensitivity in healthy men and women: the KANWU Study. *Diabetologia*, 44(3), 312–19.

34 J. Tuomilehto, J. Lindström, J. G. Eriksson, T. T. Valle, H. Hämäläinen, P. Ilanne-Parikka, … M. Uusitupa (2001). Prevention of type 2 diabetes mellitus by changes in lifestyle among subjects with impaired glucose tolerance. *New England Journal of Medicine*, 344(18), 1343–50. doi:10.1056/nejm200105033441801

35 Diabetes Prevention Program Research Group (2002). Reduction in the incidence of type 2 diabetes with lifestyle intervention or metformin. *New England Journal of Medicine*, 346(6), 393–403. doi:10.1056/NEJMoa012512

36 P. Pietinen, E. Vartiainen, R. Seppänen, A. Aro & P. Puska (1996). Changes in diet in Finland from 1972 to 1992: impact on coronary heart disease risk. *Preventive Medicine*, 25(3), 243–50. doi:https://doi.org/10.1006/pmed.1996.0053

37 L. Eyres, M. F. Eyres, A. Chisholm & R. C. Brown (2016). Coconut oil consumption and cardiovascular risk factors in humans. *Nutrition Reviews*, 74(4), 267–80. doi:10.1093/nutrit/nuw002

38 National Health and Medical Research Council (2011). *A Modelling System to Inform the Revision of the Australian Guide to Healthy Eating*. Canberra: NHMRC.

39 Food Standards Australia New Zealand (2012). *NUTTAB 2010*. Canberra: FSANZ.

40 L. Van Horn, J. A. S. Carson, L. J. Appel, L. E. Burke, C. Economos, W. Karmally, … P. Kris-Etherton (2016). Recommended dietary pattern to achieve adherence to the American Heart Association/American College of Cardiology (AHA/ACC) guidelines: a scientific statement from the American Heart Association. *Circulation*. doi:10.1161/cir.0000000000000462

41 Australian Bureau of Statistics (2014). *Australian Health Survey: Nutrition First results—Foods and nutrients, 2011–12—Discretionary food*. Canberra: ABS.

42 A. Sala-Vila, M. Guasch-Ferré, F. B. Hu, A. Sánchez-Tainta, M. Bulló, M. Serra-Mir, … E. Ros (2016). Dietary α-linolenic acid, marine ω-3 fatty acids, and mortality in a population with high fish consumption: findings from the PREvención con DIeta MEDiterránea (PREDIMED) Study. *Journal of the American Heart Association*, 5(1). doi:10.1161/jaha.115.002543

43 National Health and Medical Research Council (2013). *Australian Guide to Healthy Eating*. Canberra: NHMRC.

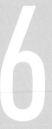

CHAPTER 6

PROTEIN: MAJOR COMPONENTS OF ANIMAL FOODS, LEGUMES, NUTS AND SEEDS

LINDA TAPSELL

CHAPTER OBJECTIVES

This chapter will enable the reader to:

- describe the chemical structure of protein and the roles of amino acids and proteins in the human body
- discuss the relative effects of dietary protein on health and disease
- identify the best food and beverage choices to ensure healthy intakes of protein.

KEY TERMS

Amino acids	Protein
High-protein diets	Protein-rich foods

KEY POINTS

- Protein is a macronutrient that is broken down into peptides and amino acids that address fundamental roles in human biology.
- The health effects of protein are addressed by meeting requirements to maintain nitrogen balance in the body and providing a proportion of protein in the diet that is associated with optimal health.
- Protein-rich foods are derived from animal and plant sources, which also deliver other important micronutrients, notably iron and calcium.

OXFORD UNIVERSITY PRESS

INTRODUCTION

Dietary protein is a macronutrient made up of amino acids that are needed for maintaining body composition and essential functions. Many of the structural components of the human body, such as muscle, are based on protein and are subject to regular turnover, but this reflects the 'tip of the iceberg' in understanding the role of protein in the human body, which is extensive (Table 6.1). The body itself produces protein through a complex system linked to genetic expression. Dietary protein needs to meet the requirements for protein turnover and growth in the human body, but not all amino acids are essential.

TABLE 6.1   RANGE OF FUNCTIONS OF PROTEIN IN THE HUMAN BODY

Structural roles	Facilitation of transport and communication	Barrier and immune functions	Enzymatic functions
Skeletal and muscle tissues, skin, epithelia, connective tissue	Plasma transport (e.g. albumin, transferrin, apolipiproteins)	Defence structures (e.g. keratin (hair), skin, tears, mucin)	Functional processes (e.g. digestion, clotting)
Cellular architecture	Hormonal systems (e.g. insulin, glucagon, growth hormone)	Inflammation and immune responses	Metabolic pathways (e.g. glycolysis, protein synthesis, citric acid and urea cycles)
	Intracellular communications (receptors)		

The scientific understanding of protein is very complex, working from molecular levels through to protein balance in the body and how food sources of protein and other nutrients serve to maintain that balance and enhance functionality. Beyond the individual, there are also ecological perspectives on the delivery of protein to populations and the implications this has for the relationship between humans and their environment. Translating across these levels is challenging, but it also reflects the breadth and depth of nutrition as an interdisciplinary science.

The protein content of foods will reflect the physiology and metabolism of the original plant or animal that forms the basis of the food [1; 2]. The protein content of this original food will be reflected in its protein content. Thus, some foods are higher in protein than others and the types of amino acids present in those foods will vary. The media may espouse various high-protein diets for weight loss and the use of protein-rich supplements in sports, but the scientific evidence for these approaches is often limiting. On the other hand, ensuring adequate intakes of protein is an important public health measure, with implications for the types of foods that are available and the dietary combinations that are encouraged. This chapter begins with the basic chemistry of protein, considers the health implications of protein consumption and identifies food sources of protein in the Australian diet.

Visit Oxford Ascend for more on protein.

STOP AND THINK

- Why is protein a fundamental macronutrient in diet?
- How has protein come to be referred to in health debates in an everyday sense?
- What would a discerning individual need to know to be able to evaluate information on protein and make food choices informed by sound science?

WHAT IS THE STRUCTURE AND FUNCTION OF PROTEIN IN HUMAN HEALTH?

Amino acids

structural units of protein, based on a carbon skeleton, with attachments of hydrogen, oxygen and nitrogen. Some (cysteine and methionine) also contain sulphur (S).

Protein is a macromolecule or polymer made up of amino acid units. Like the building blocks of carbohydrates and fats, the amino acids in protein have a carbon skeleton, with oxygen and hydrogen, but their chemical structure is further distinguished by the presence of nitrogen. Proteins are a very complex set of molecules with a three-dimensional structure. There are four levels for describing protein structure: primary, secondary, tertiary and quaternary (Table 6.2 and Figure 6.1). Primary refers to the sequence of amino acids held together in the polypeptide chain (Figure 6.2). Branch chain **amino acids** (leucine, isoleucine and valine) have side chains where one of the carbon atoms has three or more carbons attached. The secondary level describes the three-dimensional nature of the helix form, and tertiary takes this further to describe a more globular structure for proteins. The quaternary level acknowledges the presence of more complex, lattice-like structures within proteins and helps us to understand the important connection between structure and function in human biological proteins such as haemoglobin.

TABLE 6.2   STRUCTURE OF PROTEIN

Category	Description	Example
Primary	Sequence of amino acids	Polypeptide chains
Secondary	Regular structures of protein chains	Alpha helix (coils), beta strand
Tertiary	Shape of protein molecule	Folding
Quaternary	Combination of protein units	Haemoglobin

FIGURE 6.1   IMAGES OF PRIMARY, SECONDARY, TERTIARY AND QUATERNARY LEVELS OF PROTEIN

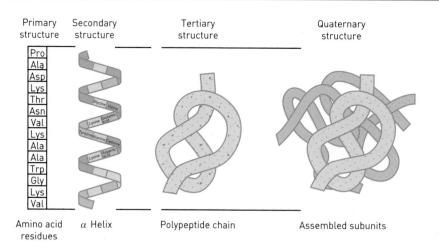

Source: D. L. Nelson & M. M. Cox (2008). *Lehninger Principles of Biochemistry*, 5th edn. New York: W.H. Freeman & Co (Figure 3.23)

FIGURE 6.2   CHEMICAL STRUCTURE OF THE AMINO ACID: METHIONINE

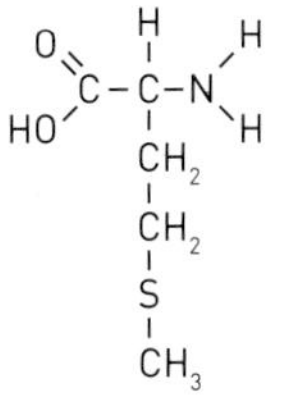

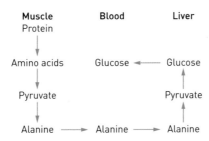

Source: https://commons.wikimedia.org/wiki/File:L-Methionine.png

Protein from the diet is broken down in the gut by enzymes (proteases and peptidases) into amino acids and peptides for further use in the body. When required, certain amino acids can provide a secondary source of glucose, which is then used for energy. Recall from Chapter 3 that amino acids delivered from muscle protein can be converted to glucose through the pathway of gluconeogenesis. Glucogenic amino acids can enter the pathway of energy metabolism via conversion to pyruvate, whereas ketogenic amino acids produce acetyl CoA through β oxidation. The shuttling of pyruvate and alanine between the liver and muscle tissue, known as the glucose-alanine cycle, represents an important function of amino acids in fuel and blood glucose delivery (Figure 6.3).

> See Chapter 3 on amino acids and peptides in consuming food.

FIGURE 6.3   PATHWAY OF AMINO ACID BREAKDOWN IN MUSCLE TO DELIVER BLOOD GLUCOSE

Muscle	Blood	Liver
Protein		
↓		
Amino acids	Glucose ←	Glucose
↓		↑
Pyruvate		Pyruvate
↓		↑
Alanine →	Alanine →	Alanine

When metabolised, protein metabolites produce carbon dioxide and water, but there is another end product, urea, which contains the nitrogen component (Figure 6.4) and is excreted in the kidney.

The nitrogen component of amino acids means it cannot be replaced by carbohydrate or fat [3], demonstrating the unique importance of protein for survival. The term '**nitrogen balance**' refers to the relationship between nitrogen being removed from the environment to support the human body and then returned to the environment [4]. The relevance of this balance is not lost in considering the position of human nutrition in environmental ecology [5].

> **Nitrogen balance**
> a condition where nitrogen intake equals nitrogen losses.

Twenty amino acids have been identified associated with dietary protein. Like other constituents in the diet, some amino acids can be converted into other types of amino acids through metabolic processes, so the requirements for each can be somewhat relative, but they are all utilised in human metabolism. An understanding of the functions of amino acids in the body has enabled scientists to characterise amino acids in terms of dietary essentiality. Indispensable amino acids must be provided in adequate amounts to retain the normal functioning of the human system, whereas non-essential amino acids can be produced by the body by other means (Table 6.3).

FIGURE 6.4　THE UREA CYCLE

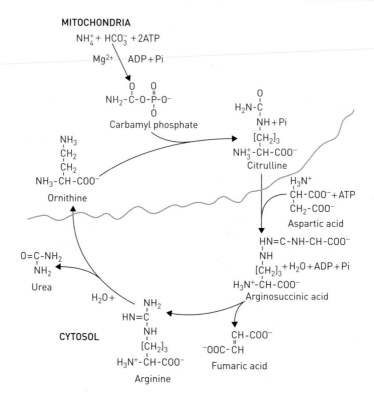

Source: A. A. Jackson & S. Truswell (2012). Chapter 5: Protein. In J. Mann & S. Truswell (eds), *Essentials of Human Nutrition*, 4th edn. Oxford University Press, Incorporated

TABLE 6.3　AMINO ACIDS CATEGORISED BY STATUS OF ESSENTIALITY

Indispensable (essential)	Conditionally indispensable (essential)	Dispensable (non-essential)
Leucine (Leu)	Tyrosine (Tyr)	Glutamic acid (Glu)
Isoleucine (Ile)	Glycine (Gly)	Alanine (Ala)
Valine (Val)	Serine (Ser)	Aspartic acid (Asp)
Phenylalanine (Phe)	Cysteine (Cys)	
Threonine (Thr)	Arginine (Arg)	
Methionine (Met)	Glutamine (Gln)	
Tryptophan (Trp)	Asparagine (Asn)	
Lysine (Lys)	Proline (Pro)	
	Histidine (His)	

The interrelationship between amino acids means that the amount of one amino acid consumed can influence the requirements for another, creating a position of amino acid balance. The amino acid profile of the diet reflects the sum of the foods consumed, so when restrictions on foods are applied, the amino acid profile may need to be considered. For example, strict vegetarian diets exclude animal foods (a major source of protein), so careful attention needs to be paid to creating dietary amino acid balance with other mixed sources of protein. The concept of **limiting amino acids**—that is, those likely to be inadequately consumed—also needs consideration. In plant-based diets these can be lysine, methionine, tryptophan, threonine and possibly also cysteine, and glycine, as the amounts delivered may not meet human requirements (hence the term, 'incomplete proteins').

> **Limiting amino acids**
> amino acids found in low amounts in 'incomplete proteins' of plant foods.

In some rare clinical cases of metabolic abnormalities, attention to dietary amino acids is also important. These include inborn genetic conditions where pathways relating to amino acid metabolism are compromised. For example, the disease known as phenylketonuria (PKU) requires carriers to avoid foods with high levels of the amino acid phenylalanine, as these people lack enzymes for the related metabolic pathways.

Amino acid metabolism is also studied in the development of cardiovascular disease. For example, epidemiological research suggests that higher blood levels of homocysteine may be associated with increased risk of cardiovascular disease [6]. Homocysteine forms the sulphur-containing amino acids cysteine and methionine. The proposed pathophysiology is complex, as there are links with the metabolism of B group vitamins (folate and vitamin B12) as well as the production of taurine, another amino acid required for the production of bile salts [7], which is implicated in cholesterol transport. Further research in this area will work to expose how these pathways come to bear on the homocysteine–heart disease hypothesis, but the dietary implications will take some time to be clarified.

A further more recent consideration is that proteins in foods are not fully digested, with some making their way to the large intestine, as is the case for dietary fibre [8]. This adds another layer of complexity in translating metabolic requirements to dietary standards.

STOP AND THINK

- What is the value of understanding the chemical structure of protein?
- What types of physiological changes would influence protein needs?
- How does our knowledge of protein requirements help us to categorise different types of foods?

WHAT ROLE DOES PROTEIN PLAY IN HUMAN HEALTH AND DISEASE?

The main considerations for dietary protein requirements are ensuring adequacy of amino acid intakes to meet metabolic and physiological requirements, and the relative amount of protein in the overall diet that may help prevent the development of chronic disease. Meeting amino acid requirements is addressed by the inclusion of 'high quality' protein in the diet. Traditionally qualitative rankings of protein were defined by Food and Agriculture Organization of the United Nations (FAO)/World Health Organization (WHO) standards, with the latest being the Digestible Indispensable Amino Acid Score (DIAAS) [9], based on the proportion and profile of the essential amino acids and the ileal digestibility of the protein. Most dietary protein is absorbed in the small intestine as smaller units (peptides) or amino acids, but some does make it to the large intestine, and there is some interaction with the microbiota, although the nutritional implications for humans are unclear [8]. Protein sourced from animals is considered more digestible and of higher quality, the latter because the proportions of amino acids better reflect human tissues. As stated earlier, the limiting amino acids in plant-sourced proteins tend to be lysine, methionine, cysteine, tryptophan, threonine and glycine [3].

Protein requirements have traditionally been based on nitrogen balance experiments, where the aim has been to at least prevent nitrogen loss. The approach is an indirect measure of protein turnover and is dependent on complete urine measurements and accurate measurements of energy intake and energy balance. A further limitation is that protein sparing may occur with low protein intakes, which may result in underestimations [10]. More recently, however, there has been a call to consider the optimisation of lean body mass (LBM) to the extent that it ensures functionality, including strength and conditioning [11]. This is considered particularly relevant in older adults and where other roles for protein may be considered—for example, with respect to managing inflammation. Thus, requirements for protein vary depending on a number of factors including age, sex and physiological status (see www.nrv.gov.au), but for adults generally it is about 0.8 g/kg body weight.

TRY IT YOURSELF

Estimate the amount of protein (in grams) required by a 75 kg adult. What percentage of total dietary energy would this account for in a 8700 kJ diet?

>> RESEARCH AT WORK

EFFECTS OF DIETARY PROTEIN INTAKE IN HEALTHY ADULTS

As part of the reviews for the fifth version of the Nordic Nutrition Recommendations, a systematic literature review was conducted to assess the evidence dietary requirements for protein based on nitrogen balance studies and for health effects of dietary protein on health based on epidemiological studies in humans in the period 2000–11 [10]. Ratings were given as *convincing*, *probable*, *suggestive* or *inconclusive*. Of the original 5718 abstracts identified after searching PubMed, 64 were found to be of sufficient quality for full review. Nitrogen balance studies produced *probable* evidence supporting an estimated average requirement of 0.66 g high quality protein/kg body weight. Limitations of the nitrogen studies were discussed, along with the short-term nature of studies using new techniques such as stable isotope methodology. Furthermore, there was a lack of studies on the dynamics of muscle protein turnover, and in the context of muscle strength and endurance.

The evidence for a relationship between a long-term low-carbohydrate/high-protein diet and increased all-cause mortality risk was rated *suggestive*, but *inconclusive* for this relationship with protein intake *per se*. There was *suggestive* evidence of an inverse relationship between cardiovascular mortality and intake of vegetable protein, but this was *inconclusive* for total protein intake. Limitations of these studies related to the dietary assessment methodology and the difficulty in separating out the effects of protein from other nutrients in protein-rich foods. The review also indicated that research was still required on potential adverse effects of high-protein diets (20–23% energy).

The use of protein as an energy source is carefully controlled. It depends on the relative amount consumed and reflects the kinetics of the relevant enzymes. When excess amounts of amino acids are available they are oxidised for energy, but this is at a minimum when the optimal amount for protein synthesis is present. 'Protein sparing' occurs when the level of amino acids is below requirements. There are also interrelationships between the oxidation of different amino acids depending on their relative supply [3].

Because amino acids are involved in the production of metabolites in cells they have a substantial impact. The effects of protein undernutrition are wide-ranging, from stunted growth to anaemia, vascular dysfunction and poor immunity [3]. In extreme cases, conditions such as kwashiorkor (severe deficiency of protein) and marasmus (severe deficiency of both protein and energy) can be seen, usually in populations subjected to famine. The other main group at risk of protein malnutrition are the elderly, particularly institutionalised and housebound older people with chronic conditions.

The position of protein in the prevention of chronic lifestyle-related diseases such as obesity, cardiovascular disease and diabetes is much more predicated on the total diet. Disease end points and disease biomarkers have been studied in relation to the relative proportion of the total energy in the diet provided by protein rather than the absolute amount of protein *per se*. Where protein, fat and carbohydrate contribute 100% of dietary energy, it has been suggested that about half of this could be flexibly delivered by any combination of these three macronutrients [11]. This is because the energy delivered from meeting physiological requirements for macronutrients may not fully account for total energy requirements. If the proportion of protein were to be increased, this would be at the expense of either carbohydrate or fat. In addition, adequate delivery of micronutrients in the same combination of foods delivering macronutrients needs to be addressed. The Australian Nutrient Reference Values (NRVs) documents indicate that protein requirements would be met with a cost of about 10% energy, but dietary modelling to ensure the concurrent delivery of micronutrients results in a greater percentage of energy from protein in the total diet. The acceptable macronutrient distribution range (AMDR) for protein was thus set at between 15 and 25% energy [12].

Increasing the protein content of weight-loss diets has been driven by mechanistic understandings that the thermic effect (metabolic energy cost) of protein is greater than carbohydrate or fat, protein may act through hormones in the gut to have greater satiety effects, and the delivery of higher levels of amino acids preserves LBM [13], although the effect on LBM is largely seen when coupled with resistance exercise [14]. Whether these mechanisms readily translate to more effective treatments is still the subject of debate. One of the challenges in reviewing this research is that participants' diets may not comply with the macronutrient profiles being tested, leading to conclusions that emphasising a reduction in calories rather macronutrient proportions is more efficacious [15]. However, the European Union's DIOGENES study did demonstrate additive effects on weight loss where compliance to a higher protein regime combined with low glycaemic index (GI) carbohydrate-rich foods was achieved, particularly in those with responsive genetic profiles [13]. More recently, greater weight loss in diet adherers was confirmed in a similar study from Mexico, even though the intention to treat analysis showed no significant effects between groups (0.8 vs 1.34 g protein/kg body weight) [16]. A further meta-analysis also argued that small shifts from carbohydrate to protein in weight-loss diets can make a difference [17]. The potential increased health risk of high protein intakes for adults is part of the debate, relating high protein intakes (>2 g/kg body weight) to increased loads of nitrogen to the gut, liver and kidneys [3]. Excessive amounts of protein under conditions of low energy demand can also result in gluconeogenesis and the formation of ketone bodies. The need to store these excessive sources of energy is counter to the goals of weight loss. Other caveats include consideration for the food sources of protein; many of these are high in saturated fat, which is linked to high blood cholesterol levels, a risk factor for cardiovascular disease [18].

>> **CASE 6.1**

THE IMPLICATIONS OF MACRONUTRIENT PROFILES VERSUS DIETARY PATTERNS IN WEIGHT LOSS

While macronutrient profiles reflect the combinations of foods consumed in the total diet, these combinations reflect patterns of food choices. A vegetarian diet, for example, is based on a pattern of food choices limited to plant-based foods. Because the main macronutrient in plants is generally carbohydrate, and in animals it is generally protein (and fat), vegetarian diets are more likely to be lower in protein and higher in carbohydrate. In a study of 74 overweight individuals with type 2 diabetes, the vegetarian test diet comprised 60% carbohydrate, 15% protein and 25% fat, whereas the conventional diet was 50% carbohydrate, 20% protein and <30% fat [19]. The test diet was twice as effective over three and six months, not just from a weight-loss perspective but also adherence to the dietary pattern.

- How significant is protein content in studies testing effects of diets in individuals for weight loss?
- How might cuisine influence better adherence to dietary recommendations?
- Which foods remain important in these studies, and why?

TRY IT YOURSELF

Examine the summary provided in *Health News* from the NHS (www.nhs.uk/news/food-and-diet/vegetarian-dieting-may-lead-to-greater-weight-loss). Which aspects of reporting in the study design and results demonstrated the scientific rigour with which the questions were addressed? What further research would strengthen the evidence for the effects seen here?

STOP AND THINK

- How has knowledge about the effects of protein on health evolved?
- How does basic science and epidemiology contribute to developing recommendations on protein consumption?
- What is the role of health and related government agencies in establishing positions on protein and health?

WHAT ARE THE BEST FOOD AND BEVERAGE CHOICES TO ENSURE HEALTHY INTAKES OF PROTEIN?

Foods sourced from animal flesh (as well as milk and eggs) and from the significant regenerative components of plants (nuts, seeds, legumes) are high in protein. Thus protein-rich foods include meat, fish, eggs, cheese, yoghurt, legumes (including soy) and nuts [20], but the digestibility of these proteins varies (Table 6.4).

TABLE 6.4   HUMAN DIGESTIBILITY OF PROTEIN IN FOODS

Food	True digestibility (%)	Food	True digestibility (%)
Beans	78	Peanuts	94
Corn, whole	87	Pea	88
Egg	97	Rice, white	88
Fish	94	Soy flour	86
Milk, cheese	95	Sunflower seed flour	90
Oatmeal	86	Wheat flour, white	96
Peanut butter	95	Wheat, whole	86

Source: Adapted from World Health Organization (2007). WHO Technical Report Series 935, *Protein and Amino Acids Requirements in Human Nutrition*. Geneva: WHO

TABLE 6.5   COMPLEMENTARY PROTEIN FOODS IN VEGETARIAN DIETS

Limiting amino acid	Plant foods	Complementary protein source
Methionine	Vegetables, beans	Grains, nuts
Lysine	Grains, corn	Legumes
Tryptophan	Corn	Legumes

As different plant foods have different limiting amino acids, plant food combinations can help overcome any concerns for inadequacies in vegetarian diets. In particular, legumes and grains are good to combine (Table 6.5). Of course, plant-based diets can also include some food sources of animal protein.

By nature, most animal-based protein-rich foods are also high in fat, but the type of fat may vary. For example, saturated fat predominates in animal-based foods such as meat and cheese, whereas unsaturated fats are found in plant foods such as nuts and seeds. Unlike cheese, milk and yoghurt also contain significant amounts of carbohydrate in the form of lactose (and possibly added sugars in flavoured varieties). Cereal foods also contain reasonable amounts of protein, but not compared with these other foods by weight (Table 6.6).

Recall that foods contain multiple nutrients (e.g. meat is not protein, it is a food). In the Australian food supply, high-protein foods also deliver important key nutrients. For example, red meat is an important dietary source of iron which is in a highly bioavailable form, but is low in calcium. Milk, cheese and yoghurt also provide significant amounts of calcium, but are low in iron. Given the significance of these two nutrients, protein-rich foods have been treated in separate categories in dietary modelling that translates to healthy eating guides. Within these categories, distinctions may be made in high-protein animal food groups, based on their saturated fat content—for example, lean versus fatty meat, full-fat or low-fat milk.

The choice of individual protein-rich foods in the diet is not limited to nutritional concerns. There is significant cultural use of these foods. For example, there can be selective inclusion or exclusion of different meats such as beef, lamb, pork, poultry and game meats [21], or excluding animal flesh entirely and replacing them with nuts, seeds and soy-based products. Across the globe, the FAO report on protein quality provides a broader perspective [9].

TABLE 6.6   PROTEIN CONTENT OF SELECTED FOODS

Food	Serving size*	g of protein per serve**
Grilled beef rump steak (trimmed)	65–130 g	20.6–41.2
Roast leg lamb (trimmed)	65–130 g	19.3–38.6
Poached egg(s)	2 large eggs (120 g)	7.93
Roast leg pork	65–130 g	20.3–40.6
Grilled chicken breast (no skin)	65–130 g	19.37–38.74
Steamed/poached basa (fish)	100 g	18.5
Pink salmon (canned, drained)	1 small can (80 g)	18.24
Chickpeas (canned, drained)	170 g/1 cup	10.71
Lentils (dried, boiled, drained)	170 g/1 cup	11.56
Soya beans (dried, boiled, drained)	170 g/1 cup	22.95
Baked beans (in tomato sauce)	170 g/1 cup	8.3
Tofu (firm)	170 g	20.4
Cheddar cheese (reduced fat)	40 g	12.44
Almonds (raw with skin)	30 g/⅔ cup	5.85
Walnuts (raw)	30 g	4.32
Sunflower seeds	30 g	8.04

*Based on the Australian Dietary Guidelines [20].
**Calculated from *NUTTAB 2010* [22].

>> CASE 6.2

TRANSLATING FOOD GUIDANCE

Using the Australian Guide to Healthy Eating tool (www.eatforhealth.gov.au/page/eat-health-calculators/calculated/1504843086), the food guidance on protein-rich foods for a non-pregnant or lactating 25-year-old female is 2.5 serves/day of protein-iron foods and 2.5 serves/day of protein-calcium foods (Figure 6.5). The sizes of a single serve for foods in these categories are: meat (65 g), poultry (80 g), fish (100 g), eggs (2 large), legumes (1 cup), tofu (170 g), nuts (30 g), milk (1 cup), cheese (2 slices) and yoghurt (200 g).

- How do these foods translate to actual foods seen in meals and dishes based on various cuisines?
- Where do soy and nut beverages fit? Are their calcium contents equivalent to milk?
- What are the nutritional advantages of choosing from the full range of foods identified in each group?

FIGURE 6.5   ONE SERVE OF PROTEIN-RICH FOODS FROM THE AUSTRALIAN DIETARY GUIDELINES

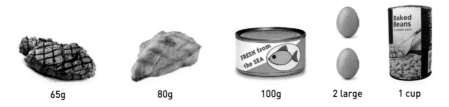

| 65g | 80g | 100g | 2 large | 1 cup |

Source: Adapted from National Health and Medical Research Council (2013). *Australian Dietary Guidelines*. Canberra: NHMRC.
© Commonwealth of Australia

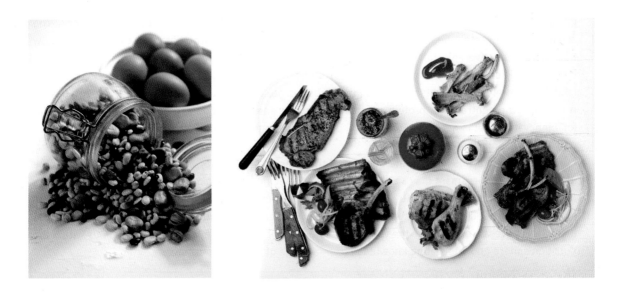

» RESEARCH AT WORK

USING PROTEIN SUPPLEMENTS FOR WEIGHT MAINTENANCE

In a randomised controlled trial, 220 overweight and obese adults were given protein supplements based on whey or soy protein, or a maltodextrin control during a 24-week weight maintenance period following an eight-week weight-loss period [23]. They also had meal tests to examine potential benefits from diet-induced thermogenesis (DIT) and satiety effects. Urinary nitrogen was measured for a 24-hour period to assess compliance with the supplements.

Compared with normal protein intakes (~0.8 g/kg body weight), supplementation with additional protein did not produce any differences in weight management. A higher DIT (~30 kJ/2.5h) resting energy expenditure (243 kJ/d) and a reduced appetite sensation were recorded for supplemented groups, but this did not convert to differences in body weight.

The study exemplifies the problems in translating known mechanistic effects of dietary protein to clinically relevant outcomes in population samples.

TRY IT YOURSELF

Record all the foods and beverages you consumed in the last 24 hours. Estimate the protein content of your diet. How does it compare to the requirement of 0.8 g/kg body weight?

» RESEARCH AT WORK

AN ECOLOGICAL PERSPECTIVE ON CONSUMPTION OF PROTEIN-RICH FOODS AND HEALTH

A novel approach to understanding the links between global eating behaviours and the rising prevalence of obesity has been provided through an approach called 'nutritional geometry'. This involves modelling interactions between patterns of consumption of nutrients in a nutritional ecology framework. The consumption of protein lies at the heart of this investigation. Using large datasets, the analyses show that there is an inverse relationship between the percentage of energy from protein and total energy intake. The Protein Leveraging Hypothesis [5] proposes that overconsumption of energy occurs in a food environment where protein is diluted (by carbohydrate and/or fat) in food products. This hypothesis recognises the centrality of protein for human survival and poses questions around the influence of food innovation that is not tied to theoretical positions on nutrition and the fundamental value of food in nutritional ecology [24].

An extension of this work is the concept of the biological efficiency of foods, whereby the genome information of an organism may be used to define its specific amino acid requirements [25]. This comes from research showing that while protein intakes are critical in early life, and have been shown to play a role in satiety (and possibly influence weight loss), higher protein intakes appear to come at a cost to lifespan. This research points to the value of maintaining a broad picture of health and ecology within the nutrition sphere and integrating knowledge from a range of scientific pursuits.

STOP AND THINK

- Why is it incorrect to refer to meat as protein?
- How are animal-sourced protein-rich foods different from those from plants? What are the implications for human nutrition?
- Which foods might be difficult to classify as animal- or plant-sourced protein-rich foods? How would their nutritional value be determined?
- How might cuisine influence the macronutrient profile of an eating pattern?

SUMMARY

- Amino acids from protein provide nitrogen in the body and their essential nature forms part of a critical parameter in health known as 'nitrogen balance'. There are 20 amino acids with varying degrees of essentiality and varying availability from foods.
- Nutritional requirements are based on maintaining nitrogen balance and providing a proportion of protein in the diet for which there is evidence of protection against chronic disease risk.

- The protein content of foods varies substantially and there is a wide range of foods that can help meet nutritional requirements for protein.
- Protein nutrition is dependent on usual dietary patterns and the choices of foods that characterise those patterns.
- Research on dietary protein has many facets, reflecting the complex features of this macronutrient and its functions in the body.

PATHWAYS TO PRACTICE

- Protein-rich foods play a critical role in maintaining the health of nutritionally at-risk groups, in particular institutionalised elderly individuals. People working in those areas should be able to identify these foods and encourage their consumption.

- The evidence base for nutritional standards on protein is built on scientific research that addresses all aspects of the effects of proteins (and amino acids and peptides) on health. Research from the laboratory to clinical and public health contexts can contribute to this evidence base.
- The position of protein in the food supply is an important consideration for those involved in developing new food products, particularly for at-risk groups.

DISCUSSION QUESTIONS

1 Why is chemical structure important in understanding the significance of dietary protein to health?
2 How is protein different from the other macronutrients, and what are the implications for health?
3 Why is protein considered the fundamental nutrient in human health?
4 What are the issues in considering the interdependence between nutrients, foods and whole diets in relation to protein?
5 What are the implications for the environment in meeting world population needs for dietary protein?

USEFUL WEBLINKS

Australian Guide to Healthy Eating tool:
www.eatforhealth.gov.au/page/eat-health-calculators/calculated/1504843086

Eat for Health:
www.eatforhealth.gov.au

FAO Dietary protein quality evaluation in human nutrition:
www.fao.org/documents/card/en/c/ab5c9fca-dd15-58e0-93a8-d71e028c8282

Food Composition Tables—Food Standards Australia New Zealand:
www.foodstandards.gov.au/science/monitoringnutrients/Pages/default.aspx

Food Standards Australia New Zealand:
www.foodstandards.gov.au

Health Direct:
www.healthdirect.gov.au

Nutrient Reference Values for Australia and New Zealand—Protein:
www.nrv.gov.au/nutrients/protein

Nutrient Reference Values for Australia and New Zealand—Macronutrient balance:
www.nrv.gov.au/chronic-disease/macronutrient-balance

Vegetarian dieting may lead to greater weight loss:
www.nhs.uk/news/food-and-diet/vegetarian-dieting-may-lead-to-greater-weight-loss

FURTHER READING

Appleby, P. N., Crowe, F. L., Bradbury, K. E., Travis, R. C. & Key, T. J. (2016). Mortality in vegetarians and comparable nonvegetarians in the United Kingdom. *American Journal of Clinical Nutrition*, 103(1), 218–30. doi:10.3945/ajcn.115.119461

Carreiro, A. L., Dhillon, J., Gordon, S., Higgins, K. A., Jacobs, A. G., McArthur, B. M., … Mattes, R. D. (2016). The macronutrients, appetite, and energy intake. *Annual Review of Nutrition*, 36(1), 73–103. doi:10.1146/annurev-nutr-121415-112624

Herber-Gast, G. C. M., Biesbroek, S., Verschuren, W. M. M., Stehouwer, C. D. A., Gansevoort, R. T., Bakker, S. J. L. & Spijkerman, A. M. W. (2016). Association of dietary protein and dairy intakes and change in renal function: results from the population-based longitudinal Doetinchem cohort study. *American Journal of Clinical Nutrition*, 104(6), 1712–19. doi:10.3945/ajcn.116.137679

Kamper, A.-L. & Strandgaard, S. (2017). Long-term effects of high-protein diets on renal function. *Annual Review of Nutrition*, 37(1), 347–69. doi:10.1146/annurev-nutr-071714-034426

Kim, J. E., O'Connor, L. E., Sands, L. P., Slebodnik, M. B. & Campbell, W. W. (2016). Effects of dietary protein intake on body composition changes after weight loss in older adults: a systematic review and meta-analysis. *Nutrition Reviews*, 74(3), 210–24. doi:10.1093/nutrit/nuv065

Kumar, P., Chatli, M. K., Mehta, N., Singh, P., Malav, O. P. & Verma, A. K. (2017). Meat analogues: health promising sustainable meat substitutes. *Critical Reviews in Food Science and Nutrition*, 57(5), 923–32. doi:10.1080/10408398.2014.939739

Mangano, K. M., Sahni, S., Kiel, D. P., Tucker, K. L., Dufour, A. B. & Hannan, M. T. (2017). Dietary protein is associated with musculoskeletal health independently of dietary pattern: the Framingham Third Generation Study. *American Journal of Clinical Nutrition*, 105(3), 714–22. doi:10.3945/ajcn.116.136762

Marinangeli, C. P. F. & House, J. D. (2017). Potential impact of the digestible indispensable amino acid score as a measure of protein quality on dietary regulations and health. *Nutrition Reviews*, 75(8), 658–67. doi:10.1093/nutrit/nux025

Paddon-Jones, D., Campbell, W. W., Jacques, P. F., Kritchevsky, S. B., Moore, L. L., Rodriguez, N. R. & Van Loon, L. J. C. (2015). Protein and healthy aging. *American Journal of Clinical Nutrition*, 101(6), 1339S–1345S. doi:10.3945/ajcn.114.084061

Pezeshki, A., Zapata, R. C., Singh, A., Yee, N. J. & Chelikani, P. K. (2016). Low protein diets produce divergent effects on energy balance. *Scientific Reports*, 6. doi:10.1038/srep25145

Shams-White, M. M., Chung, M., Du, M., Fu, Z., Insogna, K. L., Karlsen, M. C., … Weaver, C. M. (2017). Dietary protein and bone health: a systematic review and meta-analysis from the National

Osteoporosis Foundation. *American Journal of Clinical Nutrition*, 105(6), 1528–43. doi:10.3945/ajcn.116.145110

Shang, X., Scott, D., Hodge, A. M., English, D. R., Giles, G. G., Ebeling, P. R. & Sanders, K. M. (2016). Dietary protein intake and risk of type 2 diabetes: results from the Melbourne Collaborative Cohort Study and a meta-analysis of prospective studies. *American Journal of Clinical Nutrition*, 104(5), 1352–65. doi:10.3945/ajcn.116.140954

Witard, O. C., Wardle, S. L., Macnaughton, L. S., Hodgson, A. B. & Tipton, K. D. (2016). Protein considerations for optimising skeletal muscle mass in healthy young and older adults. *Nutrients*, 8(4). doi:10.3390/nu8040181

REFERENCES

1   D. R. Jacobs, Jr & L. C. Tapsell (2007). Food, not nutrients, is the fundamental unit in nutrition. *Nutrition Reviews*, 65(10), 439–50.

2   D. R. Jacobs & L. C. Tapsell (2013). Food synergy: the key to a healthy diet. *Proceedings of the Nutrition Society*, 72(2), 200–6. doi:10.1017/S0029665112003011

3   G. Wu (2016). Dietary protein intake and human health. *Food & Function*, 7(3), 1251–65. doi:10.1039/C5FO01530H

4   W. M. Rand, P. L. Pellett & V. R. Young (2003). Meta-analysis of nitrogen balance studies for estimating protein requirements in healthy adults. *American Journal of Clinical Nutrition*, 77(1), 109–27.

5   S. Simpson & D. Raubenheimer (2012). *The Nature of Nutrition: A unifying framework from animal adaptation to human obesity*. Princeton, NJ: Princeton University Press.

6   D. S. Wald, M. Law & J. K. Morris (2002). Homocysteine and cardiovascular disease: evidence on causality from a meta-analysis. *British Medical Journal*, 325(7374), 1202. doi:10.1136/bmj.325.7374.1202

7   G. J. Hankey & J. W. Eikelboom (1999). Homocysteine and vascular disease. *The Lancet*, 354(9176), 407–13. doi:http://dx.doi.org/10.1016/S0140-6736(98)11058-9

8   N. van der Wielen, P. J. Moughan & M. Mensink (2017). Amino acid absorption in the large intestine of humans and porcine models. *Journal of Nutrition*. doi:10.3945/jn.117.248187

9   Food and Agriculture Organization of the United Nations (2013). *Dietary Protein Quality Evaluation in Human Nutrition: Report of an FAO Expert Consultation. Food and Nutrition Paper 92*. Rome: FAO. Retrieved from: www.fao.org/documents/card/en/c/ab5c9fca-dd15-58e0-93a8-d71e028c8282.

10 A. N. Pedersen, J. Kondrup & E. Børsheim (2013). Health effects of protein intake in healthy adults: a systematic literature review. *Food & Nutrition Research*, 57(1), 21245. doi:10.3402/fnr.v57i0.21245

11 R. R. Wolfe, A. M. Cifelli, G. Kostas & I.-Y. Kim (2017). Optimizing protein intake in adults: interpretation and application of the recommended dietary allowance compared with the acceptable macronutrient distribution range. *Advances in Nutrition: An International Review Journal*, 8(2), 266–75. doi:10.3945/an.116.013821

12 National Health and Medical Research Council (2014). *Nutrient Reference Values for Australia and New Zealand—Macronutrient balance*. Canberra: NHMRC. Retrieved from: www.nrv.gov.au/chronic-disease/macronutrient-balance.

13 A. Astrup, A. Raben & N. Geiker (2015). The role of higher protein diets in weight control and obesity-related comorbidities. *International Journal of Obesity*, 39(5), 721–6. doi:10.1038/ijo.2014.216

14 A. M. Verreijen, M. F. Engberink, R. G. Memelink, S. E. van der Plas, M. Visser & P. J. M. Weijs (2017). Effect of a high protein diet and/or resistance exercise on the preservation of fat free mass during weight loss in overweight and obese older adults: a randomized controlled trial. *Nutrition Journal*, 16(1), 10. doi:10.1186/s12937-017-0229-6

15 F. M. Sacks, G. A. Bray, V. J. Carey, S. R. Smith, D. H. Ryan, S. D. Anton, ... D. A. Williamson (2009). Comparison of weight-loss diets with different compositions of fat, protein, and carbohydrates. *New England Journal of Medicine*, 360(9), 859–73. doi:10.1056/NEJMoa0804748

16 I. Campos-Nonato, L. Hernandez & S. Barquera (2017). Effect of a high-protein diet versus standard-protein diet on weight loss and biomarkers of metabolic syndrome: a randomized clinical trial. *Obesity Facts*, 10(3), 238–51.

17 P. M. Clifton, D. Condo & J. B. Keogh (2014). Long term weight maintenance after advice to consume low carbohydrate, higher protein diets—a systematic review and meta analysis. *Nutrition, Metabolism and Cardiovascular Diseases*, 24(3), 224–35. doi:http://dx.doi.org/10.1016/j.numecd.2013.11.006

18 D. H. Pesta & V. T. Samuel (2014). A high-protein diet for reducing body fat: mechanisms and possible caveats. *Nutrition & Metabolism*, 11(1), 53. doi:10.1186/1743-7075-11-53

19 H. Kahleova, M. Klementova, V. Herynek, A. Skoch, S. Herynek, M. Hill, ... T. Pelikanova (2017). The effect of a vegetarian vs conventional hypocaloric diabetic diet on thigh adipose tissue distribution in subjects with type 2 diabetes: a randomized study. *Journal of the American College of Nutrition*, 36(5), 364–9. doi:10.1080/07315724.2017.1302367

20 National Health and Medical Research Council (2013). *Australian Dietary Guidelines*. Canberra: NHMRC.

21 Food and Agriculture Organization of the United Nations (1992). *Meat Quality: Meat and meat products in human nutrition in developing countries. Food and Nutrition Paper 53.* Rome: FAO.

22 Food Standards Australia New Zealand (2012). *NUTTAB 2010.* Canberra: FSANZ.

23 L. Kjølbæk, L. B. Sørensen, N. B. Søndertoft, C. K. Rasmussen, J. K. Lorenzen, A. Serena, ... L. H. Larsen (2017). Protein supplements after weight loss do not improve weight maintenance compared with recommended dietary protein intake despite beneficial effects on appetite sensation and energy expenditure: a randomized, controlled, double-blinded trial. *American Journal of Clinical Nutrition*, 106(2), 684–97. doi:10.3945/ajcn.115.129528

24 D. Raubenheimer, A. K. Gosby & S. J. Simpson (2015). Integrating nutrients, foods, diets, and appetites with obesity and cardiometabolic health. *Obesity*, 23(9), 1741–2. doi:10.1002/oby.21214

25 M. D. W. Piper, G. A. Soultoukis, E. Blanc, A. Mesaros, S. L. Herbert, P. Juricic, ... L. Partridge (2017). Matching dietary amino acid balance to the in silico-translated exome optimizes growth and reproduction without cost to lifespan. *Cell Metabolism*, 25(3), 610–21. doi:https://doi.org/10.1016/j.cmet.2017.02.005

CHAPTER 7

ENERGY INTAKE AND WEIGHT MANAGEMENT: GETTING THE BALANCE RIGHT

LINDA TAPSELL

CHAPTER OBJECTIVES

This chapter will enable the reader to:

- outline the prevalence and pathophysiology of overweight and obesity
- outline the principle of energy balance and identify ways in which dietary composition influences energy balance and weight loss
- describe how healthy diets can be developed for effective and sustained weight management.

KEY TERMS

Energy balance

Overweight and obesity

Weight management

KEY POINTS

- Overweight and obesity are global public health problems significantly linked to the pathophysiology and development of cardiovascular disease and type 2 diabetes.
- The concept of energy balance underpins weight management, but the situation is complex and influenced by diet composition, physical activity and changing body composition.
- Healthy diets for effective weight management are based on patterns of food choices that assist various stages of weight management throughout the lifecycle while meeting nutritional requirements.

INTRODUCTION

See Chapter 1 for the concept of balance.

Obesity

the condition of excess body fat, measured as a BMI greater than 30 kg/m².

Body mass index (BMI)

a ratio of the measure of body weight (in kilograms) divided by height (in metres) squared.

The concept of balance is a critical tenet of nutrition science. Today, the lack of energy balance in the diets of populations is creating public health problems across the globe. Put simply, overconsumption of energy in relation to actual energy needs results in overweight and **obesity**. The 2014 report of the Australian National Preventive Health Agency noted that the life expectancy of obese individuals is shorter than for normal weight adults, and they are more likely to develop chronic debilitating disease (such as cardiovascular disease, type 2 diabetes and forms of cancer). The report also noted the rates of obesity have increased dramatically in the last 30 years, there is a socioeconomic gradient to overweight, and Indigenous Australians are much more likely to be obese than non-Indigenous Australians (1.7 higher in women and 1.4 higher in men) [1].

Population obesity statistics are assessed using a measure of **body mass index (BMI)**, where a healthy weight is defined with a BMI 18.5 to 25 kg/m² given that people in this weight range are less likely to die prematurely from health issues related to body weight [1] (Table 7.1). Observational studies of overweight (BMI 25–30 kg/m²) and obesity (>30 kg/m²) utilise this index to examine associations between overweight and environmental exposures such as dietary habits and nutritional intakes. These studies also expose other environmental influencers such as the food supply, physical environments and socioeconomic conditions. In clinical contexts and related research, more specific measures of body fat may be undertaken with varying strengths and limitations [2].

TABLE 7.1   ASSESSMENT OF OVERWEIGHT AND OBESITY

Method	Definition	Benefit	Limitations
BMI (body mass index)	Weight (kg) divided by height squared (m)²	Quick method Value in large epidemiological studies	Does not account for amount, types or distribution of body fat
Waist circumference	Tape measure from midway between lower rib and iliac crest	Gives an indication of total and visceral fat	Measurement techniques can vary
Body composition analysis	Differential measurements of body fat (density about 0.7 g/mL) vs fat free mass (about 1.0 g/mL) Estimation of total body water (bio-impedance) Imaging of fat deposits (e.g. magnetic resonance)	More detailed information on body fat	Cost, specialised equipment required and limited accuracy

TRY IT YOURSELF

Measure your weight in kilograms and your height in centimetres and calculate your BMI. Which BMI category aligns with this value?

Visit Oxford Ascend for more on understanding and calculating ratios.

Research on the pathophysiology of obesity has exposed a number of mechanisms through which excess body fat exerts a negative effect on systems within the human body. This contributes to possible explanations of the relationship between obesity and chronic disease. It also helps us to understand how energy balance itself may also be affected, and how nutritional interventions need to consider these complexities. As scientific inquiry continues, more is understood about weight loss and energy balance that can be applied to obesity management.

Weight loss occurs as a result of energy deficit. Recall from previous chapters that when fuel supplies run short, glycogen (stored carbohydrate) in the liver and muscles is mobilised, as is muscle protein and, finally, stored fat. Achieving this energy deficit, however, is the challenge. Losing weight is dependent on changes to dietary habits that have a long-term weight effect and ensure nutritional requirements are met. Not everyone is the same. When trying to lose weight it is unlikely that people will eat the same food every day; they may exercise at various levels and possibly compensate for that exercise. Metabolic rate may change depending on the degree of energy restriction and the subsequent changes in body composition. In this sense, body weight has been described as more of a 'settling point' than a '**set point**' as the various components of energy balance interact [3].

> See Chapters 3–6 on energy and carbohydrates.
>
> **Set point**
> hypothetical weight defended by the body in any given individual.

Weight-loss effects tend to plateau after one year and this is likely due to the body's inability to sustain a negative energy balance. While lowered energy expenditure does occur, it is not the cause of obesity. Weight loss tends to be slowed by passive compensatory effects that occur over long periods [3]. Because this is a long-term problem, different dietary approaches may be taken at different stages of weight loss, but establishing a healthy dietary pattern that sustains a healthy weight is the ultimate goal. There is ample evidence from the scientific literature indicating the best ways forward, both in terms of dietary effects and types of support for behaviour change.

STOP AND THINK

- Why is BMI a useful parameter for studying obesity? What are its limitations?
- How might the concept of a set point help explain weight regain?
- What more do we need to know about energy metabolism to help manage obesity in the community?

WHY IS OVERWEIGHT AND OBESITY A PROBLEM?

From a physiological perspective, overweight and obesity are problems because excess body fat can have a negative effect on the functioning of the metabolic and musculoskeletal systems. At centre stage is the fat cell, which is now understood to be responsible for a number of deleterious consequences, including inflammation. Rather than being inert storage units, we now know that fat cells (adipocytes) are highly active: they respond to the metabolic circumstance of the body and secrete signalling molecules that influence metabolic pathways.

> **Leptin**
> a hormone-like protein that is released by fat cells sending signals to the brain to reduce food intake.

Unlike other signalling molecules that are associated with inflammation, two that have been recently identified and may have promise are **leptin** (which helps appetite control) and **adiponectin** (which inhibits inflammation). Both of these molecules are being researched in depth in the hope of discovering new therapies for the management of obesity and its consequences. The complexity of the actions of the adipocyte-secreted molecules cannot be understated, but research in this area provides a greater understanding of why there are differences between individuals, and why it remains important to keep an open mind on obesity management (Figure 7.1).

> **Adiponectin**
> a protein secreted by fat cells with multiple actions, including protection from inflammation.

FIGURE 7.1   HORMONAL AND OTHER REGULATORY RESPONSES TO ALTERATIONS IN ADIPOSE
TISSUE MASS

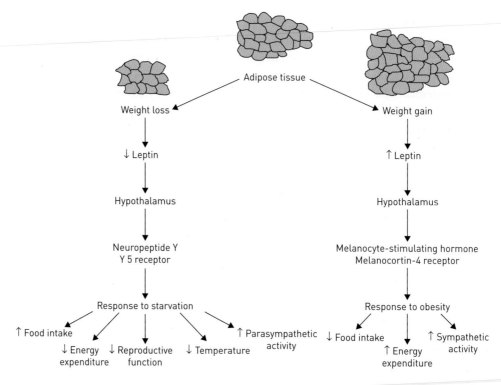

Source: S. Rössner (2012). Chapter 17: Overweight and obesity. In J. Mann & S. Truswell (eds),
Essentials of Human Nutrition, 4th edn. Oxford University Press, Incorporated

---

» RESEARCH AT WORK

NOT ALL BODY FAT IS THE SAME

Research on fat cells (adipocytes) has shown that even they can have varying degrees of 'healthiness'
depending on a number of factors, including how well they are able to cope with expansion. A poor ability
of fat cells to survive can be associated with inflammation and, thereby, insulin resistance. This also has
implications for the body's ability to manage the delivery of macronutrients.

In addition, there are different types of fat cells: white adipocytes, which are more common, and brown
adipocytes, which are associated with heat generation and tend to be activated by cold temperatures.
(Heat generation occurs when fat is oxidised for energy rather than stored, and this may occur with the
help of uncoupling proteins also present in the fat cells.) Generally, newborn humans have more brown
fat cells than adults.

Researching the profile and types of adipocytes in people of varying weight is another area of obesity
research that may help to understand individual differences in weight management, including dietary
approaches [4].

As various proteins are involved in the signalling pathways associated with fat cells, the genetic basis for obesity is another consideration. However, while the risk of obesity (and individual responsiveness to management) may be influenced by genetics, attention is being drawn more to the obesogenic environment [1]. In guidelines for paediatric obesity management, for example, genetic screening is only recommended for rare syndromes and only indicated where there is evidence of specific historical or physical features [5].

Understanding cell signalling mechanisms is helpful at the metabolic level, but studies of appetite regulation bring us closer to appreciating the impact of eating food. Research has exposed the impact of hormonal pathways that control appetite, particularly those that are also secreted by the gut (Figure 7.2). Two such hormones are *ghrelin*, which acts in opposition to leptin to stimulate appetite, and *PYY* (Peptide YY), which is released after a meal and acts to suppress appetite. Research in this area includes experimental work where participants are given meals and hormone responses are tested. As shown in Figure 7.3, however, the cessation of eating is subject to a number of factors, not just hormones, so the task of research is to piece these elements together to understand the significance of each component part.

Energy intake is regulated by a number of mechanisms in the body that influence satiation (the cessation of eating) and satiety (the feeling of fullness). Satiation determines the size of the meal and satiety controls eating between meals [6]. Much of the knowledge of these processes has been conducted under controlled experimental conditions, but in reality people consume foods in more complex and variable circumstances. Nevertheless, the concepts of satiety and satiation are useful in

FIGURE 7.2   HORMONAL REGULATION OF METABOLISM IN THE ABSORPTIVE
AND POST-ABSORPTIVE STATE

An overview of the hormonal regulation of plasma glucose concentration. During the absorptive state insulin promotes the uptake of glucose by the liver, and by muscle and adipose tissue. In the postabsorptive state, glucose levels are maintained by glycogenolysis in the liver (which is stimulated by glucagon and epinephrine) and by gluconeogenesis, which is regulated by cortisol and glucagon. Lipolysis makes fatty acids available for oxidation, and this process is promoted by growth hormone, glucagon, and epinephrine.

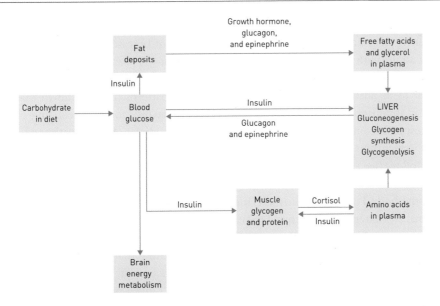

Source: G. Pocock & C. D. Richards (2006). *Human Physiology: The basis of medicine*, 3rd edn. Oxford University Press

FIGURE 7.3   MAP OF INTEGRATED FUNCTIONS INFLUENCING SATIETY AFTER EATING

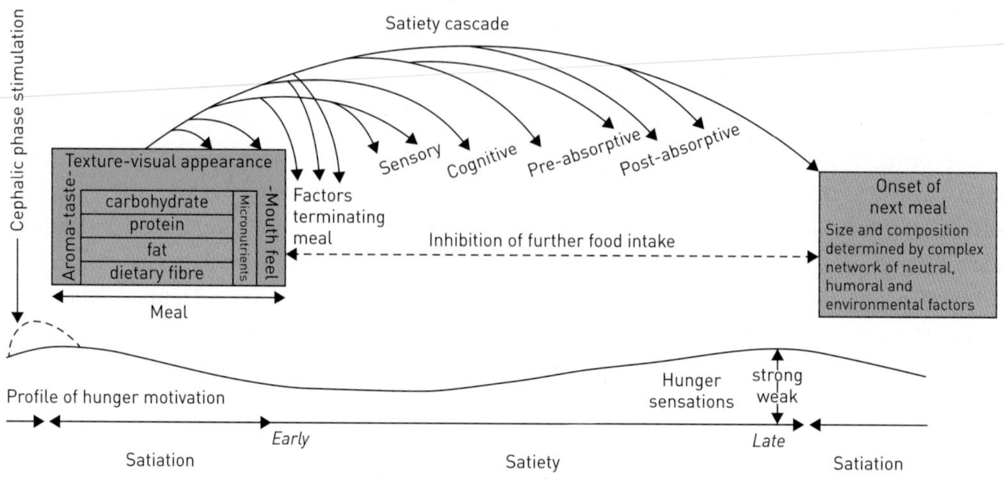

Source: S. Rössner (2012). Chapter 17: Overweight and obesity. In J. Mann & S. Truswell (eds), *Essentials of Human Nutrition*, 4th edn. Oxford University Press, Incorporated

Visit Oxford Ascend for more on portion sizes.

identifying foods that might be helpful to include in a dietary pattern for weight management. While we know how consuming some foods may influence appetite-control mechanisms, the consumption of these foods does not appear to be particularly powerful in controlling energy intake. Large portion sizes of food have been implicated in the obesity epidemic [7; 8], and studies have shown that manipulating energy density and portion sizes can be beneficial for weight loss under the right dietary conditions [9].

At a population level, however, the increasing prevalence of obesity and its related conditions has turned the tide of attention to environmental conditions that are exposing large numbers of people to excessive energy consumption levels. The Global Burden of Disease Study 2013 reported that the proportion of adults with BMI ≥25 kg/m² increased by about 8% worldwide in the period 2008–13. While increases had slowed in developed countries, this was not the case elsewhere, and the trend did not appear to be abating [10]. Analyses of global eating patterns has also shown that even where healthy food is abundantly available, consumption of poor-quality foods is reducing overall dietary quality, and Australia is one of those countries [11]. As excess body fat sets up a pathway to endogenous inflammation, concurrent increases in chronic disease, in particular cardiovascular disease and type 2 diabetes, will follow (see also Figure 7.4).

In summary, in order to lose weight, the energy value of the total diet needs to be less than the energy expended by the body. Food choice is the critical issue in energy balance and this can be considered from an internal and external perspective. From an internal perspective, the control mechanisms related to energy balance are being gradually exposed. The areas of the body that are implicated are the brain, the gut and adipose tissue. As stated earlier, we now know that adipose tissue is not inert fat; rather, it secretes hormones that can influence energy balance itself. From an external perspective, there are many other factors that influence food ingestion at a given point in time. Whether a person

FIGURE 7.4   ADIPOSE–IMMUNE INTERACTIONS DURING OBESITY

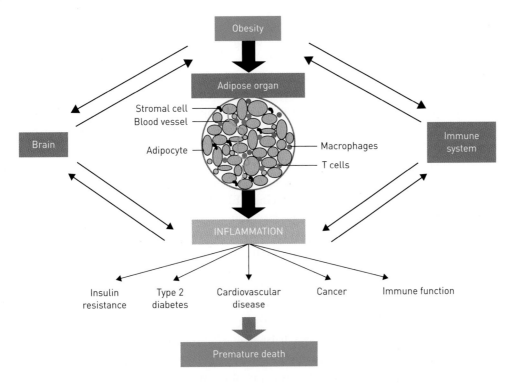

Source: D. Dixit (2008). Adipose-immune interactions during obesity and caloric restriction: reciprocal mechanisms regulating immunity and health span. *Journal of Leukocyte Biology*, 84(4), 882–92

chooses to continue eating, and how much, is also subject to various external influences. Even without considering social and environmental factors, understanding the control of appetite requires a broad view of influences and the relationships between them.

STOP AND THINK

- What are the implications of the association between obesity and chronic diseases such as cardiovascular disease and type 2 diabetes?
- How can different areas of nutrition research contribute to addressing the obesity epidemic?
- What are some of the obesogenic elements in your local environment?

HOW DOES DIET INFLUENCE ENERGY BALANCE?

Energy balance is a fundamental principle of nutrition and metabolism [12]. It means that body weight changes when there is an imbalance between dietary energy and the combined cost of physical activity and basal metabolic processes. Thus, diet is a critical component of energy balance, but there are many intricacies to appreciate. A better understanding of how diet influences energy

Metabolisable energy (ME)

the difference between ingested energy and energy losses through excretion and other processes.

Resting energy expenditure (REE)

energy expenditure required to support basal human metabolism at rest; about two-thirds of energy output.

Activity energy expenditure (AEE)

energy cost of physical activity (exercise and non-exercise). Energy expenditure = REE + TEF + AEE.

Thermic effect of food (TEF)

energy cost of food digestion and absorption (greatest for protein, then carbohydrate, then fat components).

balance may be achieved by considering the components of energy balance, and these can relate to food and the individual. Components related to the characteristic of the food are referred to as ingested or gross energy, and **metabolisable energy (ME)** of the food. Those related to the characteristics of the person are **resting energy expenditure (REE)** (basal metabolism, basal metabolic rate (BMR)) and **activity energy expenditure (AEE)**. The component that relates to the effects of a person eating a food is known as the **thermic effect of food (TEF)**. These are reported using the metric unit of energy, kilojoules (4.184 kJ = 1 kcal). Theoretically, energy balance occurs when energy consumed (ME) equates to energy expenditure (REE + TEF + AEE).

The cost of energy expenditure in a person is thus compartmentalised into three main areas: basal metabolism (influencing REE), diet-induced thermogenesis (producing the TEF) and physical activity (producing AEE). The physiological demands of accelerated body growth and pregnancy and lactation add slightly to these parameters. REE refers to the amount of energy expended in normal physiological processes, such as digestion, cell transport, circulation and so on. It constitutes about 70% of energy used. It can be a focus for those wanting to increase energy expenditure, but it is affected by a number of things, most significantly by body composition, which changes with weight loss. Muscle mass (or lean body mass, LBM) is the main determinant of BMR. Differences in LBM explain the differences in BMR seen in men compared with women and/or older people. A negative energy balance is associated with a drop in BMR, which is one of the problems associated with 'weight cycling'. Consuming some foods may influence BMR, although more research is required to consider the 'dose' required, and whether a regular dose is feasible or sufficient to affect overall energy balance over time [13]. Dietary patterns may be more important.

>> CASE 7.1

METABOLIC ADAPTATION TO WEIGHT LOSS

During periods of dieting, the body adapts to energy restriction and weight loss by reducing the BMR. This is referred to as 'metabolic adaptation'. Attempts to understand metabolic adaptation help us to understand why choices in diet and physical activity always remain important.

In a follow-up of 14 competitors six years after the weight loss reality television competition, *The Biggest Loser*, researchers reported that metabolic adaptations were persisting over time [14]. The reduction in metabolic rate (or REE) after weight loss at the end of the competition was not related to weight regain after six years, but there was ongoing slowing of the resting metabolic rate and this was seen among those maintaining the greater weight loss. The authors concluded that weight loss is an ongoing task for people who have been obese, requiring continued efforts with managing energy balance.

In another study, researchers examined how variations in diet composition may influence metabolic adaptations. They fed 21 overweight and obese adults with three diets of varying composition after they had lost 10–15% body weight over 12 weeks [15]. Decreases in REE were observed, but the reductions were greatest with the low-fat diet and least with the very low carbohydrate diet. These researchers concluded that diet composition can affect metabolic rate after weight loss, as well as other metabolic markers of weight regain such as leptin levels.

- Following attempts at weight loss, what are the implications of a persistent slowing of metabolic rate for long-term weight management and health?
- What are the limitations of weight maintenance diets defined by nutrient composition?
- How might knowledge of nutrient effects on metabolic parameters be useful in testing healthy dietary patterns for weight-loss maintenance?

Diet-induced thermogenesis (DIT) results in energy being expended from consuming a meal (TEF). This appears to be associated with certain food components such as capsaicin (in chillies) [16] and dietary protein, where there is an increased energy cost of metabolism. The latter has generated interest in the possible advantages of high-protein diets for weight loss, but generally DIT has only a relatively small effect on overall energy expenditure. Physical activity results in the most variable of the energy expenditure components and the energy cost of various physical activities such as walking, running and cycling have been assessed. However, dietary change remains the most potent contender for creating a difference in energy balance, due to the relative amount of time and effort required (see the Body Weight Planner, discussed later in this chapter). Another term, the physical activity level (PAL), represents the cost of the activity (e.g. kJ/min) expressed as a multiple of BMR. The PAL of most people in sedentary environments is about $1.55 \times$ BMR. This parameter is often used in research on energy balance in populations.

The metabolisable energy consumed by a person represents the other side of the equation and, likewise, the availability of energy from food can vary. In the laboratory setting, a bomb calorimeter can assess heat generated by combusting a food in oxygen determining the gross energy (GE) of the food, but the human gut is different from a bomb calorimeter. A quantum of energy does make it across the gut barrier (digestible energy) but there is still some energy lost, notably through biochemical pathways for protein, leaving metabolisable energy as the most accurate term for available energy. The absorption of fat, carbohydrate and protein from foods does not always reflect the absolute amounts in these foods, and thereby their metabolisable energy. Losses occur in the gut and some may pass through to the faeces. The extent to which this occurs can depend on the amount of fibre in the food or meal, the gut microbiota (which utilise fuels for themselves) and the degree of food processing. Based on a series of experiments, standardised values for energy from macronutrients (often referred to as Atwater factors, after the scientist who established them) have been derived and are used in tables of food composition. There are also conventions to report the macronutrient content of foods and calculate the food energy value based on the nutrient energy densities (17 kJ/g for carbohydrate and protein; 37 kJ/g for fat; 8 kJ/g for unavailable carbohydrate including dietary fibre), but it must be stressed that these values are approximations only (see also Figure 7.5).

FIGURE 7.5   EXAMPLE FOODS AND PERCENTAGE OF ENERGY CONTENT OVERESTIMATION OF A WESTERN DIET AND MEDITERRANEAN DIET

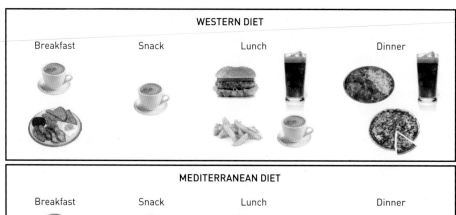

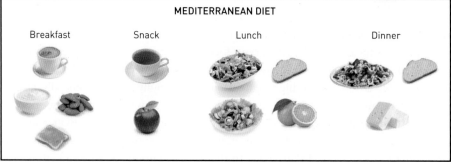

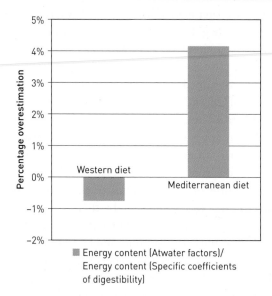

■ Energy content (Atwater factors)/
Energy content (Specific coefficients
of digestibility)

Source: E. Capuano, T. Oliviero, V. Fogliano & N. Pellegrini (2018). Role of the food matrix and digestion on calculation of the actual energy content of food. *Nutrition Reviews*, 76(4), 274–89. doi:10.1093/nutrit/nux072

TRY IT YOURSELF

Consider the diet of a young woman provided with a known composition over seven days in a metabolic suite. Bomb calorimetry of duplicate portions of the diet shows the energy value to be 9900 kJ/day (a). Energy lost through analyses of faecal samples is 710 kJ/day (b), and that lost through urine samples is 420 kJ/day (c).

Report the:
- gross energy of the diet: a
- digestible energy: a – b
- digestibility coefficient: 100(a – b)/a
- metabolisable energy: a – b – c.

≫ CASE 7.2

AVAILABLE ENERGY IN FOODS AND FOOD PROCESSING

New research is showing that the energy value attributed to foods may need to be reconsidered based on the degree of processing.

An energy balance study in which 18 healthy adults were given three different amounts of almonds to consume found that the energy content of the amounts was about 19 kJ/g, which was significantly less than that determined by Atwater factors of about 25 kJ/g [17]. Thus, not all the available energy in these foods, based on their composition, made it through to contribute energy (kilojoules/calories). A similar study using pistachios also found a 5% discrepancy in metabolisable energy compared with the Atwater-derived value of about 24 kJ/g [18].

A study comparing more highly processed meals with those containing whole foods showed that the processed food meal provided 9.7% more energy than would be expected by simply examining the attributed energy values to the foods. The authors in this study suggested that more highly processed foods might be less advantageous for overweight people [19]. A recent analysis of the National Health and Nutrition Examination Survey (NHANES) 2009–10 showed high levels of ultra-processed foods were indicative of excessive intake of added sugars (with high levels of metabolisable energy) in the diet [20]. Indeed, it is argued that food processing needs to be taken into account in food classifications as it has an impact on nutrient density and food structure that will influence availability of energy and nutrients [21]. From the perspective of meals, it also appears that a meal consisting of highly processed foods may also have a much lower thermic effect than one comprising whole foods [19]. Given the nature of the food supply, there is need to focus on means of optimising food processing to better support human health [22].

- Which food categories need particular attention when considering within category differences in metabolisable energy?
- What are the common characteristics of foods that are likely to have a high nutrient value for a reasonable level of metabolisable energy?
- How might the issue of metabolisable energy create problems for identifying best options for healthy weight-loss diets ?

Energy expenditure involves the utilisation of macronutrient fuels (fat, protein, carbohydrate). In accordance with the principles of the first law of thermodynamics, the rate of change of macronutrient stores would equal the difference between energy intake minus energy output [12]. In other words, when energy expenditure is greater than energy intake, the composition of the body will change and the energy imbalance leads to weight loss. Often this is just thought of as fat loss, but in reality the body also utilises it minimal carbohydrate stores and loses some of its protein stores (such as muscle). This change in body composition has implications for the BMR and other aspects of human metabolism.

See Chapters 4, 5 and 6 on carbohydrates and phytochemicals, fats and lipids, and protein.

≫ RESEARCH AT WORK

WORKING WITH COMPONENTS OF ENERGY BALANCE TO PLAN WEIGHT LOSS

Given the obesity epidemic and the need for effective weight-loss strategies, substantial research has been conducted on weight-loss trajectories. Research on weight-loss patterns has enabled the estimation of incremental predicted weight loss over long periods [23]. As weight loss occurs, the expected results from cutting back on a set amount of dietary energy will also change. Using weight-loss data, Hall and colleagues from the US National Institutes of Health developed a mathematical model that took into account the changes in energy requirements as weight loss occurs. In the initial study, they took data from eight weight-loss studies involving 157 people with stable weight losses between 7 and 54 kg [24]. The tool was further validated in a more recent study with 140 people in a weight-loss trial over two years [25].

This model has been used to forecast the impact of changing diet and exercise habits on weight. The resultant Body Weight Planner, now available online, enables planning for a given weight loss over a defined period of time with inputs for diet and exercise (see www.niddk.nih.gov/health-information/health-topics/weight-control/body-weight-planner/Pages/bwp.aspx). The model shows that for any given weight change and any given time period, decisions need to be made on how much dietary energy needs to be reduced and physical activity increased. The trade-offs between these four factors soon become apparent, making for more realistic planning.

TRY IT YOURSELF

Launch the Body Weight Planner from the website and enter details where a 5% body weight loss might be achieved. Keep the diet energy to no less than about 6000 kJ (or 1500 calories). Decide on a reasonable level of exercise. How long will the weight change likely take to achieve?

STOP AND THINK

- How do the different components of the energy balance equation help us better understand the problem of obesity and overweight?
- How can these components be used to plan and maintain weight-loss efforts?
- What are the ways in which diet influences energy balance?

HOW CAN A HEALTHY DIET BE DEVELOPED FOR WEIGHT LOSS?

In order to lose weight, energy consumed needs to be less than energy expended. In this context, a healthy diet has the added pressure of limited energy content alongside meeting requirements for nutrients. From a nutritional perspective, the identification of **core foods** is all the more critical when there are energy restrictions, but there may be other factors to consider. From a physiological perspective, understanding the control mechanisms operating in the brain, gut and adipose tissue helps to identify characteristics of foods and diets that may help or hinder weight loss. This may create added distinctions between types of foods and the way they are consumed in combinations.

Core foods

nutrient-dense foods that deliver significant amounts of nutrients in a healthy diet.

Much of the work that has focused on these physiological parameters addressed the macronutrient composition of the diet within a given energy value. This research was common in previous decades, where theoretical positions for studies addressed substrate utilisation and associated metabolic pathways. However, the diets for these studies had to be constructed from foods, so the effects seen were also food effects. This is because the energy content of the diet is the sum of the energy content of foods, and the energy content of foods is the sum of the energy delivered by fat, carbohydrate and protein (Figure 7.6).

FIGURE 7.6   SCHEMATIC OVERVIEW OF ENERGY INTAKE REGULATION

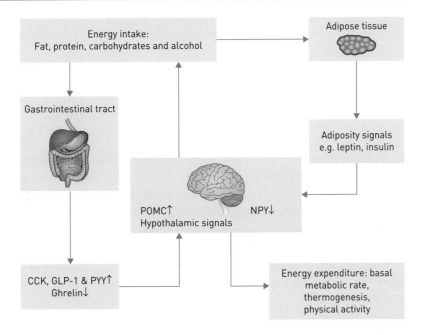

Source: H. Du & E. J. Feskens (2010). Dietary determinants of obesity. *Acta Cardiologica*, 65(4), 377–86

Plant foods such as vegetables, fruits and grains tend to be higher in carbohydrate, and contain some protein and only a little fat, while animal foods such as meats, eggs and milk products tend to be higher in protein and fat. More dense plant foods, such as nuts, seeds and legumes, are also higher in protein, whereas plant foods such as seeds and fruits that deliver oils (e.g. sunflower seeds, olives and avocado) are higher in fats. Diets commonly defined by nutrient composition, such as low fat, high protein and low carbohydrate, would all have to be constructed with varying amounts of plant and animal foods (with varying degrees of processing). Given the food sources of nutrients, a high-carbohydrate diet would tend to be based on vegetable foods. A high-protein diet (if containing full-fat animal foods) could also be a high-fat, low-carbohydrate diet.

TRY IT YOURSELF

Use the following table to estimate the total protein (a), fat (b) and carbohydrate (c) content in the following diet. Recalling the standard energy values for macronutrients, determine the energy contribution of each macronutrient (d = a × 17; e = b × 17; f = c × 37). Calculate the total energy of the diet (g = d + e + f). Calculate the proportion of energy contributed by each of the macronutrients (d/g × 100; e/g × 100; f/g × 100). Using the energy standards for high fat diet >30%, high protein >20% and high carbohydrate >50%, what would you label this diet? Which food categories need to be manipulated to modify the macronutrient profile of the diet?

Food category	Protein (g)	Fat (g)	Carbohydrate (g)
A	90	35	–
B	10	10	17
C	2	–	15
D	4	–	60
F	–	20	–
Total (g)	a	B	c
Energy (kJ)	d	e	f

The theoretical reasons for adjusting macronutrient composition have come from understandings of substrate utilisation and metabolic pathways; however, translating these positions to practice have proven difficult. In addition to theoretical positions from metabolic studies, the low-fat diet has been championed because fat has the greatest energy density (kilojoules per gram), so it has been assumed that low-fat foods may contain fewer kilojoules per gram of food and a low-fat diet may end up being lower in energy. However, these assumptions are incorrect if, for example, fat is replaced with sugar. In addition, the energy density of single foods is not the only factor in managing weight loss, as the total energy value of the diet is what counts. The debate on low-fat diets continues to be argued in the literature [26; 27].

Likewise, theoretical reasons for focusing on dietary protein comes from a mechanistic understanding of the higher metabolic cost of protein, which has led to the theory that higher-protein meals may be more advantageous in obtaining negative energy balance via the TEF [28] in addition to their satiating power [29]. However, the impact of these attributes has not proven substantial in practice [30].

Changing the macronutrient content of the diet actually means changing the balance in food choices. For people who do not normally eat this way, changing food choice patterns may be quite beneficial in reaching the target of eating fewer kilojoules. Studies of energy balance in weight loss have consistently shown that body fat loss is the result of energy imbalance, and the amount of fat lost is proportional to body composition [31]. Research has shown that changing the type of dietary fat does not have any advantage [32], nor does advising people on diets varying in protein, fat or carbohydrate content [33]. A landmark study in the United States [33] compared the effects of advising participants on four diets with varying amounts of protein, fat and carbohydrate in 811 overweight adults over two years (Figure 7.7). The researchers found that reducing energy in the diet regardless of the macronutrient target resulted in meaningful weight loss. Of interest in this study was that the groups did not reach the theoretical targets for macronutrient intakes, but they did reduce energy intakes.

OXFORD UNIVERSITY PRESS

FIGURE 7.7   THE NUTRIENT GOALS OF FAT, PROTEIN AND CARBOHYDRATE OF FOUR DIETS
FOR WEIGHT LOSS

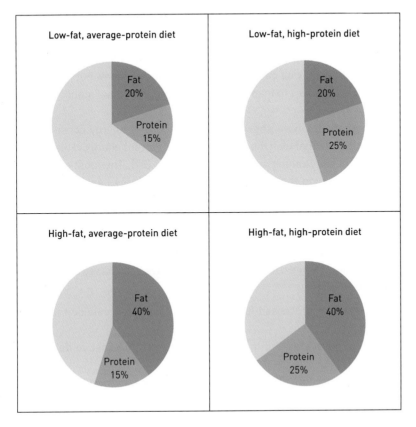

Source: Adapted from F. M. Sacks, G. A. Bray, V. J. Carey, S. R. Smith, D. H. Ryan, S. D. Anton, … D. A. Williamson (2009).
Comparison of weight-loss diets with different compositions of fat, protein, and carbohydrates.
New England Journal of Medicine, 360(9), 859–73. doi:10.1056/NEJMoa0804748

Research on dietary behaviours that influence body weight go beyond the simple testing of diet. It is recognised that the control of **food ingestion** reflects a complex interplay between neurophysiological, behavioural and environmental factors [35]. This also may be connected to the characteristics of individual foods, but whether a person continues to eat in a meal, and how much they eat in a day, can also be subject to more general external influences, such **portion sizes**, the energy density of food, and broader issues relating to the **food environment**, such as cuisine influences, food availability, nutrition promotion and food marketing. Individual foods and beverages are important, but the position of these foods needs to be considered in context. For example, vegetables could be a key food group for lowering dietary energy density because they can contain a large volume for fewer kilojoules, but they need to replace energy-dense foods, not be added to them in the diet [36].

Food ingestion
the act of consuming food.

Portion size
The amount of food consumed (or provided) in a regular serving.

Food environment
the context in which food is presented for consumption.

» CASE 7.3

ARE LARGE PORTION SIZES AND BEVERAGES MAKING PEOPLE FAT?

Because food is a commodity sold to consumers, traditional marketing approaches that provide more of the purchase for the same price can also be seen in various settings, so the consumer may feel they are getting a better deal. They may be getting more food for their money, but not for their health. Large portion sizes mean people are likely to inadvertently eat more than they intended and not balance their energy intakes.

Experimental feeding studies have shown that the amount of energy consumed by adults can be manipulated by providing foods that look the same but have different energy values, and by using various portion sizes and energy density values over a two-day period [37]. The most energy consumed usually occurs with the meals containing the foods with the highest energy density and largest portion size, and the least amount of energy is consumed in meals with the smallest portion sizes and lowest energy density (Figure 7.8).

Beverages can add to the problem and lead to overconsumption of energy, partly because liquids appear to bypass appetite sensing systems [32]. Sugar-sweetened beverages (SSBs) in particular have been associated with obesity [38] and calls for a tax on SSBs have been based on modelling for reductions in healthcare costs [39].

- Why might portion sizes for processed foods and meals prepared outside the home be larger than necessary?
- How can public health advocates and the food industry work together to deliver food services that support health?
- How can individuals take account of portion sizes and manage their own food and beverage intakes to promote health?

Bearing in mind the relationship between obesity and chronic disease, the effects of the diet on metabolic parameters in addition to body weight such as insulin response, inflammatory biomarkers and lipid levels is another consideration. The evidence for these effects is provided through randomised controlled trials and observational studies of relationships between dietary factors and health outcomes. The feasibility and sustainability of interventions supporting dietary patterns for weight management at the clinical and population health levels are further considerations.

Thus, there are many areas of nutrition research to distil in developing a healthy diet for weight loss. In the end, however, it boils down to identifying appropriate foods to consume in amounts that will support weight loss, forming a dietary pattern that is feasible, sustainable and enjoyable. Despite numerous studies addressing various forms of dietary restriction, the relationship of nutrient composition and weight maintenance remains unclear and energy restriction is still the primary target of weight-loss regimes [40].

See Chapter 2 for dietary patterns analyses.

More recent research on the effectiveness of diet in weight loss has been to focus on the development of dietary patterns. Food choices, cuisines and food combinations are all components of dietary patterns analyses.

FIGURE 7.8   MEAN CUMULATIVE ENERGY INTAKES BY MEAL

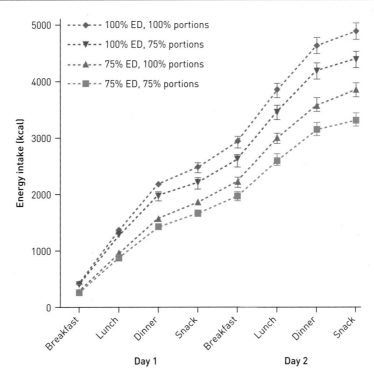

Source: B. J. Rolls, L. S. Roe & J. S. Meengs (2006). Reductions in portion size and energy density of foods are additive and lead to sustained decreases in energy intake. *American Journal of Clinical Nutrition*, 83(1), 11–7

In relation to weight change, one major study of 120,877 US women and men showed that four-year weight change was inversely associated with foods such as vegetables, wholegrains, fruits, nuts and yoghurt. Conversely, weight gain was associated with intakes of potato chips, potatoes, SSBs, processed meats and unprocessed red meats [41]. These foods reflect the food environment of the study population, but it is also easy to see the differentiation between processed and core foods. A systematic review of dietary patterns and weight loss in clinical trials identified challenges for evidence review, not least due to the considerable variation in study designs [42]. Dietary patterns were reported via studies emphasising core foods (such as the Mediterranean diet and the low-fat diet), or food exclusions (vegetarian diets) or retrospective analyses of food choices in lifestyle interventions. Mediterranean, low-fat and vegetarian dietary patterns appeared to sustain weight loss under energy deficit conditions but, importantly, all of these referred to core foods such as fruit, vegetables, legumes and wholegrains. More recently, a pre-specified secondary analysis of the PREDIMED trial showed that the receiving Mediterranean diet advice (which included substantial use of olive oil) was associated with a decrease in body weight and less regain in central adiposity compared with the control advice on a low-fat diet [43]. The PREDIMED study focused on cuisine elements that included the culinary use of oil and the inclusion of nuts, both of which added substantially to dietary fat. In a Greek Mediterranean diet study of weight-loss maintenance, only men who were maintaining weight loss showed evidence of adherence to the healthy pattern [44]. This study also commented on

See Chapters 1, 2, 5 and 7 on the PREDIMED trial and Mediterranean diet.

aspects of the environmental contexts of successful maintenance such as meal preparation, slower eating rate and higher meal frequency. Food patterns reflecting choices of low-energy-density foods was also shown to be an effective element of weight-loss maintenance after two years in a trial in the southern United States [45].

Intermittent fasting can be seen as another 'whole of diet' approach to limiting energy intake, and in some ways it has a background in cultural food practices. There are long-standing traditions of religious fasting, for example, which limit food intakes over short periods of time, often for spiritual well-being. Fasting regimes have also been used medically, with or without food supplements, or they can be part of a deliberate weight management pattern. A recent comprehensive review of intermittent fasting regimes suggested there may be promise in applying intermittent fasting, but more research is required on any effects of rebound eating, as well as a greater exposure of the physiological benefits that may arise [46].

≫ RESEARCH AT WORK

DIET, EXERCISE AND BEHAVIOURAL SUPPORT KEY TO WEIGHT LOSS AT INDIVIDUAL LEVEL

A recent review and meta-analysis of 72 studies and over a million people worldwide found that 42% of general populations reported trying to lose weight and 23% reported efforts to maintain weight [47]. The greatest prevalence was seen during 2000–09 (48.2%) in European and Central Asian populations (61.3%) among overweight/obese individuals and in women. The main strategies were dieting (restrained eating) and exercise (to compensate energy expenditure). Respondents were motivated to attempt weight loss for reasons of well-being and long-term health.

The National Health and Medical Research Council (NHMRC) clinical practice guidelines for the management of overweight and obesity in adults indicates there is the highest level for evidence for interventions that address diet, physical activity and behaviour change. Research on models of care that integrate the professional capacities of accredited practising dietitians, exercise physiologists and psychologists demonstrate and test ways in which this evidence can be translated to practice [48; 49].

Better integrated models of care extend to surgical treatments also sought for the management of obesity. A critical review of bariatric surgery, medically supervised diets and behavioural interventions recently argued that while bariatric surgery may offer greater benefits, it also offers greater risks, complications and costs compared with support for lifestyle changes. These reviews also argued that people's experiences appear to be mixed and possibly not well understood. There are benefits to all in teamwork and shared decision making [50].

TRY IT YOURSELF

Each year the US News and World Report pulls together a number of experts in the scientific literature (see http://health.usnews.com/best-diet/experts) to rate the best diet for health and fitness according a scale (5 = extremely effective, to 1 = ineffective) for a set of criteria: short-term weight loss, long-term weight loss, effectiveness for preventing or managing diabetes and heart disease, ease of compliance, nutritional completeness and health risks (including malnourishment).

A separate evaluation was done for weight-loss diets and those highly ranked were the Weight Watchers diet, Jenny Craig diet and Volumetrics diet.

- Consider the reviews for each diet and discuss how you would rank them according to the criteria.
- Which principles of energy imbalance and support for behaviour change do you see emerging in these diets?
- How important are the food and behaviour elements of these diets for long-term weight loss?

STOP AND THINK

- What influence does the food supply have on people's ability to lose weight?
- What kinds of support would benefit those in the community who want to lose weight?
- What is the limitation of the term 'diet' when discussing food and nutritional approaches to weight loss?

SUMMARY

- Overweight and obesity reflect excess body fat, which itself can lead to inflammation underpinning chronic disease, and excess weight than can impede physical functionality.
- Diet is at the cornerstone of energy balance and reducing dietary energy is a critical component of losing weight. Understanding food composition and the energy density of foods is an important first step in reducing energy intakes.
- Weight loss can lead to adaptations in energy balance, meaning adjustments may be required as weight loss progresses. Achieving effective support for changes in food choices at both the individual and broader social and environmental levels is necessary to support weight loss.

See Chapter 1 on food supply and communications.

PATHWAYS TO PRACTICE

- Understanding the basic principles of energy balance and the significance of individual foods is a key starting point for supporting people in the community trying to lose weight.
- There is a great deal of information readily available on weight-loss diets in the community. Critical review from qualified experts using valid criteria is helpful in differentiating between programs and so-called diets.
- Public health policies that address the food supply, food communications and primary-care interventions continue to develop to support efforts at managing obesity in the population through multipronged strategies.

DISCUSSION QUESTIONS

1 What does energy balance mean?
2 Why is diet the frontline approach for initiating weight loss?
3 Which types of foods are likely to be best to focus on while attempting weight loss?
4 Why do fad diets not work in the long run?

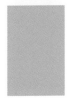

USEFUL WEBLINKS

Australian Institute of Health and Welfare—Overweight and obesity:
www.aihw.gov.au/overweight-and-obesity

Centers for Disease Control and Prevention—Overweight and obesity:
www.cdc.gov/obesity

Department of Health—A Healthy and Active Australia:
www.healthyactive.gov.au

Department of Health—Healthy Weight Guide:
http://healthyweight.health.gov.au

Dr Philipp Scherer—Adiponectin: The Body's Fat Controller:
www.scientia.global/dr-philipp-scherer-adiponectin-bodys-fat-controller

Health Direct—Obesity and Diet:
www.healthdirect.gov.au/obesity-and-diet

National Health and Medical Research Council—Obesity and overweight:
www.nhmrc.gov.au/health-topics/obesity-and-overweight

National Institute of Diabetes and Digestive and Kidney Diseases—Body Weight Planner:
www.niddk.nih.gov/health-information/health-topics/weight-control/body-weight-planner/Pages/bwp.aspx

NSW Healthy Eating and Active Living Strategy:
https://www.health.nsw.gov.au/heal/publications/nsw-healthy-eating-strategy.pdf

The US News and World Report:
http://health.usnews.com/best-diet; Experts who reviewed the diets:
http://health.usnews.com/best-diet/experts

World Health Organization—Obesity and Overweight:
www.who.int/mediacentre/factsheets/fs311/en

FURTHER READING

ENERGY BALANCE

Bartelt, A. & Heeren, J. (2014). Adipose tissue browning and metabolic health. *Nature Reviews Endocrinology*, 10, 24–36.

Benite-Ribeiro, S. A., Putt, D. A., Soares-Filho, M. C. & Santos, J. M. (2016). The link between hypothalamic epigenetic modifications and long-term feeding control. *Appetite*, 107, 445–53.

Blundell, J. E., Gibbons, C., Caudwell, P., Finlayson, G. & Hopkins, M. (2015). Appetite control and energy balance: impact of exercise. *Obesity Reviews*, 16, 67–76.

Clamp, L., Hehir, A. P. J., Lambert, E. V., Beglinger, C. & Goedecke, J. H. (2015). Lean and obese dietary phenotypes: differences in energy and substrate metabolism and appetite. *British Journal of Nutrition*, 114, 1724–33.

OXFORD UNIVERSITY PRESS

Clayton, D. J., Burrell, K., Mynott, G., Creese, M., Skidmore, N., Stensel, D. J. & James, L. J. (2016). Effect of 24-h severe energy restriction on appetite regulation and ad libitum energy intake in lean men and women. *American Journal of Clinical Nutrition*, 104, 1545–53.

Després, J. P. (2015). Exercise and energy balance: going to extremes to show that body weight is not the best outcome. *American Journal of Clinical Nutrition*, 102, 1303–4.

Gatta-Cherifi, B. & Cota, D. (2016). New insights on the role of the endocannabinoid system in the regulation of energy balance. *International Journal of Obesity*, 40, 210–19.

Gonnissen, H. K. J., Hulshof, T. & Westerterp-Plantenga, M. S. (2013). Chronobiology, endocrinology, and energy- and food-reward homeostasis. *Obesity Reviews*, 14, 405–16.

Hall, K. D. (2012). Modeling metabolic adaptations and energy regulation in humans. *Annual Review of Nutrition*, 32, 35–54.

Hall, K. D., Sacks, G., Chandramohan, D., Chow, C. C., Wang, Y. C., Gortmaker, S. L. & Swinburn, B. A. (2011). Quantification of the effect of energy imbalance on bodyweight. *The Lancet*, 378, 826–37.

Hume, D. J., Yokum, S. & Stice, E. (2016). Low energy intake plus low energy expenditure (low energy flux), not energy surfeit, predicts future body fat gain. *American Journal of Clinical Nutrition*, 103, 1389–96.

Hussain, S. S. & Bloom, S. R. (2013). The regulation of food intake by the gut–brain axis: implications for obesity. *International Journal of Obesity*, 37, 625–33.

Müller, M. J., Enderle, J., Pourhassan, M., Braun, W., Eggeling, B., Lagerpusch, M., … Bosy-Westphal, A. (2015). Metabolic adaptation to caloric restriction and subsequent refeeding: the Minnesota Starvation Experiment revisited. *American Journal of Clinical Nutrition*, 102, 807–19.

Rachid, B., Van De Sande-Lee, S., Rodovalho, S., Folli, F., Beltramini, G. C., Morari, J., … Velloso, L. A. (2015). Distinct regulation of hypothalamic and brown/beige adipose tissue activities in human obesity. *International Journal of Obesity*, 39, 1515–22.

Thomas, D. M. & Westerterp, K. (2017). Energy balance, energy turnover, and risk of body fat gain. *American Journal of Clinical Nutrition*, 105, 540–1.

Westerterp, K. R. (2013). Metabolic adaptations to over- and underfeeding: still a matter of debate? *European Journal of Clinical Nutrition*, 67, 443–5.

WEIGHT MANAGEMENT

Barlow, P., Reeves, A., McKee, M., Galea, G. & Stuckler, D. (2016). Unhealthy diets, obesity and time discounting: a systematic literature review and network analysis. *Obesity Reviews*, 17, 810–19.

Bray, G. A., Frühbeck, G., Ryan, D. H. & Wilding, J. P. H. (2016). Management of obesity. *The Lancet*, 387, 1947–56.

Brown, R. E. & Kuk, J. L. (2015). Consequences of obesity and weight loss: a devil's advocate position. *Obesity Reviews*, 16, 77–87.

De Git, K. C. G. & Adan, R. A. H. (2015). Leptin resistance in diet-induced obesity: the role of hypothalamic inflammation. *Obesity Reviews*, 16, 207–24.

Gibson, A. A., Seimon, R. V., Lee, C. M. Y., Ayre, J., Franklin, J., Markovic, T. P., … Sainsbury, A. (2015). Do ketogenic diets really suppress appetite? A systematic review and meta-analysis. *Obesity Reviews*, 16, 64–76.

Gortmaker, S. L., Swinburn, B. A., Levy, D., Carter, R., Mabry, P. L., Finegood, D. T., … Moodie, M. L. (2011). Changing the future of obesity: science, policy, and action. *The Lancet*, 378, 838–47.

Hall, K. D., Chen, K. Y., Guo, J., Lam, Y. Y., Leibel, R. L., Mayer, L. E. S., … Ravussin, E. (2016). Energy expenditure and body composition changes after an isocaloric ketogenic diet in overweight and obese men. *American Journal of Clinical Nutrition*, 104, 324–33.

Heymsfield, S. B. & Wadden, T. A. (2017). Mechanisms, pathophysiology, and management of obesity. *New England Journal of Medicine*, 376, 254–66.

Hill, J. O., Peters, J. C. & Blair, S. N. (2015). Reducing obesity will require involvement of all sectors of society. *Obesity*, 23, 255.

Leidy, H. J., Clifton, P. M., Astrup, A., Wycherley, T. P., Westerterp-Plantenga, M. S., Luscombe-Marsh, N. D., … Mattes, R. D. (2015). The role of protein in weight loss and maintenance. *American Journal of Clinical Nutrition*, 101, 1320S–1329S.

Livingstone, M. B. E. & Pourshahidi, L. K. (2014). Portion size and obesity. *Advances in Nutrition*, 5, 829–34.

Lowe, M. R., Feig, E. H., Winter, S. R. & Stice, E. (2015). Short-term variability in body weight predicts long-term weight gain. *American Journal of Clinical Nutrition*, 102, 995–9.

Raynor, H. A. & Champagne, C. M. (2016). Position of the Academy of Nutrition and Dietetics: interventions for the treatment of overweight and obesity in adults. *Journal of the Academy of Nutrition and Dietetics*, 116, 129–47.

Sanders, T. A. B. (2012). Role of dairy foods in weight management. *American Journal of Clinical Nutrition*, 96, 687–8.

Schoenfeld, B. J., Aragon, A. A. & Krieger, J. W. (2015). Effects of meal frequency on weight loss and body composition: a meta-analysis. *Nutrition Reviews*, 73, 69–82.

Soltani, S., Shirani, F., Chitsazi, M. J. & Salehi-Abargouei, A. (2016). The effect of dietary approaches to stop hypertension (DASH) diet on weight and body composition in adults: a systematic review and meta-analysis of randomized controlled clinical trials. *Obesity Reviews*, 17, 442–54.

St-Onge, M. P. (2017). Sleep–obesity relation: underlying mechanisms and consequences for treatment. *Obesity Reviews*, 18, 34–9.

Thomas, D. M., Ivanescu, A. E., Martin, C. K., Heymsfield, S. B., Marshall, K., Bodrato, V. E., … Bray, G. A. (2015). Predicting successful long-term weight loss from short-term weight-loss outcomes: new insights from a dynamic energy balance model (the POUNDS Lost study). *American Journal of Clinical Nutrition*, 101, 449–54.

Volkow, N. D., Wang, G. J., Tomasi, D. & Baler, R. D. (2013). Obesity and addiction: neurobiological overlaps. *Obesity Reviews*, 14, 2–18.

Walter, S., Mejia-Guevara, I., Estrada, K., Liu, S. Y. & Glymour, M. M. (2016). Association of a genetic risk score with body mass index across different birth cohorts. *JAMA—Journal of the American Medical Association*, 316, 63–9.

Wang, S., Moustaid-Moussa, N., Chen, L., Mo, H., Shastri, A., Su, R., ... Shen, C. L. (2014). Novel insights of dietary polyphenols and obesity. *Journal of Nutritional Biochemistry*, 25, 1–18.

Yu, Y. H., Vasselli, J. R., Zhang, Y., Mechanick, J. I., Korner, J. & Peterli, R. (2015). Metabolic vs. hedonic obesity: a conceptual distinction and its clinical implications. *Obesity Reviews*, 16, 234–47.

Zylke, J. W. & Bauchner, H. (2016). The unrelenting challenge of obesity. *JAMA—Journal of the American Medical Association*, 315, 2277–8.

REFERENCES

1   Australian National Preventive Health Agency (2014). *Obesity: Prevalence trends in Australia*. Canberra: ANPHA.

2   T. S. Han, N. Sattar & M. Lean (2006). Assessment of obesity and its clinical implications. *British Medical Journal*, 333(7570), 695–8. doi:10.1136/bmj.333.7570.695

3   J. R. Speakman, D. A. Levitsky, D. B. Allison, M. S. Bray, J. M. de Castro, D. J. Clegg, ... M. S. Westerterp-Plantenga (2011). Set points, settling points and some alternative models: theoretical options to understand how genes and environments combine to regulate body adiposity. *Disease Models & Mechanisms*, 4(6), 733–45. doi:10.1242/dmm.008698

4   P. Scherer (2017). Adiponectin: the body's fat controller. Retrieved from: www.scientia.global/dr-philipp-scherer-adiponectin-bodys-fat-controller.

5   D. M. Styne, S. A. Arslanian, E. L. Connor, I. S. Farooqi, M. H. Murad, J. H. Silverstein & J. A. Yanovski (2017). Pediatric obesity—assessment, treatment, and prevention: an endocrine society clinical practice guideline. *Journal of Clinical Endocrinology & Metabolism*, 102(3), 709–57. doi:10.1210/jc.2016-2573

6   J. M. Brunstrom (2011). The control of meal size in human subjects: a role for expected satiety, expected satiation and premeal planning. *Proceedings of the Nutrition Society*, 70(2), 155–61. doi:10.1017/S002966511000491X

7   N. M. Reily, C. P. Herman & L. R. Vartanian (2016). Portion-size preference as a function of individuals' body mass index. *Obesity Science & Practice*, 2(3), 241–7. doi:10.1002/osp4.59

8   C. P. Herman, J. Polivy, L. R. Vartanian & P. Pliner (2016). Are large portions responsible for the obesity epidemic? *Physiology & Behavior*, 156, 177–81. doi:https://doi.org/10.1016/j.physbeh.2016.01.024

9   B. J. Rolls (2009). The relationship between dietary energy density and energy intake. *Physiology & Behavior*, 97(5), 609–15. doi:https://doi.org/10.1016/j.physbeh.2009.03.011

10   M. Ng, T. Fleming, M. Robinson, B. Thomson, N. Graetz, C. Margono, ... E. Gakidou (2014). Global, regional, and national prevalence of overweight and obesity in children and adults during 1980–2013: a systematic analysis for the Global Burden of Disease Study 2013. *The Lancet*, 384(9945), 766–81. doi:10.1016/S0140-6736(14)60460-8

11   F. Imamura, R. Micha, S. Khatibzadeh, S. Fahimi, P. Shi, J. Powles & D. Mozaffarian (2015). Dietary quality among men and women in 187 countries in 1990 and 2010: a systematic assessment. *The Lancet Global Health*, 3(3), e132–e142. doi:10.1016/S2214-109X(14)70381-X

12   K. D. Hall, S. B. Heymsfield, J. W. Kemnitz, S. Klein, D. A. Schoeller & J. R. Speakman (2012). Energy balance and its components: implications for body weight regulation. *American Journal of Clinical Nutrition*, 95(4), 989–94. doi:10.3945/ajcn.112.036350

13   K. R. Westerterp & A. M. W. J. Schols (2008). Basics in clinical nutrition: energy metabolism. *European e-Journal of Clinical Nutrition and Metabolism*, 3(6), e281–e284. doi:10.1016/j.eclnm.2008.06.009

14 E. Fothergill, J. Guo, L. Howard, J. C. Kerns, N. D. Knuth, R. Brychta, ... K. D. Hall (2016). Persistent metabolic adaptation 6 years after 'The Biggest Loser' competition. *Obesity*, 24(8), 1612–19. doi:10.1002/oby.21538

15 C. B. Ebbeling, J. F. Swain, H. A. Feldman, W. W. Wong, D. L. Hachey, E. Garcia-Lago & D. S. Ludwig. (2012). Effects of dietary composition on energy expenditure during weight-loss maintenance. *JAMA— Journal of the American Medical Association*, 307(24), 2627–34. doi:10.1001/jama.2012.6607

16 P. L. H. R. Janssens, R. Hursel, E. A. P. Martens & M. S. Westerterp-Plantenga (2013). Acute effects of capsaicin on energy expenditure and fat oxidation in negative energy balance. *PLOS ONE*, 8(7), e67786. doi:10.1371/journal.pone.0067786

17 J. A. Novotny, S. K. Gebauer & D. J. Baer (2012). Discrepancy between the Atwater factor predicted and empirically measured energy values of almonds in human diets. *American Journal of Clinical Nutrition*, 96(2), 296–301. doi:10.3945/ajcn.112.035782

18 D. J. Baer, S. K. Gebauer & J. A. Novotny (2012). Measured energy value of pistachios in the human diet. *British Journal of Nutrition*, 107(1), 120–5. doi:10.1017/S0007114511002649

19 S. B. Barr & J. C. Wright (2010). Postprandial energy expenditure in whole-food and processed-food meals: implications for daily energy expenditure. *Food and Nutrition Research*, 54.

20 E. Martínez Steele, L. G. Baraldi, M. L. d. Costa Louzada, J.-C. Moubarac, D. Mozaffarian & C. A. Monteiro (2016). Ultra-processed foods and added sugars in the US diet: evidence from a nationally representative cross-sectional study. *BMJ Open*, 6(3). doi:10.1136/bmjopen-2015-009892

21 A. Fardet, E. Rock, J. Bassama, P. Bohuon, P. Prabhasankar, C. Monteiro, ... N. Achir (2015). Current food classifications in epidemiological studies do not enable solid nutritional recommendations for preventing diet-related chronic diseases: the impact of food processing. *Advances in Nutrition*, 6(6), 629–38. doi:10.3945/an.115.008789

22 D. Mozaffarian, E. J. Benjamin, A. S. Go, D. K. Arnett, M. J. Blaha, M. Cushman, ... M. B. Turner (2015). Heart disease and stroke statistics: 2016 update. *A Report From the American Heart Association*. doi:10.1161/cir.0000000000000350

23 D. M. Thomas, A. E. Ivanescu, C. K. Martin, S. B. Heymsfield, K. Marshall, V. E. Bodrato, ... G. A. Bray (2015). Predicting successful long-term weight loss from short-term weight-loss outcomes: new insights from a dynamic energy balance model (the POUNDS Lost study). *American Journal of Clinical Nutrition*, 101(3), 449–54. doi:10.3945/ajcn.114.091520

24 K. D. Hall & P. N. Jordan (2008). Modeling weight-loss maintenance to help prevent body weight regain. *American Journal of Clinical Nutrition*, 88(6), 1495–503. doi:10.3945/ajcn.2008.26333

25 A. Sanghvi, L. M. Redman, C. K. Martin, E. Ravussin & K. D. Hall (2015). Validation of an inexpensive and accurate mathematical method to measure long-term changes in free-living energy intake. *American Journal of Clinical Nutrition*, 102(2), 353–8. doi:10.3945/ajcn.115.111070

26 V. L. Veum, J. Laupsa-Borge, Ø. Eng, E. Rostrup, T. H. Larsen, J. E. Nordrehaug, ... G. Mellgren (2017). Visceral adiposity and metabolic syndrome after very high–fat and low-fat isocaloric diets: a randomized controlled trial. *American Journal of Clinical Nutrition*, 105(1), 85–99. doi:10.3945/ajcn.115.123463

27 D. S. Ludwig (2016). Lowering the bar on the low-fat diet. *JAMA—Journal of the American Medical Association*, 316(20), 2087–8. doi:10.1001/jama.2016.15473

28 H. J. Leidy, P. M. Clifton, A. Astrup, T. P. Wycherley, M. S. Westerterp-Plantenga, N. D. Luscombe-Marsh, ... R. D. Mattes (2015). The role of protein in weight loss and maintenance. *American Journal of Clinical Nutrition*, 101(6), 1320S–1329S. doi:10.3945/ajcn.114.084038

29 A. Astrup (2005). The satiating power of protein: a key to obesity prevention? *American Journal of Clinical Nutrition*, 82(1), 1–2. doi:10.1093/ajcn/82.1.1

30 T. L. Halton & F. B. Hu (2004). The effects of high protein diets on thermogenesis, satiety and weight loss: a critical review. *Journal of the American College of Nutrition*, 23(5), 373–85. doi:10.1080/07315724.2004.10719381

31 C. E. Hallgreen & K. D. Hall (2007). Allometric relationship between changes of visceral fat and total fat mass. *International Journal of Obesity*, 32, 845. doi:10.1038/sj.ijo.0803783

32 L. Tapsell, M. Batterham, X. F. Huang, S. Y. Tan, G. Teuss, K. Charlton, ... E. Warensjö (2010). Short term effects of energy restriction and dietary fat sub-type on weight loss and disease risk factors. *Nutrition, Metabolism and Cardiovascular Diseases*, 20(5), 317–25. doi:10.1016/j.numecd.2009.04.007

33 F. M. Sacks, G. A. Bray, V. J. Carey, S. R. Smith, D. H. Ryan, S. D. Anton, ... D. A. Williamson (2009). Comparison of weight-loss diets with different compositions of fat, protein, and carbohydrates. *New England Journal of Medicine*, 360(9), 859–73. doi:10.1056/NEJMoa0804748

34 M. Binks, C. N. Kahathuduwa & T. Davis (2017). Challenges in accurately modeling the complexity of human ingestive behavior: the influence of portion size and energy density of food on fMRI food-cue reactivity. *American Journal of Clinical Nutrition*, 105(2), 289–90. doi:10.3945/ajcn.116.150813

35 L. C. Tapsell, A. Dunning, E. Warensjo, P. Lyons-Wall & K. Dehlsen (2014). Effects of vegetable consumption on weight loss: a review of the evidence with implications for design of randomized controlled trials. *Critical Reviews in Food Science and Nutrition*, 54(12), 1529–38. doi:10.1080/10408398.2011.642029

36 B. J. Rolls, L. S. Roe & J. S. Meengs (2006). Reductions in portion size and energy density of foods are additive and lead to sustained decreases in energy intake. *American Journal of Clinical Nutrition*, 83(1), 11–17. doi:10.1093/ajcn/83.1.11

37 V. S. Malik, B. M. Popkin, G. A. Bray, J.-P. Després & F. B. Hu (2010). Sugar-sweetened beverages, obesity, type 2 diabetes mellitus, and cardiovascular disease risk. *Circulation*, 121(11), 1356–64. doi:10.1161/circulationaha.109.876185

38 J. L. Veerman, G. Sacks, N. Antonopoulos & J. Martin (2016). The impact of a tax on sugar-sweetened beverages on health and health care costs: a modelling study. *PLOS ONE*, 11(4), e0151460. doi:10.1371/journal.pone.0151460

39 G. A. Bray, S. R. Smith, L. de Jonge, et al. (2012). Effect of dietary protein content on weight gain, energy expenditure, and body composition during overeating: a randomized controlled trial. *JAMA—Journal of the American Medical Association*, 307(1), 47–55. doi:10.1001/jama.2011.1918

40 D. Mozaffarian, T. Hao, E. B. Rimm, W. C. Willett & F. B. Hu (2011). Changes in diet and lifestyle and long-term weight gain in women and men. *New England Journal of Medicine*, 364(25), 2392–404. doi:10.1056/NEJMoa1014296

41 L. C. Tapsell, E. P. Neale & D. J. Nolan-Clark (2014). Dietary patterns may sustain weight loss among adults. *Current Nutrition Reports*, 3(1), 35–42. doi:10.1007/s13668-013-0072-0

42 R. Estruch, M. A. Martínez-González, D. Corella, J. Salas-Salvadó, M. Fitó, G. Chiva-Blanch, ... E. Ros (2016). Effect of a high-fat Mediterranean diet on bodyweight and waist circumference: a prespecified secondary outcomes analysis of the PREDIMED randomised controlled trial. *The Lancet Diabetes & Endocrinology*, 4(8), 666–76. doi:10.1016/S2213-8587(16)30085-7

43 E. Karfopoulou, D. Brikou, E. Mamalaki, F. Bersimis, C. A. Anastasiou, J. O. Hill & M. Yannakoulia (2017). Dietary patterns in weight loss maintenance: results from the MedWeight study. *European Journal of Nutrition*, 56(3), 991–1002. doi:10.1007/s00394-015-1147-z

44 L. F. Greene, C. Z. Malpede, C. S. Henson, K. A. Hubbert, D. C. Heimburger & J. D. Ard (2006). Weight maintenance 2 years after participation in a weight loss program promoting low-energy density foods. *Obesity*, 14(10), 1795–801. doi:10.1038/oby.2006.207

45 R. E. Patterson, G. A. Laughlin, A. Z. LaCroix, S. J. Hartman, L. Natarajan, C. M. Senger, ... L. C. Gallo (2015). Intermittent fasting and human metabolic health. *Journal of the Academy of Nutrition and Dietetics*, 115(8), 1203–12. doi:10.1016/j.jand.2015.02.018

46 I. Santos, F. F. Sniehotta, M. M. Marques, E. V. Carraça & P. J. Teixeira (2017). Prevalence of personal weight control attempts in adults: a systematic review and meta-analysis. *Obesity Reviews*, 18(1), 32–50. doi:10.1111/obr.12466

47 L. C. Tapsell & E. P. Neale (2015). The effect of interdisciplinary interventions on risk factors for lifestyle disease: a literature review. *Health Education & Behavior*, 43(3), 271–85. doi:10.1177/1090198115601092

48 L. C. Tapsell, M. Lonergan, A. Martin, M. J. Batterham & E. P. Neale (2015). Interdisciplinary lifestyle intervention for weight management in a community population (HealthTrack study): study design and baseline sample characteristics. *Contemporary Clinical Trials*, 45, 394–403. doi:https://doi.org/10.1016/j.cct.2015.10.008

49 J. Beaulac & D. Sandre (2016). Critical review of bariatric surgery, medically supervised diets, and behavioural interventions for weight management in adults. *Perspectives in Public Health*, 137(3), 162–72. doi:10.1177/1757913916653425

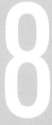

CHAPTER 8

WATER, ALCOHOL AND BEVERAGES

VINODKUMAR GOPALDASANI AND REBECCA THORNE

CHAPTER OBJECTIVES

This chapter will enable the reader to:

- describe the significance of water in maintaining overall nutritional health
- distinguish between the nutritional quality of beverages in the diet
- appreciate the impact of alcohol consumption on health.

KEY TERMS

Alcohol

Electrolytes

Hydration

Sugar

Water

KEY POINTS

- Water is a critical part of the composition of the body and adequate hydration is essential for life.
- Water is obtained from various sources including drinking water and foods consumed.
- Beverages can contribute excess sugar, fat and sodium to the diet as well as providing water and essential minerals such as calcium.
- Alcohol is a term used to describe a class of chemical compounds consumed as beverages, such as wine, beer, spirits and liqueurs, which need to be consumed with caution.

INTRODUCTION

This chapter will outline the main fluids consumed as beverages in the diet and their effects and contributions to overall health. Beverages such as water play an important role in regulating an individual's body water content to maintain normal bodily functions. While beverages such as milk and juice can add essential minerals and nutrients to the diet (e.g. calcium and vitamin C), some varieties can contribute to excess calories, sugar and fat. Individuals need to take care when including alcohol in the diet, as research has shown potential psychological and physiological side effects associated with alcohol consumption.

The most commonly consumed beverages in Australia are: water (87% of population); coffee (46%) and tea (38%); flavoured mineral waters and soft drinks (29%); and alcoholic beverages (25%) [1].

STOP AND THINK

- Why are beverages important in the diet?
- What do you recall about the relative proportion of different types of beverages offered in vending machines in public places, such as railway stations?
- How could you monitor your beverage intake and consider its adequacy and potential impact on your health?

WHAT IS THE SIGNIFICANCE OF WATER CONSUMPTION IN MAINTAINING OVERALL HEALTH?

Water
a naturally occurring fluid containing molecules of two hydrogen atoms and one oxygen atom (H_2O).

Water is the prime requirement by the body to function effectively, as it serves as the universal medium or solution in the body where all metabolic and biochemical reactions take place. It is the base molecule for a number of chemical functions within the body and gives form and structure to cells and tissues.

The human body is made up primarily of water, with 60–65% of the body weight in adult males and 50–60% of the body weight in adult females being composed of water [2]. This body water is located in two compartments (Figures 8.1 and 8.2):

- the intracellular compartment, which accounts for about 67% of the total body water
- the extracellular compartment, which accounts for the remaining 33%. The extracellular compartment is comprised of:
  - blood and plasma constituting 8%
  - intercellular (interstitial) fluids constituting 25%.

Fluid–electrolyte balance

The body's water content is tightly regulated to maintain optimum hydration, allowing normal body functions to be carried out. Body water is continually being lost through the skin (sweating), kidneys (urine), lungs (respiration) and gastrointestinal tract (digestive juices and faeces). Thus, water balance is maintained by ingestion of water through fluids or food. The primary body system that maintains water balance is the endocrine system (hypothalamic–pituitary axis) [3]. The secondary body system that maintains water balance is through the kidneys.

FIGURE 8.1   WATER CONTENT OF THE HUMAN BODY

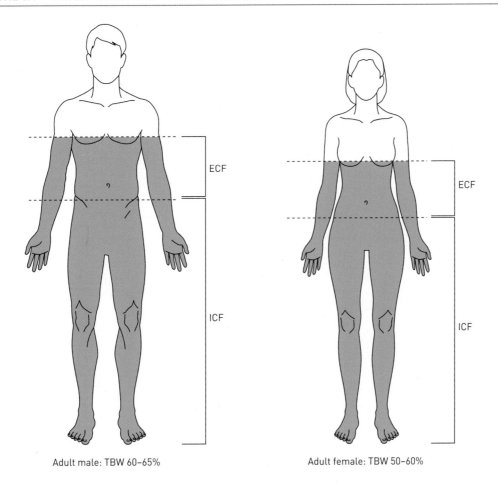

Adult male: TBW 60–65%   Adult female: TBW 50–60%

Abbreviations: TBW: total body water, ECF: extracellular fluid, ICF: intracellular fluid

Electrolytes are substances that are found in extracellular and intracellular fluid and have a significant role in maintaining homeostasis. To maintain homeostasis, the human body will continually shift water and electrolytes within it (Figure 8.3). The main electrolytes in extracellular fluid are sodium and chloride, while potassium is predominant in intracellular fluid [4].

Body fluid homeostasis

When the body is deprived of water either through inadequate intake or through loss from the body, the blood volume (specifically plasma volume) decreases. This causes the electrolytes in the plasma to become highly concentrated (increased **osmolality**). The increased osmolality is detected by specialised cells in the hypothalamus called osmoreceptors. These cells then send excitatory stimuli to the hypothalamus to increase the sensation of thirst and the

Osmolality
measure of electrolytes (mols) per kilogram of water.

FIGURE 8.2   WATER COMPOSITION OF INDIVIDUAL ORGANS

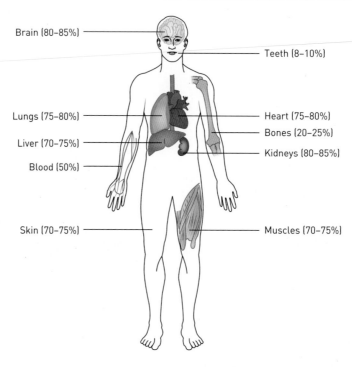

Source: 'File:2701 Water Content in the Body' by OpenStax College. Available at https://commons.wikimedia.org/wiki/File:2701_Water_Content_in_the_Body-01.jpg under a Creative Commons Attribution 2.0. Full terms at http://creativecommons.org/licenses/by/2.0

FIGURE 8.3   ELECTROLYTE CONCENTRATION IN INTRACELLULAR AND EXTRACELLULAR FLUIDS (mOsm/L H_2O)

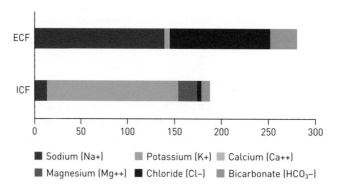

Source: J. E. Hall (2016). Unit V, Chapter 25 in *Guyton and Hall Text of Medical Physiology*, 13th edn. Philadelphia, PA: Elsevier (p. 308, Table 25.2)

secretion of anti-diuretic hormone (ADH), which signals the kidneys to increase water reabsorption. The end point is to increase the plasma volume and thus normalise osmolality. Conversely, when the plasma volume is high, osmolality decreases. This is sensed by osmoreceptors, which send inhibitory stimuli to the hypothalamus to reduce or end the secretion of ADH (Figure 8.4).

FIGURE 8.4 FEEDBACK LOOP INVOLVING KIDNEYS

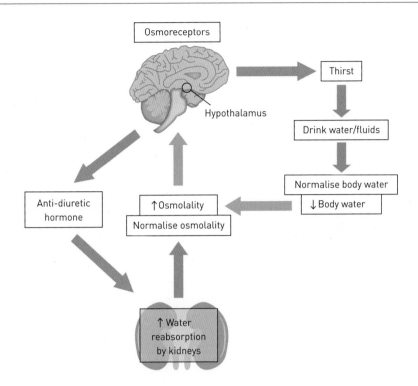

It is thought that consumption of water prevents the onset of chronic kidney disease by improving kidney function and enabling the clearance of toxins, but research in this area is ongoing. One study of 12 subjects found that increased water intake decreased the kidney's filtration rate over the three-hour duration of the study [5]. A cross-sectional analysis of older people in Australia found that those who had the highest quintile of fluid consumption compared with the lowest quintile of fluid consumption had a 50% decreased risk of chronic kidney disease [6]. Further investigations of this protective effect of fluids are still required in longitudinal studies.

Adequate hydration involves the body's ability to manage water at different levels: organ, tissue and cellular. **Dehydration** results from excessive loss of body water. **Hypotonic** and **hypertonic dehydration** occur in disease states. The most common form of dehydration is **isotonic dehydration**. Dehydration can be recognised by symptoms of light-headedness, dizziness, tiredness, irritability, headache, lapses in attention and concentration, impaired short-term memory, sunken features (particularly the eyes), flushed skin, dry mouth, throat and eyes, skin that is loose and lacks elasticity, burning sensations in the stomach, and reduced and darker urine.

Shock is also associated with water loss, specifically through plasma or blood loss. Rapid fluid loss, usually due to haemorrhage, leads to shock resulting in poor perfusion of tissues and organs, and eventually culminating in multiple organ failure. Shock is treated with rapid replacement of fluids and blood intravenously. Acute kidney injury occurs as a result of severe volume depletion and hypotension. The nephron is still

Dehydration
a condition resulting from excessive loss of body water.

Hypotonic dehydration
loss of electrolytes in excess of water.

Hypertonic dehydration
loss of water in excess of electrolytes.

Isotonic dehydration
a condition resulting from loss of both water and electrolytes.

VINODKUMAR GOPALDASANI AND REBECCA THORNE

Hyponatraemia

a condition of low levels of sodium in the blood. Resulting symptoms can range in severity and include headache, nausea, confusion, seizures and coma.

intact with normal tubular and glomerular function, so it is reversible provided it is recognised and treated early. Water intoxication is a rare condition associated with overhydration. It is mostly seen in the clinical setting of **hyponatraemia**—for example, infusion of hypotonic saline or nasogastric tube feeding with water in excess of solutes. It can also occur with the excessive use of tap water as a nasogastric tube irrigant or enema [7].

The Nutrient Reference Values (NRVs) for Australia and New Zealand [8] provide a guide to fluid requirements, with an estimated guide for adequate intake (AI) (Table 8.1). An AI was recommended rather than estimated average requirement (EAR) because it is difficult to determine actual fluid requirements, as these are so variable for each individual. The AI is based on median population intakes.

TABLE 8.1   AUSTRALIAN RECOMMENDATIONS FOR WATER CONSUMPTION

		Adequate intake (AI) fluid component only	Adequate intake (AI) food and fluid
Men	19–70 years	2.6	3.4
	>70 years	2.6	3.4
Women	19–50 years	2.1	2.8
	>50 years	2.1	2.8
Pregnancy	14–18 years	1.8	2.4
	18–50 years	2.3	3.1
Lactation	14–18 years	2.3	2.9
	18–50 years	2.6	3.5

Source: National Health and Medical Research Council (2006). *Nutrient Reference Values for Australia and New Zealand, Including Recommended Dietary Intakes*. Canberra: NHMRC. © Commonwealth of Australia

TRY IT YOURSELF

- How much water have you drunk today?
- How much fluid (juice, soft drink, alcohol, etc.) have you consumed today?
- Compare the amount you calculated with the AI for your age and gender.

In order to understand fluid/water requirements, it is important to consider the basics of water loss. About 2–2.5 L of water is lost per day with 60% in urine, 30% in exhaled air, 5% in faeces and 5% in basal sweating. These losses are calculated for sedentary activity and serve as a guide to basic fluid loss. Other conditions involving mild, moderate or strenuous activity require more fluid, as water loss will be greater compared with basic requirements. The water requirement is also influenced by environmental temperatures—for example, working in hot environments will lead to more water loss and increased fluid requirements.

Replacement of an equal amount of fluid to that lost is recommended. This considers the water estimated to be provided from metabolism (10%), ingested food (30%) and ingested fluids (60%). According to the 2011–12 National Nutrition and Physical Activity Survey [9], water contributed to 50% of total beverage consumption of Australians, with 21% from soft drinks, alcohol and cordial, 15% from tea and coffee, and 13% from juice and milk drinks. It has been suggested that for work in hot environments exceeding four hours, water may be supplemented with 7 g/100 mL of carbohydrate containing fluid and/or electrolyte containing fluids [10].

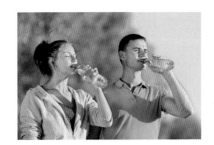

Water consumption has been linked to improved bowel function, relieving constipation [11; 12]. It contributes to improved oral health, with the provision of both fluoride (in fluoridated water supplies) and saliva production [13].

» CASE 8.1

HOW MUCH WATER DO WE REALLY NEED?

We commonly hear phrases such as 'drink eight glasses of water a day' or 'drink two litres every day'. Is there any scientific basis for this recommendation? 'Hydropathists' in the nineteenth century believed that water had the power to cure any disease and were the first to recommend consumption of large quantities of water. The first scientific support for water consumption appeared in 1945 when the National Academy of Science in the United States recommended a daily intake of 2500 mL. Some researchers believe this amount is an overestimation of individual requirements, while other researchers believe it is not enough [14; 15]. An analysis of water and beverage consumption in the Australian population showed that water consumption is below the recommended adequate intake across the population [16]. It is evident that the exact amount of water required to stay healthy is still debatable.

Drinking water in excess of what the body can pass out causes a condition called dilutional hyponatraemia, also known as water intoxication. The symptoms are the same as dehydration, including fatigue, irritability, headache and confusion. In this condition, the brain swells up due to fluid shifting into the brain cells and causing an increase in pressure inside the skull. This can rapidly progress, resulting in death. Overemphasis of increased water intake to prevent dehydration and heat illness has resulted in water intoxication and death in military personnel and was reported in the media for a worker in a remote mining site [17; 18]. These examples highlight the potential dangers associated with overhydration, requiring a balance in promoting increased water intake commensurate with water loss.

- What kind of research is needed to provide evidence-based statements on the amount of water we need to consume each day?
- Is it possible to consume too much water?
- What else do we need to know in establishing positions on hydration for the general public?

STOP AND THINK

- Why is it difficult to assess how much water a person needs to consume each day?
- What factors would you need to consider in addressing the hydration requirements of individuals?
- How would the hydration requirements of an elderly female living in a retirement village differ from those of an elite male athlete in his early 20s?

VINODKUMAR GOPALDASANI AND REBECCA THORNE

HOW DO BEVERAGES DIFFER IN TERMS OF NUTRITIONAL QUALITY?

A number of non-alcoholic beverages also serve to provide water, but care must be taken when using these as a source of body water replenishment. Non-alcoholic beverages may be considered as an addition to drinking water rather than a replacement for drinking water. They often have a high electrolyte, high sugar and high carbohydrate content, all of which provide more energy than may be required. Non-alcoholic beverages include energy and sports drinks, sugar-sweetened beverages (SSBs), fruit juice, milk, tea and coffee.

Given its high nutrient content, in particular protein and calcium, milk is both a food and a beverage. A variety of milk alternatives have emerged in recent years, including beverages made from almond, soy, coconut, rice and oats.

TRY IT YOURSELF

Using the nutrition information panel on packages, determine how non-dairy alternative milk drinks compare to cow's milk as a calcium and protein source.

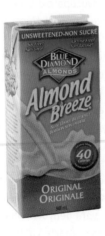 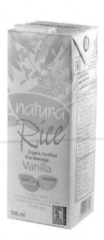

Some classes of non-alcoholic beverages provide essential nutrients such as calcium (from milk and milk alternatives) and antioxidants such as flavonols (from tea) [19]. On the other hand, sugar-sweetened soft drinks are emerging as problematic, with research showing that Australians are consuming the greatest proportion of added sugar in their diet from these products [20]. Considerations must be made in association with their consumption in the diet to assess the risk these beverages will contribute to excess energy in the diet, leading to overweight and obesity.

Tea and coffee are the most commonly consumed non-alcoholic beverages in Australia. Apart from their high-energy content, they are also high in caffeine content. The average Australian adult consumes 232 mg/day of caffeine through mainly tea and coffee [21]. Caffeine consumption is recognised as having a diuretic action, leading to fluid loss. However, a systematic literature review has shown that habitual consumption of tea and coffee as part of a daily lifestyle does not result in fluid loss in excess of what is consumed, as tolerance is quickly developed for the diuretic effects of tea and coffee [22].

» CASE 8.2

SUGAR-SWEETENED BEVERAGES IN THE DIET

The most recent Australian Health Survey found that over half (52%) of all free sugars were consumed by Australians from beverages, with soft drinks, sports and energy drinks being the most common (19%) [23].

The Rethink Sugary Drink (www.rethinksugarydrink.org.au) alliance is supported by a partnership of 13 health and community organisations, including the Heart Foundation, Diabetes Australia and Cancer Council, seeking to target a reduction in the overconsumption of sugar from SSBs [24]. The alliance is concerned with the association between SSBs and increased energy intake, which can lead to obesity and weight gain. In March 2017, a position statement was released by the alliance recommending that the Australian Government introduce a health levy on SSBs.

A report published by the World Health Organization (WHO) in 2016 illustrated evidence that reductions in consumption of SSBs could result from suitably constructed taxes on such beverages [25].

- What is the public health significance of high consumption of SSBs in the Australian population?
- What approaches could be taken to reduce consumption of SSBs where it is a problem?
- How can research in food and nutrition contribute to this debate?

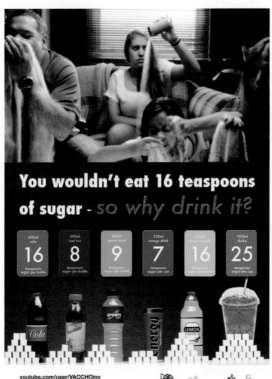

VINODKUMAR GOPALDASANI AND REBECCA THORNE

Sports drinks have been developed and heavily researched as products to assist athletes in improving their fluid intake and sporting performance. These beverages can contain carbohydrate and protein, allowing refuelling, and electrolytes to promote hydration (Table 8.2). Consuming these products can cause problems, including hyponatraemia and gastrointestinal discomfort, if over-consumed or consumed with sedentariness or low levels of activity. In addition, sports drinks, as well as SSBs, have been shown to contribute to dental erosion [26].

TABLE 8.2   ENERGY AND ELECTROLYTE CONTENTS OF SOME POPULAR SPORTS BEVERAGES

	Carbohydrate (g/100 mL)	Protein (g/L)	Sodium (mmol/L)	Potassium (mg/L)	Additional ingredients
Gatorade	6	0	21	230	
Gatorade Endurance	6	0	36	150	
Accelerade	6	15	21	66	Calcium, iron, vitamin E
Powerade No Sugar	n/a	0.5	23	230	
Powerade Isotonic	7.6	0	12	141	
Powerade Energy Edge	7.5	0	22	141	
Powerade Recovery	7.3	17	13	140	
Staminade	7.2	0	12	160	Magnesium
PB Sports Electrolyte Drink	6.8	0	20	180	
Mizone Rapid	3.9	0	10	0	B vitamins, vitamin C
Powerbar Endurance Formula	7	0	33		
Sqwincher	9	0	30.8	25	Magnesium
Aqualyte	3.7	0	12	120	
Propel Fitness Water	3.8	0	0.8	5	Vitamins B3, B5, B6, B12, folic acid (B9), vitamin E
Mizone Water	2.5	0	2	0	B vitamins, vitamin C
Lucozade Sport Body Fuel Drink	6.4	Trace	20.5	90	Vitamins B3, B5, B6, B12
Endura	6.4		34.7	160	

Source: V. Gopaldasani (2016). Supporting healthy lifestyles in the mining industry: a focus on nutrition, physical activity, hydration and heat stress. (Doctor of Philosophy), University of Wollongong, NSW

STOP AND THINK

- What considerations would need to be made when determining an individual's hydration requirements?
- Why is water the preferable source of hydration for most people?
- Among other non-alcoholic beverages, which categories may have nutritional benefits and which carry risks for overall health? Why?

HOW DOES ALCOHOL CONSUMPTION AFFECT HEALTH?

In consumer terms, 'alcohol' generally refers to beverages such as wine, beer, spirits and liqueurs. These beverages contain the chemical ethanol (C_2H_5OH), which is produced by fermenting sugar with yeast. Alcohol differs from other nutrients in beverages in that it does not require any digestion. Once ingested, alcohol can be absorbed into the bloodstream via the stomach and small intestines. The brain can be affected by alcohol within five minutes of ingestion, with blood alcohol concentration (BAC) peaking around 30–45 minutes after consumption of a standard drink [27]. The rate of absorption will differ between individuals and can be slowed by having a meal or snack. Alcohol is primarily metabolised in the liver, with small amounts expelled via urine, breath and sweat. The average rate an individual can metabolise alcohol is around 5–10 g per hour, and this will differ depending on an individual's genetic background, gender, ethnicity, body weight and composition, liver size, health status, alcohol tolerance, level and rate of ingestion, and food intake [28].

Ethanol is oxidised by the enzyme alcohol dehydrogenase to create acetaldehyde, which is then converted to acetate by acetaldehyde dehydrogenase. Higher levels of acetaldehyde in the blood, brain and tissues can have damaging effects and cause illness [29]. This can be seen in populations where inactive enzyme expression is present; the build-up of levels in the body causes facial flushing and headache [30]. Some research has shown that low to moderate intakes of alcoholic drinks may lower the incidence of cardiovascular disease and total mortality, increase high-density lipoprotein (HDL) cholesterol, improve insulin sensitivity, and reduce incidence of dementia and Alzheimer's disease, but the area is still insufficiently researched [31].

> **Alcohol**
> an organic compound characterised by a hydroxyl compound. Alcoholic drinks are classed as ethyl alcohol.

≫ RESEARCH AT WORK

WINE AND THE MEDITERRANEAN DIET

The PREDIMED trial was a large intervention trial conducted in Spain promoting the Mediterranean diet and its role in the primary prevention of many major chronic diseases. Results from this study found that a moderate intake of alcohol (5–15 g/day), specifically wine, was significantly associated with lower rates of depression [32]. However, this should not be taken out of the context of meal consumption, noting, for example, that heavy drinking appears to be associated with a higher risk of depression.

Alcohol consumption has been linked to the development and/or cause of a variety of injuries, diseases and mortality (Figure 8.5) [33; 34]. Individuals need to consider the risks associated when considering alcohol consumption.

The NHMRC guidelines were designed to establish and communicate evidence for the development of future policies for the Australian community in relation to the consumption of alcohol [35]. The 2009 guidelines particularly highlight age of consumption and vulnerable groups such as pregnant and lactating women. These national guidelines have been under revision, with updated guidelines planned for release in late 2018 (for future updates, see https://nhmrc.gov.au).

> See Chapters 1, 2, 5 and 7 on the PREDIMED trial and Mediterranean diet.

VINODKUMAR GOPALDASANI AND REBECCA THORNE

FIGURE 8.5   ALCOHOL-ATTRIBUTABLE DISEASES AND MORTALITY

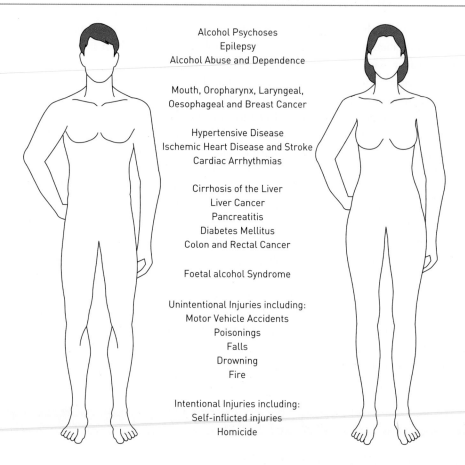

Alcohol Psychoses
Epilepsy
Alcohol Abuse and Dependence

Mouth, Oropharynx, Laryngeal,
Oesophageal and Breast Cancer

Hypertensive Disease
Ischemic Heart Disease and Stroke
Cardiac Arrhythmias

Cirrhosis of the Liver
Liver Cancer
Pancreatitis
Diabetes Mellitus
Colon and Rectal Cancer

Foetal alcohol Syndrome

Unintentional Injuries including:
Motor Vehicle Accidents
Poisonings
Falls
Drowning
Fire

Intentional Injuries including:
Self-inflicted injuries
Homicide

The 2012 Australian Dietary Guidelines recommend that Australians who choose to consume alcohol should limit intake [36]. The guidelines and the Australian Guidelines to Reduce Health Risks from Drinking Alcohol both promote that not drinking is the safest option for women planning a pregnancy, are pregnant or are breastfeeding. For the general population, the guidelines recommend that healthy men and women drink no more than two standard drinks (20 g of alcohol) on any day and no more than four on a single occasion to reduce the risk of alcohol-related disease or injury [35; 36] (Figure 8.6).

TRY IT YOURSELF

Calculate how many standard drinks you have per week. How does this rate against the NHMRC guidelines?

FIGURE 8.6   THE NUMBER OF STANDARD DRINKS IN A VARIETY OF ALCOHOLIC BEVERAGES
AND SIZES

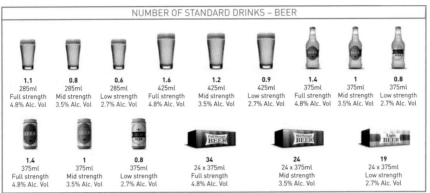

These are only an approximate number of standard drinks. Always read the container for the exact number of standard drinks.

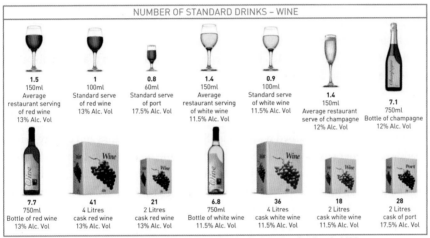

These are only an approximate number of standard drinks. Always read the container for the exact number of standard drinks.

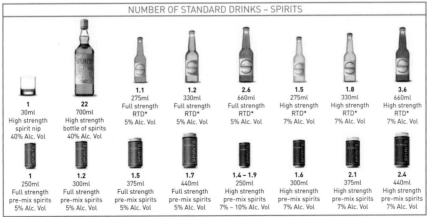

These are only an approximate number of standard drinks. Always read the container for the exact number of standard drinks.   * Ready-to-drink

Source: National Health and Medical Research Council (2009). *Australian Guidelines to Reduce Health Risks from Drinking Alcohol.*
Image taken from: Appendix A6: Number of standard drinks in various beverages. © Commonwealth of Australia

From an international perspective, data shows that a standard drink size can vary between 8 and 20 g of alcohol with low-risk guidelines ranging from 10 to 42 g per day (98–140 g per week) for women and 10 to 56 g per day (150–280 g per week) for men [37]. Research published out of Europe determined that to reduce risk of mortality, low-risk alcohol guidelines should be set at 8–10 g/day of alcohol for women and 15–20 g for men [38].

» RESEARCH AT WORK

ALCOHOL CONSUMPTION IN AUSTRALIA

The Australian Health Survey 2011–12 found that alcoholic beverages were found to be the largest contributor to dietary energy from discretionary foods [1]. In relation to total energy intake, median alcohol consumption contributed 13.7% and 12.9% for males and females, respectively, with 38.8% higher prevalence of consumption on Fridays, Saturdays and Sundays [39]. Considering Australia's growing rates of overweight and obesity, alcohol needs to be included in targets that reduce energy intake from discretionary foods.

Alcohol has also been found to be the leading contributor to the burden of disease and injury for individuals aged 0–44 years [40]. Estimates from previous years calculated that alcohol-related problems cost Australian society around $14 billion per year [41].

Alcoholic beverages can be consumed with other SSBs such as soft drinks and energy drinks, which will contribute to additional energy, sugar, caffeine and taurine in the diet. Energy drink consumption, popular in adolescent and young adult populations, is associated with additional health complications that can result in hospitalisation [42]. Individuals who recreationally ingest caffeinated 'energy drinks' have reported having a number of side effects [42], including palpitations and tachycardia, tremor/shaking, agitation and restlessness, chest pain, dizziness, insomnia, respiratory distress, headache and gastrointestinal upset.

STOP AND THINK

- What are the controversial issues relating to the risks and benefits of alcohol consumption?
- How would research on the context of drinking (e.g. during meals, at the pub) be useful for public health campaigns?
- What strategies could be developed to ensure better community management of alcohol consumption?

SUMMARY

- Beverages are an important part of the diet as they provide a source of hydration.
- Water is the most important beverage due to its functional and physiological properties associated with the human body.
- When choosing beverages consideration must be given to the nutrient and energy value that they can contribute to the diet.
- Alcohol is readily absorbed and taken up by the body, affecting the brain within minutes of consumption, and metabolised in the liver.

PATHWAYS TO PRACTICE

- Community health initiatives and projects can support vulnerable communities to target a reduction in risk of developing lifestyle diseases via minimising added sugar consumption.

- In the food industry, a broad range of health relevant initiatives includes the areas of mandatory labelling, advertising and health claims on beverages.

- Nutrition communications includes the dissemination of the new alcohol guidelines for Australians that comes from a national (e.g. the NHMRC or the Dietitians Association of Australia), state (state government) and local level (general practitioners, community projects or local health professionals).

- In public health, the importance of oral health and recommendations from the Australian Dental Association are associated with beverage consumption.

- The pre-health professional can consider the role of water consumption in promoting optimal kidney health (see www.kidney.org.au).

- Nutrition science continues research in sports science associated with optimal hydration and electrolyte balance in athletes.

DISCUSSION QUESTIONS

1   Should there be an age limit on the sale of energy drinks?
2   If the Australian Government developed non-alcoholic beverage guidelines for Australians, what would you recommend be included in the guidelines? Would the guidelines target specific groups such as children and adolescents?
3   What would be the benefits to public health if Australian schools only supplied water as a beverage and Australians were encouraged to have alcohol-free days?
4   What are the potential environmental issues associated with Australia's current beverage culture? Consider also waste issues, such as discarded coffee cups, plastic water bottles and other beverage containers.

USEFUL WEBLINKS

Healthy Kids—An initiative of NSW Ministry of Health, NSW Department of Education, Office of Sport and the Heart Foundation:

  www.healthykids.nsw.gov.au/kids-teens/stats-and-facts-teens/teens-nutrition/drinks-for-hydration.aspx

Kidney Health Australia:

  http://kidney.org.au

Mayo Clinic—Water: How much should you drink every day?:

  www.mayoclinic.org/healthy-lifestyle/nutrition-and-healthy-eating/in-depth/water/art-20044256

National alcohol guidelines: reducing the health risk:
www.nhmrc.gov.au/health-topics/alcohol-guidelines

National alliance targeting reduced consumption of sugar-sweetened beverages:
www.rethinksugarydrink.oru.au

Water—Nutrient Reference Values:
www.nrv.gov.au/nutrients/water

FURTHER READING

Armstrong, L. E. (2005). Hydration assessment techniques. *Nutrition Reviews*, 63(6 Pt 2), S40–54.

Kalinowski, A. & Humphreys, K. (2016). Governmental standard drink definitions and low-risk alcohol consumption guidelines in 37 countries. *Addiction*, 111(7), 1293–8. doi:10.1111/add.13341

Lippincott, W. W. (2010). *Fluid and Electrolytes: An incredibly easy pocket guide.* Ambler, PA: Lippincott, Williams & Wilkins.

Rehm, J. & Imtiaz, S. (2016). A narrative review of alcohol consumption as a risk factor for global burden of disease. *Substance Abuse Treatment, Prevention, and Policy*, 11(1), 37. doi:10.1186/s13011-016-0081-2

REFERENCES

1   Australian Bureau of Statistics (2014). *Australian Health Survey: Nutrition First results—Foods and nutrients, 2011–12.* Canberra: ABS. Retrieved from: www.abs.gov.au/ausstats/abs@.nsf/PrimaryMainFeatures/4364.0.55.007?OpenDocument.

2   L. E. Armstrong, I. Rosenberg, L. Armstrong, F. Manz, A. Dal Canton, D. Barclay, ... M. Ferry (2005). Hydration assessment techniques. *Nutrition Reviews*, 63(6 II), S40–S54.

3   E. N. Marieb & K. Hoehn (2012). *Human Anatomy and Physiology*, 9th edn. San Francisco, CA: Pearson Benjamin Cummings.

4   J. Terry (1994). The major electrolytes: sodium, potassium, and chloride. *Journal of Intravenous Nursing*, 17(5), 240–7.

5   P. Anastasio, M. Cirillo, L. Spitali, A. Frangiosa, R. M. Pollastro & N. G. De Santo (2001). Level of hydration and renal function in healthy humans. *Kidney International*, 60(2), 748–56. doi:10.1046/j.1523-1755.2001.060002748.x

6   G. F. M. Strippoli, J. C. Craig, E. Rochtchina, V. M. Flood, J. J. Wang & P. Mitchell (2011). Fluid and nutrient intake and risk of chronic kidney disease. *Nephrology*, 16(3), 326–34.

7   W. W. Lippincott (2010). *Fluid and Electrolytes: An incredibly easy pocket guide.* Ambler, PA: Lippincott, Williams & Wilkins.

8   National Health and Medical Research Council (2006). *Nutrient Reference Values for Australia and New Zealand, Including Recommended Dietary Intakes.* Canberra: NHMRC.

9   Australian Bureau of Statistics (2016). *National Nutrition and Physical Activity Survey, 2011–12: Water.* Canberra: ABS. Retrieved from: www.abs.gov.au/ausstats/abs@.nsf/Lookup/by%20Subject/4364.0.55.012~2011-12~Main%20Features~Water~10001.

10 R. Di Corleto, I. Firth & J. Mate (2013). *A Guide to Managing Heat Stress: Developed for use in the Australia environment*. Melbourne: Australian Institute of Occupational Hygienists.

11 R. Cuomo, R. Grasso, G. Sarnelli, G. Capuano, E. Nicolai, G. Nardone, ... E. Ierardi (2002). Effects of carbonated water on functional dyspepsia and constipation. *European Journal of Gastroenterology and Hepatology*, 14(9), 991–9.

12 K. Murakami, S. Sasaki, H. Okubo, Y. Takahashi, Y. Hosoi & M. Itabashi (2007). Association between dietary fiber, water and magnesium intake and functional constipation among young Japanese women. *European Journal of Clinical Nutrition*, 61(5), 616–22.

13 J. A. Ship & D. J. Fischer (1997). The relationship between dehydration and parotid salivary gland function in young and older healthy adults. *Journals of Gerontology—Series A Biological Sciences and Medical Sciences*, 52(5), M310–M319.

14 S. Tsindos (2012). What drove us to drink 2 litres of water a day? *Australian and New Zealand Journal of Public Health*, 36(3), 205–7.

15 H. Valtin (2002). 'Drink at least eight glasses of water a day.' Really? Is there scientific evidence for '8 × 8'? *American Journal of Physiology—Regulatory Integrative and Comparative Physiology*, 283(552–5), R993–R1004.

16 Z. Sui, M. Zheng, M. Zhang & A. Rangan (2016). Water and beverage consumption: analysis of the Australian 2011–2012 National Nutrition and Physical Activity Survey. *Nutrients*, 8(11). doi:10.3390/nu8110678

17 J. W. Gardner (2002). Death by water intoxication. *Military Medicine*, 167(5), 432.

18 *The Courier-Mail.* (2016). Inquest finds heat killed FIFO worker Glenn Newport but a new code of practice will need to differentiate between dehydration and dilutional hyponatremia. 8 May.

19 A. Crozier, D. Del Rio & M. N. Clifford (2010). Bioavailability of dietary flavonoids and phenolic compounds. *Molecular Aspects of Medicine*, 31(6), 446–67. doi:https://doi.org/10.1016/j.mam.2010.09.007

20 L. Lei, A. Rangan, V. M. Flood & J. C. Y. Louie (2016). Dietary intake and food sources of added sugar in the Australian population. *British Journal of Nutrition*, 115(5), 868–77. doi:10.1017/S0007114515005255

21 M. A. Heckman, J. Weil & E. Gonzalez de Mejia (2010). Caffeine (1, 3, 7-trimethylxanthine) in foods: a comprehensive review on consumption, functionality, safety, and regulatory matters. *Journal of Food Science*, 75(3), R77–87. doi:10.1111/j.1750-3841.2010.01561.x

22 R. J. Maughan & J. Griffin (2003). Caffeine ingestion and fluid balance: a review. *Journal of Human Nutrition and Dietetics*, 16(6), 411–20.

23 Australian Bureau of Statistics (2016). *Australian Health Survey: Consumption of added sugars, 2011–2012*. Canberra: ABS.

24 Cancer Council Victoria (2017). Rethink sugary drink. Retrieved from: www.rethinksugarydrink.org.au.

25 World Health Organization. (2016). *Fiscal Policies for Diet and Prevention of Noncommunicable Diseases: Technical meeting report*. Geneva: WHO.

26 AIS Sports Nutrition. (2009). Fluid: who needs it? *Sports Nutrition*. Retrieved from: www.ausport.gov.au/ais/nutrition/fact_sheets/fluid_-_who_needs_it.

27 S. Truswell (2012). Alcohol. In J. Mann & A. S. Truswell (eds), *Essentials of Human Nutrition*, 4th edn. New York: Oxford University Press.

28 A. I. Cederbaum (2012). Alcohol metabolism. *Clinics in Liver Disease*, 16(4), 667–85. doi:10.1016/j.cld.2012.08.002

29 J. Caballería (2003). Current concepts in alcohol metabolism. *Annual of Hepatology*, 2(2), 60–8.

30 T. K. Li, S. J. Yin, D. W. Crabb, S. O'Connor & V. A. Ramchandani (2001). Genetic and environmental influences on alcohol metabolism in humans. *Alcoholism: Clinical and Experimental Research*, 25(1), 136–44.

31 J. Rehm, G. E. Gmel, G. Gmel, O. S. M. Hasan, S. Imtiaz, S. Popova, ... P. A. Shuper (2017). The relationship between different dimensions of alcohol use and the burden of disease—an update. *Addiction*. doi:10.1111/add.13757

32 A. Gea, J. J. Beunza, R. Estruch, A. Sánchez-Villegas, J. Salas-Salvadó, P. Buil-Cosiales, ... M. A. Martínez-González (2013). Alcohol intake, wine consumption and the development of depression: the PREDIMED study. *BMC Medicine*, 11, 192. doi:10.1186/1741-7015-11-192

33 J. Rehm, G. E. Gmel, Sr, G. Gmel, O. S. M. Hasan, S. Imtiaz, S. Popova, ... P. A. Shuper (2017). The relationship between different dimensions of alcohol use and the burden of disease—an update. *Addiction (Abingdon, England)*. doi:10.1111/add.13757

34 J. Rehm & S. Imtiaz (2016). A narrative review of alcohol consumption as a risk factor for global burden of disease. *Substance Abuse: Treatment, Prevention, and Policy*, 11(1). doi:10.1186/s13011-016-0081-2

35 National Health and Medical Research Council (2009). *Australian Guidelines to Reduce Health Risks from Drinking Alcohol*. Canberra: NHMRC.

36 National Health and Medical Research Council (2013). *Australian Dietary Guidelines*. Canberra: NHMRC.

37 A. Kalinowski & K. Humphreys (2016). Governmental standard drink definitions and low-risk alcohol consumption guidelines in 37 countries. *Addiction (Abingdon, England)*, 111(7), 1293–8. doi:10.1111/add.13341

38 K. D. Shield, G. Gmel, G. Gmel, P. Mäkelä, C. Probst, R. Room & J. Rehm (2017). Lifetime risk of mortality due to different levels of alcohol consumption in seven European countries: implications for low-risk drinking guidelines. *Addiction (Abingdon, England)*. doi:10.1111/add.13827

39 B. S. Wymond, K. M. Dickinson & M. D. Riley (2016). Alcoholic beverage intake throughout the week and contribution to dietary energy intake in Australian adults. *Public Health Nutrition*, 19(14), 2592–602. doi:10.1017/S136898001600063X

40 Australian Institute of Health and Welfare (2016). *Australian Burden of Disease Study: Impact and causes of illness and death in Australia 2011* (no. 3). Canberra: AIHW.

41 M. Manning, C. Smith & P. Mazerolle (2013). *The Societal Costs of Alcohol Misuse in Australia*. Canberra: Australian Government.

42 N. Gunja & J. A. Brown (2012). Energy drinks: health risks and toxicity. *Medical Journal of Australia*, 196(1), 46–9.

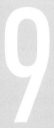

CHAPTER 9

FAT-SOLUBLE VITAMINS: A, D, E AND K

OLIVIA WRIGHT, VICKI FLOOD AND LINDA TAPSELL

CHAPTER OBJECTIVES

This chapter will enable the reader to:

- describe the chemical nature of the class of compounds known as fat-soluble vitamins
- briefly outline key functions of these chemical entities in the human body
- describe the types of foods and food patterns that would enable intakes of fat-soluble vitamins to support health.

KEY TERMS

Vitamin A, carotenoids and retinol

Vitamin D

Vitamin E and tocopherols

Vitamin K

KEY POINTS

- Vitamin A is a fat-soluble vitamin, but the nutrient class refers to a range of compounds classed together, and comes in a number of forms: retinol, retinal, retinoic acid, retinyl ester, carotenoids and xenophills. Vitamin A is important for growth, reproduction, immunisation and eye health. Some forms of vitamin A are found predominantly in animal foods, but dietary carotenoids are found in plant foods, mainly fruits and vegetables.
- Vitamin D is a fat-soluble vitamin essential for maintaining healthy bones and the optimum functioning of multiple body systems. It is primarily synthesised from cholesterol in the skin and absorbed into the circulation. It is activated by metabolic processes in the liver to form 25(OH)D and in the kidney to form the hormonally active 1,25(OH)2D. The hormonally active form can also be produced in numerous tissues throughout the body for local action on target tissues. About 5–10% of vitamin D is absorbed from foods such as oily fish (e.g. sardines, salmon), cheese, liver, and milk and margarine fortified with vitamin D2 or D3.
- Vitamin E is a principal antioxidant compound in the human body which comes in a number of forms as tocopherols or tocotrienols. Deficiency is rare. Vitamin E helps to retain the stability of polyunsatured fatty acids and is found in foods with high proportions of these, such as nuts and vegetable oils.
- Vitamin K plays a role in the formation of clotting factors and is required for normal blood coagulation. It is found in dark green, leafy vegetables, but is also synthesised by bacteria in the large bowel. The anticoagulant drug warfarin works in an antagonistic way to vitamin K.

INTRODUCTION

Visit Oxford Ascend for more on vitamins.

Vitamins are bioactive molecules that serve metabolic processes both in the original foods consumed (plants or animals) [1]. Vitamins are essential for health and are referred to as micronutrients because they are required in very small amounts. Food delivers vitamins in biological doses and often in combination with other micronutrients with which they share metabolic pathways or purposes. Historically, a knowledge of vitamins emerged from observations of clinical deficiencies, their isolation from foods and the characterisation of their chemical structure. Specific functions in human physiology and metabolism were identified in association with deficiency disorders. Further categorisation of vitamins into fat-soluble and water-soluble entities was helpful in developing an understanding of requirements. Thus, fat-soluble and water-soluble vitamins have different locations and pathways for absorption in the gut and there is a difference in the ability to excrete excessive amounts. While excess water-soluble vitamins may be excreted via the kidney, this is not the case for fat-soluble vitamins where serious toxicity states have been observed. The most well-known of these is that of early Arctic explorers who consumed polar bear liver, with the subsequent illness attributed to vitamin A toxicity.

The fat-soluble vitamins are known as vitamins A, D, E and K. Vitamin A is required for the formation of visual pigments and deficiency is associated with night blindness; vitamin D is required for normal bone formation and deficiency results in rickets in children or osteomalacia in adults; vitamin E has powerful antioxidant capacities, protecting cell membranes, so deficiency may lead to damage in these areas, but research is required; and vitamin K is associated with the formation of clotting factors, and deficiency can lead to bleeding and bruising.

With advances in food and nutritional sciences, fat-soluble vitamins have come to be known as classes of chemical compounds rather than single entities, and their health benefits have been considered beyond the prevention of overt deficiency, to maximising the functionality of the human system and preventing chronic disease. The availability of published research that provides a body of evidence for micronutrient health effects varies considerably. Among the fat-soluble vitamins, vitamin D has perhaps received the most attention, with recent research moving beyond bone health to areas such as metabolic dysfunction [2]. Not only does it remain important for the maintenance of healthy bones, but new research is also linking it to numerous other essential processes in the body, including inflammation, immune system function, cardiovascular function, blood glucose regulation and cognition.

In providing an introductory overview of fat-soluble vitamins, this chapter focuses on the structure and function of the chemical entities that represent fat-soluble vitamins, and identifies the major food sources for delivering these nutrients in their naturally occurring context with other nutrients in a food matrix within an overall healthy diet.

STOP AND THINK

- Why would solubility in fat be relevant to the action of a vitamin?
- How does the solubility help to identify food sources?
- Do all forms of these vitamins have the same chemical properties?

WHAT ARE THE STRUCTURES AND FUNCTIONS OF VITAMIN A AND CAROTENOIDS?

Vitamin A is a term that refers to a collection of chemical compounds that can broadly be described as carotenoids or retinoids (Figure 9.1). Both are found in plants and animals, but carotenoids are mostly found in plants and retinoids in animals. Preformed vitamin A is made up of retinyl esters and retinol, and some carotenoids are known as pro-vitamin A carotenoids, and contribute to trans-retinol compounds (β-carotene, α-carotene and β-cryptoxanthin). While categorised as a fat-soluble vitamin, vitamin A requirements actually refer to a group of compounds defined by their biological activity. The measurement term 'retinol equivalence' refers to the biological activity of 1 µg of all trans-retinol compounds.

Other carotenoids found in foods (such as lycopene, lutein and zeaxanthin) are not converted to trans-retinol compounds, but there is increasing evidence that these carotenoids are important for good health. The stability of the vitamin A class of compounds, in particular the carotenoids, can be compromised under certain conditions, especially at high temperatures. Chemical changes such as oxidation, isomerisation and polymerisation can occur [3].

See Chapter 4 on phytonutrients.

Vitamin A compounds are first released from binding proteins in the stomach. Their absorption in the gut is associated with dietary fat, as micelles are formed through the action of bile and digestive enzymes. Within the mucosal cells in the duodenum, retinyl esters and carotenoids (provitamin A) are converted to retinol. About 70–90% of retinol is absorbed, but this is less (30–50%) for carotenoids [4]. There are a number of factors that may influence the relative availability of retinol and carotenoids in the body, including the ingested food (e.g. raw or cooked in a fat such as olive oil), genetics and control systems (e.g. higher carotenoid levels in the body lowers bioavailability). Hypercarotenaemia (showing as yellow/orange skin colouring) is a condition that can occur when there is overly excessive consumption of orange fruit or vegetables such as carrots. Retinol is transported to the liver via chylomicron packages and converts to retinal and retinoic acid, the form in which vitamin A is eventually stored in the liver. Most digested vitamin A is stored in the liver and these stores can last several months and toxicity can occur. Transport to tissues is facilitated by binding proteins [5]. Once digested, the duodenal mucosal cells (cells of the intestine) are involved in the absorption and conversion of retinyl esters and provitamin A carotenoids to retinol in the body. Retinol is then further oxidised to retinal and then to retinoic acid. Once digested, the majority (~90%) of vitamin A is stored as retinoic acid in the liver, creating reserves for several months' requirements. The storage in the liver occurs via chylomicron transportation of the vitamin. Following storage, retinol can be further transported using retinol-binding proteins to the tissues requiring it.

Vitamin A serves a number of functions in the body. It enables night vision and colour perception, supports reproduction and immunity and is involved in the maturation of cells [6]. Requirement levels vary depending on age and state of health, including the functioning of the liver, the presence of disease and the ability to absorb fat. Inadequate intakes can lead to eye disease such as xeropthalmia (where bacterial infection can emerge from poor mucus production in the eye) and night blindness [7]. Other areas of the body that can be affected include skin and hair where growth and cell regeneration are important. Table 9.1 lists vitamin A requirements.

FIGURE 9.1   STRUCTURES OF THE RETINOIDS AND CAROTENOIDS

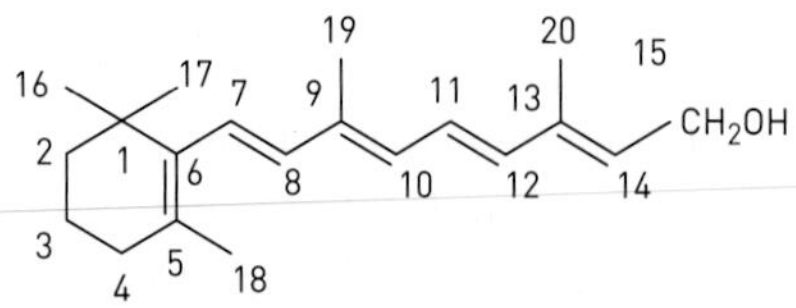

All-*trans* retinol (vitamin A, vitamin A$_1$)

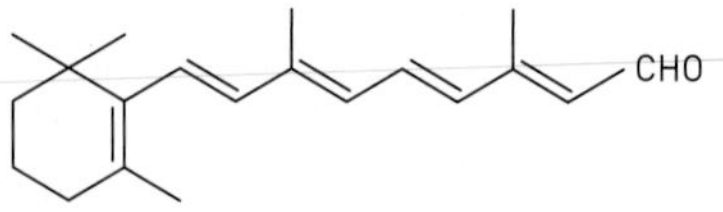

All-*trans* retinal

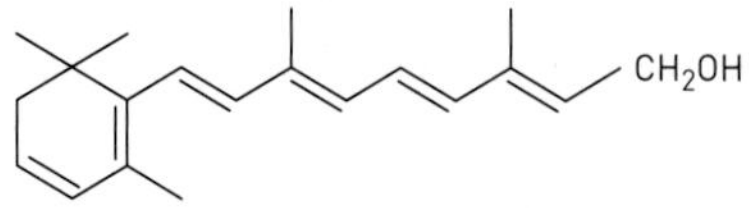

3-Dehydroretinol (vitamin A$_2$)

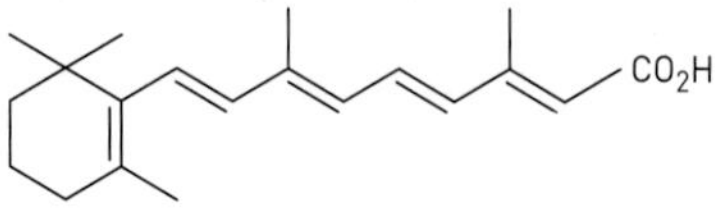

All-*trans* retinoic acid

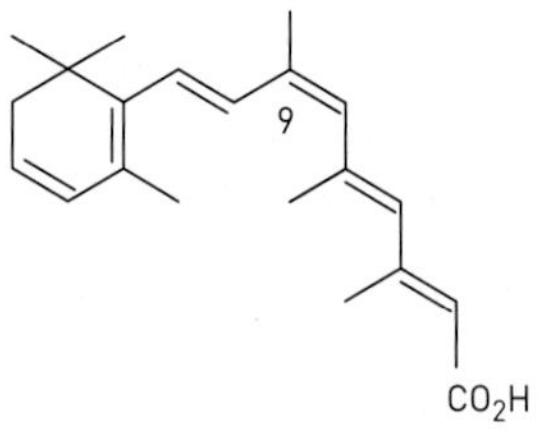

9-*cis* retinoic acid

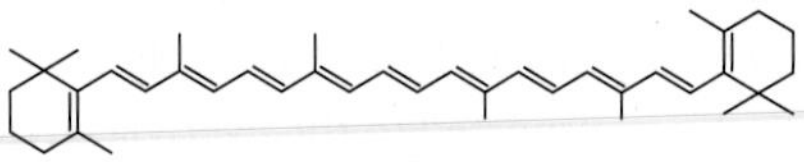

β-Carotene

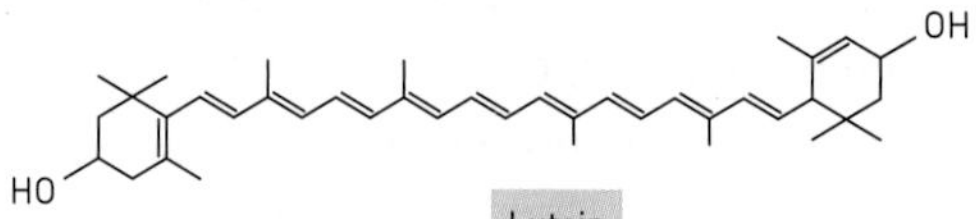

Lutein

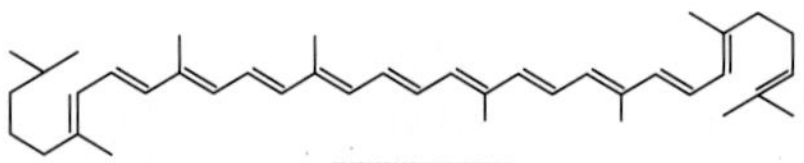

Lycopene

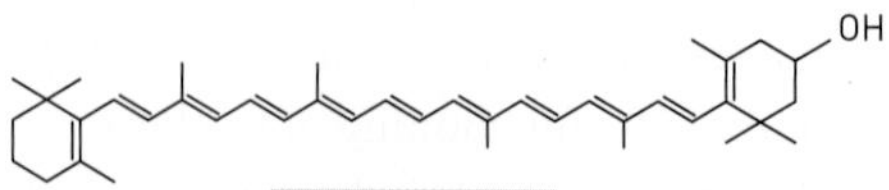

β-Cryptoxanthin

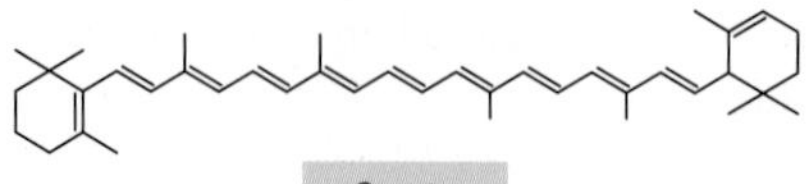

α-Carotene

Source: D. I. Thurnham (2012). Chapter 12: Vitamin A and carotenoids. In J. Mann & S. Truswell (eds), *Essentials of Human Nutrition*, 4th edn. Oxford University Press, Incorporated

TABLE 9.1   VITAMIN A (RETINOL EQUIVALENTS) REQUIREMENTS

Recommended intakes of vitamin A (µg/day)	Estimated average requirement (EAR)	Recommended dietary intake (RDI)	Upper level of intake (UL)
Men			
19–70 years	625	900	3000
>70 years	625	900	3000
Women			
19–50 years	500	700	3000
>50 years	500	700	3000
Pregnancy			
14–18 years	530	700	2800
18–50 years	550	800	3000
Lactation			
14–18 years	780	1100	2800
18–50 years	800	1100	3000

Source: National Health and Medical Research Council (2006). *Nutrient Reference Values for Australia and New Zealand, including Recommended Dietary Intakes*. Canberra: NHMRC. © Commonwealth of Australia

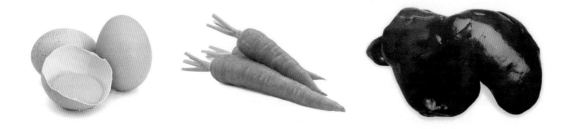

STOP AND THINK

- Why is vitamin A classed together with carotenoids?
- Why would a vitamin delivered in plant foods be different from that in an animal?
- Why would these compounds convert into each other?

WHAT ARE THE MAJOR FOOD SOURCES OF VITAMIN A AND CAROTENOIDS?

Given its biological roles, good dietary sources of vitamin A tend to be foods originating from animals and associated vitamin A storage sites, including liver, fish and eggs. Milk can be fortified with vitamin A and it will also exist in oils. In contrast, precursors of vitamin A, such as the carotenoids, are pigments in yellow fruits and vegetables and in dark green leafy vegetables.

     OLIVIA WRIGHT, VICKI FLOOD AND LINDA TAPSELL

Retinol equivalents

1 µg retinol equivalent = 1 µg all trans-retinol or 6 µg all trans-beta-carotene or 12 µg alpha-carotene, beta-cryptoxanthin and other provitamin carotenoids. 1 IU = 0.3 µg retinol equivalents [4].

Vitamin A is an antioxidant fat-soluble nutrient that may be found naturally or added to foods during fortification. It is added to margarines (creating the yellow colouring) and occurs naturally in meats and dairy products (fat-containing foods). It is only in trace amounts in nuts and seeds. **Retinol equivalents** include the collection of provitamin A carotenoid nutrients (mainly α- and β-carotene) that form the yellow or orange colour of fruits and vegetables. Carrots are a commonly identified example of a food rich in β-carotene, as are mangoes (Table 9.2).

TABLE 9.2   VITAMIN A (RETINOL EQUIVALENTS AND β-CAROTENE) CONTENT OF FOODS

Food	Serving size[1]	µg of vitamin A (retinol equivalents) per serve[3]	µg of β-carotene per serve[3]
Orange (navel), peeled	150 g	21	108
Carrot (raw)	75 g	987	4497
Mango (raw) peeled	150 g	549	2149.5
Orange sweet potato (baked) peeled	75 g	929.25	5433
Grilled lamb liver	65 g	21669	29.9
Polyunsaturated margarine	10 g[2]	79.3	50
Cream cheese	40 g	140	76.4

[1]Based on the Australian Dietary Guidelines [8].
[2]Based on modelling of the Australian Dietary Guidelines [9].
[3]Calculated from *NUTTAB 2010* [10].

Age-related macular degeneration (AMD)

degeneration of the macular component of the eye leading to blindness.

Lutein and zeaxanthin are two fat-soluble carotenoids known as xanthophylls. Kale and spinach are a particularly rich source of lutein and zeaxanthin (Table 9.3). They are major constituents of the macular pigment in the eye, which is concentrated in the macula of the retina. The retina is responsible for fine feature visions, and there has been a focus in recent years about how the accumulation of these carotenoids in the pigment may prevent or slow the progression of **age-related macular degeneration (AMD)**, a leading cause of blindness in older adults. These nutrients are likely to play an antioxidant role, important in eye health, which is readily exposed to light and oxygen, and additionally provide blue light-filtering properties, which are also likely to be important to protect the eye. There is also evidence that bioavailability of these carotenoids may be decreased due to competition with other carotenoids when consumed in the same meal, but that area of research requires further development [11].

TRY IT YOURSELF

Provide a sample day's dietary intake that includes a range of vitamin A food sources, and calculate the intake of retinol equivalents, beta-carotene, and lutein and zeaxanthin.

» RESEARCH AT WORK

LUTEIN AND AGE-RELATED EYE DISEASE

In a randomised clinical trial of people with AMD, known as the AREDS-2 trial [12], 10 mg of lutein and 2 mg of zeaxanthin supplements slowed the progression of the AMD only when their diets were low in lutein and zeaxanthin, and the supplement did not have an impact on the progression of AMD when they consumed higher amounts of lutein and zeaxanthin. This implies there may be a threshold level of intake that is important for good eye health. In this study, the threshold level was approximately 1134 µg/per 1000 calorie diet (interquartile range of 1030–1244 µg/1000 cals). If we assume a 2000-calorie diet that implies dietary intakes of at least 2268 µg of L/Z (interquartile range of 2069-2488 µg), this may provide protection against late AMD [13]. Other observation studies have also reported a protective effect of L/Z from AMD. In a study of older people in Australia, known as the Blue Mountains Eye Study, people who consumed diets with the highest tertile of L/Z had a 65% reduced risk of developing AMD (cases known as neo-vascular AMD) (RR: 0.35, 95% CI (0.13–0.92) [14].

TABLE 9.3   LUTEIN AND ZEAXANTHIN CONTENT OF COMMON FOODS

Food item	Serve	Lutein and zeaxanthin (µg/100g)	Amount per serve
Kale, cooked	75 g	18,246	13,684.5
Spinach, raw	75 g	12,197	9147.7
Parsley	5 g	5562	278.1
Peas, green, boiled	75 g	2593	1944.7
Pistachio nuts, raw	30 g	1404	421.2
Egg yolk, raw	2 eggs, 50 g each	1094	1094
Frozen corn, boiled from frozen	75 g	684	513

Source: US Department of Agriculture Agricultural Research Service (2018). USDA National Nutrient Database for Standard Reference. Retrieved from https://ndb.nal.usda.gov/ndb

STOP AND THINK

• Why would the plant-based compounds (carotenoids) and the animal-based compounds (retinoid) be classed together as a vitamin category?
• What is the significance of vitamin A nutrition for older people in the community? Why would they be at risk of health problems related to this vitamin?
• How would advice to consume adequate vitamin A fit with other advice to consume a healthy diet?

WHAT ARE THE STRUCTURES AND FUNCTIONS OF VITAMIN D?

Rickets

brittle bone disease due to vitamin D deficiency.

Vitamin D is a fat-soluble vitamin, or secosteroid, historically associated with development of strong and healthy bones. This knowledge evolved from studies showing that vitamin D deficiency in childhood was associated with the improper mineralisation of bones during growth and development. The condition was called **rickets**, or brittle bone disease, and resulted in bowed legs, knocked knees and curved spines as children grew. In adults, vitamin D deficiency impairs calcium and phosphorous absorption, resulting in poor bone remineralisation and subsequent bone pain, osteomalacia (osteo = bone; malacia = softening) and increased risk of fractures [15].

Vitamin D has been linked to numerous essential processes within the human body beyond bone metabolism, including inflammation, immune system function, cardiovascular function, blood glucose regulation and cognition [16–18]. There is also a link between maternal vitamin D intake and the health of offspring, particularly mental health [19]. Vitamin D has a hormonal mechanism of action by binding to its receptor, the vitamin D receptor (VDR), in target tissues. Classical physiological roles for vitamin D include calcium homeostasis and bone metabolism [20]. Vitamin D helps to increase calcium absorption from the intestine by promoting the synthesis of proteins essential for calcium absorption. The hormonally active form of vitamin D is increasingly being identified as important across multiple body systems, particularly in relation to reducing systemic inflammation associated with chronic disease [21], improving immune function and cognitive function [22; 23]. Beyond disruptions to calcium homeostasis, impaired bone metabolism and osteoporosis, inadequate levels have been associated with cancer, insulin resistance, obesity, diabetes, infertility, musculoskeletal disorders, adverse pregnancy outcomes, cognitive dysfunction, depression and cardiovascular disease [24–28].

Vitamin D is produced cutaneously—that is, in the skin—on exposure to sunlight. Exposure of around 15% of the body's surface area (e.g. arms and hands) in the midday sun produces around 25 µg vitamin D (or 1000 international units [IU]) [29]. Vitamin D is therefore different from other dietary nutrients. It requires two steps to become biologically active, so is sometimes referred to as a prohormone [30]. The vitamin D production process commences with the conversion of cholesterol in the skin to 5,7-cholesteradienol, or 7-dehydrocholesterol (7-DHO). Exposure to a specific wavelength range of ultraviolet B (UVB) rays from the sun (280–315 nm) causes 7-DHO to be converted to pre-vitamin D3. Isomerisation caused by heat then converts pre-vitamin D3 into vitamin D3, or cholecalciferol. Vitamin D3 is released from the skin bound to vitamin D binding protein (DBP) and travels to the liver where it is hydroxylated (an hydroxyl or OH group is added) to form 25-hydroxyvitamin D [25(OH)D], or calcidiol, by microsomal cytochrome P450 enzyme CYP2R1 (25-hydroxylase) and mitochondrial cytochrome P450 CYP27A1 (27-hydroxylase). 25(OH)D bound to DBP is released into the circulation and taken up by the kidneys via megalin or cubilin endocytosis [31]. 25(OH)D is converted to the hormonally active form of 1,25–dihydroxyvitamin D [1,25(OH)$_2$D], or calcitriol, in the kidneys by the enzyme CYP27B1 (1a-hydroxylase). This is the form of vitamin D associated with physiological functions. If levels of 1,25(OH)$_2$D are sufficient, excess 25(OH)D is inactivated to 24,25(OH)$_2$D by CYP24A1 (24-hydroxylase), as part of a five-step catabolism process [32; 33]. See also Table 9.4.

Vitamin D2 and the small amount of vitamin D3 found in dietary sources are absorbed from micelles through passive diffusion in the small intestine. Fat and bile salts assist the absorption process. The vitamin D and fat is incorporated into chylomicrons for absorption into the lymphatic system prior to entering the bloodstream. Around 40% of the vitamin D is transported in the blood via

TABLE 9.4   SUMMARY OF VITAMIN D CHEMICAL FORMS AND METABOLITES

Vitamin D chemical subtype	Source and role	Properties
7-dehydrocholesterol	Produced in the skin on contact with sunlight (UVB 280–315 nm); cholesterol precursor	Provitamin D; no reported clinical utility
Vitamin D2, ergocalciferol	Plant foods	Produced by irradiation of ergosterol by ultraviolet (UV) light
Vitamin D3, cholecalciferol	Animal foods	Produced by irradiation of 7-DHO by UV light
25-hydroxyvitamin D, 25(OH)D	Produced by the liver after hydroxylation of 7-dehydroxycholesterol; pre-hormone	Half life: 3 weeks; good clinical utility
1,25-dihydroxyvitamin D, 1,25(OH)$_2$D	Produced by the kidneys and in intestinal cells after hydroxylation of 25(OH)D; active hormone—binds to vitamin D receptor throughout body; regulated by parathyroid hormone	Half life: 4 hours; elevated in bone disease; poor clinical utility
24,25-dihydroxyvitamin D, 24,25(OH)$_2$D	Inactivated form of 1,25(OH)$_2$D once calcium homeostasis restored [34]	Suppresses apoA-I gene expression [35]

Source: G. Peter, R. Colin, J. John, H. Stuart, L.-D. Lilia & D. Colin (2004). Global Solar UV Index: Australian measurements, forecasts and comparison with the UK. *Photochemistry and Photobiology*, 79(1), 32–9. doi:10.1111/j.1751-1097.2004.tb09854.x

chylomicrons, where the rest is transferred to vitamin D binding protein for transport to extrahepatic tissues. New research has suggested a role for cholesterol membrane transporters in transporting vitamin D across the epithelial cells of the intestines [36].

Vitamin D exerts genomic effects in the cell through the vitamin D receptor. In the human body, most cells and organs have VDRs, which explains the multitude of effects of vitamin D on body systems [37]. The VDR is termed a 'nuclear receptor'. This means that when activated by the binding of its ligand, vitamin D, the VDR heterodimerises (i.e. joins together) with the retinoid X receptor (RXR) and binds to specific vitamin D response elements (VDRE) on DNA strands, leading to expression of certain genes. Genome-wide studies using microarray technology have shown that genes related to immune function are 'switched on' in the presence of vitamin D, and therefore vitamin D may play a vital role in protection from the onset of disease [38]. Vitamin D also exerts non-genomic effects through the vitamin D membrane receptor, another VDR but in a different location. The most well-characterised effect is calcium influx, which has multiple effects throughout the cell—for example, cell cycle progression, cell proliferation and cell division [39].

The liver is a major storage site for both vitamin D3 and 25(OH)D, and adipose tissue also stores large amounts of vitamin D3 and smaller amounts of 25(OH)D [40]. Skeletal muscle is another potential storage site for 25(OH)D [41]. Several other tissues, including the brain, skin, placenta, ovaries, endometrium, testis, spermatozoa, pituitary gland, prostate gland, breast and parathyroid glands have been identified as containing 1a-hydroxylase, providing evidence for extra-renal production of 1,25(OH)$_2$D [42]. The VDR has also been characterised in these tissues [28; 43]. This suggests that these tissues and organs are utilising active vitamin D for physiological functioning.

>> CASE 9.1

VITAMIN D AND EXPOSURE TO SUNLIGHT

Despite sun exposure being the best way to maintain adequate vitamin D levels, caution is needed. The UV Index is an internationally standardised ranking for the potential of the sun's UV rays to burn the skin. It ranges from 1, 2 (low), 3, 4, 5 (moderate), 6, 7 (high), 8, 9, 10 (very high) to 11+ (extreme). The UV Index is moderate to extreme in most parts of Australia throughout the year, leading to a high risk of skin cancer. A position statement about the risks and benefits of sun exposure has been developed by the Australian and New Zealand Bone and Mineral Society (ANZBMS), the Australian College of Dermatologists, Cancer Council Australia, Endocrine Society of Australia and Osteoporosis Australia. When the UV Index is 3 or above during summer in Australia, sun exposure to arms and hands for only a few minutes in the mid-morning or afternoon is recommended on most days of the week. Sun protection (broad-brimmed hat, protective clothing, sunscreen, sunglasses and shade) is recommended if exposure is any more than a few minutes. When the UV Index is less than 3 in autumn and winter in Australia, it is recommended people go outside in the middle of the day with some skin exposure on most days of the week. Table 9.5 shows the UV Index in selected Australian cities averaged over the days in each month and is obtained from the position statement document. The highlighting shows the months and locations where the UV Index is less than 3. It can be seen that the UV Index rarely drops below 3 in Australia and this only occurs in the autumn/winter months.

- Table 9.5 presents an average UV Index for each state for each month of the year. How does the UV Index vary across the day? Visit the UV Index website and determine the average UV Index and its daily variation for the state you live in: www.arpansa.gov.au/services/monitoring/ultraviolet-radiation-monitoring/ultraviolet-radiation-index.
- How can recommendations for sun exposure during the peak of summer be developed for people living in different states?

TABLE 9.5   UV INDEX* IN SELECTED AUSTRALIAN CITIES AVERAGED OVER THE DAYS IN EACH MONTH

Location	Jan	Feb	Mar	Apr	May	Jun	Jul	Aug	Sep	Oct	Nov	Dec
Darwin	12.3	12.6	12.5	11.1	9.2	8.2	8.7	10.2	11.9	12.6	12.4	12.0
Brisbane	11.8	11.2	9.5	6.9	4.8	3.7	4.1	5.4	7.4	8.9	10.5	11.3
Perth	11.8	11.0	8.6	5.8	3.8	2.8	3.0	4.3	6.1	8.1	9.8	11.4
Sydney	10.5	9.5	7.5	5.2	3.2	2.3	2.5	3.6	5.3	7.1	8.7	10.0
Canberra	10.7	7.7	6.9	4.8	2.9	1.9	2.2	3.3	5.0	6.8	8.5	10.6
Adelaide	11.2	10.1	7.8	5.1	3.0	2.1	2.3	3.4	5.2	7.2	9.2	10.7
Melbourne	10.3	9.0	7.0	4.4	2.4	1.6	1.7	2.8	4.3	6.3	8.3	9.8
Hobart **	8	7	4	3	1	1	1	2	3	4	6	7

*The UV Index is a measure of the amount of UV radiation from the sun at the earth's surface at solar noon on a particular day.
**Hobart data is supplied from personal communication from the Australian Radiation Protection and Nuclear Safety Agency.

Source: Australian and New Zealand Bone and Mineral Society, Australasian College of Dermatologists, Cancer Council Australia & Endocrine Society of Australia and Osteoporosis Australia (2016). *Position Statement: Sun exposure and vitamin D—Risks and benefits.* Cancer Council Australia. Retrieved from: http://wiki.cancer.org.au/policy/Position_statement_-_Risks_and_benefits_of_sun_exposure

Those considered most at risk of vitamin D insufficiency or deficiency are the housebound elderly (poor skin synthetic function), hospital patients in long-term care, those with malabsorption syndromes or on total parenteral nutrition (TPN), babies and infants of vitamin D deficient mothers, those with skin cancer or at a high risk of skin cancer, people with dark skin pigmentation or those who constantly wear sun protective clothing or veils [44–46]. It is suggested adults aged >70 years have around 75% lower capacity to synthesise the precursors for vitamin D production in the skin [47].

According to current definitions of insufficiency (25(OH)D <50 nmol/L) and deficiency (25(OH)D <25 nmol/L) based on the maintenance of calcium homeostasis [48] (Table 9.6), 37–67% of Australian women are estimated to be insufficient in vitamin D [49], along with billions of people worldwide [50]. It is possible to maintain adequate vitamin D status from sun exposure alone; however, this increasing prevalence of vitamin D insufficiency and deficiency suggests this may not be occurring. Changes to more inactive, indoor lifestyles may have contributed to reduced levels. Vitamin D levels are also known to be lower in the winter months when skin production is lower since a higher proportion of the skin loses contact with the sun through greater clothing coverage.

TABLE 9.6   DEFINITIONS OF VITAMIN D STATUS

Definition	Range (nmol/l)
Deficient	<30
Insufficient	30–50
Sufficient	>50

Source: A. C. Ross (2010). *Dietary Reference Intakes for Calcium and Vitamin D*. Washington, DC: National Academies Press

» CASE 9.2

MEASUREMENT OF VITAMIN D STATUS

Measurement of vitamin D status has increased around tenfold in the past 10 years [51]. The values shown in Table 9.6 are typically used to define vitamin D status [52]; however, the definition of vitamin D deficiency varies between countries and institutes. This is due to the use of different outcomes as cut-offs for serum 25(OH)D levels—for example, the recommendation of >60 nmol/l to prevent falls in the elderly [53], or >82.5 nmol/l to reduce colorectal cancer risk by 50% [22].

Serum 25(OH)D is used as a biomarker for vitamin D status as it is more stable, more abundant and easier to assay than the active form, or 1,25(OH)$_2$D. There is no universal consensus on appropriate reference ranges for vitamin D for bone health [54] or insufficiency/deficiency [55], and no empirical evidence for reference ranges for other conditions [56] or racial variations. Levels between 50 and 82.5 nmol/l are recommended [57–59]. A wide range of assays have been developed to test serum 25(OH)D, including competitive binding protein assays, radioimmunoassays and liquid chromatography. There is no national or international standardisation for the assay/s and cross-validation between methods is not standard practice [60]. Most disagreement between the assays occurs at the highest and lowest quartiles of vitamin D status [60–62], which reduces confidence in any clinical definitions of insufficiency/deficiency. Considering that emerging clinical vitamin D research is focused on supplementation to determine its effects across a range of diseases/conditions, the ability to accurately and reliably measure vitamin D status is essential in order to measure appropriate clinical outcomes, and further research and investigation is warranted.

- Consider the case of Mr Davis, a hypothetical elderly man who was vitamin D deficient (25 nmol/L) and had his vitamin D status tested in 2016. His doctor prescribed a vitamin D supplement and would like him to have his vitamin D level re-tested six months later. Unfortunately, the laboratory analysis provider has changed. What are the implications for interpretations of results?
- What level of vitamin D should Mr Davis aim for, and why?

Conversion factors for vitamin D

1 µg cholecalciferol = 0.2 µg 25(OH)D; 1 international unit (IU) = 0.025 µg cholecalciferol or 0.005 µg 25(OH)D.

Serum parathyroid hormone (PTH) levels are usually elevated in vitamin D deficiency due to the coinciding disturbances in serum calcium homeostasis. A combination of $1,25(OH)_2D$ and PTH increase to rectify this by increasing calcium absorption from the intestine, mobilising calcium from bone and increasing calcium reabsorption from the distal tubule of the kidney [63]. The greater risk of osteoporosis in those with vitamin D deficiency is due to the increased calcium mobilisation from bone. **Conversion factors for vitamin D** are important when considering vitamin D status (see www.nrv.gov.au/nutrients/vitamin-d).

The recommended intake for vitamin D varies internationally, but in Australia the adequate intake (AI) for cholecalciferol is 5 µg/day (or 200 IU) for infants, children, adolescents and adults, 10 µg/day (or 400 IU) for adults 51–70 years and 15 µg/day (or 600 IU) for adults >70 years. The AI level is set higher for older adults in an attempt to compensate for poorer absorption with age and to reduce the risk of fractures. As vitamin D is a fat-soluble vitamin, excess may be toxic. The upper level (UL) of intake is set at 25 µg/day for infants and 80 µg/day for children, adolescents and all adults. The largest risk of toxicity is from consumption of fish liver oils. The estimated dietary intake of vitamin D in Australia is largely unknown as current food databases are limited. Fortification of edible oil spreads with vitamin D is mandatory in Australia. Fortification of modified and skim milk products, powdered milks, yoghurts, table confections and cheese is voluntary [4].

>> RESEARCH AT WORK

NEONATAL VITAMIN D STATUS AND RISK OF SCHIZOPHRENIA

Researchers from the Department of Psychiatry and the Queensland Brain Institute, University of Queensland, Australia, and the University of Aarhus and the Statens Serum Institut, Denmark, investigated the association between neonatal vitamin D status and the risk of developing schizophrenia later in life [64]. The study design was an individually matched case-control study drawn from a population-based cohort. It included 424 individuals with schizophrenia and 424 controls matched for sex and birth date. Records were sourced from Danish national health registers and a Newborn Screening Biobank. Dried blood spots were analysed for 25(OH)D3 and 25(OH)D2 to determine neonatal vitamin D status. 25(OH)D3 levels were divided into quintiles, or five equal proportions, to allow in-depth investigation of the results. The study authors calculated the population attributable fraction (PAF), which is defined as the contribution of a risk factor to a disease or a death (for the equation, see www.who.int/healthinfo/global_burden_disease/metrics_paf/en), and this was 44%. A large proportion of the sample, particularly those born earlier, was excluded due to an inadequate amount of blood in the blood spots for analysis, but since date of birth was a matching criteria in the study, the researchers ensured this did not bias the findings. Data analysis was also controlled for potential confounding variables, including parental history of mental illness, migrant status, age of parents and urbanisation of place of birth.

Dietary 25(OH)D2 was detected in less than 5% of the samples, suggesting this was not a significant source of vitamin D. There was significant seasonal variation in 25(OH)D3, which was expected, given the reliance on sunlight exposure for its production. It was interesting that children of migrant women had significantly lower 25(OH)D3 levels than children of non-migrant women. The results indicated that neonates in the lower three quintiles of 25(OH)D3 had a twofold elevated risk of schizophrenia than those in the fourth quintile (25(OH)D3 concentrations between 40.5 and 50.9 nmol/L). The 25(OH)D3 levels for the fourth quintile were low and in the insufficient range according to the definition of vitamin D status. In this study, the relationship between neonatal vitamin D levels and risk of schizophrenia was non-linear—that is, it did not progress in a straight line. The researchers had another surprising finding: neonates in the highest quintile of 25(OH)D3 had a significantly increased risk of schizophrenia. The authors concluded that both low and high concentrations of 25(OH)D3 are associated with the risk of developing schizophrenia later in life. This result is consistent with evidence that the relationship between 25(OH)D3 levels and disease or mortality is U-shaped—that is, deficiency and excess are not good for health [37]. The study did not examine any genetic differences, or single nucleotide polymorphisms (SNPs), in genes responsible for the metabolism of 25(OH)D3 to 1,25(OH)2D, or SNPs for the VDR or DBP, but the authors indicated that this work is planned. The researchers also cautioned against several potential confounders to the interpretation of findings that may also be associated with vitamin D status, including heat stress, maternal fish intake and maternal body mass index. Further work is needed to encompass these factors and determine optimal levels of vitamin D for pregnant women to optimise neonatal levels. There is also a need for ongoing research exploring the impact of 25(OH)D3 status on brain development and mental health.

STOP AND THINK

- How many different forms of vitamin D are there and how are they sourced by the body?
- What are the implications of exposure to sunlight in establishing adequate vitamin D status?
- Why is vitamin D such a challenging and significant nutrient on which to conduct research?

WHAT ARE THE MAJOR FOOD SOURCES OF VITAMIN D?

Around 5–10% of vitamin D levels in humans result from dietary intake [29]. Vitamin D2, or ergosterol, is a fungal type of vitamin D found in plant sources only (e.g. mushrooms and yeast). It can be activated to ergocalciferol through irradiation with UV light [65]. Vitamin D3, or cholecalciferol, is found in animal foods, particularly those with a high fat content, including oily fish (e.g. sardines, salmon), egg yolk, cheese, liver, as well as milk and margarine fortified with vitamin D2 or D3. These food sources are similar to those for retinol.

Table 9.7 shows the main food sources of vitamin D and their content in micrograms (µg) per 100 grams. A large amount of these foods would need to be consumed to be considered a substantial source of vitamin D. A limitation of the current Australian Food Databases (AUSNUT 2011–13) is the lack of information on vitamin D content of foods. AUSNUT 2007 included vitamin D content and a summary is included in Table 9.7.

     OLIVIA WRIGHT, VICKI FLOOD AND LINDA TAPSELL

TABLE 9.7   FOOD SOURCES OF VITAMIN D

Food	Vitamin D content (µg/100g)
Non-fortified	
Cod liver oil	210
Butter	0.65
Egg, chicken, whole, poached	0.67
Milk, yoghurt, reduced-regular fat	0.2–0.6
Cheese, non-specified	3
Liver	0.1–0.2
Beef, lamb, chicken, kangaroo, lean, grilled	0.12
Pork, lean, grilled	0.5–0.8
Oyster, baked or grilled	0.14
Squid or calamari, baked or grilled	0.13
Anchovy, canned in oil, drained	2
Sardine, canned in tomato sauce, undrained	8
Salmon, pink, canned in brine	1
Salmon, red, canned in brine	4
Salmon, grilled or smoked	7
Trout, rainbow, aquacultured, steamed or poached	8
Hoki, steamed or poached	4
Tuna, canned in brine	0.8
Tuna, yellowfin steaks, grilled or barbecued with olive oil	3
Fortified	
Milk	0.6–2.0
Margarine	4.5

Source: Food Standards Australia New Zealand (2012). *AUSNUT 2007*. Canberra: FSANZ

TRY IT YOURSELF

Using Table 9.7, analyse your average daily vitamin D intake. Assess your intake and devise two strategies for how you could improve your intake if needed. This may or may not involve supplements. Consider how to achieve optimum absorption.

In Australia, around 51% of dietary vitamin D intake is obtained from meat, fish, eggs and meat substitutes, with the majority coming from canned fish (28%) [66]. Supplementation contributes to 8% of vitamin D intake for men and 4% of intake for women [66]. Evidence suggests better absorption of vitamin D is achieved when it is consumed with the largest meal of the day [67], and in combination with mono-unsaturated fatty acids [68]. Improvement in accuracy of assessment of vitamin D intake may be achieved by taking the content of the preliminary metabolite, 25-hydroxyvitamin D [25(OH)D], in foods into account [69].

≫ CASE 9.3

VITAMIN D DEFICIENCY AND SUPPLEMENTATION

In addition to the traditional groups at risk of vitamin D deficiency due to limited sun exposure, poor absorption or poor synthetic function in the skin, new groups of at-risk individuals are thought to be emerging. This is occurring in line with the rising rates of lifestyle-related conditions and chronic disease.

Vitamin D deficiency is common in people who are obese [70] and patients undergoing bariatric surgery for obesity [71]. The cause for low serum 25(OH)D levels in obese individuals has not been confirmed. A popular theory is sequestration, where fat-soluble vitamin D is stored, but inaccessible, in adipose tissue in obese individuals [40]. Reduced sun exposure in the obese population has been studied [70], as well as potential differences in vitamin D synthesis and release from the skin [70]. Non-alcoholic fatty liver disease, a common condition in obese subjects, has also been suggested as inhibiting production of 25(OH)D [72]. A recent theory is that volumetric dilution can explain the majority of differences in serum 25(OH)D levels between obese and lean subjects [73]. Patients due to undergo bariatric surgery as a treatment for obesity often present with deficient or insufficient vitamin D status before surgery [71; 74]. Low serum 25(OH)D also persists postoperatively and requires regular monitoring and supplementation to achieve sufficiency [75].

Vitamin D status is also implicated in osteoporosis and hip fracture. Whether vitamin D supplementation is effective in preventing hip fracture in older people is controversial. A recent meta-analysis of several randomised controlled trials indicated vitamin D alone appears to have no significant effect on hip fracture reduction; however, in combination with calcium, fracture risk is lowered [76]. This is not surprising, as the food sources most rich in vitamin D3 also provide a source of calcium (e.g. cheese, oily fish). The complex interplay between individual genetic risk for low bone mineral density and response to vitamin D and calcium supplementation may contribute to the efficacy of supplementation and requires further investigation [77].

Supplementation of vitamin D can be in the form D2 or D3, and there have been conflicting reports regarding whether these forms are equally potent. An estimation of the average effect of vitamin D supplementation on serum 25OHD levels suggests every 1000 IU vitamin D3 (25 µg) increases serum 25(OH)D by 25 nmol/l [78]. Several studies have reported vitamin D3 supplements are more effective than vitamin D2 in raising serum 25(OH)D levels [79–83]; however, there appears to be no significant difference in $1,25(OH)_2D$ levels post-supplementation with either D2 or D3 [83]. Lehmann and colleagues [79] noted a large decrease in 25(OH)D in vitamin D2 supplemented patients. There are several possible reasons why vitamin D3 may be more effective in raising serum 25(OH)D levels than vitamin D2. Vitamin D3 and its metabolites have higher affinity for VDR, DBP and hepatic 25-hydroxylase, compared with vitamin D2 and its metabolites [84]. Additionally, metabolism of $1,25(OH)_2D$ by 24-hydroxylase produces $1,24,25(OH)_3D3$, which is biologically active and binds to the VDR. Metabolism of $1,25(OH)_2D2$ leads to the production of $1,24,25(OH)_3D2$, which is not biologically active [84]. Vitamin D2 became popular as a supplement and food fortification agent as it cured rickets in infants during the 1930s; however, D3 is considered more effective on the basis of the 25(OH)D marker of nutritional status. It is recommended not to use vitamin D2 as a supplement [84].

OLIVIA WRIGHT, VICKI FLOOD AND LINDA TAPSELL

There is a body of evidence debating the value of oral versus other routes of vitamin D supplementation. The efficiency of utilisation of oral vitamin D supplements is dependent on the liver. The liver is responsible for synthesising 25(OH)D, but it is also responsible for inactivating excess vitamin D2 or D3 and excreting the by-products through the bile [85]. Oral supplements of vitamin D3 are rapidly absorbed through hepatic (portal) circulation and activated to 25(OH)D, followed by a rapid inactivation process for the unused vitamin D3. Greater efficiency is achieved when vitamin D3 is absorbed through the skin into the circulation, as this process occurs more slowly. The liver receives a more gradual supply of vitamin D3 and converts this to 25(OH)D over a longer period of time, providing a constant supply of 25(OH)D and avoiding the rapid inactivation process associated with oral intake [85]. There is an opportunity for future research to investigate an alternative mode of delivering vitamin D supplements via the skin. Vitamin D creams and sunscreens already exist and may be an acceptable option to improve vitamin D status.

- What is the difference between classical vitamin D deficiency seen in rickets and the new emerging areas of concern for vitamin D status?
- What are the main issues regarding the choices of supplementation?
- What other strategies may be put in place to improve vitamin D status in those at risk of vitamin D deficiency?

TRY IT YOURSELF

Research online and evaluate the variety of non-oral vitamin D supplements available—for example, creams and sprays. Go to a chemist or health-food shop and collect information about all of their different types of vitamin D supplements, noting whether they provide vitamin D2 or D3 and the dosage. Review the variety of supplements available.

STOP AND THINK

- Why is there controversy around the management of vitamin D status in humans?
- How relevant are food sources of vitamin D in meeting population requirements?
- How has research broadened the debate on vitamin D?

WHAT ARE THE STRUCTURES AND FUNCTIONS OF VITAMIN E AND VITAMIN K?

Vitamin E is a principal antioxidant in the human body. Like vitamin A, vitamin E also refers to a group of related compounds, this time known as tocopherols and tocotrienols, differing by the number of C=C double bonds in their chemical structure (Figure 9.2). In all, there are a number of different forms of these two categories of compounds (including four forms of tocopherols and numerous stereoisomers). Vitamin E activity is measured as α tocopherol equivalents (αTE). Isomers of this compound are the most numerous in the human diet, and it is also the most biologically active form. Like vitamin A, vitamin E absorption is linked to fat absorption, but the proportion absorbed can reduce if saturation is achieved. As in other fat-soluble vitamins, excessive intake of vitamin E may lead to toxicity.

FIGURE 9.2   STRUCTURE OF TOCOPHEROLS AND TOCOTRIENOLS

	R$_1$	R$_2$	
Tocopherol	CH$_3$	CH$_3$	α-tocopherol
	CH$_3$	H	β-tocopherol
	H	CH$_3$	γ-tocopherol
	H	H	δ-tocopherol
Tocotrienol	CH$_3$	CH$_3$	α-tocotrienol
	CH$_3$	H	β-tocotrienol
	H	CH$_3$	γ-tocotrienol
	H	H	δ-tocotrienol

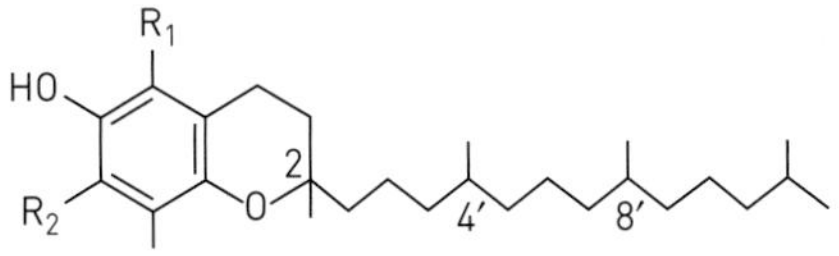

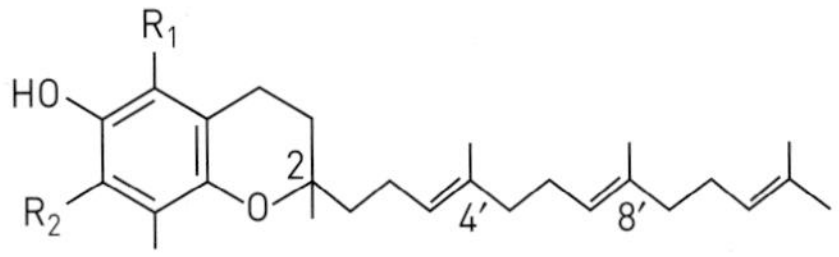

Source: S. Truswell & J. Mann (2012). Chapter 14: Vitamins C and E. In J. Mann & S. Truswell (eds), *Essentials of Human Nutrition*, 4th edn. Oxford University Press, Incorporated

Deficiency of vitamin E is rare and an AI (based on median population intakes) is the nutrient reference value set for Australians, as shown in Table 9.8.

Vitamin K acts in the liver to synthesise gamma-carboxyglutamic acid, an amino acid that forms part of coagulation factors that act in a cascade in the formation of clots. A deficiency of vitamin K can lead to bleeding but, on the other hand, the anticoagulant drug warfarin acts antagonistically to

TABLE 9.8   VITAMIN E REQUIREMENTS

Recommended intakes of vitamin E (mg/day)	Adequate intake (AI)	Upper level of intake (UL)
Men		
19–50 years	10	300
51–70 years	10	300
>70 years	10	300
Women		
19–50 years	7	300
51–70 years	7	300
>70 years	7	300
Pregnancy		
14–18 years	8	300
18–50 years	7	300
Lactation		
14–18 years	12	300
18–50 years	11	300

Source: National Health and Medical Research Council (2006). *Nutrient Reference Values for Australia and New Zealand, including Recommended Dietary Intakes*. Canberra: NHMRC. © Commonwealth of Australia

vitamin K. A recent review of vitamin K summarises current knowledge on the vitamin and considers the evidence on its potential role in the development of cardiovascular disease [86].

WHAT ARE THE MAJOR FOOD SOURCES OF VITAMIN E AND VITAMIN K?

Vitamin E, with powerful antioxidant capacities, exists in nature alongside unsaturated fatty acids, which are prone to oxidation. For example, walnuts are unique in the tree nut food group for their high levels of polyunsaturated fatty acids, but they also contain high levels of γ tocopherol. In fact, vegetable oils and nuts are good sources of vitamin E. This natural combination of nutrients suggests there may be an interdependence in requirements for vitamin E and essential fatty acids.

The vitamin E content of a food refers to the value of α-, β- and γ-tocopherol, not just the most common form of α-tocopherol. Vitamin E is found in nuts and seeds, oils and fats. Other foods include meats and avocados (Table 9.9).

Vitamin K is found in dark green leafy vegetables and some organ meats. It is also synthesised by bacteria in the large bowel, where some absorption also occurs. Recently, multiple forms of vitamin K have been found in dairy foods [2].

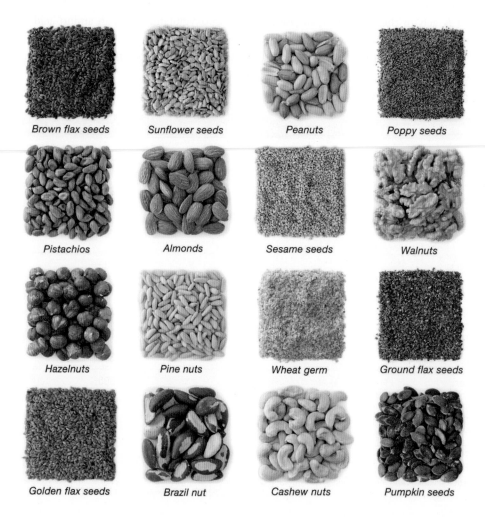

Brown flax seeds   Sunflower seeds   Peanuts   Poppy seeds

Pistachios   Almonds   Sesame seeds   Walnuts

Hazelnuts   Pine nuts   Wheat germ   Ground flax seeds

Golden flax seeds   Brazil nut   Cashew nuts   Pumpkin seeds

OXFORD UNIVERSITY PRESS

TABLE 9.9 VITAMIN E CONTENT OF FOODS

Food	Serving size[1]	mg of vitamin E per serve[3]
Almond (with skin)	30 g	8.442
Pine nuts (raw)	30 g	3.882
Sesame seeds	30 g	58.104
Sunflower seeds	30 g	11.739
Tahini	30 g	64.071
Sunflower oil	7 g[2]	3.609
Polyunsaturated margarine	10 g[2]	3.468

[1]Based on the Australian Dietary Guidelines [8].
[2]Based on modelling of the Australian Dietary Guidelines [9].
[3]Sourced from NUTTAB 2010 [10].

STOP AND THINK

- Why is deficiency in vitamin E rare?
- What does the presence of vitamin E in nuts and oils tell us about the interconnections between nutrients in foods?
- Why might malabsorption of fats and prolonged treatment with antibiotics affect vitamin K status?

SUMMARY

- Vitamin A is a fat-soluble vitamin composed of many elements, predominantly carotenoids (found in fruits and vegetables) or retinoids (found in animal foods). Provitamin A compounds (β-carotene, α-carotene and β-cryptoxanthin) are converted to retinol. Vitamin A is essential for eye health and other areas of growth and development. The xenophills lutein and zeaxanthin that accumulate in the macula of the eye are particularly important.

- Vitamin D is represented in many chemical forms: from 7-dehydrocholesterol (provitamin D, formed under the skin), to 25 hydroxyvitamin D (pre-hormone, produced in the liver), 1-25 dihydroxyvitamin D (active hormone produced by the kidney and intestinal cells) to 24,25 dihyrdoxyvitamin D (inactivated hormone), alongside the dietary sources of vitamin D2 (ergocalciferol found in plants) and vitamin D3 (cholecalciferol found in animal foods). Thus, vitamin D is essentially produced cutaneously (i.e. in the skin) on exposure to sunlight. Exposure of around 15% of the body's surface area (e.g. arms and hands) in the midday sun produces around 25 µg vitamin D (or 1000 international units [IU]). Vitamin D has a hormonal mechanism of action by binding to its receptor, the vitamin D receptor (VDR), in target tissues. The relationship between 25(OH)D3 levels and disease or mortality is U-shaped—that is, deficiency and excess are not good for health.

- The AI for cholecalciferol in Australia is 5 µg/day (or 200 IU) for infants, children, adolescents and adults, 10 µg/day (or 400 IU) for adults 51–70 years and 15 µg/day (or 600 IU) for adults >70 years. Those most at risk of vitamin D deficiency are the housebound elderly with poor skin synthetic function, hospital patients in long-term care, those with malabsorption syndromes or on total parenteral nutrition (TPN), babies and infants of vitamin D deficient mothers, those with skin cancer or at a high risk of skin cancer, people with dark skin pigmentation or those who constantly wear sun-protective clothing or veils.

- Vitamin E presents as a set of tocopherols and tocotrienols and is found in plant foods with high polyunsaturated fatty acid contents such as nuts, seeds and oils. More research is required on human deficiency but the compounds have potent antioxidant activity, which is likely to be protective from the negative effects of oxidative stress.
- Vitamin K acts in the liver to produce clotting factors. It is produced by bacteria in the gut and is contained in green leafy vegetables.

PATHWAYS TO PRACTICE

- As large subgroups of the general population consume inadequate serves of fruit and vegetables, intakes of vitamin A components such as lutein are at risk. Public health approaches that support intakes of fruits and vegetables (with some focus on different types and colour) would help address this problem. Likewise, Vitamin D requires consideration. While is important that safe sun exposure messages are maintained given the high risk of skin cancer during most of the year in Australia, when the UV Index is 3 or above in Australia, sun exposure to arms and hands for only a few minutes in the mid-morning or afternoon is still recommended on most days of the week.
- All health workers would benefit from awareness of vitamin D nutrition, particularly those caring for elderly or institutionalised individuals. People should be encouraged to consume a variety of food sources rich in vitamin D3 as part of a healthy diet, even though it represents only around 5–10% of vitamin D levels. In older adults, vitamin D3 supplements should be taken with calcium to improve prevention of bone fractures. Evidence suggests vitamin D3, or cholecalciferol, is the optimum form of vitamin D for food fortification, as it is more effective at raising 25(OH)D than vitamin D2, or ergocalciferol. Practitioners working in antenatal care may encourage pregnant women and women thinking of becoming pregnant to have their vitamin D levels tested given the significant implications for neonatal brain development and the child's future mental health. Health professionals should be encouraged to order 25(OH)D analyses from the same laboratory consistently, and to find out which method of testing is being used. Further research in this area will remain informative.

DISCUSSION QUESTIONS

1   What type of evidence would be required to determine a Nutrient Reference Value for carotenoids such as lutein and zeaxanthin? What would be the practical challenges in ensuring most people in the population consumed adequate amounts of these vitamin A components?
2   Outline the pathways to producing adequate Vitamin D in the body for the maintenance of health. What does this tell you about the roles and functions of vitamins in the body?
3   What might be effective strategies for people living in your state to maintain their vitamin D status? Who would benefit most from exposure to sunlight rather than oral vitamin D supplements?
4   Which subgroups in the community may need to be concerned about their intakes of vitamin E and vitamin K? Give reasons.

USEFUL WEBLINKS

Macular Disease Foundation:
    www.mdfoundation.com.au

Metrics: Population Attributable Fraction (PAF)—Quantifying the contribution of risk factors to the Burden of Disease:
    www.who.int/healthinfo/global_burden_disease/metrics_paf/en

Michael Holick—The D-lightful vitamin D for good health:
    www.youtube.com/watch?v=hiGBVDcbFVk

Nutrient Reference Values—Vitamin D:
    www.nrv.gov.au/nutrients/vitamin-d

Understanding vitamin D:
    www.youtube.com/watch?v=onSPZ0aBUKM

US Department of Agriculture, for comprehensive nutrient database of carotenoids:
    www.ars.usda.gov/northeast-area/beltsville-md/beltsville-human-nutrition-research-center/nutrient-data-laboratory

UV Index website:
    www.arpansa.gov.au/services/monitoring/ultraviolet-radiation-monitoring/ultraviolet-radiation-index

World Health Organization—Global vitamin A deficiency:
    www.who.int/nutrition/topics/vad/en

FURTHER READING

Feldman, D., Pike, J. W. & Adams & J. S. (eds). (2011). *Vitamin D. Volume 1*, 3rd edn. San Diego, CA: Elsevier Science Publishing Co Inc.

Fu, X., Harshman, S. G., Shen, X., Haytowitz, D. B., Karl, J. P., Wolfe, B. E. & Booth, S. L. (2017). Multiple vitamin K forms exist in dairy foods. *Current Developments in Nutrition*, 1(6), e000638. doi:10.3945/cdn.117.000638

Johnson, E. J. (2014). Role of lutein and zeaxanthin in visual and cognitive function throughout the lifespan. *Nutrition Reviews*, 72(9), 605–12. doi:10.1111/nure.12133

Kryscio, R. J., Abner, E. L., Caban-Holt, A., Lovell, M., Goodman, P., Darke, A. K., ... Schmitt, F. A. (2017). Association of antioxidant supplement use and dementia in the prevention of Alzheimer's disease by vitamin E and selenium trial (PREADViSE). *JAMA Neurology*, 74(5), 567–73. doi:10.1001/jamaneurol.2016.5778

Manzi, F., Flood, V., Webb, K. & Mitchell, P. (2002). The intake of carotenoids in an older Australian population: the Blue Mountains Eye Study. *Public Health Nutrition*, 5(2), 347–52. doi:10.1079/phn2002258

Tripkovic, L., Wilson, L. R., Hart, K., Johnsen, S., de Lusignan, S., Smith, C. P., ... Lanham-New, S. A. (2017). Daily supplementation with 15 µg vitamin D2 compared with vitamin D3 to increase wintertime 25-hydroxyvitamin D status in healthy South Asian and white European women: a 12-wk randomized, placebo-controlled food-fortification trial. *American Journal of Clinical Nutrition*, 106(2), 481–90. doi:10.3945/ajcn.116.138693

REFERENCES

1   D. R. Jacobs, Jr & L. C. Tapsell (2007). Food, not nutrients, is the fundamental unit in nutrition. *Nutrition Reviews*, 65(10), 439–50.

2   T. J. Wang (2016). Vitamin D and cardiovascular disease. *Annual Review of Medicine*, 67(1), 261–72. doi:10.1146/annurev-med-051214-025146

3   J. A. Olson (1996). Biochemistry of vitamin A and carotenoids. In A. Sommer & K. P. W. Jr (eds), *Vitamin A Deficiency: Health, survival and vision*. New York: Oxford University Press.

4   National Health and Medical Research Council (2006). *Nutrient Reference Values for Australia and New Zealand, including Recommended Dietary Intakes*. Canberra: NHMRC.

5   D. I. Thurnham (2012). Vitamin A and carotenoids. In J. Mann & A. S. Truswell (eds), *Essentials in Human Nutrition*, 4th edn. Oxford University Press.

6   S. A. Tanumihardjo (2011). Vitamin A: biomarkers of nutrition for development. *American Journal of Clinical Nutrition*, 94(2), 658s–665s. doi:10.3945/ajcn.110.005777

7   K. B. Feroze & E. J. Kaufman (2017). Xerophthalmia. In *StatPearls [Internet]*. Treasure Island, FL: StatPearls Publishing. Retrieved from: www.ncbi.nlm.nih.gov/books/NBK431094.

8   National Health and Medical Research Council (2013). *Australian Dietary Guidelines*. Canberra: NHMRC.

9   National Health and Medical Research Council (2011). *A Modelling System to Inform the Revision of the Australian Guide to Healthy Eating*. Canberra: NHMRC.

10 Food Standards Australia New Zealand (2012). *NUTTAB 2010*. Canberra: FSANZ.

11 E. Reboul, S. Thap, F. Tourniaire, M. Andre, C. Juhel, S. Morange, ... P. Borel. (2007). Differential effect of dietary antioxidant classes (carotenoids, polyphenols, vitamins C and E) on lutein absorption. *British Journal of Nutrition*, 97(3), 440–6. doi:10.1017/s0007114507352604

12 Age-Related Eye Disease Study 2 Research Group (2013). Lutein + zeaxanthin and omega-3 fatty acids for age-related macular degeneration: the age-related eye disease study 2 (areds2) randomized clinical trial. *JAMA—Journal of the American Medical Association*, 309(19), 2005–15. doi:10.1001/jama.2013.4997

13 B. Eisenhauer, S. Natoli, G. Liew & V. M. Flood (2017). Lutein and zeaxanthin-food sources, bioavailability and dietary variety in age-related macular degeneration protection. *Nutrients*, 9(2). doi:10.3390/nu9020120

14 J. S. L. Tan, J. J. Wang, V. Flood, E. Rochtchina, W. Smith & P. Mitchell (2008). Dietary antioxidants and the long-term incidence of age-related macular degeneration. *Ophthalmology*, 115(2), 334–41. doi:http://dx.doi.org/10.1016/j.ophtha.2007.03.083

15 R. Y. H. Leung, B. M. Y. Cheung, U.-S. Nguyen, A. W. C. Kung, K. C. B. Tan & C.-L. Cheung (2017). Optimal vitamin D status and its relationship with bone and mineral metabolism in Hong Kong Chinese. *Bone, in press*. doi:http://dx.doi.org/10.1016/j.bone.2017.01.030

16 S. Afzal, P. Brøndum-Jacobsen, S. E. Bojesen & B. G. Nordestgaard (2014). Vitamin D concentration, obesity, and risk of diabetes: a mendelian randomisation study. *The Lancet Diabetes & Endocrinology*, 2(4), 298–306. doi:http://dx.doi.org/10.1016/S2213-8587(13)70200-6

17 M. F. Holick (2004). Sunlight and vitamin D for bone health and prevention of autoimmune diseases, cancers, and cardiovascular disease. *American Journal of Clinical Nutrition*, 80(6), 1678S–1688S.

18 T. J. Wang, M. J. Pencina, S. L. Booth, P. F. Jacques, E. Ingelsson, K. Lanier, ... R. S. Vasan. (2008). Vitamin D deficiency and risk of cardiovascular disease. *Circulation*, 117(4), 503–11. doi:10.1161/circulationaha.107.706127

19 J. J. McGrath, F. P. Féron, T. H. J. Burne, A. Mackay-Sim & D. W. Eyles (2004). Vitamin D3—implications for brain development. *Journal of Steroid Biochemistry and Molecular Biology*, 89–90, 557–60. doi:http://dx.doi.org/10.1016/j.jsbmb.2004.03.070

20 P. H. Anderson, A. G. Turner & H. A. Morris (2012). Vitamin D actions to regulate calcium and skeletal homeostasis. *Clinical Biochemistry*, 45(12), 880–6. doi:10.1016/j.clinbiochem.2012.02.020

21 E. K. Calton, K. N. Keane & M. J. Soares (2015). The potential regulatory role of vitamin D in the bioenergetics of inflammation. *Current Opinion in Clinical Nutrition and Metabolic Care*, 18(4), 367–73.

22 E. D. Gorham, M. F. Holick, C. F. Garland, F. C. Garland, W. B. Grant, S. B. Mohr, ... M. Wei (2007). Optimal vitamin D status for colorectal cancer prevention: a quantitative meta analysis. *American Journal of Preventive Medicine*, 32(3), 210–16. doi:10.1016/j.amepre.2006.11.004

23 P. Szodoray, M. Zeher, E. Bodolay, B. Nakken, J. Gaal, R. Jonsson, ... R. Gesztelyi (2008). The complex role of vitamin D in autoimmune diseases. *Scandinavian Journal of Immunology*, 68(3), 261–70.

24 M. F. Holick (2004). Vitamin D: importance in the prevention of cancers, type 1 diabetes, heart disease, and osteoporosis. *American Journal of Clinical Nutrition*, 79(3), 362–71.

25 A. K. Saenger, T. J. Laha, D. E. Bremmer & S. M. H. Sadrzadeh (2006). Quantification of serum 25-hydroxyvitamin D2 and D3 using HPLC-tandem mass spectrometry and examination of reference intervals for diagnosis of vitamin D deficiency. *American Journal of Clinical Pathology*, 125(6), 914–20.

26 D. Teegarden & S. S. Donkin (2009). Vitamin D: emerging new roles in insulin sensitivity. *Nutrition Research Reviews*, 22(01), 82–92.

27 O. R. L. Wright, I. J. Hickman, W. G. Petchey, C. M. Sullivan, C. Ong, F. J. Rose, ... T. M. O'Moore-Sullivan (2013). The effect of 25-hydroxyvitamin D on insulin sensitivity in obesity: is it mediated via adiponectin? *Canadian Journal of Physiology and Pharmacology*, 91(6), 496–501. doi:10.1139/cjpp-2012-0436

28 P. Pludowski, M. F. Holick, S. Pilz, C. L. Wagner, B. W. Hollis, W. B. Grant, ... M. Soni (2013). Vitamin D effects on musculoskeletal health, immunity, autoimmunity, cardiovascular disease, cancer, fertility, pregnancy, dementia and mortality: a review of recent evidence. *Autoimmunity Reviews*, 12(10), 976–89. doi:http://dx.doi.org/10.1016/j.autrev.2013.02.004

29 C. A. Nowson, J. J. McGrath, P. R. Ebeling, A. Haikerwal, R. M. Daly, K. M. Sanders, ... R. S. Mason (2012). Vitamin D and health in adults in Australia and New Zealand: a position statement. *Medical Journal of Australia*, 196(11), 686–7.

30 G. Jones (2013). Extrarenal vitamin D activation and interactions between vitamin D2, vitamin D3, and vitamin D analogs. *Annual Review of Nutrition*, 33, 23–44.

31 R. Kaseda, M. Hosojima, H. Sato & A. Saito (2011). Role of megalin and cubilin in the metabolism of vitamin D-3. *Therapeutic Apheresis and Dialysis*, 15, 14–17. doi:10.1111/j.1744-9987.2011.00920.x

32 G. Makin, D. Lohnes, V. Byford, R. Ray & G. Jones (1989). Target cell metabolism of 1,25-dihydroxyvitamin D3 to calcitroic acid. Evidence for a pathway in kidney and bone involving 24-oxidation. *Biochemistry Journal*, 262(1), 173–80.

33 G. S. Reddy & K. Y. Tserng (1989). Calcitroic acid, end product of renal metabolism of 1,25-dihydroxyvitamin D3 through C-24 oxidation pathway. *Biochemistry*, 28(4), 1763–9. doi:10.1021/bi00430a051

34 R. St-Arnaud & F. H. Glorieux (1998). Editorial: 24, 25-dihydroxyvitamin D—active metabolite or inactive catabolite? *Endocrinology*, 139(8), 3371–4. doi:10.1210/en.139.8.3371

35 K. R. Wehmeier, A.-R. Alamir, S. Sultan, M. J. Haas, N. C. W. Wong & A. D. Mooradian (2011). 24, 25-dihydroxycholecalciferol but not 25-hydroxycholecalciferol suppresses apolipoprotein A-I gene expression. *Life Sciences*, 88(1–2), 110–16. doi:10.1016/j.lfs.2010.11.005

36 E. Reboul, A. Goncalves, C. Comera, R. Bott, M. Nowicki, J.-F. Landrier, … P. Borel (2011). Vitamin D intestinal absorption is not a simple passive diffusion: evidences for involvement of cholesterol transporters. *Molecular Nutrition & Food Research*, 55(5), 691–702. doi:10.1002/mnfr.201000553

37 M. T. Drake (2014). Vitamin D and the goldilocks principle: too little, too much, or just right? *Journal of Clinical Endocrinology and Metabolism*, 99(4), 1164–6.

38 K. Standahl Olsen, C. Rylander, M. Brustad, L. Aksnes & E. Lund (2013). Plasma 25 hydroxyvitamin D level and blood gene expression profiles: a cross-sectional study of the Norwegian Women and Cancer Post-genome Cohort. *European Journal of Clinical Nutrition*, 67(7), 773–8. doi:10.1038/ejcn.2013.53

39 T. Capiod (2011). Cell proliferation, calcium influx and calcium channels. *Biochimie*, 93(12), 2075–9. doi:http://dx.doi.org/10.1016/j.biochi.2011.07.015

40 E. B. Mawer, J. Backhouse, C. A. Holman, G. A. Lumb & S. W. Stanbury (1972). The distribution and storage of vitamin D and its metabolites in human tissues. *Clinical Science*, 43(3), 413–31.

41 M. Abboud, C. Gordon-Thomson, A. J. Hoy, S. Balaban, M. S. Rybchyn, L. Cole, … R. S. Mason (2014). Uptake of 25-hydroxyvitamin D by muscle and fat cells. *Journal of Steroid Biochemistry and Molecular Biology*, 144, Part A(0), 232–6. doi:http://dx.doi.org/10.1016/j.jsbmb.2013.10.020

42 D. D. Bikle (2009). Extra renal synthesis of 1,25-dihydroxyvitamin D and its health implications. *Clinical Reviews in Bone and Mineral Metabolism*, 1–12. doi:10.1007/s12018-009-9033-y

43 D. W. Eyles, S. Smith, R. Kinobe, M. Hewison & J. J. McGrath (2005). Distribution of the vitamin D receptor and 1 alpha-hydroxylase in human brain. *Journal of Chemical Neuroanatomy*, 29(1), 21–30. doi:10.1016/j.jchemneu.2004.08.006

44 K. Tai, A. G. Need, M. Horowitz & I. M. Chapman (2008). Vitamin D, glucose, insulin, and insulin sensitivity. *Nutrition*, 24(3), 279–85.

45 D. Wolpowitz & B. A. Gilchrest (2006). The vitamin D questions: how much do you need and how should you get it? *Journal of the American Academy of Dermatology*, 54(2), 301–17.

46 Australian and New Zealand Bone and Mineral Society, Australasian College of Dermatologists, Cancer Council Australia & Endocrine Society of Australia and Osteoporosis Australia (2016). *Position Statement: Sun exposure and vitamin D—Risks and benefits*. Cancer Council Australia. Retrieved from: http://wiki.cancer.org.au/policy/Position_statement_-_Risks_and_benefits_of_sun_exposure.

47 M. F. Holick & T. C. Chen (2008). Vitamin D deficiency: a worldwide problem with health consequences. *American Journal of Clinical Nutrition*, 87(4), 1080S–1086S.

48 M. Kimlin, S. Harrison, M. Nowak, M. Moore, A. Brodie & C. Lang (2007). Does a high UV environment ensure adequate vitamin D status? *Journal of Photochemistry and Photobiology B: Biology*, 89(2–3), 139–47.

49 I. A. F. van der Mei, A.-L. Ponsonby, O. Engelsen, J. A. Pasco, J. J. McGrath, D. W. Eyles, … G. Jones (2007). The high prevalence of vitamin D insufficiency across Australian populations is only partly explained by season and latitude. *Environmental Health Perspectives*, 115(8).

50 M. F. Holick (2007). Vitamin D deficiency. *New England Journal of Medicine*, 357, 266–81.

51 B. W. Hollis (2008). Measuring 25-hydroxyvitamin D in a clinical environment: challenges and needs. *American Journal of Clinical Nutrition*, 88(2), 507S–510S.

52 A. C. Ross (2010). *Dietary Reference Intakes for Calcium and Vitamin D.* Washington, DC: National Academies Press.

53 H. A. Bischoff-Ferrari, J. Henschkowski, B. Dawson-Hughes, H. B. Staehelin, J. E. Orav, A. E. Stuck, ... D. P. Kiel (2009). Fall prevention with supplemental and active forms of vitamin D: a meta-analysis of randomised controlled trials. *British Medical Journal,* 339(7725), 843–6. doi:10.1136/bmj.b3692

54 E. Cavalier, E. Rozet, R. Gadisseur, A. Carlisi, M. Monge, J. P. Chapelle, ... P. Delanaye (2010). Measurement uncertainty of 25-OH vitamin D determination with different commercially available kits: impact on the clinical cut offs. *Osteoporosis International,* 21(6), 1047–51. doi:10.1007/s00198-009-1052-5

55 R. J. Singh (2008). Are clinical laboratories prepared for accurate testing of 25-hydroxy vitamin D? *Clinical Chemistry,* 54(1), 221–3. doi:10.1373/clinchem.2007.096156

56 P. Glendenning, M. Taranto, J. Noble, A. Musk, C. Hammond, P. Goldswain, ... S. Vasikaran (2006). Current assays overestimate 25-hydroxyvitamin D3 and underestimate 25-hydroxyvitamin D2 compared with HPLC: need for assay-specific decision limits and metabolite-specific assays. *Annals of Clinical Biochemistry,* 43(1), 23–30. doi:10.1258/000456306775141650

57 W. B. Grant & M. F. Holick (2005). Benefits and requirements of vitamin D for optimal health: a review. *Alternative Medicine Review,* 10(2), 94–111.

58 R. P. Heaney (2005). The vitamin D requirement in health and disease. *Journal of Steroid Biochemistry and Molecular Biology,* 97(1), 13–19. doi:10.1016/j.jsbmb.2005.06.020

59 R. Vieth, J. J. McGrath, A. W. Norman, R. Scragg, S. J. Whiting, W. C. Willett, ... C. Lamberg-Allardt (2007). The urgent need to recommend an intake of vitamin D that is effective. *American Journal of Clinical Nutrition,* 85(3), 649–50.

60 P. Lips, M. C. Chapuy, B. Dawson-Hughes, H. A. P. Pols & M. F. Holick (1999). An international comparison of serum 25-hydroxyvitamin D measurements. *Osteoporosis International,* 9(5), 394–7. doi:10.1007/s001980050162

61 N. Binkley, D. Krueger, C. S. Cowgill, L. Plum, E. Lake, K. E. Hansen, ... M. K. Drezner (2004). Assay variation confounds the diagnosis of hypovitaminosis D: a call for standardization. *Journal of Clinical Endocrinology and Metabolism,* 89(7), 3152–7. doi:10.1210/jc.2003-031979

62 G. Snellman, H. Melhus, R. Gedeborg, L. Byberg, L. Berglund, L. Wernroth & K. Michaëlsson (2010). Determining vitamin D status: a comparison between commercially available assays. *PLOS ONE,* 5(7), e11555.

63 S. Christakos, P. Dhawan, A. Porta, L. J. Mady & T. Seth (2011). Vitamin D and intestinal calcium absorption. *Molecular and Cellular Endocrinology,* 347(1–2), 25–9. doi:http://dx.doi.org/10.1016/j.mce.2011.05.038

64 J. J. McGrath, D. W. Eyles, C. Anderson, P. Ko, T. H. J. Burne, B. Norgaard-Pedersen, ... P. B. Mortensen (2010). Neonatal vitamin D status and risk of schizophrenia. *Archives of General Psychiatry,* 67(9), 889–94.

65 P. K. Kamweru & E. L. Tindibale (2016). Vitamin D and vitamin D from ultraviolet-irradiated mushrooms (review). *International Journal of Medicinal Mushrooms,* 18(3), 205–14. doi:10.1615/IntJMedMushrooms.v18.i3.30

66 N. Jayaratne, M. C. B. Hughes, T. I. Ibiebele, S. van den Akker & J. C. van der Pols (2013). Vitamin D intake in Australian adults and the modeled effects of milk and breakfast cereal fortification. *Nutrition,* 29(7–8), 1048–53. doi:http://dx.doi.org/10.1016/j.nut.2013.02.011

67 G. B. Mulligan & A. Licata (2010). Taking Vitamin D with the largest meal improves absorption and results in higher serum levels of 25-hydroxyvitamin D. *Journal of Bone and Mineral Research*, 25(4), 928–30. doi:10.1002/jbmr.67

68 S. Niramitmahapanya, S. S. Harris & B. Dawson-Hughes (2011). Type of dietary fat is associated with the 25-hydroxyvitamin D-3 increment in response to vitamin D supplementation. *Journal of Clinical Endocrinology & Metabolism*, 96(10), 3170–4. doi:10.1210/jc.2011-1518

69 C. L. Taylor, K. Y. Patterson, J. M. Roseland, S. A. Wise, J. M. Merkel, P. R. Pehrsson & E. A. Yetley (2014). Including food 25-hydroxyvitamin D in intake estimates may reduce the discrepancy between dietary and serum measures of vitamin D status. *Journal of Nutrition*, 144(5), 654–9. doi:10.3945/jn.113.189811

70 J. Wortsman, L. Y. Matsuoka, T. C. Chen, Z. Lu & M. F. Holick (2000). Decreased bioavailability of vitamin D in obesity. *American Journal of Clinical Nutrition*, 72(3), 690–3.

71 M. Blum, G. Dolnikowski, E. Seyoum, S. S. Harris, S. L. Booth, J. Peterson, … B. Dawson-Hughes (2008). Vitamin D 3 in fat tissue. *Endocrine*, 33(1), 90–4.

72 M. Eliades, R. Hernaez, E. Spyrou, N. Agrawal, M. Lazo, F. L. Brancati, … E. Guallar (2013). Meta-analysis: vitamin D and non-alcoholic fatty liver disease. *Alimentary Pharmacology and Therapeutics*, 38(3), 246–54. doi:10.1111/apt.12377

73 A. T. Drincic, L. A. G. Armas, E. E. Van Diest & R. P. Heaney (2012). Volumetric dilution, rather than sequestration best explains the low vitamin D status of obesity. *Obesity (Silver Spring, Md.)*, 20(7), 1444–8.

74 E. Lin, D. Armstrong-Moore, Z. Liang, J. F. Sweeney, W. E. Torres, T. R. Ziegler, … N. Gletsu-Miller (2011). Contribution of adipose tissue to plasma 25-hydroxyvitamin D concentrations during weight loss following gastric bypass surgery. *Obesity*, 19(3), 588–94.

75 C. F. Dix, J. D. Bauer & O. R. L. Wright (2017). A systematic review: vitamin D status and sleeve gastrectomy. *Obesity Surgery*, 27(1), 215–25. doi:10.1007/s11695-016-2436-1

76 S. Boonen, P. Lips, R. Bouillon, H. A. Bischoff-Ferrari, D. Vanderschueren & P. Haentjens (2007). Need for additional calcium to reduce the risk of hip fracture with vitamin D supplementation: evidence from a comparative metaanalysis of randomized controlled trials. *Journal of Clinical Endocrinology and Metabolism*, 92(4), 1415–23.

77 Y. Wang, J. Wactawski-Wende, L. E. Sucheston-Campbell, L. Preus, K. M. Hovey, J. Nie, … H. M. Ochs-Balcom (2017). The influence of genetic susceptibility and calcium plus vitamin D supplementation on fracture risk. *American Journal of Clinical Nutrition*, 105(4), 970–9.

78 E. Romagnoli, J. Pepe, S. Piemonte, C. Cipriani & S. Minisola (2013). Value and limitations of assessing vitamin D nutritional status and advised levels of vitamin D supplementation. *European Journal of Endocrinology*, 169(4), R59–R69.

79 U. Lehmann, F. Hirche, G. I. Stangl, K. Hinz, S. Westphal & J. Dierkes (2013). Bioavailability of vitamin D-2 and D-3 in healthy volunteers, a randomized placebo-controlled trial. *Journal of Clinical Endocrinology & Metabolism*, 98(11), 4339–45. doi:10.1210/jc.2012-4287

80 R. P. Heaney, R. R. Recker, J. Grote, R. L. Horst & L. A. G. Armas (2011). Vitamin D3 is more potent than vitamin D2 in humans. *Clinical Endocrinology and Metabolism*, 96(3), E447–E452. doi:10.1210/jc.2010-2230

81 N. Binkley, D. Gemar, J. Engelke, R. Gangnon, R. Ramamurthy, D. Krueger & M. K. Drezner (2011). Evaluation of ergocalciferol or cholecalciferol dosing, 1,600 IU daily or 50,000 IU monthly in older adults. *Journal of Clinical Endocrinology and Metabolism*, 96(4), 981–8.

82 L. Tripkovic, H. Lambert, K. Hart, C. P. Smith, G. Bucca, S. Penson, ... S. Lanham-New (2012). Comparison of vitamin D2 and vitamin D3 supplementation in raising serum 25-hydroxyvitamin D status: a systematic review and meta-analysis. *American Journal of Clinical Nutrition*, 95(6), 1357–64. doi:10.3945/ajcn.111.031070

83 J. B. Wetmore, C. Kimber, J. D. Mahnken & J. R. Stubbs (2016). Cholecalciferol v. ergocalciferol for 25-hydroxyvitamin D (25(OH)D) repletion in chronic kidney disease: a randomised clinical trial. *British Journal of Nutrition*, 116(12), 2074–81. doi:10.1017/S000711451600427X

84 L. A. Houghton & R. Vieth (2006). The case against ergocalciferol (vitamin D2) as a vitamin supplement. *American Journal of Clinical Nutrition*, 84(4), 694–7.

85 D. R. Fraser (1983). The physiological economy of vitamin D. *The Lancet*, 30 April, 969–71.

86 A. J. van Ballegooijen & J. W. Beulens (2017). The Role of Vitamin K Status in Cardiovascular Health: Evidence from Observational and Clinical Studies. *Current Nutrition Reports*, 6, 197. https://doi.org/10.1007/s13668-017-0208-8

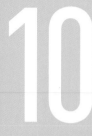

WATER-SOLUBLE VITAMINS: B AND C

LINDA TAPSELL

CHAPTER OBJECTIVES

This chapter will enable the reader to:

- describe the chemical structure of the B group vitamins and vitamin C
- briefly describe the function of these vitamins in the human body
- recognise the major food sources of the B group vitamins and vitamin C.

KEY TERMS

B group vitamins   Vitamin C

Citrus fruits   Wholegrains

KEY POINTS

- The chemical classification of water-soluble vitamins has implications for the body's ability to excrete excessive amounts of these vitamins.
- B group vitamins generally act as coenzymes in metabolic processes and to an extent are interdependent, whereas vitamin C has strong antioxidant properties, with an integral role in collagen formation.
- The identification of deficiency diseases reflects a period of concentrated scientific investigation linking clinical observations and resultant trials with chemical identification and synthesis of vitamins.
- Dietary modelling for the Australian Guide to Healthy Eating ensures adequate intakes of the water-soluble vitamins from core foods, but food fortification has been necessary for thiamin and folic acid, and supplements are recommended for some subgroups such as pregnant women.

OXFORD UNIVERSITY PRESS

INTRODUCTION

The differentiation between fat-soluble and water-soluble vitamins refers to this basic chemical property, but like all nutrients, they play particular roles in human physiology and biochemistry. The B group vitamins have distinctive roles in a range of areas, particularly in human metabolism, and while vitamin C also has enzymatic roles, it has been best known for its involvement in the synthesis of collagen, which is interrupted in the presentation of **scurvy**. The classification of 'water soluble' means that these vitamins can be excreted in the urine and this distinction has helped to differentiate the risk of toxicity compared with fat-soluble vitamins, which are less able to be excreted. In addition, the water solubility feature helps to appreciate the need for skill in preparation and cooking of foods, as water-soluble vitamins can be lost without due care [1]. In general, nutrient retention factors are an important consideration in determining the availability of nutrients from foods [2].

Historically, observations of food intake were critical in uncovering the essentiality of water-soluble vitamins. The discovery of vitamin C has its origins in observations of scurvy in long-distance seafarers from as early as the fifteenth century. The first scientific publication, James Lind's *Treatise on the Scurvy*, appeared in the eighteenth century and demonstrated the link between citrus fruit consumption and the protection of collagen formation that was needed to prevent the associated bleeding gums and painful death [3]. During the first half of the twentieth century, chemists identified the chemical compounds linked to the prevention of the disease, and described the chemical structure that has been synthesised in the **vitamin supplements** we know today.

> **Scurvy**
> a clinical state of vitamin C deficiency characterised by bleeding gums and loss of teeth through poor connective tissue.

> **Vitamin supplements**
> generally containing chemically derived compounds equivalent in structure and function to the compounds naturally occurring in foods.

TRY IT YOURSELF

Consider the global significance placed on discoveries relating to vitamins in the twentieth century. How many Nobel Prize winners have been associated with vitamin-related research?

The history of vitamin B is similar [4], but rather than being linked to citrus fruit consumption, the clinical and dietary observations of thiamin deficiency and subsequent trials revolved around the consumption of polished rice versus wholegrain components. In due course, as with vitamin C, the chemical structure of thiamin was also determined and synthesised. In the process, the name of the vitamin was originally spelt 'thiamine', but this changed when it became apparent the chemical structure of the vitamin was not in the amine class.

Thiamin was originally named B1 (and continues to be recognised as such). The B group vitamins were discovered and chemically identified one after the other, so they were differentiated by number (B1, B2, B3). In time, it became more common practice to refer to them by name, such as thiamin. The Nutrient Reference Values (NRVs) for Australia and New Zealand (www.nrv.gov.au) refer to nine B group vitamins: thiamin (vitamin B1), niacin (vitamin B2), riboflavin (vitamin B3), pyridoxine, and related compounds known as vitamin B6, pantothenic acid, biotin, folate and cobalamins, known as vitamin B12.

Before the chemical characterisation of vitamins, it appears the significance of food in the prevention of deficiency states took some time to be operationalised in health protective strategies (especially for seafarers), but today the nutritional value of wholegrain cereals and fresh fruit and vegetables is well recognised. The dietary modelling for national dietary guidelines, for example, demonstrates how these

Visit Oxford Ascend for more on vitamins.

LINDA TAPSELL

food groups contribute to meeting requirements for vitamins and minerals in the general population [5]. While food sources of these individual nutrients can be identified, it is not surprising to see the same foods emerge time and again. This reflects the natural synergy that occurs between these nutrients and other components within foods, where the sum of the parts is greater than the individual nutrients [6].

There are other interesting matters to ponder about foods and nutrients in this setting. For example, given the vast array of chemical compounds operating in the body's complex physiological and biochemical systems, why are these particular chemicals required in the diet while others are not? Could this be a consequence of long-standing environmental conditions, namely available and consumed food? A case in point is vitamin C, which the human body is not able to synthesise and must access through food, even though this is not the case for most animals. Our knowledge of water-soluble vitamins and their relationship to food remains incomplete, albeit continually being advanced by rigorous and disciplined scientific investigation.

STOP AND THINK

- How has the science of chemistry influenced our understanding of B and C group vitamins? What are the strengths and limitations of this knowledge with respect to public health?
- Why would the food sources of vitamin C be limited to an apparently small category of foods such as fruits?
- Why do so many classes of B group vitamins exist? What might they have in common besides their name?

WHAT ARE THE STRUCTURES AND FUNCTIONS OF THE B GROUP VITAMINS?

As a class of chemical compounds essential for human physiology and metabolism, the B group vitamins are all linked to significant metabolic pathways (Table 10.1). Vitamin deficiency thus presents with a range of clinical symptoms, and treatment generally responds to dietary correction. Preventive health lies in ensuring an adequate supply of these nutrients through key foods, identified as providing significant amounts of the nutrient class. Problems emerge when the food supply is inadequate, including a limited number of available foods and nutrient-depleting food practices, but they can also arise when nutritious food are plentiful but compete with poor-quality foods for choices made by the community. This is often the case in Western societies such as Australia [7], where so-called 'discretionary foods' are consumed in significant proportions.

See Chapter 2 on discretionary foods.

Thiamin (vitamin B1) has a chemical structure consisting of 2,5-dimethyl-6-aminopyrimidine (a pyrimidine ring) and 4-methyl-5-hydroxy ethyl thiazole (a thiazolium ring) with a methylene bridge in between (Figure 10.1). The main form of thiamin is thiamin pyrophosphate, a coenzyme. It also occurs as thiamin triphosphate in the brain. Thiamin status is tested by measuring levels of the enzyme transketolase in red blood cells.

Thiamin is generally not stable to heat and other components in the diet can interfere with thiamin absorption. It is absorbed in the gut mainly in the jejunum. The dynamics of absorption depend on the amount present, and is more passive with higher concentrations. Like other water-soluble vitamins, there is no major storage site for thiamin in the body and excess is excreted in the urine. There is no

TABLE 10.1   FUNCTIONS OF B GROUP VITAMINS

Vitamin	Function	Clinical condition	Note
Thiamin (B1)	Coenzyme • CHO metabolism • BCAA catabolism	Beri beri	Wernicke's encephalopathy in alcoholism
Riboflavin (B2)	Coenzyme • protein metabolism—fat metabolism	Ariboflavinosis	Unstable to ultraviolet light
Niacin (B3)	Coenzyme • oxidative phosphorylation • fatty acid synthesis	Pellagra	Tryptophan also a source (calculated as niacin equivalents)
Pantothenic acid (B5)	Coenzyme • TCA cycle (CHO,PTN) • fatty acid elongation	No reported deficiency states	
Pyridoxine (B6)	Coenzyme • AA synthesis • glucose from glycogen Bile acid, lecithin production	Toxic neural symptoms have been observed	Group of compounds
Biotin (B7)	Coenzyme • TCA cycle • PTN, fat CHO metabolism		May also be produced by microbiota
Cobalamin (B12)	Coenzyme • metabolism S-AA (homocysteine to MET)	Pernicious anaemia (lack intrinsic factor (IF)) Macrocytic anaemia (B12 deficiency)	Requires IF in stomach Synthesised by bacteria
Folate	Single carbon transfer (methyl group donation) • DNA synthesis, cell division	Megaloblastic/macrocytic anaemias	Neural tube defects associated with insufficiency

FIGURE 10.1   STRUCTURE OF THIAMINE

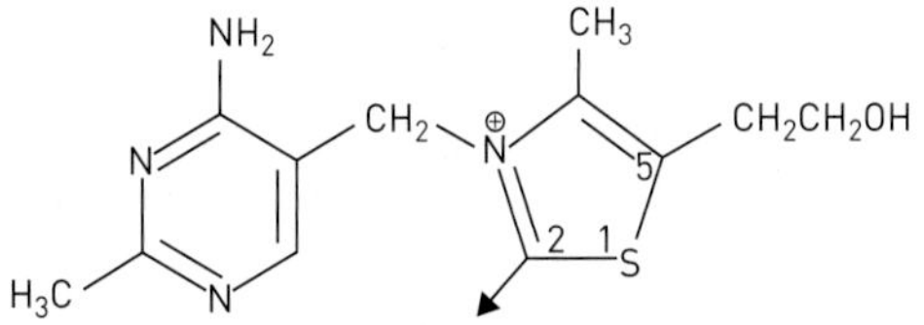

Thiamin

known toxicity for thiamin, as beyond 5 mg/day it tends to be excreted, but that does not rule out the possibility that very high doses could have adverse effects [8].

Thiamin is involved in amino acid metabolism and carbohydrate metabolism, notably gluconeogenesis. It serves as a coenzyme in carbohydrate metabolism (citric acid cycle and hexose monophosphate shunt) as well as catabolism of branched chain amino acids [9]. Carbohydrate metabolism is lessened with insufficient thiamin (notably impaired glucose metabolism and accumulation of pyruvate and lactate) and reduced catabolism of branched chain amino acids. How this translates to clinical signs

FIGURE 10.2 STRUCTURE OF RIBOFLAVIN

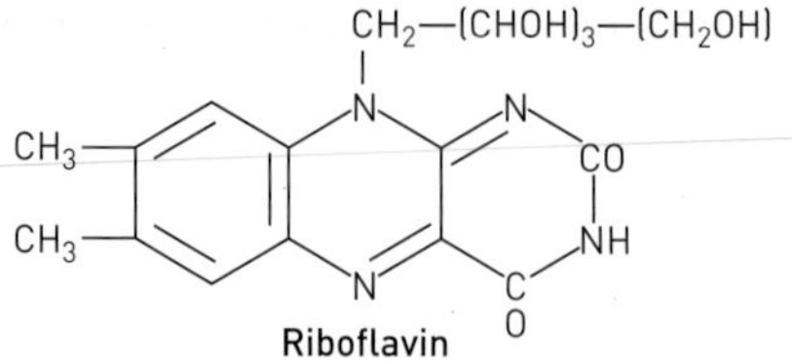

Riboflavin

and symptoms is complex, but there can be negative effects on the nervous system and difficulties with memory retention. After 25–30 days of inadequate intake, a state of deficiency emerges with symptoms including swelling (oedema), a weakened heart muscle and symptoms associated with the nervous system. Seen in the acute and chronic phases respectively, this condition is known as **beri beri**. It is mainly seen in people suffering from alcoholism or those in extreme states of poverty. As thiamin is utilised in alcohol metabolism, a condition known as **Wernicke's encephalopathy** (or Wernicke-Korsakoff syndrome) can result from the compounded nature of high alcohol consumption and lack of thiamin in food. For unknown reasons, the two clinical conditions of Wernicke-Korsakoff syndrome and beri beri rarely occur together. Thiamin is not known to be toxic.

Beri beri

a thiamin deficiency disease presenting as heart failure (acute/wet) or neuropathy (chronic/dry).

Wernicke's encephalopathy

a thiamin deficiency state seen in people suffering from alcoholism, with features of confusion, paralysis of the eye and memory loss.

The chemical name for *riboflavin (vitamin B)* is 7,8–dimethyl-10-('D-ribityl) isoallaxazine. It consists of a ribose alcohol joined to an aloxazine ring. The active form includes the addition of a ribityl side chain (Figure 10.2). Most of the riboflavin is lost after a mere four hours' exposure to the ultraviolet in sunlight.

The amount of riboflavin consumed influences the level of metabolism, but it has a high bioavailability. In the first place, it is absorbed with the help of a carrier system in the small intestine but is taken up in the blood in its free form. Riboflavin is transported within the body as free riboflavin, its coenzyme form (flavin mononucleatide [FMN] involved in oxidation in mitochondria and in energy-related pathways) or bound with plasma albumin. It can be found in muscle as flavin adenine dinucleotide (FAD) [10]. FAD and FMN are the bioactive forms of the nutrient.

Like thiamin, riboflavin is central to protein and fat metabolism, also serving as a coenzyme rather than carbohydrates. The main role is in energy production, but it also has roles in the immune and nervous systems. In particular, it is involved in a number of chemical conversions such as converting pyridoxine to its bioactive form, tryptophan to niacin, and methylenetetrahydrofolate to methyl tetrahydrofolate. As energy production and the metabolic pathways of macronutrients are connected, deficiency (**ariboflavinosis**) is often seen in conjunction with deficiencies of other vitamins. Symptoms of deficiency include inflammation of the tongue or the mouth and eye disorder. Toxicity has not been reported for riboflavin, presumably due to the tight controls on absorption in the gut and its water-soluble nature enabling excretion via the urine.

Ariboflavinosis

deficiency of riboflavin involving inflammation of the tongue, most commonly seen with other vitamin B deficiencies.

Niacin equivalents

the amount of niacin (mg) calculated as (niacin (mg) plus tryptophan(mg)/60) mg.

Niacin (vitamin B3) is defined by its biological activity and occurs as two compounds in the acid form as nicotinic acid (full chemical name pyridine 3-carboxylic acid) and the amine form, nicotinamide. The amino acid tryptophan can also convert to niacin. Thus, the amount of niacin is referred to as **niacin equivalents**. It is calculated as the sum of preformed niacin (mg) and a fraction of the tryptophan present ($\times$/60), reflecting the conversion ratio.

Human absorption of niacin occurs in the stomach and the small intestine to be later transported in the plasma, but minimal amounts are stored in the body. As a B group vitamin, it is a component of coenzymes, this time nicotinamide-adenine-dinucleotide (NAD) and nicotinamide-adenine-dinucleotide phosphate (NADP), both of which are involved in oxidative phosphorylation, part of the energy production process in the mitochondria. Its hydrogen donor capacity is featured in fatty acid synthesis.

The amount of niacin required reflects the physiological interdependence between nutrients, which is biologically determined. Niacin requirements largely depend on that for the amino acid tryptophan. Given the complex interplay between nutrients within human metabolism, the amount of niacin required is linked to the needs for and status of other nutrients, namely tryptophan, riboflavin, pyridoxine and iron. The deficiency disease is called **pellagra** (with symptoms of dermatitis, diarrhoea, delirium and dementia) and deficiency can occur after about 45 days of insufficiency.

> **Pellagra**
> a niacin deficiency disease presenting with dermatitis, diarrhoea, delirium and dementia.

≫ RESEARCH AT WORK

NIACIN IN THE PREVENTION OF DISEASE

Niacin has been considered for coronary heart disease risk reduction by increasing HDL cholesterol concentrations via effects on APO-A1 cholesterol ester transfer protein and an ATP binding transporter, having a modest effect on LDL cholesterol levels and reducing triglyceride levels. However, its use in favour of other therapies has been in question for some time, in addition to concerns that it may cause adverse effects in the high doses required [11].

In more recent times, animal model studies targeting congenital malformations examined enzymes associated with the kynurenine pathway (in which tryptophan is converted to NAD) and demonstrated that niacin supplementation during gestation prevented malformations in mice [12]. This research, however, can only produce hypotheses for later testing in humans. The main limitation of this research is that the way in which the body processes and utilises niacin in mice may be very different from its metabolism in humans.

The knowledge inherent in this research, however, continues to support the significance of a diet providing adequate amounts of niacin for maintaining health.

Pantothenic acid (vitamin B5) has a butyryl-beta-alanine structure, otherwise known as 3-[[(2R)-2,4-dihydroxy-3, 3-dimethylbutanoyl]amino] propanoic acid. It is essential for the formation of coenzyme A, a fundamental unit in the tricarboxylic acid metabolic cycle (concerned with carbohydrate and amino acid disposal). Pantothenic acid also produces acyl carrier protein (ACP), which assists the elongation of fatty acids. This makes pantothenic acid an important co-factor in macronutrient (and thereby energy) metabolism, but it is distinguished by delivering acyl chemical groups into the processes.

As with other nutrients, there is some degree of control of absorption of pantothenic acid, ranging from it being actively absorbed at low concentrations and changing to passive absorption at high concentrations. It is transported by red blood cells in the CoA form and is actively taken up in cells with the help of a carrier protein. Specific reported deficiency has not been found.

Pyridoxine (vitamin B6) refers to a number of chemical compounds, namely pyridoxal, pyridoxine, pyridoxamine and the phosphate compounds of each of these. The main chemical entity in the body and in food is pyridoxal-5'-phosphate (PLP), which acts as a coenzyme, this time in transferring amine units in the production of essential amino acids and the breakdown of others, and assisting decarboxylation in various functional areas. Requirements are linked to protein intake.

Pyridoxine is absorbed passively by the mucosal cells of the small intestine. It also occurs in different chemical forms that interconvert. The pyridoxal and pyridoxamine forms are better absorbed than pyridoxine. Transport occurs via attachment to albumin and haemoglobin. It is diffused into liver cells and undergoes rephosphorylation. This bioactive form pyridoxine (pyridoxal phosphate) works alongside riboflavin.

Given its biochemical roles, pyridoxine has many functions. It is vital to neurotransmitter and haemoglobin synthesis and in almost all stages of amino acid metabolism. It is found with the enzyme that releases glucose from glycogen stores (glycogen phosphorylase), is associated with bile acid function and is involved in the synthesis of lecithin. Deficiency can lead to anaemia, vomiting, an appearance of flaky skin, convulsions, headache and a sore tongue. Toxicity is related to destruction of the nerves observed through taking high-dose supplements.

Biotin (vitamin B7) is a heterocyclic compound, 5-(2-oxo-1,3,3a,4,6,6a-hexahydrothieno[3,4-d] imidazol-4-yl)pentanoic acid found in free form or bound to proteins. As with the other B group vitamins, biotin serves as a coenzyme in metabolic cycles (e.g. the tricarboxylic acid (TCA) cycle). It is involved in macronutrient metabolism, notably fatty acid synthesis, glucose production and the breakdown of amino acids. Biotin is an enzyme cofactor in mitochondria. While there is unknown toxicity, deficiency is mainly seen in the presence of alcoholism. It may also result in anaemia, depression and dermatitis, mainly in persons suffering from alcoholism. Given these roles, biotin can be found in most cells, and is most abundant in the organs with a significant metabolic role such as the liver, kidneys and pancreas.

Digestion begins at the protein level of biocytin and the biotin-containing oligopeptides releasing and converting to biotin. Biotin is absorbed in both the small and large intestine via a carrier-mediated process (human sodium dependent multivitamin transporter, hSMVT), which is also used for pantothenic acid. Biotin can also be produced by the intestinal microbiota, an area of ongoing research interest [13]. A recent review of studies indicates a number of areas in which the study of biotin is expanding and notes an emerging use of biotin therapy in some conditions [14].

Cobalamin is actually referred to more often in the numbered form—that is, *vitamin B12*. Again, it reflects a number of chemical compounds including hydroxycobalamin, methylcobalamin and deoxyadenosylcobalamin. The chemical structure is three-dimensional, compromising four pyrole rings (corrinoid ring). At the centre is cobalt. The coenzyme functions of vitamin B12 concern propionate catabolism in the mitochondria, and the metabolism of sulphur-containing amino acids, converting homocysteine to methionine. Other distinguishing features of vitamin B12 are that an intrinsic binder in the stomach is required for absorption and the vitamin itself is synthesised by bacteria.

Vitamin B12 is found bound to animal protein. It is first released then bound to a binder produced in the saliva. A significant component of cobalamin digestion and absorption is the involvement of binding proteins. In food, cobalamin is bound to animal protein, which is first released to allow a binding protein secreted in the stomach to attach and carry it through the gut. Binding proteins are digested in the small intestine (duodenum), and the cobalamin is absorbed in the ileum. Cobalamin is then transported in the blood, again attached to protein (transcobalamin II), and stored long term in the liver. Methylcobalamin and 5-deoxyadenosylcobalamin are the active forms.

Cobalamin acts as a coenzyme in folate metabolism, so the deficiency states can be confounded and tests are required to distinguish between them. Deficiency of dietary cobalamin results in **macrocytic anaemia**. Deficiency due to the additional inability

Macrocytic anaemia
anaemia caused by vitamin B12 deficiency characterised by large, lower density red blood cells.

to absorb vitamin B12 (through lack of intrinsic Factor) is termed **pernicious anaemia**. It has additional functions relating to the nervous system, via involvement in fatty acid synthesis within myelin. Deficiency leads to macrocytic anaemia, occurring in those at risk of inadequate intakes such as older adults and people following a vegan diet. Toxicity is also unknown. There are advantages in using an array of assessments in monitoring vitamin B12 status (serum B12, holoTC, MMA), particularly in the early stages of pregnancy in at-risk groups [15].

> **Pernicious anaemia**
> an intractable anaemia caused by a lack of vitamin B12 (extrinsic factor) and its binding protein (intrinsic factor).

» RESEARCH AT WORK

VITAMIN B12 AND DISEASE PREVENTION

While deficiency disease is itself an issue, whether subclinical vitamin B12 status affects disease risk or reduced functionality has provided other directions for research. This has been the case for research in cardiovascular disease and the maintenance of cognition.

Vitamin B12 is involved in the conversion of homocysteine to methionine. Inadequate vitamin B12 intakes have also been implicated in the risk of cardiovascular disease, through high homocysteine (Hcy) levels [16]. The latter are seen to act as permissive agents in endothelial damage as well as causing enhanced lipid peroxidation and the production of free radicals. In addition to clinical studies, this relationship was observed in a largely vegetarian population with existing coronary artery disease [17], supporting further investigative work in this area. The concept, however, underpins the importance of food choices and dietary intakes that attend to nutritional composition, particularly in vulnerable populations.

Given the role of vitamin B12 in neurological pathways, its status has also been implicated in studies of cognitive decline. In one German cross-sectional study of 100 patients (50–80 years) with mild cognitive impairment, low (but not deficient) vitamin B12 status was associated with poor memory performance [18]. In a later trial, of 201 mildly vitamin B12–deficient older patients (>75 years) from seven primary care practices in the United Kingdom, correction of this deficiency did not have any beneficial effects on neurologic or cognitive function [19]. This was examined in the absence of signs or symptoms of vitamin B12 deficiency (anaemia, neurological or cognitive signs and symptoms). While these two studies demonstrate the important interrelationships between observational and clinical studies, the latter indicates that focusing on a single nutrient for broader health outcomes may not be appropriate. Again, however, it is likely that vitamin B12 plays an important role in cognitive function and adequate intakes in the diet will be significant in contributing to its continuance.

Folate (tetrahydrofolate) is the naturally occurring vitamin found in food (such as foliage—green leafy vegetables), whereas folic acid (pteroyl glutamic acid, PGA) is the form used in vitamin supplements and the fortification of food as it is more stable than folate. Folate can also appear as 5,10-methylene tetrahydrofolate. In chemical terms, this means a methyl group may be attached to nitrogen in the 5 or 10 position. It can also be attached between the two positions.

Folate in food usually appears in a polyglutamate form. Once consumed, the gut enzymes hydrolyse this compound into a monoglutamate ready for absorption. Folate appears as 5-methyl tetrahydrofolate in blood. In cells, it appears in the polyglutamate form. Folic acid consumed as supplements or in enriched foods converts to tetrahydrofolate prior to absorption (Figure 10.3). Within cells it returns to the polyglutamate form. Genetic profiles have implications for the levels of enzymes required for folate

LINDA TAPSELL

FIGURE 10.3 FOLATE MECHANISM

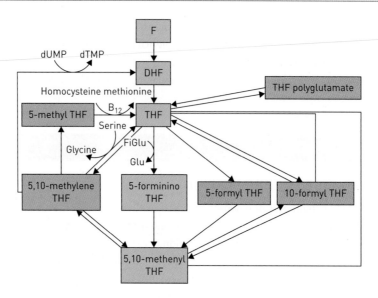

Source: S. Truswell (2012). Chapter 13: The B vitamins. In J. Mann & S. Truswell (eds), *Essentials of Human Nutrition*, 4th edn. Oxford University Press, Incorporated (Figure 13.8, p. 231)

metabolism. This means some people require more folate than others. The liver is the storage site for folate. There is some excretion in bile but very little in urine [20].

Folate plays an important role in single carbon transfer donating methyl groups. This occurs during purine and pyrimidine synthesis of DNA (in its 5,10-methylene tetrahydrofolate form), and is implicated in cell division. At this point we see another instance of synergy between nutrients. DNA synthesis is strongly linked to vitamin B12 status. A deficiency of vitamin B12 means that folate remains in a 5-methyl tetrahydrofolate form and this has implications for the pathways in which the folate group act.

Like vitamin B12, folate also serves as a coenzyme in the re-methylation of homocysteine to methionine, and the megablastic (or macrocytic) anaemia symptoms of folate deficiency can emerge similarly to that of vitamin B12. There is also a proposed role in the development of neurotransmitters in the brain [21]. Other signs of folate deficiency are inadequate growth, neural tube defects in infants, inflammation of the tongue and diarrhoea. Pregnant women and their developing babies are at risk. In those on particular medications, secondary deficiency can occur with alcohol dependence.

» RESEARCH AT WORK

B GROUP VITAMINS AND CANCER

The interest in folate and cancer prevention stems from its significant role in DNA methylation, synthesis and repair. This role has implications for gene expression and gene stability, and cancer research has long focused on genetic intervention. In this review, scientists examine and discuss the potential for folate supplementation to help reduce the risk of childhood leukaemia [22]. They outline the role of folate in the cell and explain how damage occurs. They review the positions on folate and cancer (including expressed concerns for excessive folate intake) and take the case of the risk of childhood leukaemia as an example of how knowledge of folate metabolism could be applied in disease prevention. This narrative form of review is different from systematic evidence-based reviews, but it serves to help develop arguments and hypotheses that can drive research to better understand the relationship between nutrients, foods, diets and health.

The significance of one carbon transfer in cell metabolism and high prevalence of use of vitamin B supplements indicated a need to consider relative risk with cancer. In the VITAL cohort (>77,000 participants aged 50–76 years), the 10-year average daily dose of multivitamin supplements and incidence of lung cancer were considered [23]. In women there was no association between use of vitamin B6, folate and B12 supplements and lung cancer. However, associations were found in men for vitamin B6 and B12 supplements, and this was even higher if they were smokers at baseline. The authors concluded that the association between B6 and B12 supplement use and lung cancer was sex specific and related to the type of supplements (single or multivitamin). This study confirmed that, rather than providing added benefit, vitamin supplementation could potentially be harmful.

STOP AND THINK

- How has the role of the B group vitamins emerged alongside the developing science of the biochemistry? Which related significant scientific developments occurred in the mid-twentieth century?
- Using examples of research in the B group vitamins, what different considerations need to be made between understanding deficiency states versus the prevention of disease and maintenance of functionality?
- How has the understanding of B group vitamin deficiency informed public health strategies to support well-being in the population?

WHAT ARE THE MAJOR FOOD SOURCES OF THE B GROUP VITAMINS?

Because of their multiple roles in energy metabolism, and significant impacts on functional systems operating in the body, the B group vitamins are well distributed in humans and the foods they consume of animal origin (with similar processes). They are also found in relatively unprocessed plant foods, particularly where there is significant genetic carriage and/or nutrient density (seeds, wholegrains, leafy vegetables) [24]. Many processed foods have added B group vitamins, and in the case of thiamin and folic acid, this also arises from the **mandatory fortification of foods**.

The requirements for B group vitamins are defined in the NRVs (www.nrv.gov.au). Requirements are higher in pregnant women and folic acid supplements are advised (Table 10.2). As a group, B vitamins are delivered in the total diet, with varying amounts coming from different foods that together meet requirements. This combination of relative amounts and types of foods underpins the recommended food choices outlined in the Australian Guide to Healthy Eating [25].

There are two ways to consider food sources of B group vitamins: the relative amount of vitamin per gram of food, and the relative amount of vitamin consumed from a particular food source. Both are useful in translating requirements to food sources, but both also need to be considered in dietary

Mandatory fortification of foods
addition of a nutrient to a defined level in specific foods as stipulated by legislation in the food standards code.

TABLE 10.2   VITAMIN B AND FOLATE REQUIREMENTS

Recommended intakes of B vitamins and folate (mg/day and µg/day)	B1 thiamin	B2 riboflavin	B3 niacin	B5 pantothenic Acid	B6 pyridoxine	B7 biotin	B12 cobalamin	Folate
	RDI mg/day	RDI mg/day	RDI mg/day)	AI mg/day	RDI mg/day	AI µg/day	RDI µg/day	RDI µg/day
Men								
19–70 years	1.2	1.3	16	6.0	1.3 1.7 (>50yr)	30	2.4	400
>70 years	1.2	1.6	16	6.0	1.7	30	2.4	400
Women								
1–50 years	1.1	1.1	14	4.0	1.3	25	2.4	400
>50 years	1.1	1.1 1.3 (>70yr)	14	4.0	1.5	25	2.4	400
Pregnancy								
1–18 years	1.4	1.4	18	5.0	1.9	30	2.6	600
1–50 years	1.4	1.4	18	5.0	1.9	30	2.6	600
Lactation								
1–18 years	1.4	1.6	17	5.0	2.0	35	2.8	500
1–50 years	1.4	1.6	17	5.0	2.0	35	2.8	500

Source: National Health and Medical Research Council (2006). *Nutrient Reference Values for Australia and New Zealand, Including Recommended Dietary Intakes*. Canberra: NHMRC. © Commonwealth of Australia

modelling for an adequate diet. For example, organ meats like liver, and green leafy vegetables contain high levels of folate, but health surveys indicate they are not consumed regularly in significant amounts. Thus, the position of the food in the average cultural eating pattern is an important consideration.

In line with their biological functions, foods that comprise animal flesh (in particular organ meats), milk or fruit/seed-like properties of plants are also higher in protein and, for meats, the whole B group of vitamins. Red meat and offal (liver) have the best vitamin B12 content.

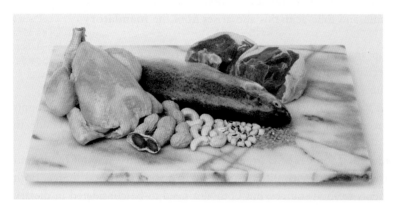

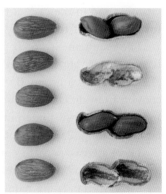

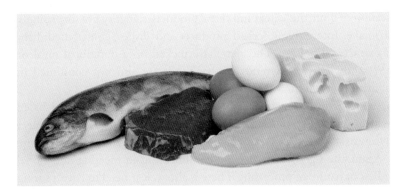

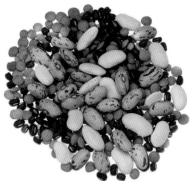

Nuts and seeds are also a good source of thiamin, while more riboflavin is found in milk, eggs, meat and offal, and niacin in fish. The biotin in meat and beans is more bioavailable than in other foods. This is because it is present in a cellular or free form rather than a bound form. Biotin is found in almonds, peanuts and organ meats, and to some degree in egg yolks.

'Meat, poultry and game products and dishes' were the second highest contributors (11%) to reported thiamin intakes, and the majority (29%) of vitamin B12 on the day reported in the Nutrition First results [26]. The category of 'Fish and seafood products and dishes' delivered 8.8% of vitamin B12.

In Australia, bread and cereals are **staple foods**, so they are consumed in relatively large amounts. This means that their contribution to the delivery of nutrients can end up being significant, even if they have relatively lower quantities of a nutrient than foods more concentrated with that nutrient. In Australia, bread and flour are fortified with the **limiting B group vitamins**, folate and thiamin (www.foodstandards.gov.au) to ensure adequate intakes in the population, particularly in at-risk groups, such as women of childbearing age, where adequate intakes can help prevent health problems such as neural tube defects in the infant.

Australia is a leading producer of wheat, oats and many other grains that are both exported and delivered into the food supply [27]. Because humans do not have the capabilities to digest cereals grains such as wheat straight from the field, they have developed cultural techniques of milling and processing (cooking) that enable consumption and enjoyment. Processing, however, can remove important nutrients, which is a real consideration for differentiating between grain foods, in particular, and introducing the need to value **wholegrains** [28; 29].

Forms of processing now produce a wide range of products, from relatively unprocessed grain products, such as rolled oats, to highly processed cereal-based products such as extruded snack foods delivered in snack packs. Analyses from the Australian National Health Survey [26], distinguishes these two categories as 'cereal products' and 'cereal based products and dishes', respectively. The Nutrition First results [26] note that bread and cereals appeared as significant contributors of B group vitamins in the Australian diet, as summarised below.

- *Folate:* Most (57%) of the folate was reportedly consumed in 'cereal products', as well as the more processed category of 'cereal based products and dishes'. This reflects the recent fortification of bread with folate.

Staple foods

foods that deliver essential nutrients and also form the foundation of a cuisine in a particular cultural context.

Limiting B group vitamins

vitamins likely to be under-consumed and thereby increasing the risk of public health problems.

See Chapter 4 on dietary fibre and plant-based nutrients.

Wholegrains

foods that retain essential components of the entire grain.

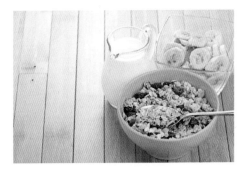

- *Thiamin:* Given thiamin fortification of flour, the 'cereal and cereal products' category not surprisingly contributed 41% of reported intake. Interestingly, 'cereal products and dishes' contributed 12%, alongside vegetable and meat extracts (also 12%). This may have picked up a traditional meal or snack, the Vegemite™ sandwich, and reminds us that foods are also not consumed in isolation but in combinations in cultural cuisines.

See Chapter 2 on planning a healthy diet.

- *Vitamin B12:* Rather than the basic grain products, the more processed category of 'cereal-based products and dishes' were classed among the main sources of vitamin B12 (13%). This would reflect the contribution of other, likely animal-sourced food ingredients in the products and dishes that were nonetheless 'based' on cereals. Again, the significance of food combinations in meeting nutritional requirements is apparent, regardless of nature of processing. There is also a clear need to have a strong understanding of food composition and the relative position of nutrients in foods when working with nutrition and food.

≫ CASE 10.1

FOLIC ACID FORTIFICATION OF BREAD

Since 2009, Australian millers have been required to add folic acid to wheat flour that is used for bread making (see www.foodstandards.gov.au). This was due to the public health need to ensure adequate folic acid intakes in women preparing for a pregnancy. Intakes one month before and three months after conception can prevent neural tube defects (NTD), such as spina bifida, which occurs when the neural tube does not close and fuse in early pregnancy when it should. The foods that need to be fortified include all wheat breads, rolls, buns, flatbreads, muffins and bread-making flour, but exclude organic bread and those made with only other grains. Other countries that have undertaken this strategy include the United States and Canada.

See the information on folic acid/folate and pregnancy at: www.foodstandards.gov.au/consumer/generalissues/pregnancy/folic/Pages/default.aspx.

- What kind of evidence base was required before this fortification strategy was put in place?
- How would monitoring the effects of this strategy be undertaken?
- Why is bread a good food to choose for fortification, and why are organic breads excluded?

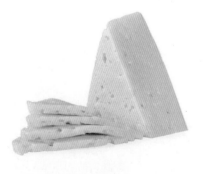

Breads and cereals were also the main source of thiamin consumed on the day of the Nutrition First Results, with the 'cereal and cereal products' category contributing 41% and the 'cereal products and dishes' contributing 12%. Again, yeast, vegetable and meat extracts were also the second main source (12%), reflecting traditional eating patterns and the significance of a cultural food, such as Vegemite™, in delivering a key nutrient within the population.

The main B group vitamins provided by milk and milk products are riboflavin (primarily found in dairy products) and vitamin B12 ('Milk products and dishes' provided 30% of this vitamin in the Nutrition First results of the

AHS [26]). Niacin is another significant B group vitamin delivered through this food group. Cow's milk has lower levels of niacin compared with breast milk. Unprocessed foods deliver foods as nicotinamide compounds.

Leafy green vegetables, legumes and citrus fruit provide greater proportions of folate than meat and some riboflavin is found in mushrooms and spinach. Niacin and vitamin B6 in particular are also found in vegetables.

TRY IT YOURSELF

Write down a list of the foods you consumed in the last 24 hours. Which of these were major sources of B group vitamins? Were any of them foods fortified with B group vitamins? Which of the B vitamins do you think you may not be consuming enough of, and how could you fix that?

STOP AND THINK

- Why do whole food categories rather than single foods present as major sources of B group vitamins?
- Why is fortification with thiamin and folate necessary to protect public health in Australia. Why is bread a fortified food?
- How is food fortification managed by food standards and can any food be fortified to increase the nutrient content?

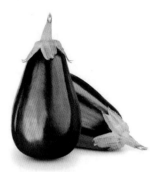

WHAT IS THE STRUCTURE AND FUNCTION OF VITAMIN C?

Vitamin C is a molecule related to glucose, but primates are missing the enzyme that enables conversion from glucose. Hence, the vitamin is essential. Vitamin C comes in a number of chemical forms, namely L-ascorbic acid, D-ascorbic acid, L-isoascorbic acid and D-isoascorbic acid (Figure 10.4). In human metabolism, vitamin C acts as a cofactor for enzymes and is thus involved in conversion processes—for

FIGURE 10.4 STRUCTURE OF VITAMIN C

Source: https://pubchem.ncbi.nlm.nih.gov/image/imagefly.cgi?cid=54670067&width=500&height=500

Collagen
a main structural protein in connective tissue.

See Case 17.2 in Chapter 17 on vitamin C deficiency.

example, converting ferric iron (Fe^{3+}) to ferrous iron (Fe^{2+}) and lysine (an amino acid) to carnitine. It is also necessary for the beta-oxidation of long chain fatty acids and the synthesis of **collagen**. Insufficient intakes of L-ascorbic acid found in foods leads to the deficiency disease of scurvy.

The bioavailability of vitamin C is high and absorption occurs via active transport mechanisms in the small intestine; however, excess amounts (more than 1 g/day) are excreted.

Requirements vary across individuals in a population, and the main concern for adequate intakes is to prevent scurvy. By consuming fresh fruit and vegetables, it is not difficult to achieve requirements for vitamin C (Table 10.3). Surprisingly, deficiencies are emerging in healthy Western societies, including Australia (see Case 17.3), underlining the need for better nutrition practices in the community and heightened awareness among healthcare workers. As vitamin C is a water-soluble vitamin, excessive circulating levels are lost in the urine. High doses of vitamin C supplements are unable to further increase circulating vitamin C levels.

In deficient states of the production of vitamin C, normal collagen is compromised, meaning areas containing collagen fibre become fragile and the repair is hindered, leading to such things as bleeding gums and even haemorrhaging.

Certain groups in the population may be at risk of insufficient vitamin C intakes. Convalescence from illness and poor appetite indicate times where needs may be higher. Increased vitamin C intake can be achieved with more fruit or vegetables, or via supplements.

TABLE 10.3 VITAMIN C REQUIREMENTS

Recommended intakes of vitamin C (mg/day)	Estimated average requirement (EAR)	Recommended dietary intake (RDI)	Upper level of intake (UL)*
Men			
19–70 years	30	45	1000
>70 years	30	45	1000
Women			
19–50 years	30	45	1000
>50 years	30	45	1000
Pregnancy			
14–18 years	38	55	1000
18–50 years	40	60	1000
Lactation			
14–18 years	58	80	1000
18–50 years	60	85	1000

*Unable to establish upper limit, thus a prudent limit is suggested.

Source: National Health and Medical Research Council (2006). *Nutrient Reference Values for Australia and New Zealand, Including Recommended Dietary Intakes*. Canberra: NHMRC. © Commonwealth of Australia

>> CASE 10.2

DOES TAKING EXTRA VITAMIN C HAVE HEALTH BENEFITS?

Beyond the prevention of scurvy, vitamin C has been considered for potential protective roles in cancer prevention, influenza prevention or minimisation, and eye health, particularly given its antioxidant functions. Supporting immune function may be a new consideration for vitamin C given its location in immune reactive cells and in glands and parts of the eye, but this will require more research. In addition, the presence of ascorbic acid may protect against the formation of carcinogenic compounds such as nitrosamines in the stomach. The evidence, however, has not been forthcoming.

- A major trial in the United Kingdom testing the effects of 250 mg/day vitamin C plus vitamin E and β-carotene showed no benefits in total mortality, coronary heart disease, strokes or cancer mortality [30]. While the EPIC-Norfolk cohort study did demonstrate an inverse association between plasma ascorbate levels and deaths from all causes of cardiovascular diseases, this may rather reflect high intakes of fruits and vegetables [31].
- An early World Cancer Research evidence review stated that vitamin C 'possibly' protected against stomach cancer [32], but this was revised and the new recommendation stated 'do not use supplements for cancer prevention' [33]. Reviews of trials have not consistently indicated protective effects and nutrients can be obtained from a healthy diet [34].
- Randomised controlled trials on immune function have nearly all shown no reduced incidence of colds; they may possibly be of shorter duration [35; 36].
- A large cohort study found that women who took vitamin C tablets in the long term had a significantly lower incidence of cataract operations [27], but there remained the possibility of confounding— for example, people who take vitamin supplements may have worn sunglasses. The nutritional composition of ongoing studies in the prevention of vision loss in the elderly is an ongoing area of research [37].

Vitamin C is added to beverages and supplements are commonly available at doses of 50, 100, 250, 500 and 1000 mg, partly as sodium ascorbate. Given the ability to excrete vitamin C, doses above 500 mg/day are questionable [38].

- How do assumptions arise on the additional health benefits of higher vitamin C intakes?
- What kind of research is required to produce a body of research providing adequate evidence?
- How likely is it that individuals in the population will have inadequate vitamin C intakes?

STOP AND THINK

- Why do humans need vitamin C?
- Which groups in the community are most at risk of inadequate vitamin C intakes, and why?
- What other components of foods have functions related to vitamin C?

LINDA TAPSELL

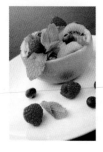

WHAT ARE THE MAJOR FOOD SOURCES OF VITAMIN C?

The major food sources of vitamin C are fresh fruits and vegetables, although there is a wide range in content (from <10 mg per 100 g to >200 mg per 100 g; see Table 10.3). Vitamin C can be easily lost with heating, as well as in alkaline conditions and the presence of copper, issues to be taken into account when considering cooking methods and utensils.

STOP AND THINK

- Why could vitamin C be considered a natural ingredient with a functional role in food preservation?
- Why do fruits and vegetables need to be fresh to ensure adequate intakes of vitamin C?
- What are the implications of eating a variety of fruits and vegetables for ensuring adequate intakes of vitamin C?

SUMMARY

- The water-soluble vitamins have important roles in human metabolism and health protection; excess consumption is excreted; and deficiency states have been characterised.
- Consuming the types and amounts of food groups outlined in the Australian Guide to Healthy Eating will generally ensure adequate intakes of these vitamins in the population.
- Further research on the impacts of food processing and food fortification will expand understanding of these nutrients, especially following their consumption in their naturally occurring contexts.

PATHWAYS TO PRACTICE

- An inadequate consumption of foods prepared to preserve water-soluble vitamins can place individuals at risk of nutrient deficiencies. Healthcare workers in a range of roles need to be aware of these risk conditions and consider signs of deficiency.
- Food service operations, particularly those delivering to elderly adults, need to meet standards for food preparation that ensure adequate water-soluble vitamin retention.
- Monitoring dietary intakes at the population level remains an important public health activity; in particular, in assessing the impact of fortification of B group vitamins.

DISCUSSION QUESTIONS

1 With respect to water-soluble vitamins in foods, what is the difference between food innovation at the industry level and food fortification for public health purposes?
2 What does the history of research in water-soluble vitamins tell us about the connection between scientific discovery and practice in nutrition?
3 How important is the knowledge of water-soluble vitamins, their roles and sources to health practitioners across the board?

USEFUL WEBLINKS

Australian Guide to Healthy Eating:
www.eatforhealth.gov.au

Australian Health Survey 2011–12—Essential minerals:
www.abs.gov.au/ausstats/abs@.nsf/Lookup/by%20Subject/4364.0.55.008~2011-12~Main%20
Features~Essential%20minerals~400

Food Standards Australia New Zealand—AUSNUT 2011–13 food nutrient database:
www.foodstandards.gov.au/science/monitoringnutrients/ausnut/ausnutdatafiles/Pages/
foodnutrient.aspx

Food Standards Australia New Zealand—Folic acid/folate and pregnancy:
www.foodstandards.gov.au/consumer/generalissues/pregnancy/folic/Pages/default.aspx

HealthDirect—Health topics:
www.healthdirect.gov.au/health-topics

National Institutes of Health, Office of Dietary Supplements—Thiamin:
https://ods.od.nih.gov/factsheets/Thiamin-HealthProfessional

Nutrient Reference Values for Australia and New Zealand—Nutrients:
www.nrv.gov.au/nutrients

Nutrient retention factors:
www.ars.usda.gov/ARSUserFiles/80400525/Data/retn/retn06.pdf

USDA Table of Nutrient Retention Factors:
www.ars.usda.gov/ARSUserFiles/80400525/Data/retn/retn06.pdf

FURTHER READING

Al-Khudairy, L., Flowers, N., Wheelhouse, R., Ghannam, O., Hartley, L., Stranges, S. & Rees, K. (2017).
Vitamin C supplementation for the primary prevention of cardiovascular disease. *Cochrane Database
of Systematic Reviews*, 3. doi:10.1002/14651858.CD011114.pub2

Antony, A. C. (2017). Evidence for potential underestimation of clinical folate deficiency in resource-
limited countries using blood tests. *Nutrition Reviews*, 75(8), 600–15. doi:10.1093/nutrit/nux032

Ashor, A. W., Werner, A. D., Lara, J., Willis, N. D., Mathers, J. C. & Siervo, M. (2017). Effects of vitamin
C supplementation on glycaemic control: a systematic review and meta-analysis of randomised
controlled trials. *European Journal of Clinical Nutrition*, 71, 1371–80. doi:10.1038/ejcn.2017.24

Boyles, A. L., Yetley, E. A., Thayer, K. A. & Coates, P. M. (2016). Safe use of high intakes of folic
acid: research challenges and paths forward. *Nutrition Reviews*, 74(7), 469–74. doi:10.1093/nutrit/
nuw015

Gahche, J. J., Bailey, R. L., Potischman, N. & Dwyer, J. T. (2017). Dietary supplement use was very
high among older adults in the United States in 2011–2014. *Journal of Nutrition*, 147(10), 1968–76.
doi:10.3945/jn.117.255984

Gille, D. & Schmid, A. (2015). Vitamin B12 in meat and dairy products. *Nutrition Reviews*, 73(2), 106–15.
doi:10.1093/nutrit/nuu011

McBurney, M. I., Hartunian-Sowa, S. & Matusheski, N. V. (2017). Implications of US nutrition facts label changes on micronutrient density of fortified foods and supplements. *Journal of Nutrition*, 147(6), 1025–30. doi:10.3945/jn.117.247585

Merle, B. M. J., Silver, R. E., Rosner, B. & Seddon, J. M. (2016). Dietary folate, B vitamins, genetic susceptibility and progression to advanced nonexudative age-related macular degeneration with geographic atrophy: a prospective cohort study. *American Journal of Clinical Nutrition*, 103(4), 1135–44. doi:10.3945/ajcn.115.117606

Meyer-Ficca, M. & Kirkland, J. B. (2016). Niacin. *Advances in Nutrition*, 7(3), 556–8. doi:10.3945/an.115.011239

Mills, J. L. (2017). Strategies for preventing folate-related neural tube defects supplements, fortified foods, or both? *JAMA—Journal of the American Medical Association*, 317(2), 144–5. doi:10.1001/jama.2016.19894

Minto, C., Vecchio, M. G., Lamprecht, M. & Gregori, D. (2017). Definition of a tolerable upper intake level of niacin: a systematic review and meta-analysis of the dose-dependent effects of nicotinamide and nicotinic acid supplementation. *Nutrition Reviews*, 75(6), 471–90. doi:10.1093/nutrit/nux011

Molloy, A. M., Pangilinan, F. & Brody, L. C. (2017). Genetic risk factors for folate-responsive neural tube defects. *Annual Review of Nutrition*, 37(1), 269–91. doi:10.1146/annurev-nutr-071714-034235

Qin, B., Xun, P., Jacobs, D. R., Zhu, N., Daviglus, M. L., Reis, J. P., … He, K. (2017). Intake of niacin, folate, vitamin B-6, and vitamin B-12 through young adulthood and cognitive function in midlife: the Coronary Artery Risk Development in Young Adults (CARDIA) study. *American Journal of Clinical Nutrition*, 106(4), 1032–40. doi:10.3945/ajcn.117.157834

Schandelmaier, S., Briel, M., Saccilotto, R., Olu, K. K., Arpagaus, A., Hemkens, L. G. & Nordmann, A. J. (2017). Niacin for primary and secondary prevention of cardiovascular events. *Cochrane Database of Systematic Reviews*, 2017(6). doi:10.1002/14651858.CD009744.pub2

Sechi, G., Sechi, E., Fois, C. & Kumar, N. (2016). Advances in clinical determinants and neurological manifestations of B vitamin deficiency in adults. *Nutrition Reviews*, 74(5), 281–300. doi:10.1093/nutrit/nuv107

Smith, A. D. & Refsum, H. (2016). Homocysteine, B vitamins, and cognitive impairment. *Annual Review of Nutrition*, 36(1), 211–39. doi:10.1146/annurev-nutr-071715-050947

Stanhewicz, A. E. & Kenney, W. L. (2017). Role of folic acid in nitric oxide bioavailability and vascular endothelial function. *Nutrition Reviews*, 75(1), 61–70. doi:10.1093/nutrit/nuw053

Struijk, E. A., Lana, A., Guallar-Castillón, P., Rodríguez-Artalejo, F. & Lopez-Garcia, E. (2018). Intake of B vitamins and impairment in physical function in older adults. *Clinical Nutrition*, 37(4), 1271–8. doi:10.1016/j.clnu.2017.05.016

Truswell, S. (2017). Chapter 12: B vitamins. In J. Mann & S. Truswell (eds), *Essentials of Human Nutrition*, 5th edn. Oxford University Press, Incorporated.

Young, J. I., Züchner, S. & Wang, G. (2015). Regulation of the epigenome by vitamin C. *Annual Review of Nutrition*, 35(1), 545–64. doi:10.1146/annurev-nutr-071714-034228

REFERENCES

1 A. D. T. Fabbri & G. A. Crosby (2016). A review of the impact of preparation and cooking on the nutritional quality of vegetables and legumes. *International Journal of Gastronomy and Food Science*, 3(suppl. C), 2–11. doi:https://doi.org/10.1016/j.ijgfs.2015.11.001

2 US Department of Agriculture (2007). USDA Table of Nutrient Retention Factors. Retrieved from: www.ars.usda.gov/ARSUserFiles/80400525/Data/retn/retn06.pdf.

3 M. Bartholomew (2002). James Lind's treatise of the scurvy (1753). *Postgraduate Medical Journal*, 78(925), 695–6. doi:10.1136/pmj.78.925.695

4 D. Lonsdale (2006). A review of the biochemistry, metabolism and clinical benefits of thiamin(e) and its derivatives. *Evidence-based Complementary and Alternative Medicine*, 3(1), 49–59. doi:10.1093/ecam/nek009

5 National Health and Medical Research Council (2011). *A Modelling System to Inform the Revision of the Australian Guide to Healthy Eating*. Canberra: NHMRC.

6 D. R. Jacobs & L. C. Tapsell (2013). Food synergy: the key to a healthy diet. *Proceedings of the Nutrition Society*, 72(2), 200–6. doi:10.1017/S0029665112003011

7 F. Imamura, R. Micha, S. Khatibzadeh, S. Fahimi, P. Shi, J. Powles & D. Mozaffarian (2015). Dietary quality among men and women in 187 countries in 1990 and 2010: a systematic assessment. *The Lancet Global Health*, 3(3), e132–e142. doi:10.1016/S2214-109X(14)70381-X

8 US National Institutes of Health (2018). Thiamin: Fact sheet for professionals. Retrieved from: https://ods.od.nih.gov/factsheets/Thiamin-HealthProfessional.

9 J. C. Kerns & J. L. Gutierrez (2017). Thiamin. *Advances in Nutrition: An International Review Journal*, 8(2), 395–7. doi:10.3945/an.116.013979

10 National Health and Medical Research Council (2014). *Nutrient Reference Values for Australia and New Zealand—Riboflavin*. Canberra: NHMRC.

11 D. M. Lloyd-Jones (2014). Niacin and HDL cholesterol—time to face facts. *New England Journal of Medicine*, 371(3), 271–3. doi:10.1056/NEJMe1406410

12 H. Shi, A. Enriquez, M. Rapadas, E. M. M. A. Martin, R. Wang, J. Moreau, … S. L. Dunwoodie (2017). NAD deficiency, congenital malformations, and niacin supplementation. *New England Journal of Medicine*, 377(6), 544–52. doi:10.1056/NEJMoa1616361

13 H. M. Said (2009). Cell and molecular aspects of human intestinal biotin absorption. *Journal of Nutrition*, 139(1), 158–62. doi:10.3945/jn.108.092023

14 D. M. Mock (2017). Biotin: from nutrition to therapeutics. *Journal of Nutrition*, 147(8), 1487–92. doi:10.3945/jn.116.238956

15 A. A. Khan, A. Krishnan, D. J. Harrington & S. Robinson (2016). Application of a multi-marker approach to assess vitamin B12 status at the end of the first trimester of pregnancy. *Blood*, 128(22), 4804.

16 S. Poloni, H. Blom & I. Schwartz (2015). Stearoyl-CoA desaturase-1: is it the link between sulfur amino acids and lipid metabolism? *Biology*, 4(2), 383.

17 N. Mahalle, M. V. Kulkarni, M. K. Garg & S. S. Naik (2013). Vitamin B12 deficiency and hyperhomocysteinemia as correlates of cardiovascular risk factors in Indian subjects with coronary artery disease. *Journal of Cardiology*, 61(4), 289–94. doi:10.1016/j.jjcc.2012.11.009

18 T. Köbe, A. V. Witte, A. Schnelle, U. Grittner, V. A. Tesky, J. Pantel, … A. Flöel (2016). Vitamin B-12 concentration, memory performance, and hippocampal structure in patients with mild cognitive impairment. *American Journal of Clinical Nutrition*, 103(4), 1045–54. doi:10.3945/ajcn.115.116970

19 A. D. Dangour, E. Allen, R. Clarke, D. Elbourne, A. E. Fletcher, L. Letley, … K. Mills (2015). Effects of vitamin B-12 supplementation on neurologic and cognitive function in older people: a randomized controlled trial. *American Journal of Clinical Nutrition*, 102(3), 639–47. doi:10.3945/ajcn.115.110775

20 S. Truswell (2017). Chapter 12: B vitamins. In J. Mann & S. Truswell (eds), *Essentials of Human Nutrition*, 5th edn. Oxford University Press, Incorporated.

21 M. K. Georgieff (2007). Nutrition and the developing brain: nutrient priorities and measurement. *American Journal of Clinical Nutrition*, 85(2), 614S–620S.

22 C. D. Cantarella, D. Ragusa, M. Giammanco & S. Tosi (2017). Folate deficiency as predisposing factor for childhood leukaemia: a review of the literature. *Genes & Nutrition*, 12(1), 14. doi:10.1186/s12263-017-0560-8

23 T. M. Brasky, E. White & C.-L. Chen (2017). Long-term, supplemental, one-carbon metabolism–related vitamin B use in relation to lung cancer risk in the Vitamins and Lifestyle (VITAL) cohort. *Journal of Clinical Oncology*, 35(30), 3440–8. doi:10.1200/jco.2017.72.7735

24 E. Ros (2010). Health benefits of nut consumption. *Nutrients*, 2(7), 652.

25 National Health and Medical Research Council (2013). *Australian Guide to Healthy Eating*. Canberra: NHMRC.

26 Australian Bureau of Statistics (2014). *Australian Health Survey: Nutrition First Results—Foods and nutrients, 2011–12*. Canberra: ABS.

27 S. Spencer & M. Kneebone (2012). *FOODmap: An analysis of the Australian food supply chain*. Canberra: Department of Agriculture, Fisheries and Forestry.

28 S. Lillioja, A. L. Neal, L. Tapsell & D. R. Jacobs (2013). Whole grains, type 2 diabetes, coronary heart disease, and hypertension: links to the aleurone preferred over indigestible fiber. *BioFactors*, 39(3), 242–58. doi:10.1002/biof.1077

29 A. Surget & C. Barron (2005). Histologie du gratin de ble. *Industrie des cereales*, 145, 3–7.

30 Heart Protection Study Collaborative Group (2002). MRC/BHF Heart Protection Study of antioxidant vitamin supplementation in 20 536 high-risk individuals: a randomised placebo-controlled trial. *The Lancet*, 360(9326), 23–33. doi:https://doi.org/10.1016/S0140-6736(02)09328-5

31 K.-T. Khaw, S. Bingham, A. Welch, R. Luben, N. Wareham, S. Oakes & N. Day (2001). Relation between plasma ascorbic acid and mortality in men and women in EPIC-Norfolk prospective study: a prospective population study. *The Lancet*, 357(9257), 657–63. doi:https://doi.org/10.1016/S0140-6736(00)04128-3

32 World Cancer Research Fund/American Institute for Cancer Research (1997). *Food Research and the Prevention of Cancer: A global perspective*. Washington, DC: American Institute for Cancer Research.

33 British Nutrition Foundation (2018). *BNF Looks at the Recommendations in the World Cancer Research Fund: 2018 Third Expert Report*. Retrieved from www.nutrition.org.uk/attachments/article/1152/WCRF%20recommendations.pdf.

34 World Cancer Research Fund/American Institute for Cancer Research (2018). *Diet, Nutrition, Physical Activity and Cancer: Third Expert Report from the World Cancer Research Fund*. Washington, DC: American Institute for Cancer.

35 A. S. Truswell (1985). ABC of nutrition. Vitamins II. *British Medical Journal (Clinical research edn)*, 291(6502), 1103.

36 H. Hemilä & E. Chalker (2013).Vitamin C for preventing and treating the common cold. *Cochrane Database of Systematic Reviews*, 1. doi:10.1002/14651858.CD000980.pub4

37 A. Gorusupudi, K. Nelson & P. S. Bernstein (2017). The Age-Related Eye Disease 2 Study: micronutrients in the treatment of macular degeneration. *Advances in Nutrition: An International Review Journal*, 8(1), 40–53. doi:10.3945/an.116.013177

38 M. Levine (1996). Vitamin C pharmacokinetics in healthy volunteers: evidence for a recommended dietary allowance. *Proceedings of the National Academy of Sciences—PNAS*, 93(8), 3704.

CHAPTER 11

MAJOR MINERALS: SODIUM, POTASSIUM, CALCIUM, MAGNESIUM AND PHOSPHORUS

LINDA TAPSELL

CHAPTER OBJECTIVES

This chapter will enable the reader to:

- describe the chemical nature of the minerals sodium, potassium, calcium, phosphorus and magnesium
- briefly outline key functions of these minerals in the human body
- describe the patterns of food choices that would enable intakes of these minerals to support health.

KEY TERMS

Calcium   Potassium

Magnesium   Sodium

Phosphorus

KEY POINTS

- Sodium and potassium act as cations in electrolytic solutions and are involved in physiological functions that relate to the management of fluid volume. Increasing sodium intake is associated with increasing blood pressure in populations.
- Calcium, magnesium and phosphorus have a range of roles in human physiology and metabolism, but all are present in significant amounts in bone, thus maintaining the skeletal system. Loss of calcium in the bone can make them thin and weak, leading to fracture.
- Excessive sodium intakes and inadequate calcium intakes during the lifecycle have implications for the development of chronic disease later in life.

OXFORD UNIVERSITY PRESS

INTRODUCTION

As discussed in earlier chapters, food is a composite of multiple chemical compounds. Descriptions of food components often begin with the nature of their chemical structure. Unlike, for example, carbohydrates that are combinations of carbon, hydrogen and oxygen, or vitamins that may belong to a class of chemically related compounds, minerals are chemical elements—that is, pure compounds made from a single type of atom. They can be found in the periodic table, along with their atomic number (see www.rsc.org/periodic-table) and are naturally occurring in the earth. From an ecological perspective, minerals may enter the food chain via absorption in the roots of plants. The plants may then be consumed and become part of an animal, which itself may become food for another animal or human. In each condition, the mineral has a specific structural and functional role, but this chapter focuses on those roles in the human body.

There are many minerals in the earth's environment, and many function significantly in human physiological systems. The focus of this chapter is on minerals known to be significant in human health and related to contemporary public health issues. Specifically we look at two main areas: sodium and potassium with a focus on their relationship with blood pressure; and calcium, magnesium and phosphorus with a focus on their importance for bone health.

See Chapter 3 on digestion, absorption and metabolism.

See Chapter 4 on carbohydrates and phytochemicals.

See Chapters 9 and 10 on vitamins.

Diet composition is important in managing the balance of intakes of all nutrients and, in particular, minerals. The food delivery system has a daily impact on the dose of minerals. Dietary intake may challenge any regulatory systems the body has in place to maintain balance, or simply be insufficient for requirements. Interactions between components in food can also interfere with the availability of the mineral for absorption. Thus, the mere presence in the food does not always equate to delivery of the mineral in those amounts to the systems requiring it. Appreciating the major food sources of key minerals and achieving balance in consumption across food groups is one of the tenets of a healthy diet.

As significant elements in the machinery of human physiology and metabolism, the minerals discussed in this chapter have multiple roles and are influenced by many factors. The focus for sodium and potassium is on the management of fluid volume, with implications for blood pressure. For calcium, magnesium and phosphate, the emphasis is on bone structure and function, with some recognition of other roles.

STOP AND THINK

- What could be some of the ecological implications for meeting mineral requirements for humans?
- How is the absorption and transport of minerals managed in the human body?
- How can changes in food composition create problems for mineral nutrition in humans?

WHAT ARE THE STRUCTURES AND FUNCTIONS OF SODIUM AND POTASSIUM WITH SIGNIFICANT IMPLICATIONS FOR NUTRITION?

Sodium (Na) and potassium (K) can be found on the periodic table with the atomic numbers of 11 and 19, respectively. Here they are classified as metals and they form positive ions in chemical reactions. In the body, they both are cations, so they carry charges that influence active transport of molecules across cell membranes.

FIGURE 11.1 REGULATION OF SODIUM AND POTASSIUM LEVELS

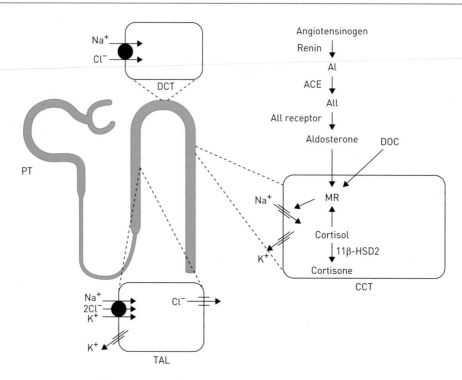

Abbreviations: AI, angiotensin I; ACE, angiotensin converting enzyme; AII, angiotensin II (AII); MR, mineralocorticoid receptor; GRA, glucocorticoid-remediable aldosteronism; PHA1, pseudohypoaldosteronism, type-1; AME, apparent mineralocorticoid excess; 11 bHSD2, 11b-hydroxysteroid dehydrogenase-2; DOC, deoxycorticosterone; and PT, proximal tubule.

Source: R. P. Lifton, A. G. Gharavi & D. S. Geller (2001). Molecular mechanisms of human hypertension. *Cell*, 104(4), 545–56. doi:10.1016/S0092-8674(01)00241-0

Sodium is found in the extracellular fluid, whereas potassium is in intracellular fluid. This balance is maintained through the sodium/potassium ATP-ase pump. This cellular machinery is fundamental to the activity of nerve and muscle cells. There are many homeostatic mechanisms that control sodium in the body, including the renin-angiotensin hormone system, the kallikrein-kinin system, the systematic nervous system, atrial natriuretic peptide and other factors that regulate blood flow in the kidneys [1]. Likewise, potassium is also tightly controlled through reabsorption via the kidneys or increased secretion following the release of the hormone aldosterone [1].

Figure 11.1 is a diagram of a nephron and shows the filtering unit of the kidney. Sodium is often consumed as sodium chloride (NaCl). Molecular pathways show Na reabsorption mediated in individual renal cells in the thick ascending limb of the loop of Henle (TAL), distal convoluted tubule (DCT) and cortical collecting tubule (CCT). The pathway of the renin-angiotensin system is shown, with the major regulator of renal **salt** reabsorption.

The actual relationship between salt intake and blood pressure has been debated for many years (Figure 11.2). Historically a physiological condition, pressure-**naturesis** [2] was termed, which described the pressure required to excrete sodium and water in the kidney.

Salt

common table salt with the chemical name sodium chloride.

Natriuresis

extraction of sodium in the urine.

FIGURE 11.2 INTERACTION OF THE MODERN WESTERN DIET AND THE KIDNEYS IN THE
PATHOGENESIS OF PRIMARY HYPERTENSION

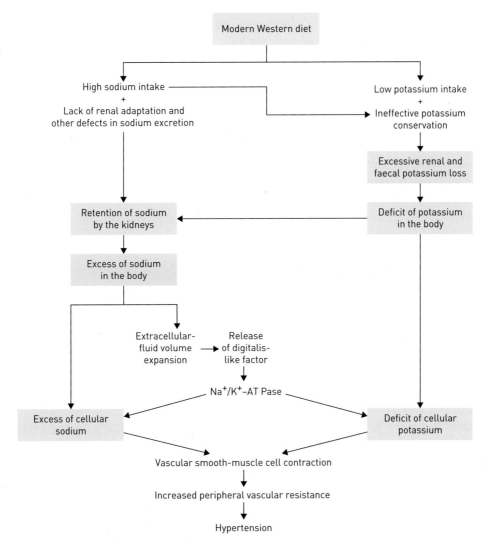

Source: H. J. Adrogué & N. E. Madias (2007). Sodium and potassium in the pathogenesis of hypertension. *New England Journal of Medicine*, 356(19), 1966–78. doi:10.1056/NEJMra064486

TRY IT YOURSELF

You may find that sodium is reported in different units, so it can be difficult to establish the relevance of the quantity. To convert:

- mg of sodium to mg of salt (sodium chloride), multiply by 2.5
- mg of salt to mg of sodium, divide by 2.5
- mmol of sodium to mg of sodium, multiply by 23
- mmol of sodium to mg of sodium chloride, multiply by 58.5.

How many grams of salt are in 2000 mg sodium? How many teaspoons of salt would this amount to? How much sodium is in a regular serve of your favourite bread or breakfast cereal?

Visit Oxford Ascend for more on understanding and converting units of measurement.

The possible link between sodium intake and blood pressure has been observed in animal model studies [3; 4]. Human observational studies indicated a similar relationship. Evidence for the effects of sodium (and potassium) intakes on blood pressure and related health outcomes has mounted over the years. Early on, there were a number of observations made of cohorts consuming 3 g salt per day [5], and in whom blood pressure did not rise with age [6].

An early ecological study, INTERSALT, gained attention not only because of its size and distribution across multiple centres, but also because it measured sodium intake using 24-hour urinary excretion, an accurate biomarker of intake [7]. Later studies confirmed the potential reduced risk from ischaemic heart disease and stroke with reduced sodium intakes [8].

The INTERSALT study also showed that higher urinary potassium was associated with lower blood pressure [9]. Thus, the sodium-to-potassium ratio (Na:K) was introduced to debate on the regulation of blood pressure [10]. An Australian study demonstrated that a one-unit decrease in the Na:K ratio was associated with a reduced systolic blood pressure (of 1.8 mm Hg). Urinary sodium and the Na:K ratio were both associated with systolic blood pressure and explained 20% of the variation in systolic blood pressure [11]. Later, a greater association was found between blood pressure and the urinary Na:K ratio than with sodium or potassium levels alone [12].

» CASE 11.1

WHAT DO WE KNOW ABOUT SALT?

A recent brief media commentary [13] suggested that a principle related to salt and 'taught to doctors' may be 'completely wrong'. The assumption of this principle was that eating too much salt leads to thirst, and this is followed by water consumption and then loss of salt and water in the urine to maintain sodium balance. The article refers to two 'dense' papers on salt management by the body in the *Journal of Clinical Investigation* [13].

The editorial commentary notes that this research focused on understanding the response to a high salt intake [14]. It is suggested that a complex regulatory process comes into play that involves hormone fluctuations, food and water consumption, as well as salt and water excretion through the kidneys.

The research reported by Kitada and colleagues [15] involved experiments with mice and humans (a water balance study on 10 participants on a simulated space flight to Mars). The studies were indeed complex and drew on an understanding of control mechanisms covered in the study of human systems' physiology and the biochemistry of energy metabolism. The other study, by Rakova and colleagues [16], did not correct a misconception that excess sodium is dealt with via mechanisms that maintain balance in extracellular fluid (ECF). Rather, this research challenged its simplicity. It suggested that ECF homeostasis *and* urine formation were under important control systems in conditions of high salt intakes. Thus, a new 'water conserving' principle related to urine concentration has been added, exposing a physiological regulatory network involving not just the kidneys but also the liver and muscle.

- How are the approaches to discussing this research different between the media report and the scientific editorial?
- What does this research tell us about how knowledge and understanding of blood pressure regulation evolves and the biological systems that are considered for nutritional interventions?
- Which aspects of diet are likely to be relevant in translating the concepts emerging from this research to practice?

Clinical trials manipulating dietary sodium and potassium provide a higher level of evidence for practice. They were justified by systematic reviews reporting that restricting sodium intake in people with hypertension reduces their blood pressure (e.g. see the report by Geleijnse and colleagues [17]). Among the first of these, the two Trials of Hypertension Prevention studies (TOHP I and II) with about 19 years follow-up showed that salt reduction reduced cardiovascular disease in adults with untreated pre-hypertension. Importantly, the Na:K ratio was also implicated in these results [18]. Nutrients such as sodium and potassium are delivered by foods, so it follows that the observations seen on dietary sodium and potassium are also reflective of the food choices made by populations and trial participants. This is not to reduce the nutritional importance of sodium and potassium, but rather to place them in a dietary context [19]. High sodium and low potassium characteristics of a diet may also be indicative of poor dietary quality in relation to health.

STOP AND THINK

- How does scientific knowledge of the way in which sodium and potassium operate in human systems translate to evidence for the effects of diet on health?
- What is the relevance of food in understanding the effects of sodium on health?
- Why are population studies useful in understanding the effects of dietary sodium and potassium on health?

WHICH PATTERNS OF FOOD CHOICES LEAD TO DIETARY LEVELS OF SODIUM AND POTASSIUM THAT SUPPORT HEALTH?

There is increasing evidence that certain patterns of food choices that have characteristic sodium and potassium levels can influence blood pressure levels in the population. The landmark set of randomised controlled trials that addressed all aspects of sodium and potassium, food choices and dietary patterns in relation to blood pressure were entitled 'Dietary Approaches to Stop Hypertension' (DASH) (Table 11.1). The DASH diet was essentially a low total and saturated fat diet based on vegetables and fruit and containing low-fat dairy products. The first trial provided strong evidence that the diet could reduce blood pressure as much as some antihypertensive drugs [20]. It showed a significant reduction in systolic and diastolic blood pressure after eight weeks compared with a typical American diet. The public health implications were calculable.

The issue of the sodium content of the diet remained a concern in the scientific community, so the follow-up DASH-sodium trial investigated the additional benefits of salt restriction [21]. This trial compared high (150 mmol/day) intermediate (100 mmol/day) and low (65 mmol/day) sodium intakes

TABLE 11.1   KEY STUDIES OF DIETARY PATTERNS TARGETING HYPERTENSION

Diet intervention	Characteristics
DASH diet	Fruit and vegetables, low-fat dairy foods, low dietary saturated fat
DASH-sodium	DASH diet with sodium restrictions
DASH-low energy (DEW-IT)	DASH diet with limited kilojoules
DASH-lifestyle (PREMIER)	DASH diet with lifestyle modifications

on the DASH diet, and compared with controls. This study demonstrated the expected graduated reduction in blood pressure, confirming the added significance of dietary sodium in this context. This set of studies demonstrates the interdependence between nutrients (e.g. sodium and potassium), foods (e.g. vegetables and fruit) and the total diet (e.g. the relative amounts of vegetables and fruits compared with high fat foods) in promoting health. While the evidence emerged from a number of different perspectives, there was a consistency in the observations, with the translation exposing a dietary pattern that may help reduce hypertension in Western communities.

Body weight also has an impact on blood pressure, so the dietary variable of energy intake also needs to be considered. This was addressed in the Diet, Exercise and Weight Loss Intervention Trial (DEW-IT) [22], which involved overweight participants with hypertension. Adding reduced energy to the DASH diet model, this study demonstrated a reduction in ambulatory blood pressure after adjusting for weight loss. Adding further lifestyle variables, the PREMIER trial combined the DASH diet with other lifestyle modifications (weight loss, exercise, sodium and alcohol limitations) [23]. Although the addition of advice to follow the DASH diet to lifestyle modification only showed small incremental decreases of blood pressure, participants were not given food and had to purchase

See Chapter 7 on energy intake and weight management.

and prepare their own food. This more 'real-life' scenario likely affected outcomes [24] and exposed the extent to which broader social and physical environments need to support lifestyle change overall.

>> RESEARCH AT WORK

INTEGRATING EVIDENCE ON THE RELATIONSHIP BETWEEN BLOOD PRESSURE AND INTAKES OF NUTRIENTS (SODIUM, POTASSIUM), FOODS AND DIETARY PATTERNS

As research in food, nutrition and health evolves, the understanding of the relationship between nutrients, foods and total diets broadens. There is an interdependence between all levels, as nutrients are delivered by foods and dietary patterns are developed by combinations of foods [25; 26]. The question of whether it is the nutrient, the food or the diet having the effect is really a moot point as it is likely all three, but with varying emphases depending on the circumstances. The sodium–blood pressure relationship appears to be most obvious in circumstances where the diet delivers a very high amount of sodium, most likely through processing [19]. There is also the issue of population versus individual effects.

See Chapter 1 on the interrelationship between food, nutrition and health.

To address the food-related issues and consider the clinical relevance of the sodium–blood pressure debate, Ndanuko and colleagues from the University of Wollongong undertook a series of studies examining the associations between diet and blood pressure, with a focus on a clinical sample of overweight individuals attending a lifestyle intervention trial. In the first study, a meta-analysis of randomised controlled trials was conducted to examine the evidence published in the scientific literature for effects of dietary patterns on blood pressure [27]. The meta-analysis showed the effect as a significant reduction in blood pressure (-4.06 mm Hg systolic and -2.30 mm Hg diastolic) resulting from dietary patterns that were characterised by predominant consumption of fruit, vegetables, wholegrains, legumes, seeds, nuts, fish and low-fat dairy foods, but relatively small amounts of meat, sweets and alcohol. (Note this reflects the DASH diet pattern, but in that research, studies were obtained from across the globe.) Importantly, this analysis exposed the foods that would comprise a healthy dietary pattern, and which in their natural form would contribute potassium in the diet but were not naturally high in sodium.

Next, the relationships between blood pressure and both nutrients (sodium and potassium) and dietary patterns (defined by foods) were examined in a relatively small clinical sample of less than 300 people [28; 29]. The analysis was done on measurements taken before people received treatment, reflecting the usual intakes of the people attending the clinic. The relationships seen in large studies remained relevant to this smaller group of overweight adults. Sodium intakes and the dietary Na:K ratio (both assessed by urinary biomarkers) significantly predicted systolic blood pressure even after controlling for age, sex, body mass index (BMI) and hypertension medication use as potential confounders.

The major contributors for sodium intake for this group of people were cereals (including products and dishes made with cereals), and products and dishes made with meat, poultry, game or milk products. The latter food groups were also major contributors for dietary potassium intake as were vegetable products and dishes. Thus, the main discriminating foods for sodium intake were cereal-based foods, whereas for potassium they were vegetable-based foods.

An analytical tool called principal component analysis was applied to the data to examine the blood pressure relationship with dietary patterns. Six dietary patterns were predominant and the pattern that had relatively higher amounts of nuts, seeds, fruit and fish was significantly associated with lower systolic blood and diastolic blood pressure. As nuts, seeds, fruit and fish are also naturally low in sodium and high in potassium than commercial foods, it was not surprising to see that this dietary pattern was also significantly associated with a lower Na:K ratio. In this set of analyses, the relationship between nutrients (sodium and potassium), foods (vegetables, nuts, seeds, fish) and diets (combinations of these foods) can be seen, and with respect to the effect of diet on blood pressure. Thus we see the complex interplay between nutritional components in understanding the relationship between diet and health, in this case in relation to blood pressure (Figure 11.3).

FIGURE 11.3 NUTRIENTS, FOODS AND DIETARY PATTERNS ASSOCIATED WITH BLOOD PRESSURE

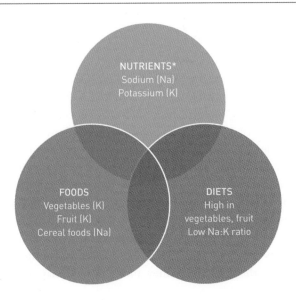

*High sodium and low potassium intakes associated with higher blood pressure.

As the scientific evidence on the relationship between sodium intakes and health continues to build, recommended intakes for sodium are continually updated by the World Health Organization (WHO) and national health authorities. Australian and New Zealand authorities updated the Nutrient Reference Values (NRVs) for sodium in 2017 using a new purpose-specific methodological framework [30]. Given the public health implications of the established relationship between sodium intakes and blood pressure, sodium was identified as a priority for review, with the relevant NRVs being the suggested dietary target (SDT) and upper level of intake (UL). The review noted the abundance of sodium in the food supply, particularly through processed foods and takeaway meals. Following extensive review of the literature and a consideration of current population intakes, the SDT for adults was set as a target of 2000 mg/day, which is about half the current average consumption (3600 mg/day). This means that most individuals need to reduce their sodium intakes. From a public health perspective, a reduction in average blood pressure would be anticipated [31]. To support these types of public health initiatives at a global level, WHO has set up salt reduction collaborative centres (WHO-CC SALT), including the George Institute in Sydney (www.georgeinstitute.org.au), which provides monthly updates of the literature and activities being undertaken in this area.

STOP AND THINK

- How many different scientific disciplines can you identify as contributing to our understanding of the nutritional aspects of sodium and potassium?
- How has the scientific investigation into the effects of dietary sodium and potassium on blood pressure evolved over time?
- How does this translate to action at the public health level?

WHAT ARE THE STRUCTURES AND FUNCTIONS OF CALCIUM, MAGNESIUM AND PHOSPHORUS WITH SIGNIFICANT IMPLICATIONS FOR NUTRITION?

Visit Oxford Ascend for more on calcium.

Like sodium and potassium, calcium (Ca) and magnesium (Mg) are also classified as metals, appearing on the periodic table with atomic weights of 20 and 12, respectively (www.rsc.org/periodic-table). Phosphorus (P) is also in the periodic table (atomic weight 15), but it is not classed as a metal and is highly reactive in nature, presenting biologically as phosphate (a central phosphorus atom surrounded by four oxygen atoms). Calcium, magnesium and phosphate are cations with multiple cellular functions.

Given their significant roles in multiple functions, imbalances in calcium, magnesium and phosphate levels can result in serious conditions, such as cardiac arrhythmias and respiratory difficulties. Thus, tight homeostatic mechanisms control the levels in the body, with absorption by the gut balanced by renal excretion. When levels drop, absorption increases from the gut, and minerals are released from the bone and reabsorbed through the renal tubules. Fine adjustments are made to balance losses through the kidney with the calcium, magnesium and phosphate absorbed from the diet [32] (Figure 11.4). Abnormalities in homeostasis are called disorders of mineral metabolism, which can manifest at the target areas of the intestine, kidney and bone, and may involve parathyroid hormone and vitamin D [33].

FIGURE 11.4   FLUX BETWEEN BODY COMPARTMENTS FOR CALCIUM, MAGNESIUM AND PHOSPHORUS

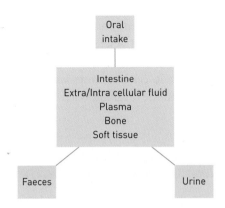

Source: Adapted from J. Blaine, M. Chonchol & M. Levi (2015). Renal control of calcium, phosphate, and magnesium homeostasis. *Clinical Journal of the American Society of Nephrology*, 10(7), 1257–72. doi:10.2215/cjn.09750913

Calcium is essential for life as it is involved in essential biochemical reactions. In the human body, 99% of the calcium can be found in the bones and teeth, with the remaining 1% found in extracellular fluids (ECF) and intracellular fluids (ICF), where it has essential roles to enable normal body functions such as muscle contraction and the activation of some enzymatic reactions. Calcium needs to be in a soluble form for absorption, and this is helped by the acidic environment in the stomach. Absorption is also facilitated by calcium binding proteins, the production of which is influenced by vitamin D. Insoluble calcium compounds can be formed through binding with other food components, such as phytates and oxalates in plant foods, inhibiting absorption.

Magnesium is an abundant intracellular cation (99% in ICF, in bone, muscle and soft tissue) with functions including bone formation, intracellular signalling, involvement in DNA synthesis and oxidative phosphorylation. Intestinal absorption can vary between 25 and 75% depending on whether the diet is magnesium rich or depleted [33].

Phosphorus is found mainly in bone. Serum phosphate levels are tightly controlled to support a number of functions including bone formation and energy metabolism, and as components of phospholipids and nucleic acids [33]. Intestinal absorption is mediated by co-transporters, managing serum phosphate levels along with renal regulatory systems [33].

Bone formation and sustainability is dependent on the supply of its component nutrients [34]. Throughout the body, about 99% of calcium and 60% of magnesium is in the bone. The majority of phosphorus is also in bone, where it plays an important role in mineralisation [33]. Other nutrients are also implicated in bone health, namely protein, vitamin D, potassium and fluoride, but calcium is the main mineral. Protein constitutes about half the volume of extracellular bone material, with calcium phosphate crystals forming the other half [35]. As there appears to be limited ability to adapt to low calcium intakes, the ratio of phosphorus to calcium appears more important that phosphorus alone, and the relationship between magnesium and bone health is less well understood [34]. Calcium requirements vary between individuals because of different physiological needs depending on factors such as age and sex. An adequate intake of calcium is essential for bone health. As growth is rapid in childhood, and peak bone mass is achieved in early adulthood, consuming adequate calcium during these periods is important. The relationship between calcium absorption and skeletal calcium accumulation remains an area of scientific research, particularly in relation to the use of calcium supplements. On average, an adult will absorb around a quarter of the calcium consumed in the diet, but this can increase can increase to up to 60% when physiological needs are high, such as following periods of inadequate calcium intakes and during pregnancy or growth where extra calcium is required for growing bones. As bones are dynamic structures, continuously losing and gaining minerals, an adequate supply of dietary calcium is required to maintain a balance in calcium stores within the body. For teeth, the turnover is not as fast, and the addition of fluorides to the drinking water also helps to protect calcium from being lost by chemical reactions.

» RESEARCH AT WORK

EVALUATING CALCIUM SUPPLEMENTATION

Given the importance of calcium for bone health, the requirement for calcium and issues around the use of calcium supplements for preventive health purposes are debated in the scientific literature. While this has included concerns around issues such as the risk of cardiovascular disease, the observed differences in responses to calcium supplementation suggest this may be an area of need for 'personalised nutrition' [36].

In the Women's Health Initiative trial, participants were given either 1000 mg elemental calcium with 400 IU vitamin D or a placebo and followed up for about 6.5 years to assess bone fractures. In the analysis of data from over 5000 postmenopausal women, the protective effect of supplementation was only seen in women with the lowest genetic risk score associated with bone mineral density. This suggested that supplementation was not having an effect in those at high genetic risk, exposing the complex interrelationships at play between bone health, genetics and nutrient action [37].

From a nutritional perspective, bone serves as a reservoir for calcium and phosphorus. When calcium delivered through the intestine falls below the amount of calcium lost (through digestive secretions, shed skin, hair, sweat, urine), parathyroid hormone is secreted, releasing calcium to maintain serum levels. Low calcium intakes are significant in periods of growth, when peak bone mass is achieved, and in older age when calcium ingested does not compensate for calcium lost. These two stages are significant in exposing the relationship between low calcium intakes and low bone mass [35]. Osteoporosis is a condition when bones fracture under normal everyday stresses and is more prevalent among post-menopausal women; the loss of oestrogen is implicated in the loss of bone mass.

STOP AND THINK

- How does understanding the chemical properties of calcium, magnesium and phosphorus help in appreciating their biological functions?
- How does the concept of bone development demonstrate the interdependence between minerals (and other compounds) in health?
- What might be the limitations of supplementation of a single mineral in this context?

WHICH PATTERNS OF FOOD CHOICES DELIVER INTAKES OF CALCIUM, MAGNESIUM AND PHOSPHORUS THAT SUPPORT HEALTH?

Just as the study of bone displayed the interrelationship between calcium, magnesium and phosphorus in nutrition, an understanding of foods means an appreciation of the multiple nutrients they deliver. Dairy foods (milk, cheese, yoghurt) have often been aligned with bone health, not least because they provide significant amounts of key nutrients associated with bone health: calcium, protein and phosphorus [38]. While the quality of the total diet always remains paramount in health, specifically including foods that are a rich source of calcium will ensure adequate calcium intakes. The DASH diet, for example, provided substantial amounts of dairy foods as well as fruits, vegetables and wholegrains [39; 40]. Vegetables such as collard greens, kale, soy beans, bok choy, okra and broccoli also provide calcium, bearing in mind the bioavailability and amount of calcium from plant sources is less than in dairy foods, with about around 250 mg/day provided from non-dairy foods [41]. Magnesium is also found in spinach, okra, tomato, potato, sweet potato and raisins.

Results from the Australian Health Survey 2011–12 (AHS) showed that milk and milk-based foods were the richest sources of calcium in Australian diets, but there were also other foods that are sources of calcium [42]. Children aged 2–3 years old were more likely to meet requirements for calcium, but more that 50% of those >2 years had inadequate intakes, particularly women. However, 21% of females reported consuming some form of calcium supplement intake some time during the survey. These data provide impetus for public health campaigns to ensure adequate calcium is consumed in the diet, and for high-quality calcium-rich foods to be available for all .

The 2011–12 AHS survey indicated that 15% of women and 3% men reported having osteoporosis (increasing in >50 years to 23% women, 6% men). The healthcare implications are seen in the 12% of institutionalised persons. There were 19,000 minimal trauma hip fractures in this time in people over 50 years old; of these, 71% were over 80 years and 72% female. Even though the rate has deceased, the number has increased, reflecting the challenges of the ageing population profile [42].

≫ CASE 11.2

CALCIUM CLAIMS ON FOODS

While the delivery of all essential nutrients for a defined energy (kilojoule) value characterises a high-quality diet, it also represents a combination of foods that together meet these requirements. This means that each food in the diet must be delivering key nutrients. Unlike other minerals, calcium is only found in significant amounts in a few foods (many foods contain small amounts), which means care must be taken in planning the total diet. This need could also be seen as an opportunity to produce calcium-fortified food products, as well as provide education for consumers on naturally calcium-rich foods.

Food Standards Australia New Zealand (FSANZ) allows two forms of health claims: general level health claims, which do not refer to serious disease or biomarkers of disease—for example, 'Calcium for healthy bones and teeth'; and high level health claims, which require approval. Calcium is among the topics with a degree of pre-approval—for example, for statements like 'Diets high in calcium may reduce the risk of osteoporosis in people aged 65 years and over' (www.foodstandards.gov.au/consumer/labelling/nutrition/Pages/default.aspx).

Because total diet quality remains a defining factor in food choice, there are caveats on the use of these claims (e.g. relating to the context of the claim—high calcium diet, age group) and conditions (e.g. the food must provide not less than 200 mg calcium per serve, and it should fit in an appropriate food category).

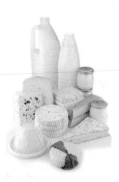

- Why do health claims need to be regulated?
- What are some of the problems that could arise with a single nutrient focus on food product development?
- How can claims on single foods influence the development of total diets of high quality?

Meeting calcium requirements involves consuming a combination of foods that together provide the total amount of calcium defined by the EAR. For example, a 25-year-old woman could get half of her calcium requirements (840 mg/day; see Table 11.2) from a cup of milk and a tub of yoghurt, and the rest from a slice of cheese, a serve of salmon and some almonds (Table 11.3).

TABLE 11.2   CALCIUM REQUIREMENTS

Recommended intakes of calcium (mg/day)	Estimated average requirement (EAR)	Recommended dietary intake (RDI)	Upper level of intake (UL)
Men			
19–70 years	840	1000	2500
>70 years	1100	1300	2500
Women			
19–50 years	840	1000	2500
>50 years	1100	1300	2500
Pregnancy			
14–18 years	1050	1300	2500
18–50 years	840	1000	2500
Lactation			
14–18 years	1050	1300	2500
18–50 years	840	1000	2500

Source: National Health and Medical Research Council (2006). *Nutrient Reference Values for Australia and New Zealand, Including Recommended Dietary Intakes.* Canberra: NHMRC. © Commonwealth of Australia

TABLE 11.3   MEETING CALCIUM REQUIREMENTS: 25-YEAR-OLD WOMAN

Food	Calcium (mg)
1 cup of skim milk (250 mL) from a skinny latte	302.5
200 g strawberry yoghurt	328
1 slice of reduced fat cheddar cheese (20 g)	199
Half a small tin of salmon (canned, drained—40 g)	140
Almonds (30 g)	75
TOTAL	1044.5

Source: Food Standards Australia New Zealand (2010). *Nutrient Tables for Use in Australia (NUTTAB).* Retrieved from: www.foodstandards.gov.au/science/monitoringnutrients/nutrienttables/nuttab/Pages/default.aspx

TRY IT YOURSELF

Record all the foods you consumed in the past 24 hours. Note the amount and rough estimation of calcium content for the following: milk (300 mg/250 mL), yoghurt (300 mg/250 g) and cheese (300 mg/45 g). Identify the calcium content of other foods from labels or food databases. If you eat four to five serves of vegetables/day, allow about 250 mg calcium from vegetable sources. How does your calcium intake compare with the recommended dietary intake (RDI)?

STOP AND THINK

- What does the study of calcium, magnesium and phosphorus tell us about nutritional homeostasis in the human body?
- Why does calcium stand out as a mineral that needs attention in a healthy diet for Australians?
- How might the prevalence of osteoporosis in the community influence the development of the food supply, especially for older women?

SUMMARY

- The major minerals discussed in this chapter have identifiable chemical structures and known functions within the body that have clear implications for nutrition practice.
- The current body of evidence indicates problems with overconsumption of sodium in relation to blood pressure and limited consumption of calcium in support of bone health and the prevention of osteoporosis.
- Food sources of the major minerals can be identified, but these need to be considered in the context of the quality of the total diet and the implications for how the food supply is being developed.

PATHWAYS TO PRACTICE

- The public health problems of hypertension and osteoporosis in the community reflect significant challenges for nutrition education and public health campaigns.
- A comprehensive knowledge of food composition, food preparation and the commercial development of food is necessary to be able to influence the delivery of key nutrients to the population.
- Food standards and health claims legislation is another area in which nutrition expertise can be applied in industry and government roles.

DISCUSSION QUESTIONS

1 How do the development of population health campaigns and the advice given to individuals differ in relation to (a) sodium and blood pressure and (b) calcium supplementation and the prevention of osteoporosis?
2 Given what we know about sodium and calcium as key nutrients in population health, what is the next set of research questions that would direct future policy and practice?
3 How important are resources that maintain up-to-date information on the composition of foods, given the rate of new product development?

USEFUL WEBLINKS

Australian Health Survey—Calcium intakes, 2011–12:
www.abs.gov.au/ausstats/abs@.nsf/Lookup/by%20Subject/4364.0.55.008~2011-12~Main%20Features~Calcium~401#2

Australian Health Survey—Sodium intakes, 2011–12:
www.abs.gov.au/ausstats/abs@.nsf/Lookup/by%20Subject/4364.0.55.008~2011-12~Main%20Features~Sodium~403

DASH diet—healthy eating to lower your blood pressure:
www.mayoclinic.org/healthy-lifestyle/nutrition-and-healthy-eating/in-depth/dash-diet/art-20048456

DASH Eating Plan:
www.nhlbi.nih.gov/health/health-topics/topics/dash

Food Standards Australia New Zealand—Nutrient tables for use in Australia (NUTTAB):
www.foodstandards.gov.au/science/monitoringnutrients/nutrientables/nuttab/Pages/default.aspx

Food Standards Australia New Zealand—Nutrition content claims and health claims:
www.foodstandards.gov.au/consumer/labelling/nutrition/Pages/default.aspx

George Institute WHO Collaborating Centre—Salt:
www.georgeinstitute.org.au/projects/world-health-organization-collaborating-centre-for-population-salt-reduction-who-cc-salt

Healthdirect—Potassium:
www.healthdirect.gov.au/potassium

Healthy Bones Australia:
www.healthybonesaustralia.org.au

National Osteoporosis Foundation 2016:
https://cdn.nof.org/wp-content/uploads/2016/04/Healthy-Bone-Brochure_FINAL.pdf

Nutrient Reference Values—Nutrients:
www.nrv.gov.au/nutrients

Royal Society of Chemistry—Periodic table:
www.rsc.org/periodic-table

The Best Diet—DASH diet:
http://health.usnews.com/best-diet/dash-diet

The Heart Foundation—Salt and health:
www.heartfoundation.org.au/healthy-eating/food-and-nutrition/salt

World Health Organization:
www.who.int/nutrition/publications/guidelines/sodium_intake/en

FURTHER READING

Adrogué, H. J. & Madias, N. E. (2017). Sodium and potassium in the pathogenesis of hypertension: focus on the brain. *Current Opinion in Nephrology and Hypertension*, 26(2), 106–13. doi:10.1097/MNH.0000000000000301

Binia, A., Jaeger, J., Hu, Y., Singh, A. & Zimmermann, D. (2015). Daily potassium intake and sodium-to-potassium ratio in the reduction of blood pressure: a meta-analysis of randomized controlled trials. *Journal of Hypertension*, 33(8), 1509–20. doi:10.1097/HJH.0000000000000611

Bolland, M. J., Leungm, W., Tai, V., Bastin, S., Gamble, G. D., Grey, A. & Reid, I. R. (2015). Calcium intake and risk of fracture: systematic review. *BMJ (Online)*, 351. doi:10.1136/bmj.h4580

Calvo, M. S., Moshfegh, A. J. & Tucker, K. L. (2014). Assessing the health impact of phosphorus in the food supply: issues and considerations. *Advances in Nutrition: An International Review Journal*, 5(1), 104–13. doi:10.3945/an.113.004861

Chandler, P. D., Wang, L., Zhang, X., Sesso, H. D., Moorthy, M. V., Obi, O., ... Song. Y. (2015). Effect of vitamin D supplementation alone or with calcium on adiposity measures: a systematic review and meta-analysis of randomized controlled trials. *Nutrition Reviews*, 73(9), 577–93. doi:10.1093/nutrit/nuv012

Chiu, S., Bergeron, N., Williams, P. T., Bray, G. A., Sutherland, B. & Krauss, R. M. (2016). Comparison of the DASH (Dietary Approaches to Stop Hypertension) diet and a higher-fat DASH diet on blood pressure and lipids and lipoproteins: a randomized controlled trial. *American Journal of Clinical Nutrition*, 103(2), 341–7. doi:10.3945/ajcn.115.123281

Chung, M., Tang, A. M., Fu, Z., Wang, D. & Newberry, S. (2016). Calcium intake and cardiovascular disease risk: an updated systematic review and meta-analysis. *Annals of Internal Medicine*, 165(12), 856–66. doi:10.7326/M16-1165

Clark, J. L., Rech, L., Chaity, N., Sihag, J., Taylor, C. G. & Aliani, M. (2015). Possible deleterious hormonal changes associated with low-sodium diets. *Nutrition Reviews*, 73(1), 22–35. doi:10.1093/nutrit/nuu003

Cogswell, M. E., Mugavero, K., Bowman, B. A. & Frieden, T. R. (2016). Dietary sodium and cardiovascular disease risk: measurement matters. *New England Journal of Medicine*, 375(6), 580–6. doi:10.1056/NEJMsb1607161

de Baaij, J. H., Hoenderop, J. G. & Bindels, R. J. M. (2015). Magnesium in man: implications for health and disease. *Physiological Reviews*, 95(1), 1–46. doi:10.1152/physrev.00012.2014

Elijovich, F., Weinberger, M. H., Anderson, C. A. M., Appel, L. J., Bursztyn, M., Cook, N. R., ... Laffer, C. L. (2016). Salt sensitivity of blood pressure: a scientific statement from the American Heart Association. *Hypertension*, 68(3), e7–e46. doi:10.1161/HYP.0000000000000047

Falkner, B. (2017). Does potassium deficiency contribute to hypertension in children and adolescents? *Current Hypertension Reports*, 19(5). doi:10.1007/s11906-017-0733-2

Foss, J. D., Kirabo, A. & Harrison, D. G. (2017). Do high-salt microenvironments drive hypertensive inflammation? *American Journal of Physiology—Regulatory Integrative and Comparative Physiology*, 312(1), R1–R4. doi:10.1152/ajpregu.00414.2016

Freedman, L. S., Commins, J. M., Moler, J. E., Willett, W., Tinker, L. F., Subar, A. F., … Prentice, R. L. (2015). Pooled results from 5 validation studies of dietary self-report instruments using recovery biomarkers for potassium and sodium intake. *American Journal of Epidemiology*, 181(7), 473–87. doi:10.1093/aje/kwu325

Gumz, M. L., Rabinowitz, L. & Wingo, C. S. (2015). An integrated view of potassium homeostasis. *New England Journal of Medicine*, 373(18), 1787–8. doi:10.1056/NEJMc1509656

Hope, S. F., Webster, J., Trieu, K., Pillay, A., Ieremia, M., Bell, C., … Moodie, M. (2017). A systematic review of economic evaluations of population-based sodium reduction interventions. *PLOS ONE*, 12(3). doi:10.1371/journal.pone.0173600

Horning, K. J., Caito, S. W., Tipps, K. G., Bowman, A. B. & Aschner, M. (2015). Manganese is essential for neuronal health. *Annual Review of Nutrition*, 35, 71–108. doi:10.1146/annurev-nutr-071714-034419

John, K. A., Maalouf, J., Barsness, C. B., Yuan, K., Cogswell, M. E. & Gunn J. P. (2016). Do lower calorie or lower fat foods have more sodium than their regular counterparts? *Nutrients*, 8(8). doi:10.3390/nu8080511

Laffer, C. L., Scott, R. C. III, Titze, J. M., Luft, F. C. & Elijovich, F. (2016). Hemodynamics and salt-and-water balance link sodium storage and vascular dysfunction in salt-sensitive subjects. *Hypertension*, 68(1), 195–203. doi:10.1161/hypertensionaha.116.07289

Li, P., Fan, C., Lu, Y. & Qi, K. (2016). Effects of calcium supplementation on body weight: a meta-analysis. *American Journal of Clinical Nutrition*, 104(5), 1263–73. doi:10.3945/ajcn.116.136242

McDonough, A. A., Veiras, L. C., Guevara, C. A. & Ralph, D. L. (2017). Cardiovascular benefits associated with higher dietary K+ vs. lower dietary Na+: evidence from population and mechanistic studies. *American Journal of Physiology—Endocrinology and Metabolism*, 312(4), E348–E356. doi:10.1152/ajpendo.00453.2016

Mozaffarian, D., Fahimi, S., Singh, G. M., Micha, R., Khatibzadeh, S., Engell, R. E., … Powles, J. (2014). Global sodium consumption and death from cardiovascular causes. *New England Journal of Medicine*, 371(7), 624–34. doi:10.1056/NEJMoa1304127

Park, J., Kwock, C. K. & Yang, Y. J. (2016). The effect of the sodium to potassium ratio on hypertension prevalence: a propensity score matching approach. *Nutrients*, 8(8). doi:10.3390/nu8080482

Pilic, L., Pedlar, C. R. & Mavrommatis, Y. (2016). Salt-sensitive hypertension: mechanisms and effects of dietary and other lifestyle factors. *Nutrition Reviews*, 74(10), 645–58. doi:10.1093/nutrit/nuw028

Protiva, P., Pendyala, S., Nelson, C., Augenlicht, L. H., Lipkin, M. & Holt, P. R. (2016). Calcium and 1,25-dihydroxyvitamin D3 modulate genes of immune and inflammatory pathways in the human colon: a human crossover trial. *American Journal of Clinical Nutrition*, 103(5), 1224–31. doi:10.3945/ajcn.114.105304

Rhee, O. J., Rhee, M. Y., Oh, S. W., Shin, S. J., Gu, N., Nah, D. Y., … Lee, J. H. (2016). Effect of sodium intake on renin level: analysis of general population and meta-analysis of randomized controlled trials. *International Journal of Cardiology*, 215, 120–6. doi:10.1016/j.ijcard.2016.04.109

Rizzoli, R. (2014). Dairy products, yogurts, and bone health. *American Journal of Clinical Nutrition*, 99(5), 1256S–1262S. doi:10.3945/ajcn.113.073056

Rooney, M. R., Pankow, J. S., Sibley, S. D., Selvin, E., Reis, J. P., Michos, E. D. & Lutsey, P. L. (2016). Serum calcium and incident type 2 diabetes: the Atherosclerosis Risk in Communities (ARIC) study. *American Journal of Clinical Nutrition*, 104(4), 1023–9. doi:10.3945/ajcn.115.130021

Rosanoff, A., Dai, Q. & Shapses, S. A. (2016). Essential nutrient interactions: does low or suboptimal magnesium status interact with vitamin D and/or calcium status? *Advances in Nutrition: An International Review Journal*, 7(1), 25–43. doi:10.3945/an.115.008631

Salomo, L., Poulsen, S. K., Rix, M., Kamper, A.-L., Larsen, T. M. & Astrup, A. (2016). The New Nordic Diet: phosphorus content and absorption. *European Journal of Nutrition*, 55(3), 991–6. doi:10.1007/s00394-015-0913-2

Sayer, R. D., Wright, A. J., Chen, N. & Campbell, W. W. (2015). Dietary Approaches to Stop Hypertension diet retains effectiveness to reduce blood pressure when lean pork is substituted for chicken and fish as the predominant source of protein. *American Journal of Clinical Nutrition*, 102(2), 302–8. doi:10.3945/ajcn.115.111757

Schwingshackl, L. & Hoffmann, G. (2015). Diet quality as assessed by the Healthy Eating Index, the Alternate Healthy Eating Index, the Dietary Approaches to Stop Hypertension score, and health outcomes: a systematic review and meta-analysis of cohort studies. *Journal of the Academy of Nutrition and Dietetics*, 115(5), 780–800. doi:10.1016/j.jand.2014.12.009

Stanhewicz, A. E. & Larry Kenney, W. (2015). Determinants of water and sodium intake and output. *Nutrition Reviews*, 73(suppl. 2), 73–82. doi:10.1093/nutrit/nuv033

Steinberg, D., Bennett, G. G. & Svetkey, L. (2017). The DASH diet, 20 years later. *JAMA—Journal of the American Medical Association*, 317(15), 1529–30. doi:10.1001/jama.2017.1628

Stone, M. S., Martyn, L. & Weaver, C. M. (2016). Potassium intake, bioavailability, hypertension, and glucose control. *Nutrients*, 8(7). doi:10.3390/nu8070444

Takeda, E., Yamamoto, H., Yamanaka-Okumura, H. & Taketani, Y. (2014). Increasing dietary phosphorus intake from food additives: potential for negative impact on bone health. *Advances in Nutrition: An International Review Journal*, 5(1), 92–7. doi:10.3945/an.113.004002

Trieu, K., Neal, B., Hawkes, C., Dunford, E., Campbell, N., Rodriguez-Fernandez, R., ... Webster, J. (2015). Salt reduction initiatives around the world: a systematic review of progress towards the global target. *PLOS ONE*, 10(7). doi:10.1371/journal.pone.0130247

Uribarri, J. & Calvo, M. S. (2014). Dietary phosphorus intake and health. *American Journal of Clinical Nutrition*, 99(2), 247–8. doi:10.3945/ajcn.113.080259

Villarroel, P., Villalobos, E., Reyes, M. & Cifuentes, M. (2014). Calcium, obesity, and the role of the calcium-sensing receptor. *Nutrition Reviews*, 72(10), 627–37. doi:10.1111/nure.12135

Webster, J., Waqanivalu, T., Arcand, J., Trieu, K., Cappuccio, F. P., Appel, L. J., ... McLean, R. (2017). Understanding the science that supports population-wide salt reduction programs. *Journal of Clinical Hypertension*. doi:10.1111/jch.12994

Xiao, Q., Murphy, R. A., Houston, D. K., Harris, T. B., Chow, W. & Park, Y. (2013). Dietary and supplemental calcium intake and cardiovascular disease mortality: the National Institutes of Health–AARP Diet and Health study. *JAMA Internal Medicine*, 173(8), 639–46. doi:10.1001/jamainternmed.2013.3283

Zganiacz, F., Wills, R. B. H., Mukhopadhyay, S. P., Arcot, J. & Greenfield, H. (2017). Changes in the sodium content of Australian processed foods between 1980 and 2013 using analytical data. *Nutrients*, 9(5). doi:10.3390/nu9050501

REFERENCES

1   National Health and Medical Research Council (2006). *Nutrient Reference Values for Australia and New Zealand, Including Recommended Dietary Intakes*. Canberra: NHMRC.

2   A. C. Guyton (1989). Dominant role of the kidneys and accessory role of whole-body autoregulation in the pathogenesis of hypertension. *American Journal of Hypertension*, 2(7), 575–85.

3   H. E. d.Wardener & G. A. MacGregor (2001). Blood pressure and the kidney. In R. W. Schrier (ed.), *Diseases of the Kidney and Urinary Tract*, 7th edn (pp. 1329–61). Philadelphia, PA: Lippincott Williams & Wilkins.

4   D. Denton, R. Weisinger, N. I. Mundy, E. J. Wickings, A. Dixson, P. Moisson, et al. (1995). The effect of increased salt intake on blood pressure of chimpanzees. *Nature Medicine*, 1(10), 1009–16.

5   D. Denton (1982). *Hunger for Salt: An anthropological, physiological and medical analysis*. Heidelberg: Springer-Verlag.

6   W. J. Oliver, E. L. Cohen & J. V. Neel (1975). Blood pressure, sodium intake, and sodium related hormones in the Yanomamo Indians, a 'no-salt' culture. *Circulation*, 52(1), 146–51.

7   INTERSALT Cooperative Research Group (1988). INTERSALT: an international study of electrolyte excretion and blood pressure. Results for 24 hour urinary sodium and potassium excretion. *British Medical Journal*, 297(6644), 319–28. doi:10.1136/bmj.297.6644.319

8   Prospective Studies Collaboration (2002). Age-specific relevance of usual blood pressure to vascular mortality: a meta-analysis of individual data for one million adults in 61 prospective studies. *The Lancet*, 360(9349), 1903–13. doi:https://doi.org/10.1016/S0140-6736(02)11911-8

9   J. Stamler, G. Rose, R. Stamler, P. Elliott, A. Dyer & M. Marmot (1989). INTERSALT study findings. Public health and medical care implications. *Hypertension*, 14(5), 570–7. doi:10.1161/01.hyp.14.5.570

10 P. Elliott, J. Stamler, R. Nichols, A. R. Dyer, R. Stamler, H. Kesteloot & M. Marmot (1996). INTERSALT revisited: further analyses of 24 hour sodium excretion and blood pressure within and across populations. *British Medical Journal*, 312(7041), 1249–53. doi:10.1136/bmj.312.7041.1249

11 C. E. Huggins, S. O'Reilly, M. Brinkman, A. Hodge, G. G. Giles, D. R. English & C. A. Nowson (2011). Relationship of urinary sodium and sodium-to-potassium ratio to blood pressure in older adults in Australia. *Medical Journal of Australia*, 195(3), 128–32.

12 V. Perez & E. T. Chang (2014). Sodium-to-potassium ratio and blood pressure, hypertension, and related factors. *Advances in Nutrition*, 5(6), 712–41. doi:10.3945/an.114.006783

13 G. Kolath (2017). Why everything we know about salt may be wrong. *New York Times*, 8 May. Retrieved from: www.nytimes.com/2017/05/08/health/salt-health-effects.html?_r=0.

14 M. Zeidel (2017). Salt and water: not so simple. *Journal of Clinical Investigation*, 127(5), 1625–6. doi:10.1172/JCI94004

15 K. Kitada, S. Daub, Y. Zhang, J. D. Klein, D. Nakano, T. Pedchenko, ... J. Titze (2017). High salt intake reprioritizes osmolyte and energy metabolism for body fluid conservation. *Journal of Clinical Investigation*, 127(5), 1944–59. doi:10.1172/JCI88532

16 N. Rakova, K. Kitada, K. Lerchl, A. Dahlmann, A. Birukov, S. Daub, ... J. Titze (2017). Increased salt consumption induces body water conservation and decreases fluid intake. *Journal of Clinical Investigation*, 127(5), 1932–43. doi:10.1172/JCI88530

17 J. M. Geleijnse, F. J. Kok & D. E. Grobbee (2003). Blood pressure response to changes in sodium and potassium intake: a metaregression analysis of randomised trials. *Journal of Human Hypertension*, 17(7), 471–80.

18 N. R. Cook, E. Obarzanek, J. A. Cutler, J. E. Buring, K. M. Rexrode, S. K. Kumanyika, ... P. K. Whelton (2009). Joint effects of sodium and potassium intake on subsequent cardiovascular disease: the Trials of Hypertension Prevention follow-up study. *JAMA Internal Medicine*, 169(1), 32–40. doi:10.1001/archinternmed.2008.523

19 L. C. Tapsell, E. P. Neale, A. Satija & F. B. Hu (2016). Foods, nutrients, and dietary patterns: interconnections and implications for dietary guidelines. *Advances in Nutrition: An International Review Journal*, 7(3), 445–54. doi:10.3945/an.115.011718

20 L. J. Appel, T. J. Moore, E. Obarzanek, W. M. Vollmer, L. P. Svetkey, F. M. Sacks, ... D. W. Harsha (1997). A clinical trial of the effects of dietary patterns on blood pressure. *New England Journal of Medicine*, 336(16), 1117–24. doi:10.1056/nejm199704173361601

21 F. M. Sacks, L. P. Svetkey, W. M. Vollmer, L. J. Appel, G. A. Bray, D. Harsha, ... J. A. Cutler (2001). Effects on blood pressure of reduced dietary sodium and the Dietary Approaches to Stop Hypertension (DASH) diet. *New England Journal of Medicine*, 344(1), 3–10. doi:10.1056/nejm200101043440101

22 E. R. Miller III, T. P. Erlinger, D. R. Young, M. Jehn, J. Charleston, D. Rhodes, ... L. J. Appel (2002). Results of the Diet, Exercise, and Weight Loss Intervention Trial (DEW-IT). *Hypertension*, 40(5), 612–18.

23 L. J. Appel, C. M. Champagne, D. W. Harsha, L. S. Cooper, E. Obarzanek, P. J. Elmer, ... D. R. Young (2003). Effects of comprehensive lifestyle modification on blood pressure control: main results of the PREMIER clinical trial. *JAMA—Journal of the American Medical Association*, 289(16), 2083–93. doi:10.1001/jama.289.16.2083

24 C. Wibisono, Y. Probst, E. Neale & L. Tapsell (2016). Impact of food supplementation on weight loss in randomised-controlled dietary intervention trials: a systematic review and meta-analysis. *British Journal of Nutrition*, 115(8), 1406–14. doi:10.1017/s0007114516000337

25 D. R. Jacobs, M. D. Gross & L. C. Tapsell (2009). Food synergy: an operational concept for understanding nutrition. *American Journal of Clinical Nutrition*, 89(5), 1543S–1548S. doi:10.3945/ajcn.2009.26736B

26 D. R. Jacobs, Jr & L. C. Tapsell (2007). Food, not nutrients, is the fundamental unit in nutrition. *Nutrient Reviews*, 65(10), 439–50.

27 R. N. Ndanuko, L. C. Tapsell, K. E. Charlton, E. P. Neale & M. J. Batterham (2016). Dietary patterns and blood pressure in adults: a systematic review and meta-analysis of randomized controlled trials. *Advances in Nutrition: An International Review Journal*, 7(1), 76–89. doi:10.3945/an.115.009753

28 R. N. Ndanuko, L. C. Tapsell, K. E. Charlton, E. P. Neale & M. J. Batterham (2017). Associations between dietary patterns and blood pressure in a clinical sample of overweight adults. *Journal of the Academy of Nutrition and Dietetics*, 117(2), 228–39. doi:10.1016/j.jand.2016.07.019

29 R. N. Ndanuko, L. C. Tapsell, K. E. Charlton, E. P. Neale, K. M. O'Donnell & M. J. Batterham (2017). Relationship between sodium and potassium intake and blood pressure in a sample of overweight adults. *Nutrition*, 33, 285–90. doi:http://dx.doi.org/10.1016/j.nut.2016.07.011

30 Department of Health (2015–17). *Methodological Framework for the Review of Nutrient Reference Values.* Canberra: Department of Health. Retrieved from: www.nrv.gov.au/file/methodological-framework-pdf-705kb.

31 Department of Health (2017). *Nutrient Reference Values for Australia and New Zealand. Revised Sodium Nutrient References Values.* Retrieved from: www.nrv.gov.au.

32 S. M. Moe (2008). Disorders involving calcium, phosphorus, and magnesium. *Primary Care,* 35(2), 215–37, v–vi. doi:10.1016/j.pop.2008.01.007

33 J. Blaine, M. Chonchol & M. Levi (2015). Renal control of calcium, phosphate, and magnesium homeostasis. *Clinical Journal of the American Society of Nephrology,* 10(7), 1257–72. doi:10.2215/cjn.09750913

34 C. Palacios (2006). The role of nutrients in bone health, from A to Z. *Critical Reviews in Food Science and Nutrition,* 46(8), 621–8. doi:10.1080/10408390500466174

35 R. P. Heaney, S. Abrams, B. Dawson-Hughes, A. Looker, A. Looker, R. Marcus, ... C. Weaver (2000). Peak bone mass. *Osteoporosis International,* 11(12), 985–1009. doi:10.1007/s001980070020

36 R. Civitelli & T. Peterson (2017). Toward personalized calcium and vitamin D supplementation. *American Journal of Clinical Nutrition,* 105(4), 777–8. doi:10.3945/ajcn.117.154278

37 Y. Wang, J. Wactawski-Wende, L. E. Sucheston-Campbell, L. Preus, K. M. Hovey, J. Nie, ... H. M. Ochs-Balcom (2017). The influence of genetic susceptibility and calcium plus vitamin D supplementation on fracture risk. *American Journal of Clinical Nutrition,* 105(4), 970–9. doi:10.3945/ajcn.116.144550

38 R. P. Heaney (2000). Calcium, dairy products and osteoporosis. *Journal of the American College of Nutrition,* 19(suppl. 2), 83S–99S. doi:10.1080/07315724.2000.10718088

39 H. J. Adrogué & N. E. Madias (2007). Sodium and potassium in the pathogenesis of hypertension. *New England Journal of Medicine,* 356(19), 1966–78. doi:10.1056/NEJMra064486

40 M. C. Houston & K. J. Harper (2008). Potassium, magnesium, and calcium: their role in both the cause and treatment of hypertension. *Journal of Clinical Hypertension,* 10(7), 3–11. doi:10.1111/j.1751-7176.2008.08575.x

41 National Osteoporosis Foundation. (2016). *Your Guide to a Bone Healthy Diet.* Retrieved from: https://cdn.nof.org/wp-content/uploads/2016/04/Healthy-Bone-Brochure_FINAL.pdf.

42 Australian Bureau of Statistics (2015). *Australian Health Survey: Usual nutrient intakes, 2011–12.* Canberra: ABS. Retrieved from: www.abs.gov.au/ausstats/abs@.nsf/Lookup/by%20Subject/4364.0.55.008~2011-12~Main%20Features~Calcium~401#2.

OXFORD UNIVERSITY PRESS

CHAPTER 12

OTHER KEY MINERALS: IODINE, FLUORIDE, IRON AND ZINC

LINDA TAPSELL AND KAREN CHARLTON

CHAPTER OBJECTIVES

This chapter will enable the reader to:

- describe the chemical nature of the minerals iodine, fluoride, iron and zinc
- briefly outline key functions of these minerals in the human body
- describe the patterns of food and beverage choices that would enable intakes of these minerals to support health.

KEY TERMS

Fluoride	Iron
Iodine	Zinc

KEY POINTS

- Iodine is an essential component of thyroid hormones, which significantly influence human metabolism.
- Fluoride is a significant structural component of bones and teeth.
- Iron is an essential component of blood enabling oxygen transport throughout the body.
- Zinc plays a number of roles in human metabolism, particularly in relation to cellular immunity.

INTRODUCTION

Minerals serve a multitude of functions in human physiology and metabolism. In the previous chapter, two groups of minerals with major health implications for the Australian population, namely blood pressure and bone health, were discussed. Overall, the Nutrient Reference Values (NRVs) for Australia and New Zealand (www.nrv.gov.au/nutrients) outline the requirements for 14 minerals and trace elements (calcium, chromium, copper, fluoride, iodine, iron, magnesium, manganese, molybdenum, phosphorus, potassium, selenium, sodium and zinc). Intakes of minerals are required in varying amounts, albeit less than the macronutrients (protein, fat and carbohydrate), which are required in amounts determined in grams; whereas, vitamins and minerals (micronutrients) are required in milligrams and micrograms. The term 'trace' element is applied when very small amounts are necessary. The amount required reflects the function of those minerals in the body, and our understanding of this varies depending on the investment that has been made in science in that area over time.

See Chapter 11 on the function of the major minerals.

» CASE 12.1

NUTRITIONAL OBSERVATIONS AND INTERVENTIONS: IODINE

The relationship between iodine intakes and goitre has been known for centuries. In the 1820s a French chemist, Jean-Baptiste Boussingault, conducting geological surveys in Central America, observed that goitre occurred in areas where salt was naturally low in iodine, and he recommended that governments use naturally iodised salt to combat goitre. However, controversy in the scientific and medical community as to the cause of goitre ensued for the next 100 years, and this recommendation was not implemented. It was the work of an American physician, Dr David Marine, who conducted a series of systematic experiments from 1907–19 in Ohio, part of the US 'goitre belt', that conclusively showed that a lack of iodine in the diet resulted in goitre. Consequently, there was renewed interest in iodisation of salt, and in the United States potassium iodide was added to table salt from 1924 [1].

In New Zealand and Australia endemic goitre in the early part of the twentieth century was due to very low levels of iodine in soils. Iodine was added to salt, but this was not legally required. At the same time, iodine entered the food supply through contamination of dairy products caused by the use of iodophors as cleaning agents to prevent mastitis in dairy herds. This resulted in a reduction of goitre incidence and adequate iodine status from the 1960s to 1980s. A re-emergence of mild iodine deficiency in New Zealand and Australia was observed in the 1990s and this coincided with a replacement of iodophors with chlorine-based sanitisers by dairy farmers and a reduction in the use of iodised salt. In the early to mid 2000s, a voluntary fortification program of iodised salt in bread was trialled in Tasmania. This program improved the iodine status of schoolchildren, but had no impact in pregnant women [2; 3].

- How does this case study demonstrate the value of observation in nutrition science?
- How many different disciplines could be seen in this case study, and what did they do?
- What are the remaining challenges for translating science to practice here?

The identification of problems associated with dietary intake of minerals also reflects current circumstances associated with the health profile of the population, the food supply and available research data. This chapter broadens the focus to another four key minerals that have current public health implications in Australia and in global nutrition. These minerals have attracted a reasonable amount of attention from nutrition science, with research focused on better understanding the systems and processes related to them. Each of these minerals is linked to functions that are significant in maintaining health. Iodine plays an important role in cognitive development; adequate fluoride is linked to dental health; iron assists in the ability to carry oxygen throughout the body; and zinc is a component of enzymes with significant functions in the body. The physiological changes that occur during particular life stages can influence requirements such as pregnancy, infancy/childhood and advanced ageing.

The significance of these minerals to the diet of Australians is reflected in a number of ways. The selective reporting of Nutrition First results of the Australian Health Survey [4] reveals the average intakes and major food sources of iodine and iron. A recent review of the NRVs for Australia and New Zealand included fluoride as a priority nutrient. From a more global perspective, zinc is a key nutrient of concern among micronutrient deficiencies, which remain a recognised problem in low–middle-income countries [5]. Zinc status may also be compromised in at-risk groups in high-income countries, including older adults and those consuming vegetarian diets [6], and zinc was one of the key nutrients reported in the modelling of the diets underpinning the Australian Guide to Healthy Eating (www.eatforhealth.gov.au). Toxicity is an issue for minerals, but the types and amounts of foods described for age and sex categories in these guidelines show how adequate intakes can be consumed with judicious food choices. However, the number and type of foods (and beverages) delivering significant amounts of these minerals can be limited. This has public health implications for monitoring intakes and assessing health-related outcomes.

STOP AND THINK

- How does knowledge of the effects of these trace minerals on health emerge?
- How do standards such as the NRVs (in Australia and New Zealand) and Dietary Reference Intakes (in the United States) relate to the trace mineral consumption of the population?
- Why would iodine, fluoride, iron and zinc be important trace minerals to consider for the Australian population?

WHAT IS THE STRUCTURE AND FUNCTION OF IODINE WITH SIGNIFICANT IMPLICATIONS FOR NUTRITION?

Iodine (I) is an elemental component with atomic number 131 found in soil, where it can enter the food chain. In the human body, iron combines with other structures to form the pro-hormone thyroxine (T_4) and the more potent active form 3,5,3' tri-iodothyronine (T_3), a key regulator of important cellular processes (Figure 12.1). Thyroid hormones are involved in many metabolic processes critical for normal growth and development, particularly of the brain and central nervous system. The **thyroid hormones** are also important for energy production and oxygen consumption in cells, thereby maintaining the body's metabolic rate.

Thyroid hormones
hormones produced by the thyroid gland that influence human metabolism.

FIGURE 12.1   STRUCTURE OF THYROXINE HORMONE SHOWING IODINE CONFIGURATION

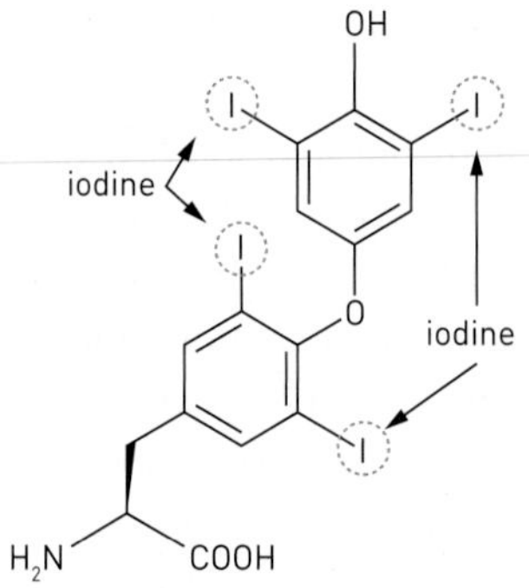

Thyroxine (T4)

Legend: Thyroid gland produces thyroxine (T_4) and triiodothyronine (T_3). The major form of thyroid hormone in blood is thyroxine (T_4) with a ratio of T_4:T_3 in blood of about 20:1. Thyroxine is converted to active T_3 (three to four times more potent than T_4) within cells.

The thyroid undergoes a number of adaptive changes when iodine intake falls, which ensures that a continual supply of thyroid hormones, in particular T_3, is available for normal growth and development. A fall in T_4 stimulates the production of TSH (thyroid-stimulating hormone), which subsequently causes an enlargement in the thyroid gland, increased uptake of iodine from the blood, increased synthesis of thyroglobulin (-Tg; a protein), and a shift in the ratio of T_4 to T_3 (preferential T_3 secretion) released into the blood.

Iodine deficiency disorders (IDD)

clinical manifestations of iodine deficiency including goitre, hypothyroidism, impairment of mental and physical development, and cretinism.

Goitre

a condition evidenced by an enlarged thyroid gland resulting from iodine deficiency.

Hashimotos disease

a chronic inflammatory disorder of the thyroid gland caused by abnormal antibodies and white blood cells that mistakenly attack and damage healthy thyroid cells.

A lack of iodine in the diet can cause a myriad of adverse effects known as **iodine deficiency disorders (IDD)**, and these include **goitre** (reflected in increased thyroid volume), hypothyroidism, impairment of mental and physical development, and in its most severe form, cretinism (Table 12.1). Abnormal thyroid function also occurs in **Hashimotos disease**, but this is an autoimmune disorder.

Goitre can be measured by palpation by trained physicians and graded according to criteria of WHO/UNICEF/ICCIDD. The presence of goitre in >5% of the population indicates iodine deficiency [7]. After long-standing exposure to iodine deficiency, it may take years or even generations to normalise thyroid volumes in the population. Endemic goitre is the most visible consequence of IDD. There may be developmental gains with correction of iodine deficiency even in older children from mildly deficient countries. A clinical trial from New Zealand demonstrated that supplementation with 150 µg/day of iodine in children aged 10–13 years resulted in significant improvements in overall cognitive function and in two subscale cognition test scores [8]. Table 12.2 lists estimated average requirements (EAR) and recommended dietary intakes (RDI) for iodine for adults.

Biomarkers to assess iodine status include urinary iodine concentration (UIC) and measures related to thyroid function (thyroid volume, thyroid hormones, TSH, thyroglobulin (Tg) and radioactive iodine uptake).

UIC provides a convenient indicator of population level iodine and can be assessed from a spot (casual) urine sample because approximately 90% of dietary iodine is excreted in the

TABLE 12.1   HEALTH CONSEQUENCES OF IODINE DEFICIENCY AT DIFFERENT LIFE STAGES

Life stages	Health consequences of iodine deficiency
Foetus and neonate	Spontaneous abortion Premature delivery and stillbirth Congenital anomalies Increased perinatal mortality Neurological cretinism
Child and adolescent	Neurological cretinism Myxedematous cretinism Impaired mental function; decreased IQ Hypothyroidism Delayed physical development Goitre
Adult	Hypothyroidism Impaired mental function Goitre Iodine-induced hyperthyroidism (in nodular goitre)
All ages	Goitre Hypothyroidism Increased susceptibility to nuclear radiation

Sources: Adapted from M. Li & C. J. Eastman (2012). The changing epidemiology of iodine deficiency. *Nature Reviews Endocrinology*, 8(7), 434–40. doi:10.1038/nrendo.2012.43; B. Hetzel (1983). Iodine deficiency disorders (IDD) and their eradication. *The Lancet*, 322(8359), 1126–9. doi:10.1016/S0140-6736(83)90636-0; C. J. Eastman (2014). Iodine deficiency disorders continue to be a problem in the Asia Pacific region. *Journal of the ASEAN Federation of Endocrine Societies*, 27(2). doi:10.15605/jafes.027.02.06

TABLE 12.2   RECOMMENDED DIETARY INTAKES OF IODINE BY AGE AND SEX

Age	EAR* µg/day	RDI** µg/day
Men		
19–30 years	100	150
31–50 years	100	150
51–70 years	100	150
>70 years	100	150
Women		
19–30 years	100	150
31–50 years	100	150
51–70 years	100	150
>70 years	100	150

*EAR: Estimated average requirement
**RDI: Recommended dietary intake

Source: National Health and Medical Research Council (2014). *Nutrient Reference Values for Australia and New Zealand—Iodine*. Canberra: NHMRC. © Commonwealth of Australia

TABLE 12.3   RECOMMENDED CUT-OFFS FOR URINARY IODINE CONCENTRATION (UIC)

Population group	UIC µg/L	Iodine status
Children	<25	Severe deficiency
Non-pregnant adults Lactating women	25–49	Moderate deficiency
	50–99	Mild deficiency
	100–299	Sufficiency
	>300	Excess
Pregnant women	<50	Deficiency
	150–250	Sufficiency
	>250	Excess

Source: Adapted from World Health Organization (2007). *Assessment of Iodine Deficiency Disorders and Monitoring Their Elimination: A guide for programme managers*, 3rd edn. Geneva: WHO

urine enabling measurement through collections of casual or spot urine samples [9]. Median UIC is determined for a population group and compared with recommended values. UIC should not be used to assess iodine status in individuals because of its high intra- and inter-individual variation. Iodine sufficiency is indicated if the median UIC for a population exceeds 100 µg/L, and if no more than 20% of the population have a UIC below 50 µg/L [7]. Table 12.3 shows the recommended cut-offs for UIC used to categorise severity of iodine deficiency across life stages, as well as values that indicate iodine excess. The recommended method of assessing success or failure of fortification programs in correcting iodine deficiency is determined by assessing median UIC in schoolchildren aged 6–12 years every five years.

Thyroid hormones (TSH, T_4, and T_3) are often measured, but are insensitive indicators of iodine status except in severe iodine deficiency and in newborns. In newborns, TSH measurement is routinely collected through a heelprick blood test, but is used to diagnose congenital hypothyroidism rather than for population-level iodine monitoring . Elevated neonatal TSH is indicated as >5 IU/mL [7]. Thyroglobulin may be a more sensitive index of current iodine status, but is yet to be used in routine monitoring of iodine status. In iodine deficiency, secretion of Tg from the thyroid gland increases and is positively correlated with thyroid volume. The use of Tg as an index of iodine status is relatively new, with the primary focus on school-aged children. It is proposed that a median Tg value >13 µg/L indicates iodine deficiency in this age group [10]. In one study of 10–13-year-old schoolchildren with mild iodine deficiency, Tg fell below the 10 ng/L cut-off indicative of adequate iodine status after seven months of iodine supplementation [8], which suggests that it responds to the correction of iodine deficiency more rapidly than thyroid volume.

Iodine deficiency is one of the most common nutrient deficiencies in the world, with almost one billion people affected. The main cause of iodine deficiency is low levels of iodine in foods grown in soils that are deplete of iodine, often as a result of glaciation and leaching from flooding. Given the serious consequences of iodine deficiency, strategies to improve iodine intakes, such as fortification and supplementation, are imperative.

STOP AND THINK

....

- How would you describe the ecology of iodine in human health?
- What are the consequences of not dealing with adequate availability of iodine for human consumption?
- How has scientific research helped us to better understand the need for iodine in the diet and how to provide it for populations?

WHICH DIETARY SOURCES SUPPORT AN ADEQUATE INTAKE OF IODINE TO MEET NUTRITIONAL REQUIREMENTS?

Foods are an important source of iodine, with problems arising when the local food supply has a low iodine content (that may reflect the soil mineral content). The mammary gland is able to concentrate iodine, so milk and dairy foods can provide iodine. As fish and other seafood are able to bioaccumulate iodine, they can be the richest food sources (Table 12.4).

People who consume diets that contain only small amounts of fish and seafood, moderate-to-low quantities of milk and dairy products, and include locally produced fruits and vegetables grown in iodine-poor soils are at risk of being iodine deficient. RDIs of iodine are increased in pregnancy and lactation to account for the additional needs of the developing foetus and the quantities of iodine supplied in breast milk.

Iodised salt has continued to be the most common food vehicle for iodine fortification globally because salt fulfils the following criteria: it is eaten in consistent amounts by a large proportion of the target population; iodine from iodised salt is well absorbed; iodised salt does not affect the sensory properties of food; salt production is usually limited to a few producers; and the cost of iodisation of salt is very low and the technology relatively simple.

Iodised salt
table salt (sodium chloride) enriched with iodine.

TABLE 12.4   DIETARY SOURCES OF IODINE

Food	Iodine (ug/day)*	Serving size
Milk (2% fat)	135	250 mL (cup)
Iodised salt	150	1/3 tsp
Morwong (steamed)	90	100 g
Snapper (steamed)	40	100 g
Crab flesh (boiled)	59	100 g
Prawns (cooked)	25	100 g
Egg (poached)	21	1 egg
Yoghurt	25	150 g
Cheese (Swiss)	15	25 g (slice)
Other hard cheeses	5	25 g (slice)

Source: Calculated from Food Standards Australia New Zealand (2014). *AUSNUT 2011–13*. Canberra: FSANZ

LINDA TAPSELL AND KAREN CHARLTON

» CASE 12.2

UNIVERSAL SALT IODISATION

The inclusion of iodine in salt (sodium chloride) presents a quandary for nutrition in societies where excess sodium is consumed and hypertension is prevalent. However, given the global public health problem of iodine deficiency and its consequences, the World Health Organization (WHO) endorses **universal salt iodisation (USI)**, whereby all salt for human and animal consumption is iodised. The introduction of iodine into areas with a history of iodine deficiency can lead to a temporary increase in the incidence of thyrotoxicosis, which gradually resolves after two to five years, and the benefits of improved iodine status outweigh the disadvantages. Nevertheless, the implementation of USI without adequate monitoring may result in iodine intakes that are considered to be more than adequate. The 2016 global estimate of iodine nutrition, based on surveys of school-age children conducted between 2002 and 2016, shows that iodine intake is insufficient in 15 countries, sufficient in 102, but excessive (MUIC >300 ug/L or 237 umol/L) in 10 countries [11; 12]. Among the 15 countries with insufficient intake, only two are classified as moderately deficient and 13 as mildly deficient. This represents a reduction in the number of countries with insufficient iodine intake from 32 in 2011, to 25 in 2015 and to 15 in 2016, which reflects continuing progress to improved coverage of iodised salt at the national level.

> **Universal salt iodisation (USI)**
>
> whereby all salt for human and animal consumption is enriched with iodine.

> See Chapter 11 on sodium and hypertension.

High iodine intakes are associated with iodine-induced hyperthyroidism and autoimmune thyroid disease. It is generally agreed that in countries with long-standing iodine deficiency, iodine intake should not exceed 500 μg/day [13]. However, there is a lack of consensus about the upper level of what constitutes an adverse risk to health. For example, the European Commission's Scientific Committee for Food had set an UL of 600 μg/day for adults and pregnant women [14], which was almost half of that recommended by the US Institute of Medicine (1100 μg/day) [15]. In its recommendations for iodine requirements in pregnancy, lactation and for young children, the WHO expressed a cautious approach regarding upper levels, stating that a daily intake >500 μg/day in pregnancy and lactation, and >180 μg/day in children younger than two years, is not necessary since it may theoretically be associated with impaired thyroid function [13]. Since the mid 1990s, the Network for the Sustained Elimination of Iodine Deficiency, a global coalition of various governmental and non-governmental agencies, has worked to eliminate iodine deficiency. Worldwide, approximately 70% of the world's population is estimated to use iodised salt in a total of 130 countries [16]. In many countries, the presence of many small and independent salt producers means it is difficult to regulate the production of adequately iodised salt; while in other countries, USI is not possible because of trade barriers (i.e. some countries prohibit the addition of iodised salt to processed foods), thereby impacting on food exports. Thus, other components in the diet have been fortified either by including iodised salt as an ingredient (e.g. in bread), feeding animals iodine-enriched feeds, which increase the iodine content of foods produced by these animals (e.g. in eggs [17]), or by the direct addition of an iodine compound to sugar [18], fish sauce [19] or water [20]. However, the International Council for the Control of Iodine Deficiency Disorders (ICCIDD) advises countries to adopt USI.

- What are the implications of USI for the global food supply?
- How can the benefits and risks of USI be managed at a country level?
- Why is nutrition monitoring and surveillance important in this scenario?

Mandatory fortification of food with iodine is one public health approach for dealing with endemic iodine deficiency. From a public health point of view, mandatory fortification is simpler because associated legislation identifies which foods can be fortified, and often provides guidelines on the permitted range of fortification. However, the decision to implement mandatory fortification or voluntary fortification is often influenced by the food industry. In Switzerland, more than 95% of household salt is iodised and 90% of food manufacturers voluntarily add iodised salt to their products, largely due to a good working relationship between the scientific community and the local food industry. Furthermore, Switzerland has a good monitoring program to ensure that the iodine status of the population remains adequate and, if necessary, adjustments are readily made to the amount of iodine in iodised salt by federal decree rather than the drawn-out parliamentary process required in many other countries. In 1952, the level of salt iodisation in Switzerland was 3.75 mg/kg, which was increased to 7.5 mg/kg in 1962, 15 mg/kg in 1980, and finally to 20 mg/kg in 1998, resulting in the adequate iodine status of both children and pregnant women [21; 22]. In later years, a lack of iodine was observed in the diets of very young children, as most weaning foods are not fortified with iodine and do not contain salt, and nutrition guidelines discourage the addition of salt to foods prepared in the home for children under one year of age [23]. This highlights the need to assess the iodine status of all segments in a population to identify the range of foods that should be fortified with iodine, as dietary patterns and habits can vary throughout the lifecycle.

>> CASE 12.3

MANDATORY FOOD FORTIFICATION WITH IODINE IN AUSTRALIA

In September 2009, the mandatory inclusion of iodised salt in bread was introduced in Australia. In order to identify the most suitable vehicle for fortification, extensive dietary modelling was undertaken to maximise the proportion of different subpopulations with intakes above the EAR, while at the same time to minimise the proportion of subpopulations above the upper limit (UL). Such modelling requires regularly updated food composition data with iodine contents, as well as dietary intake data from the target population. A major challenge was a lack of data for some foods regarding the contribution of sodium chloride to the total sodium content, which may have overestimated the effect of fortification for such foods. Reformulations of many processed foods in response to salt reduction initiatives meant older food composition data were out of date and required both indirect (via product ingredient lists) and direct analysis of the salt content of foods. Another difficulty was a lack of data on the consumption of iodised table salt, which had to be extrapolated from national sales data. Modelling data found that the increase in mean iodine intake using 45 mg/kg iodised salt in bread alone was similar if 15 mg/kg iodised salt was used in all salted foods; hence, a decision was made to only fortify bread. Bread fortification was projected to increase mean iodine intake by 54 and 84 µg/day in Australians aged two years or older and New Zealanders aged 15 years or older, respectively; the higher salt content of New Zealand bread at the time of modelling accounts for most of this difference. Undoubtedly, as the salt content of bread drops further in these countries, the legislated iodine targets will need revision. In-depth examination of food intake patterns did not reveal any foods suitable for fortification that had high, widespread consumption by adult women but not by young children. To avoid excessive intakes in young children who have UL values for iodine that are close to the RDI for pregnant women, it was not feasible to meet the substantially higher iodine requirements of pregnant and lactating women. In order to the meet the gap in iodine intakes for these women, the National Health and Medical Research Council and Department of Health Antenatal Clinical Guidelines recommend an oral supplement of 150 µg/day [24; 25]. The 2011–13 National Nutrition and Physical Activity Survey collected biomarkers of iodine status and reported that children across all states are now iodine replete [4]. Pregnant women remain at risk of suboptimal deficiency, unless they take an iodine supplement. Whether fortification is mandatory or voluntary, routine monitoring of the fortified foods and the impact of fortification on the iodine status of the population is required. An improvement in median UIC (MUIC) of primary school-aged children has been observed across all states in Australia since the introduction of the mandatory fortification scheme, with all states having a MUIC above 100 ug/L (Table 12.5). Similarly, Australian adults had a population MUIC of 124 µg/L, with 13% having a UIC <50 µg/L. The Australian Health Survey 2011–12 did not include pregnant women, so national data post-fortification is not available [4].

- What does the data described in the case study indicate with regard to ensuring adequate iodine intake in the Australian population?
- What are some of the strategies that may be needed to address subgroups of the population?
- What type of data is needed for monitoring purposes?

TABLE 12.5   COMPARISON OF MEDIAN UIC IN 8–10-YEAR-OLD AUSTRALIAN SCHOOLCHILDREN BETWEEN 2003–04 (PRE-FORTIFICATION) AND 2011–12 (POST-FORTIFICATION)

State	2003–04 NINS median UIC	2011–13 NNPAS median UIC
Queensland	137 µg/L	166 µg/L
New South Wales	89 µg/L	177 µg/L
Victoria	74 µg/L	163 µg/L
South Australia	101 µg/L	150 µg/L
Western Australia	143 µg/L	261 µg/L

Abbreviations: NINS: National Iodine Nutrition Survey; AHS-NNPAS: National Nutrition and Physical Activity Survey

Sources: M. Li, C. J. Eastman, K. V. Waite, G. Ma, et al. (2006). Are Australian children iodine deficient? Results of the Australian National Iodine Nutrition Study. *Medical Journal of Australia*, 184(4), 165–9; Australian Bureau of Statistics (2013). *Australian Health Survey: Biomedical Results for Nutrients, 2011–12—Iodine*. Canberra: ABS.

Given some of the problems associated with USI, there is merit in considering whether a more graduated approach, whereby one staple food is fortified at a time, is worth consideration, particularly in areas of mild iodine deficiency. Such an approach would allow for an incremental increase in iodine status in the population, thereby reducing the risk of thyrotoxicosis in those with excessive iodine intakes. It also would require monitoring and interim steps, such as supplementation, to ensure that groups in the population with higher iodine requirements such as pregnant or lactating women are consuming adequate amounts of iodine, while at the same time ensuring that those with lower requirements (i.e. young children) are not being exposed to excessive quantities of iodine.

>> RESEARCH AT WORK

MONITORING IODINE INTAKES IN AUSTRALIA

In Australia, the amount of iodine added to salt used in the bread-making process was modelled assuming an average intake of 100 g (2–3 slices) per day [26]. Bread, defined under the legislation, includes regular bread and bread rolls (plain/unfilled/untopped varieties); flat breads (e.g. pita bread, naan bread); focaccia and pide (Turkish bread); bagels (white, wholemeal, sweet); topped breads, buns and rolls (e.g. cheese and bacon rolls); baked English-style muffins (white, white high fibre, multigrain, wholemeal and fruit); sweet buns; and fruit breads and rolls (e.g. raisin bread). Organic bread and chemically aerated non-yeast leavened dough, such as damper and soda breads, are exempt. Secondary analysis from the 2011–12 Australian National Nutrition and Physical Activity Survey found that that only 8.6% of women of childbearing age (14–50 years) and 8% of children (2–18 years) were consuming 100 g of bread or more per day [4]. Main sources of iodine intake at the time of the survey were cereal and cereal products (including bread; 29%), followed by milk products and dishes (26%) and non-alcoholic beverages (including tap water; 15%). Fish and seafood, despite being the richest dietary source of iodine, contributed only 4% of iodine intake because of low intakes. Bread consumption at ⩾100 g/day was associated with five times greater odds of achieving an adequate iodine intake compared with lower bread consumption in women of childbearing age, and 12 times in children aged 2–18 years. This analysis demonstrates the importance of ongoing monitoring and surveillance required after introduction of a national fortification program. A change in dietary habits within the population, as in the case where bread consumption may decrease due to the popularity of low-carbohydrate diets and avoidance of gluten-containing foods, may adversely influence the effectiveness of the program. Other food vehicles that could be fortified with iodine may need to be identified, or the amount of iodine added to bread revised.

STOP AND THINK

- Why does inadequate iodine intake re-emerge in communities, and which groups are most at risk?
- In countries where well-functioning USI programs exist, there is concern that salt reduction strategies may adversely impact on population level iodine status. How could this be addressed?
- What would be the implications for the food industry of fortifying iodine in staple foods?

WHAT IS THE STRUCTURE AND FUNCTION OF FLUORIDE WITH SIGNIFICANT IMPLICATIONS FOR NUTRITION?

Fluoride is the anion (F⁻) of the non-metallic trace element fluorine (atomic number 9). Fluoride is bound in nature, presenting in water supplies in varying amounts (around 0.1 ppm; per part million), which can be higher in volcanic regions. It is also present in seawater. Plants can accumulate fluoride, in particular in tea leaves [27], so tea drinkers may have higher fluoride intakes, but well within safe ranges.

The most significant role of fluoride in nutrition is through binding calcium and stimulating bone formation. During tooth development, fluoride is taken up in tooth enamel where the fluoro apatite that forms helps to reduce the solubility or demineralisation of enamel. This occurs during repeated exposure to acidic environments (from the action of cariogenic bacteria on sugars in the mouth) where the action of gradual fluoride uptake reduces the pH level required for further damage, leaving the enamel more resistant [27]. Higher doses of fluoride can cause dental fluorosis, but even moderate levels of fluorosis are uncommon and severe cases rare in Australia and New Zealand (www.nrv.gov.au).

As in the case of iodine, the origins of fluoride use in preventive health lay in astute observations of populations. A recent review has summarised this history as beginning in the late nineteenth century where brown stains on enamel (mottling) were observed in different regions of the United States and later chemical analysis identified the causal agent as fluoride [27]. This led to the seminal epidemiological work by Dean in which dental fluorosis was described in a dose response manner, and an inverse association was observed with dental caries [28; 29]. Further work enabled Dean to determine that levels of 1 ppm prevented dental caries without negative effects on enamel [30; 31]. Systematic fluoridation followed in the cities of Grand Rapids, Evanston, Brantford and Newberg, producing convincing effects of 50% reduction in incidence of dental caries. Today, water fluoridation remains one of the mainstays of public dental health [32–34].

In 2017, the NHMRC approved revised NRVs for fluoride put forward by the Department of Health. As fluoride plays an important role in the prevention of dental caries, consuming adequate fluoride during childhood is particularly important, as new teeth are emerging. The two revised NRVs for fluoride, for children six months to eight years of age, emerged from the application of a new methodological framework for determining NRVs for Australia and New Zealand [35]. This revision confirmed the current adequate intake (AI) level of 0.05 mg/kg body weight/day. However, a review of available evidence relating to breast- and formula-fed infants noted that a preventive effect in the 0–6 months age group could not be established, so reference to this age group was withdrawn. Using the new methodology, the UL was revised to 0.20 mg/kg bw/day supported by evidence that severe dental fluorosis (adverse effect) is reduced to an acceptable level at this UL value. There were no implications for current guidelines on drinking water in Australia and New Zealand, or for infant formulation of infant formulae [58].

STOP AND THINK

- How widespread is fluoride in the food environment?
- How significant is the NRV review process for working with fluoride in health promotion?
- Why would fluoride toxicity be unlikely in the general population?

WHICH DIETARY SOURCES SUPPORT AN ADEQUATE INTAKE OF FLUORIDE TO MEET NUTRITIONAL REQUIREMENTS?

The main dietary source of fluoride is drinking water. Beverages form the main sources of fluoride in the diet, with strong tea standing out as providing extra amounts. The fluoride in bottled water depends on its source, as is the case with manufactured products.

Water fluoridation
the addition of fluoride to water.

Following the compilation of an evidence evaluation report and associated information paper, the NHMRC released a public statement in November 2017: 'NHMRC strongly recommends community **water fluoridation** as a safe, effective and ethical way to help reduce tooth decay across the population. NHMRC supports Australian states and territories fluoridating their drinking water supplies within the drinking range of 0.6 to 1.1 milligrams per litre (mg/L)' [34].

>> **CASE 12.4**

WATER, FLUORIDATION AND HEALTH EDUCATION

Health literacy is an important element in effective health promotion and disease prevention activities. To this end, health agencies prepare materials to assist communities in understanding and engaging with health promotion programs. Water fluoridation was introduced into New South Wales in the country town of Yass in 1956, and continues to provide populations access to this public health strategy across nearly all of the state's population [36]. In support of ongoing communication and health education on this topic, Water Fluoridation Q&A materials are available to the general public (see www.health.nsw. gov.au/environment/water/Documents/fluoridation-questions-and-answers-nsw.pdf).

Information provided includes:

- the basics of fluoride and water fluoridation
- how fluoride is added to the water supply—legalities, technical issues, quality assurance
- information on dental caries as a public health issue
- evidence for the benefits of fluoridation and issues around fluoride exposure
- social and environmental issues:
  - What is the value of providing this information to communities?
  - How does science underpin the information provided?
  - How do the questions reflect the broader context in which public health nutrition (and dental) programs sit?

TRY IT YOURSELF

Review the documents produced by the NHMRC and NSW Health on water fluoridation and identify the scientific evidence that was scrutinised and presented to form public health statements.

STOP AND THINK

- How is the case of fluoride in nutrition different from that of other minerals?
- What areas of further research would further benefit public health–related interventions?
- Which areas of further knowledge would assist health practitioners in providing advice on fluoride nutrition?

WHAT IS THE STRUCTURE AND FUNCTION OF IRON WITH SIGNIFICANT IMPLICATIONS FOR NUTRITION?

In chemical terms, iron (Fe) is described as a heavy metal (atomic number 26), occurring naturally in soils, and thereby taken up by plant foods, which are in turn consumed by animals. Like other nutrients, iron in food is not consumed and digested in isolation. The food delivery context for iron is categorised

FIGURE 12.2 STRUCTURE OF HAEM IRON

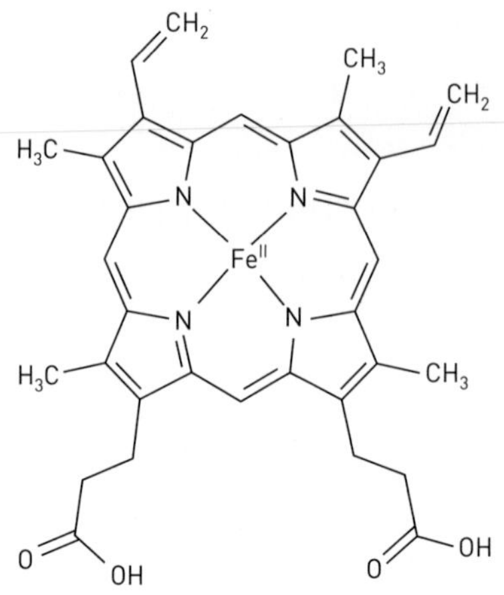

Source: https://en.wikipedia.org/wiki/Iron#/media/File:Heme_b.svg

into two forms: haem and non-haem. The haem form includes a protein found in animal meat (haemoglobin) that caries iron in the centre (Figure 12.2) and binds oxygen molecules for transport throughout the body. Another haem-molecule, myoglobin, stores oxygen in muscles. Thus iron obtained from animal meat is presented in a similar chemical packaging to which it ultimately emerges in the human system (haemoglobin and myoglobin), reflecting congruent physiological processes. In food, this chemical structure enables better availability for absorption, and in the body it serves to protect the body from the effects of iron itself as it is being transported.

The chemical packaging of other forms of iron also reflect the differences in physiological processes within the source food (plant or animal). Non-haem iron comes in a variety of forms in plants, eggs and milk (as well as animal meats). These can include other proteins (such as ferritin, lactoferrin) and iron combined with other elements to form salts. In plant foods, the iron can be bound to other compounds (such as phytates and tannins) and the availability for absorption can be lower. The absorption of non-haem iron could be increased by reducing the iron from its ferric (Fe^{3+}) state to a ferrous (Fe^{2+}) state. This can be achieved by consuming vitamin C (ascorbic acid) with non-haem iron. Vitamin C could also chelate the ferrous iron, keeping it in a more soluble form and protecting it from absorption inhibitors. By nature, however, the iron in human breast milk is much more bioavailable than the iron in cow's milk. This would be expected, given the origins of food in nature, reflecting the biological determinism and interdependence between nutrients. That said, the form of chemical delivery in a food has significant implications for programs that involve iron fortification of staple foods such as cereals.

Typically, the body maintains tight controls over iron stores. Circulating iron comes mainly from the breakdown of red blood cells, leaving a lesser dependence on absorption. The release of iron from cells is limited by the presence of the hormone *hepcidin*, which is secreted by the liver in response to a number of physiological conditions associated with oxygen supply, red blood cell status and immune function. As iron is toxic in excess but cannot be excreted, understanding the influences on hepcidin secretion and function is important in dealing with the pathogenesis of iron-related disorders [37].

The availability of iron following the digestion of food is subject to the conditions of the gut, but the final uptake reflects need, most notably the rate of formation of red blood cells. About 25% of dietary mean iron is absorbed and up to 17% of non-haem iron is absorbed, factors that need to be taken into account when considering iron requirements in the food supply.

Once delivered by mucosal cells, iron is bound to the transporter protein *transferrin*, and most is taken to the bone marrow to form *haemoglobin*, serving a major function in oxygen delivery. Excess iron is stored as *ferritin* in the cells. With this understanding, iron status can be evaluated via a range of measurements (Figure 12.3).

Serum ferritin provides an indication of depleted iron stores, but in **iron deficiency anaemia** low haemoglobin and serum hepcidin are also seen [38]. **Haemochromatosis** (an inherited condition commonly referred to as iron storage disease) shows greatly increased levels of serum ferritin, serum iron and transferrin saturation in the company of low serum hepcidin.

Iron deficiency can be considered in regard to the way in which iron is transported and stored in the body. One of the primary functions of iron is associated with the production of red blood cells. Thus, iron deficiency can be seen when red blood cell counts begin to drop. This is known as iron deficiency anaemia. Another consideration is the depletion of iron stores, and it is possible that iron stores could become depleted and this may not yet show up as reduced red blood cell counts.

See Chapter 3 on digestion, absorption and metabolism.

Iron deficiency anaemia
a medical condition caused by inadequate supply of iron to the bone marrow to produce adequate haemoglobin levels.

Haemochromatosis
an inherited condition caused by lack of hepcidin resulting in very high levels of serum iron.

FIGURE 12.3 HEPCIDIN REGULATES SYSTEMIC IRON HOMEOSTASIS

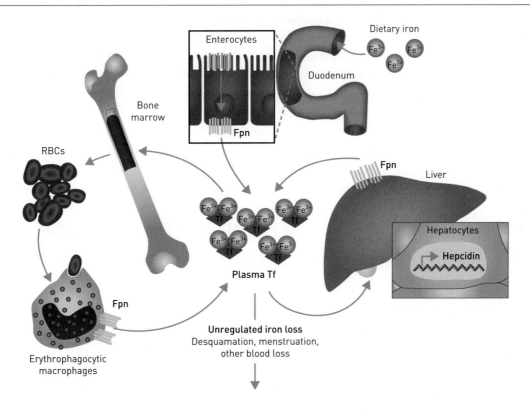

The hormone hepcidin regulates plasma iron concentrations by controlling ferroportin concentrations on iron-exporting cells, including duodenal enterocytes, recycling macrophages of the spleen and liver, and hepatocytes. Hepcidin production by hepatocytes is the main source of plasma hepcidin. Hepatocyte hepcidin synthesis is regulated at the transcriptional level by multiple stimuli.

Fpn = ferroportin; Tf = transferrin

Source: V. Sangkhae & E. Nemeth (2017). Regulation of the iron homeostatic hormone hepcidin. *Advances in Nutrition*, 8(1), 126–36 (Figure 1). doi:10.3945/an.116.013961

>> **RESEARCH AT WORK**

MITIGATING WORLDWIDE ANAEMIA PREVALENCE

Anaemia, or decreased production of red blood cells, remains a global public health nutrition problem [39]. The condition results in weakness and fatigue as well as cognitive and performance problems. A recent review noted two main categories of anaemia, relating to (1) insufficient or defective red blood cell production and (2) conditions in which red blood cells are destroyed. Dietary iron deficiency relates to inadequate red blood cell production, but other causes of anaemia include leukaemia, renal disease and other nutrient deficiencies (folate and vitamin B12). The history of prevalence of anaemia links dietary problems (dependence on cereal-based foods containing phytates and polyphenols and thereby poor iron availability) with poor sanitation and infestations that could lead to blood loss. The prevalence of iron deficiency anaemia (IDA) has been reducing, but it remains the highest in pregnant women, infants and children. The complex processes involved in iron homeostasis, managed between iron transport that responds to cellular iron levels, and the hepatic driven regulation of iron at the whole body level, are also associated with the body's response to inflammation. Understanding how this works under conditions of infection is important for correctly interpreting biomarkers of iron status and determining appropriate treatment regimens. On the other hand, meeting iron requirements during the physiological changes occurring during pregnancy and in infancy also require careful monitoring, as a lack of iron can have significant effects on brain development and cognitive function. Indeed, there is an argument for monitoring iron status throughout the lifespan, as a range of conditions can emerge, again requiring a deep understanding of iron homeostasis and how it is effected in different circumstances.

STOP AND THINK

- Why is the food source of iron an important consideration in nutrition?
- Why do disorders of iron metabolism develop?
- How would dietary behaviour be associated with the presentation of disorders of iron metabolism?

WHICH DIETARY SOURCES SUPPORT AN ADEQUATE INTAKE OF IRON TO MEET NUTRITIONAL REQUIREMENTS?

The possibility of reduced iron stores and its implications underlines the need for a regular intake of iron in the diet. While haemoglobin in red blood cells lasts about four months, iron is also recycled from old cells, so there are some efficiencies in the system. Of course, conditions such as pregnancy increase the requirements for iron as more red blood cells are produced. Requirements for iron also increase during lactation as iron is lost through breast milk. For most people, some iron can be excreted via the gut but further losses could occur in blood, through wounds or menstruation.

Given the chemical structures, the proportion of iron absorbed from haem iron is much higher than from non-haem iron. The structure of haem iron molecules also helps to overcome the influence of

Anti-nutrients

compounds in food that impede the availability and absorption of nutrients.

compounds that may block absorption. These are often found in plants and are sometimes referred to as **anti-nutrients**. They include phytates and some polyphenolic compounds. This issue needs to be considered when the diet only provides plant-based sources of iron (such as in vegan diets).

Naturally, haem iron is found in meat, in the form of haemoglobin and myoglobin. High concentrations of haem iron can be found in red meats (beef, lamb) and especially in organ meats such as liver. Other meats (pork, chicken, fish) deliver reasonable quantities, but not as much as red meat. Some haem iron can be sourced from eggs.

As stated earlier, the bioavailability of the non-haem iron is less than for haem iron, but the body may absorb more of these iron salts if there are low stores. Non-haem iron can be found in cereals, legumes (including lentils, chickpeas), green leafy vegetables and some dried fruits or other vegetables with varying degrees of bioavailability. Given the chemical nature of iron, co-consumption of foods rich in vitamin C improves absorption. Cereal-based foods containing phytate-rich husks can be problematic for accessing non-haem iron in those at risk of inadequate intakes [40; 41]. Some commercial foods can also be iron fortified, in accordance with food standards. The Nutrition First results of the Australian Health Survey 2011–12 reported cereals and cereal products as the main source of iron on the day of analysis (31%) [4]. This included 17% from ready-to-eat breakfast cereals and 10% from regular breads, and rolls. The next main sources were meat, poultry and game products and dishes (17%) and cereal-based products and dishes (16%) (Table 12.6). Compared with the 1995 survey, average iron intakes were less (1.3 per 1000 kJ vs 1.5 mg per 1000 kJ) [4].

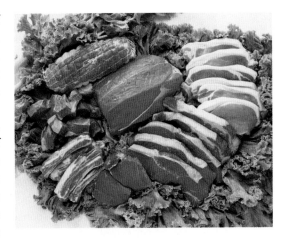

TABLE 12.6   FOOD SOURCES OF IRON

Food	Serving size[1]	mg of iron per serve[2]
Grilled lamb liver	65 g	7.25
Grilled beef rump steak (fully trimmed)	65–130 g	2.11–4.22
Roast leg lamb (fully trimmed)	65–130 g	1.61–3.22
Poached egg(s)	2 large eggs (120 g)	2.4
Roast leg pork	65–130 g	0.89–1.78
Grilled chicken breast (no skin)	65–130 g	0.26–0.52
English spinach (boiled, drained)	75 g	2.93
Dried apricots	30 g	0.93
Breakfast cereals fortified with iron	30 g	1.24–5.09

[1]Based on the Australian Dietary Guidelines [42].
[2]Calculated from Food Standards Australia New Zealand (2012). *NUTTAB 2010*. Canberra: FSANZ.

TRY IT YOURSELF

Identify the main sources of iron in your diet. How could you ensure adequate intakes of iron in an average week?

LINDA TAPSELL AND KAREN CHARLTON

≫ RESEARCH AT WORK

STUDIES OF FOODS AND IRON STATUS

Despite recent reductions in prevalence, iron deficiency anaemia (IDA) remains a global public health issue [43]. It is still commonly seen in women, and children and people consuming vegetarian diets [44]. Some of the research is outlined below.

1   Level of tannins in foods and iron absorption [45]
   • One of the food-related problems in IDA is that major plant-food sources of iron, such as sorghum, contain tannins that may lower iron availability, but the extent to which this occurs for individuals needs to be examined. In this small crossover experimental trial, researchers in the United States examined the dose response to tannin supplementation on iron bioavailability and status in a small sample of female volunteers. They also examined the effect of salivary proteins and the role of the level of astringency on responses. The results indicated a degree of responsiveness to tannin supplementation, such that iron bioavailability and status did not appear impaired but rather enzyme production was stimulated and sensations of astringency became reduced over time. This novel exploratory research suggested the need to better understand individual responses to tannins in food and questioned the general assumption that tannins need to be removed to improve iron bioavailability in this population.

2   Iron biofortified beans and cognitive performance [46]
   • Women of reproductive age are at risk of IDA, which can manifest itself in impaired cognitive performance by disrupting brain energy metabolism or neurotransmitter regulation. In this double blind trial (registered with clinicaltrials.gov NCT01594359), n = 150 low iron status women in Rwanda aged 18–27 years were randomly allocated to receive control beans (50 mg Fe ppm) or iron biofortified beans (86 mg Fe ppm) for 18 weeks. Cognitive performance, in particular efficacy of search and speed of retrieval in memory tasks, improved more in those receiving the biofortified beans.

Appreciating the food sources of iron is only one step in ensuring adequate iron intakes in any given population. The need for iron-rich or -enriched foods can be well demonstrated, but even when they are readily available, consumption is not always assured. Reasons may centre on food security, frailty and cultural eating patterns. Clinical conditions such as haemochromatosis and renal disease may also need to be considered. In addition, individual responsiveness and dietary requirements may vary. At various levels of public health, clinical nutrition, and food production and distribution at the global level, iron remains an important and challenging nutrient within research and practice.

≫ CASE 12.5

IRON SUPPLEMENTATION IN POPULATIONS AT RISK

Given the prevalence of iron deficiency, supplemental programs such as micronutrient powder programs (MNPs) have been provided in at-risk communities for some time, but they rely on ongoing research and evaluation to inform practice. Researchers from Kenya have argued that providing home iron fortification for complementary foods targeting young children was not efficacious enough [47], but a commentary suggests that iron EDTA may be required to improve effectiveness. In addition, the supplementation of iron should not be occurring in isolation from other related strategies, such as improving water and sanitation and including anti-infective treatments [48].

On the other hand, groups such as the Global Alliance for Improved Nutrition are engaged in studies that identify factors that affect adherence to recommendations on point of use fortification of MNPs [49]. They have found that cultural–ecological perspectives should be brought into programs so that evaluations are broadened beyond biological outcomes.

Another supplemental strategy is the use of fortified blended foods (FBFs) based on micronutrient fortified blends of milled cereals and pulses, such as corn, soybean, sorghum and cowpea. The Micronutrient Fortified Food Aid Pilot Project (MFFAPP) in Tanzania is conducting an efficacy study to provide information on the viability of extruded products from these foods to improve nutrition in children aged 6–53 months in the Mara region. The published study protocol provides a useful overview of the conditions and parameters that can be considered in these interventions [50].

- What issues has research exposed for supplementation programs in developing countries to address micronutrient deficiencies?
- How is the scientific understanding of iron metabolism integrated into these programs and related research?
- How can the broad social and environmental platform on which these interventions are based be described?

STOP AND THINK

- Which iron-rich foods would require particular attention for different subgroups within the population and why?
- How do iron-rich foods fit within a healthy dietary pattern for the general population?
- What contribution could new food product development make in improving iron nutrition in the population?

WHAT IS THE STRUCTURE AND FUNCTION OF ZINC WITH SIGNIFICANT IMPLICATIONS FOR NUTRITION?

Zinc (Zn) is a metallic trace element (atomic number 30) also taken up into the food chain through its origins in the earth. Zinc deficiency can occur in populations relying on grains grown in zinc-deficient soil. Its essentiality in the diet is related to its functions concerning insulin production and insulin action as well as membrane function. It also has antioxidant properties [51]. The main site of uptake is the duodenum and zinc can be lost to the body in the intestine, through renal mechanisms or via the skin. Zinc is stored throughout the body—for example, in muscles and bones.

Early reports of zinc deficiency occurred in cases where dietary intakes were limited to a few foods such as bread, potatoes and milk, or bread and beans [52]. In one report, the main symptoms were defined as growth retardation and hypogonadism that responded to zinc therapy, beyond that achieved by improving the quality of the diet and concurrent iron insufficiency commonly seen with the condition [53]. The problems with achieving adequate zinc in the diet are similar to that of iron, with benefits from consuming animal foods and limited bioavailability plant foods due to phytates. Unlike iron, however, zinc is ubiquitous in cells as it is a regular component of enzyme systems, so the physiological processes linked to zinc are more difficult to define.

During digestion, zinc emerges as free ions, which become bound following uptake by the cells in the gut that are transported to the liver. The degree of absorption appears to be linked to the zinc status of the individual, with homeostatic mechanisms working towards maintaining normal levels. Zinc is mainly found in tissue, but when transported to tissues it is bound to albumin.

Minerals such as zinc are nutrients for plants as they are for humans. Phytic acid in plants that bind zinc (and other nutrients), creating problems for humans, appears to have a role in storing minerals for plants [54]. This demonstrates how nutrients do not exist naturally in isolation, and their 'packaging' reflects the biological context in which they operate. There are also implications for food processing to improve nutrient accessibility. Given issues of bioavailability, there has been some concern as to whether other minerals, such as calcium and iron, may interfere with zinc absorption, but studies suggest this is not the case. However, zinc absorption appears to be enhanced with the consumption of animal-protein-rich foods such as meat and this may have to do with the amino acid environment [52]. Further research in this area will help to determine which foods (and food combinations) may be best to develop for communities at risk of zinc deficiency.

Adequate zinc intakes are clearly required for growth, so intakes are particularly important for pregnant and breastfeeding women, children and adolescents. Zinc nutrition is also important in old age when decreased ability to absorb nutrients may occur, and in places where diarrhoeal disease is prevalent. In the latter case, immune function may be impaired due to zinc insufficiency [52]. Zinc status is measured by blood plasma or serum levels, although variations can occur for a number of reasons.

STOP AND THINK

- What are the similarities and differences between the physiological positions of iron and zinc in human nutrition?
- Why would it be difficult to differentiate the symptoms of zinc deficiency?
- Which particular groups in the population are at risk of zinc insufficiency, and why?

WHICH DIETARY SOURCES SUPPORT AN ADEQUATE INTAKE OF ZINC TO MEET NUTRITIONAL REQUIREMENTS?

Requirements for zinc are outlined in Table 12.7. Requirements may be higher if diets are limited to certain types of plants, as bioavailability can limit the relationship between the amount if zinc present in the food and the amount that makes it through to the body's system.

As zinc has such a ubiquitous biological role, it is found in a wide range of foods, but in greater amounts in red meat and shellfish, particularly oysters. Smaller amounts are provided in grains, cereals, pulses, legumes, dairy products, nuts and seeds. Like iron, the bioavailability of zinc from plant foods is protected by other plant components. Zinc bioavailability may be improved with certain preparation techniques that reduce binding by plant components [55]. Requirements are, however, met with food intake patterns aligned with the Australian Dietary Guidelines [42].

TABLE 12.7   RECOMMENDED DIETARY INTAKE FOR ZINC

Gender/age	RDI
Men >19 years old	14 mg/day
Adolescent males 14–18 years	13 mg/day
Women >19 years old	8 mg/day
Adolescent females 14–18 years	7 mg/day

Source: National Health and Medical Research Council (2014). *Nutrient Reference Values for Australia and New Zealand—Iodine*. Canberra: NHMRC. © Commonwealth of Australia

TABLE 12.8   ZINC CONTENT OF FOODS

Food	Serving size[1]	mg of zinc per serve[3]
Oyster, raw	65–100 g (6 oysters ~90 g)	31.13–47.89
Oyster, smoked, canned in oil and drained	65–100 g	9.55–14.7
Beef rump steak, trimmed, grilled	65–130 g	5.239–10.48
Pumpkin seeds (hulled, dried)	30 g[2]	2.238

[1] Based on the Australian Dietary Guidelines [42]
[2] Based on modelling of the Australian Dietary Guidelines [56]
[3] Calculated from Food Standards Australia New Zealand (2012). *NUTTAB 2010*. Canberra: FSANZ.

TRY IT YOURSELF

Identify the major sources of zinc in your diet. How could you improve your intake of zinc and other essential minerals in the diet?

>> RESEARCH AT WORK

ZINC AND IRON STATUS IN OLDER PEOPLE

Older adults can experience decreased nutrient absorption due to age-related conditions [6]. Vegetarian-style eating patterns, characterised by the minimal consumption of meat, a major source of bioavailable iron and zinc, may add to this problem. With this in mind, researchers reviewed the literature to compare the zinc and iron status of elderly people consuming a vegetarian versus meat-containing diet. A previous systematic review and meta-analysis [57] showed evidence of lower zinc concentrations in vegetarians compared with non-vegetarians, but few studies looked at this in older people. In fact, the problem appeared to be more that older people, especially those in institutions, tended to have lower serum zinc levels. There were few studies that reported on these comparisons for iron so it was not possible to draw conclusions with confidence. Dietary data was limited and most studies did not report on biomarkers of iron status. Nevertheless, ensuring adequate zinc and iron intakes in older people presents with challenges for the types of foods made available to them. Supplements may be necessary, but the authors also noted that iron supplements should be used with caution in this age group because of the side effect of constipation.

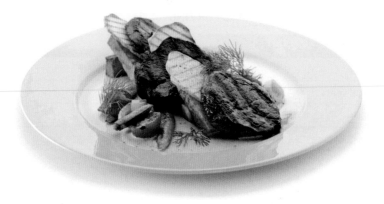

STOP AND THINK

- How can an adequate intake of zinc be assured in the current Australian diet?
- Which groups are most at risk of not consuming adequate amounts of zinc?
- Which food reparation techniques would increase bioavailability of zinc?

SUMMARY

- Iodine is an essential mineral required for thyroid hormone production, brain development in the foetus and neurocognitive development in children.
- Universal salt iodisation is a global strategy to combat widespread iodine deficiencies; in Australia, all salt used in bread-making is required by law to contain iodine, whereas pregnant and lactating women require iodine supplements to meet the increased needs of themselves and their babies.
- Fluoride is a trace mineral that helps with the prevention of tooth decay. The dietary delivery of fluoride is mainly through water fluoridation programs.
- Iron is essential for the development of red blood cells and the supply of oxygen to cells. Haem iron, found in meat flesh, is more bioavailable than iron contained in plant foods.
- Zinc is essential for the functioning of multiple enzyme and other cell systems throughout the body. It is found in varying quantities in a wide range of foods with meat and shellfish containing considerable amounts.
- Science has exposed the need for key minerals in the diet by observations of deficiency states and an understanding of the link between foods and nutritional status
- Mineral deficiency states also reflect ecological conditions; minerals are present in soils and are taken up by plants which form part of the food chain.
- Micronutrient deficiency is a risk in both developed and developing countries, and at-risk groups are readily identifiable.
- Addressing adequate intakes of micronutrients in the population may include the development and distribution of fortified food products, supplemental programs, and programs for nutritional food services, community nutrition education and community development.

PATHWAYS TO PRACTICE

- Severe micronutrient deficiencies can have significant health effects, such as mental retardation and cretinism in the case of iodine deficiency and reduced cognitive development in the case of iron deficiency. Awareness of the importance of iodine and iron consumption, particularly during pregnancy, is an issue for a range of health professionals.
- In order to prevent deficits and support functionality in children, and older adults in particular, it is essential to eradicate micronutrient deficiency on a population level through fortification of the food supply. Nutritionists working within the food industry and in developing countries can play a significant role in enabling requirements for food fortification, nutrition education and community development programs.
- Risk of both inadequate and excess micronutrient intakes requires regular monitoring to accompany fortification programs as well as strategies to address subpopulations at risk. Skills in nutritional epidemiology can be applied in public health roles involving monitoring and surveillance of iodine status in the population.

DISCUSSION QUESTIONS

1   What do health practitioners, governments and the food sector need to know about the key minerals iodine, fluoride, iron and zinc in order to appreciate their necessity in foods?
2   What are the public health strategies for addressing adequate population intakes of iodine, fluoride, iron and zinc in Australia. Why is each strategy different?
3   What are the implications for the development of the food supply of achieving adequate micronutrient intake in the population?
4   How can knowledge of micronutrient homeostasis be applied in clinical practice, particularly in groups at risk of malnutrition and/or malabsorption?

USEFUL WEBLINKS

Australian Dietary Guidelines:
www.eatforhealth.gov.au

Australian Health Survey 2011–12—Essential minerals:
www.abs.gov.au/ausstats/abs@.nsf/Lookup/by%20Subject/4364.0.55.008~2011-12~Main%20Features~Essential%20minerals~400

Australian Health Survey 2011–12—Iodine:
www.abs.gov.au/ausstats/abs@.nsf/Lookup/4364.0.55.006Chapter1202011-12

Centers for Disease Control and Prevention—Community water fluoridation:
www.cdc.gov/fluoridation/index.html

Food Standards Australia New Zealand—AUSNUT 2011–13 food nutrient database:
www.foodstandards.gov.au/science/monitoringnutrients/ausnut/ausnutdatafiles/Pages/foodnutrient.aspx

Food Standards Australia New Zealand—Iodine fortification:
www.foodstandards.gov.au/consumer/nutrition/iodinefort/pages/default.aspx

HealthDirect—Health topics:
www.healthdirect.gov.au/health-topics

National Health Medical Research Council—Water Fluoridation and human health in Australia:
www.nhmrc.gov.au/health-topics/health-effects-water-fluoridation

New South Wales Health—Water fluoridation: questions and answers:
www.health.nsw.gov.au/environment/water/Documents/fluoridation-questions-and-answers-nsw.pdf

Nutrient Reference Values for Australia and New Zealand—Nutrients:
www.nrv.gov.au/nutrients

World Health Organization—Anaemia:
www.who.int/topics/anaemia/en

World Health Organization—Inadequate or excess fluoride:
www.who.int/ipcs/assessment/public_health/fluoride/en

FURTHER READING

Agrawal, S., Berggren, K. L., Marks, E. & Fox, J. H. (2017). Impact of high iron intake on cognition and neurodegeneration in humans and in animal models: a systematic review. *Nutrition Reviews*, 75(6), 456–70. doi:10.1093/nutrit/nux015

Anderson, G. J. & Frazer, D. M. (2017). Current understanding of iron homeostasis. *American Journal of Clinical Nutrition*, 106(Suppl.6), 1559S–1566S. doi:10.3945/ajcn.117.155804

Brough, L. (2017). Global iodine status has improved: but we must not be complacent. *British Journal of Nutrition*, 117(3), 439–40. doi:10.1017/S0007114517000113

Carriquiry, A. L., Spungen, J. H., Murphy, S. P., Pehrsson, P. R., Dwyer, J. T., Juan, W. & Wirtz, M. S. (2016). Variation in the iodine concentrations of foods: considerations for dietary assessment. *American Journal of Clinical Nutrition*, 104(Suppl.3), 877S–887S. doi:10.3945/ajcn.115.110353

Ershow, A. G., Goodman, G., Coates, P. M. & Swanson, C. A. (2016). Research needs for assessing iodine intake, iodine status, and the effects of maternal iodine supplementation. *American Journal of Clinical Nutrition*, 104(Suppl.3), 941S–949S. doi:10.3945/ajcn.116.134858

Frazer, D. M. & Anderson, G. J. (2017). Is there a better way to set population iron recommendations? *American Journal of Clinical Nutrition*, 105(6), 1255–6. doi:10.3945/ajcn.117.158188

Georgieff, M. K. (2017). Iron assessment to protect the developing brain. *American Journal of Clinical Nutrition*, 106(Suppl.6), 1588S–1593S. doi:10.3945/ajcn.117.155846

Gordeuk, V. R. & Brannon, P. M. (2017). Ethnic and genetic factors of iron status in women of reproductive age. *American Journal of Clinical Nutrition*, 106(Suppl.6), 1594S–1599S. doi:10.3945/ajcn.117.155853

Hoofnagle, A. N. (2017). Harmonization of blood-based indicators of iron status: making the hard work matter. *American Journal of Clinical Nutrition*, 106(Suppl.6), 1615S–1619S. doi:10.3945/ajcn.117.155895

Huynh, D., Condo, D., Gibson, R., Makrides, M., Muhlhausler, B. & Zhou, S. J. (2017). Comparison of breast-milk iodine concentration of lactating women in Australia pre and post mandatory iodine fortification. *Public Health Nutrition*, 20(1), 12–17. doi:10.1017/S1368980016002032

Huynh, D., Condo, D., Gibson, R., Muhlhausler, B., Ryan, P., Skeaff, S., ... Zhou, S. J. (2017). Iodine status of postpartum women and their infants in Australia after the introduction of mandatory iodine fortification. *British Journal of Nutrition*, 117(12), 1656–62. doi:10.1017/S0007114517001775

Juan, W., Trumbo, P. R., Spungen, J. H., Dwyer, J. T., Carriquiry, A. L., Zimmerman, T. P., ... Murphy, S. P. (2016). Comparison of 2 methods for estimating the prevalences of inadequate and excessive iodine intakes. *American Journal of Clinical Nutrition*, 104(Suppl.3), 888S–897S. doi:10.3945/ajcn.115.110346

Knez, M., Nikolic, M., Zekovic, M., Stangoulis, J. C., Gurinovic, M. & Glibetic, M. (2017). The influence of food consumption and socio-economic factors on the relationship between zinc and iron intake and status in a healthy population. *Public Health Nutrition*, 20(14), 2486–98. doi:10.1017/S1368980017001240

Long, S. E., Catron, B. L., Boggs, A. S., Tai, S. S. & Wise, S. A. (2016). Development of Standard Reference Materials to support assessment of iodine status for nutritional and public health purposes. *American Journal of Clinical Nutrition*, 104(Suppl.3), 902S–906S. doi:10.3945/ajcn.115.110361

Low, M. S.Y., Speedy, J., Styles, C. E., De-Regil, L. M. & Pasricha, S. R. (2016). Daily iron supplementation for improving anaemia, iron status and health in menstruating women. *Cochrane Database of Systematic Reviews*, (4). doi:10.1002/14651858.CD009747.pub2

O'Brien, K. O. & Ru, Y. (2017). Iron status of North American pregnant women: an update on longitudinal data and gaps in knowledge from the United States and Canada. *American Journal of Clinical Nutrition*. doi:10.3945/ajcn.117.155986

O'Kane, S. M., Pourshahidi, L. K., Farren, K. M., Mulhern, M. S., Strain, J. J. &.Yeates, A. J (2016). Iodine knowledge is positively associated with dietary iodine intake among women of childbearing age in the UK and Ireland. *British Journal of Nutrition*, 116(10), 1728–35. doi:10.1017/S0007114516003925

Pearce, E. N. & Caldwell, K. L. (2016). Urinary iodine, thyroid function, and thyroglobulin as biomarkers of iodine status. *American Journal of Clinical Nutrition*, 104(Suppl.3), 898S–901S. doi:10.3945/ajcn.115.110395

Pearce, E. N., Lazarus, J. H., Moreno-Reyes, R. & Zimmermann, M. B. (2016). Consequences of iodine deficiency and excess in pregnant women: an overview of current knowns and unknowns. *American Journal of Clinical Nutrition*, 104(Suppl.3), 918S–923S. doi:10.3945/ajcn.115.110429

Pehrsson, P. R., Patterson, K. Y., Spungen, J. H., Wirtz, M. S., Andrews, K. W., Dwyer, J. T. & Swanson, C. A. (2016). Iodine in food- and dietary supplement-composition databases. *American Journal of Clinical Nutrition*, 104, 868S–876S. doi:10.3945/ajcn.115.110064

Prentice, A. M., Mendoza, Y. A., Pereira, D., Cerami, C., Wegmuller, R., Constable, A. & Spieldenner, J. (2017). Dietary strategies for improving iron status: balancing safety and efficacy. *Nutrition Reviews*, 75(1), 49–60. doi:10.1093/nutrit/nuw055

Ru, Y., Pressman, E. K., Cooper, E. M., Guillet, R., Katzman, P. J., Kent, T. R., ... O'Brien, K. O. (2016). Iron deficiency and anemia are prevalent in women with multiple gestations. *American Journal of Clinical Nutrition*, 104(4), 1052–60. doi:10.3945/ajcn.115.126284

Trumbo, P. R. (2016). FDA regulations regarding iodine addition to foods and labeling of foods containing added iodine. *American Journal of Clinical Nutrition*, 104(Suppl.3), 864S–867S. doi:10.3945/ajcn.115.110338

Wessling-Resnick, M. (2017). Excess iron: considerations related to development and early growth. *American Journal of Clinical Nutrition*, 106(Suppl.6), 1600S–1605S. doi:10.3945/ajcn.117.155879

Yokoi, K. & Konomi, A. (2017). Iron deficiency without anaemia is a potential cause of fatigue: meta-analyses of randomised controlled trials and cross-sectional studies. *British Journal of Nutrition*, 117(10), 1422–31. doi:10.1017/S0007114517001349

Zhang, C. & Rawal, S. (2017). Dietary iron intake, iron status, and gestational diabetes. *American Journal of Clinical Nutrition*, 106(Suppl.6), 1672S–1680S. doi:10.3945/ajcn.117.156034

REFERENCES

1   K. J. Carpenter (2005). David Marine and the problem of goiter. *Journal of Nutrition*, 135(4), 675–80.

2   J. A. Seal, Z. Doyle, J. R. Burgess, R. Taylor & A. R. Cameron (2007). Iodine status of Tasmanians following voluntary fortification of bread with iodine. *Medical Journal of Australia*, 186(2), 69–71.

3   J. R. Burgess, J. A. Seal, G. M. Stilwell, P. J. Reynolds, E. R. Taylor & V. Parameswaran (2007). A case for universal salt iodisation to correct iodine deficiency in pregnancy: another salutary lesson from Tasmania. *Medical Journal of Australia*, 186(11), 574–6.

4   Australian Bureau of Statistics (2015). *Australian Health Survey: First results, 2011–12*. Canberra: ABS.

5   S. Y. Hess (2017). National risk of zinc deficiency as estimated by national surveys. *Food and Nutrition Bulletin*, 38(1), 3–17. doi:10.1177/0379572116689000

6   M. Foster, A. Chu & S. Samman (2017). Vegetarian nutrition for the older adult: vitamin B12, iron, and zinc. *Current Nutrition Reports*, 6(2), 80–92. doi:10.1007/s13668-017-0194-x

7   World Health Organization (2007). *Assessment of Iodine Deficiency Disorders and Monitoring Their Elimination: A guide for programme managers*, 3rd edn. Geneva: WHO.

8   R. C. Gordon, M. C. Rose, S. A. Skeaff, A. R. Gray, K. M. Morgan & T. Ruffman (2009). Iodine supplementation improves cognition in mildly iodine-deficient children. *American Journal of Clinical Nutrition*, 90(5), 1264–71. doi:10.3945/ajcn.2009.28145

9   L. Patrick (2008). Iodine: deficiency and therapeutic considerations. *Alternative Medicine Review*, 13(2), 116.

10 Z. F. Ma & S. A. Skeaff (2014). Thyroglobulin as a biomarker of iodine deficiency: a review. *Thyroid*, 24(8), 1195–209. doi:10.1089/thy.2014.0052

11 The Iodine Global Network (2016). Global Iodine Nutrition Scorecard 2016. Retrieved from: www.ign.org/cmdata/Scorecard_2016_SAC_PW.pdf. Zurich: The Iodine Global Network.

12 M. Gizak, J. Gorstein & M. Andersson (2017). Epidemiology of iodine deficiency. In E. Pearce (ed.), *Iodine Deficiency Disorders and Their Elimination*. Ebook; retrieved from: https://link.springer.com/book/10.1007/978-3-319-49505-7. Springer, p. 35.

13 M. Andersson, B. de Benoist, F. Delange & J. Zupan (2007). Prevention and control of iodine deficiency in pregnant and lactating women and in children less than 2-years-old: conclusions and recommendations of the technical consultation. *Public Health Nutrition*, 10(12A), 1606–11. doi:10.1017/S1368980007361004

14 European Commission/Scientific Committee on Food (2002). *Opinion of the Scientific Committee on Food on the Tolerable Upper Intake Level of Iodine (expressed in 7 October 2002)*. Brussels: European Commission/ Scientific Committee on Food.

15 Institute of Medicine (US) Panel on Micronutrients (2001). *Dietary Reference Intakes for Vitamin A, Vitamin K, Arsenic, Boron, Chromium, Copper, Iodine, Iron, Manganese, Molybdenum, Nickel, Silicon, Vanadium and Zinc*. Washington, DC: National Academies Press.

16 United Nations System & Standing Committee on Nutrition (SCN) News (2007). *Universal Salt Iodisation*. Sudbury, UK: Lavenham Press.

17 W. Charoensiriwatana, P. Srijantr, P. Teeyapant & J. Wongvilairattana (2010). Consuming iodine enriched eggs to solve the iodine deficiency endemic for remote areas in Thailand. *Nutrition Journal*, 9(1), 68. doi:10.1186/1475-2891-9-68

18 M. Eltom, B. Elnagar, E. A. Sulieman, F. A. Karlsson, H. V. Van Thi, P. Bourdoux & M. Gebre-Medhin (1995). The use of sugar as a vehicle for iodine fortification in endemic iodine deficiency. *International Journal of Food Sciences and Nutrition*, 46(3), 281–9. doi:10.3109/09637489509012560

19 B. Chanthilath, V. Chavasit, S. Chareonkiatkul & K. Judprasong (2009). Iodine stability and sensory quality of fermented fish and fish sauce produced with the use of iodated salt. *Food and Nutrition Bulletin*, 30(2), 183–8.

20 S. Squatrito, R. Vigneri, F. Runello, A. M. Ermans, R. D. Polley & S. H. Ingbar (1986). Prevention and treatment of endemic iodine-deficiency goiter by iodination of a municipal water supply. *Journal of Clinical Endocrinology and Metabolism*, 63(2), 368–75. doi:10.1210/jcem-63-2-368

21 M. B. Zimmermann, I. Aeberli, T. Torresani & H. Bürgi (2005). Increasing the iodine concentration in the Swiss iodized salt program markedly improved iodine status in pregnant women and children: a 5-y prospective national study. *American Journal of Clinical Nutrition*, 82(2), 388–92.

22 S.Y. Hess, M. B. Zimmermann, T. Torresani, H. Bürgi & R. F. Hurrell (2001). Monitoring the adequacy of salt iodization in Switzerland: a national study of school children and pregnant women. *European Journal of Clinical Nutrition*, 55(3), 162–6.

23 M. Andersson, I. Aeberli, N. Wüst, A. M. Piacenza, T. Bucher, I. Henschen, ... M. B. Zimmermann (2010). The Swiss iodized salt program provides adequate iodine for school children and pregnant women, but weaning infants not receiving iodine-containing complementary foods as well as their mothers are iodine deficient. *Journal of Clinical Endocrinology & Metabolism*, 95(12), 5217–24. doi:10.1210/jc.2010-0975

24 National Health and Medical Research Council (2010). *NHMRC Public Statement: Iodine supplementation for pregnant and breastfeeding women*. Canberra: NHMRC. Retrieved from: www.nhmrc.gov.au/guidelines-publications/new45.

25 Australian Health Ministers' Advisory Council (2012). *Clinical Practice Guidelines: Antenatal Care—Module 1*. Canberra: Australian Government Department of Health and Ageing. Retrieved from: www.health. gov.au/internet/main/publishing.nsf/Content/phd-antenatal-care-index/$File/ANC_Guidelines_Mod1_ v32.pdf.

26 K. Charlton, Y. Probst & G. Kiene (2016). Dietary iodine intake of the Australian population after introduction of a mandatory iodine fortification programme. *Nutrients*, 8(11), 701.

27 D. Kanduti, P. Sterbenk & B. Artnik (2016). Fluoride: a review of use and effects on health. *Materia Socio-Medica*, 28(2), 133–7. doi:10.5455/msm.2016.28.133-137

28 H. T. Dean (1934). Classification of mottled enamel diagnosis. *Journal of the American Dental Association (1922)*, 21(8), 1421–6. doi:https://doi.org/10.14219/jada.archive.1934.0220

29 H. T. Dean & E. Elias (1935). Studies on the minimal threshold of the dental sign of chronic endemic fluorosis (mottled enamel). *Public Health Reports (1896–1970)*, 50(49), 1719–29. doi:10.2307/4581707

30 H. T. Dean, J. Philip, F. A. Arnold, Jr & E. Elias (1941). Domestic water and dental caries: ii. a study of 2,832 white children, aged 12-14 years, of 8 suburban Chicago communities, including lactobacillus acidophilus studies of 1,761 children. *Public Health Reports (1896–1970)*, 56(15), 761–92. doi:10.2307/4583693

31 H. T. Dean, F. A. Arnold, Jr & E. Elias (1942). Domestic water and dental caries: v. additional studies of the relation of fluoride domestic waters to dental caries experience in 4,425 white children, aged 12 to 14 years, of 13 cities in 4 states. *Public Health Reports (1896–1970)*, 57(32), 1155–79. doi:10.2307/4584182

32 World Health Organization (2018). International Programme on Chemical Safety: Inadequate or excess fluoride. Retrieved from: www.who.int/ipcs/assessment/public_health/fluoride/en.

33 Division of Oral Health National Center for Chronic Disease Prevention and Health Promotion (2016). Community water fluoridation. Retrieved from: www.cdc.gov/fluoridation/index.html.

34 National Health and Medical Research Council (2017). *Public Statement 2017: Water fluoridation and human health*. Retrieved from: www.nhmrc.gov.au/health-topics/health-effects-water-fluoridation.

35 Department of Health (2015–17). *Methodological Framework for the Review of Nutrient Reference Values*. Canberra: Department of Health. Retrieved from: www.nrv.gov.au/file/methodological-framework-pdf-705kb.

36 NSW Health (2015). *Water Fluoridation: Questions and answers*. Sydney: NSW Health. Retrieved from: www.health.nsw.gov.au/environment/water/Documents/fluoridation-questions-and-answers-nsw.pdf.

37 V. Sangkhae & E. Nemeth (2017). Regulation of the iron homeostatic hormone hepcidin. *Advances in Nutrition: An International Review Journal*, 8(1), 126–36. doi:10.3945/an.116.013961

38 A. Lopez, P. Cacoub, I. C. MacDougall & L. Peyrin-Biroulet (2016). Iron deficiency anaemia. *The Lancet*, 387(10021), 907–16. doi:https://doi.org/10.1016/S0140-6736(15)60865-0

39 K. Schümann & N. W. Solomons (2017). Perspective: what makes it so difficult to mitigate worldwide anemia prevalence? *Advances in Nutrition: An International Review Journal*, 8(3), 401–8. doi:10.3945/an.116.013847

40 R. F. Hurrell, M. B. Reddy, J. Burri & J. D. Cook (2002). Phytate degradation determines the effect of industrial processing and home cooking on iron absorption from cereal-based foods. *British Journal of Nutrition*, 88(2), 117–23. doi:10.1079/BJN2002594

41 U. Schlemmer, W. Frølich, R. M. Prieto & F. Grases (2009). Phytate in foods and significance for humans: food sources, intake, processing, bioavailability, protective role and analysis. *Molecular Nutrition & Food Research*, 53(S2), S330–S375. doi:10.1002/mnfr.200900099

42 National Health and Medical Research Council (2013). *Australian Dietary Guidelines*. Canberra: NHMRC.

43 G. A. Stevens, M. M. Finucane, L. M. De-Regil, C. J. Paciorek, S. R. Flaxman, F. Branca, … M. Ezzati (2013). Global, regional, and national trends in haemoglobin concentration and prevalence of total and severe anaemia in children and pregnant and non-pregnant women for 1995–2011: a systematic analysis of population-representative data. *The Lancet Global Health*, 1(1), e16–e25. doi:https://doi.org/10.1016/S2214-109X(13)70001-9

44 C. Camaschella (2015). Iron-deficiency anemia. *New England Journal of Medicine*, 372(19), 1832–43. doi:10.1056/NEJMra1401038

45 N. M. Delimont, N. M. Fiorentino, K. A. Kimmel, M. D. Haub, S. K. Rosenkranz & B. L. Lindshield (2017). Long-term dose-response condensed tannin supplementation does not affect iron status or bioavailability. *Current Developments in Nutrition*, 1(10). doi:10.3945/cdn.117.001081

46 L. E. Murray-Kolb, M. J. Wenger, S. P. Scott, S. E. Rhoten, M. G. Lung'aho & J. D. Haas (2017). Consumption of iron-biofortified beans positively affects cognitive performance in 18- to 27-year-old Rwandan female college students in an 18-week randomized controlled efficacy trial. *Journal of Nutrition*, 147(11), 2109–17. doi:10.3945/jn.117.255356

47 E. M. Teshome, P. E. A. Andang'o, V. Osoti, S. R. Terwel, W. Otieno, A. Y. Demir, ... H. Verhoef (2017). Daily home fortification with iron as ferrous fumarate versus NaFeEDTA: a randomised, placebo-controlled, non-inferiority trial in Kenyan children. *BMC Medicine*, 15(1), 89. doi:10.1186/s12916-017-0839-z

48 F. T. Wieringa (2017). Micronutrient powders to combat anemia in young children: does it work? *BMC Medicine*, 15(1), 99. doi:10.1186/s12916-017-0867-8

49 A. Tumilowicz, C. H. Schnefke, L. M. Neufeld & G. H. Pelto (2017). Toward a better understanding of adherence to micronutrient powders: generating theories to guide program design and evaluation based on a review of published results. *Current Developments in Nutrition*, 1(6). doi:10.3945/cdn.117.001123

50 N. M. Delimont, S. Chanadang, M. V. Joseph, B. E. Rockler, Q. Guo, G. K. Regier, ... B. L. Lindshield (2017). The MFFAPP Tanzania Efficacy Study Protocol: newly formulated, extruded, fortified blended foods for food aid. *Current Developments in Nutrition*, 1(5), e000315. https://doi.org/10.3945/cdn.116.000315

51 W. Maret (2013). Zinc biochemistry: from a single zinc enzyme to a key element of life. *Advances in Nutrition: An International Review Journal*, 4(1), 82–91. doi:10.3945/an.112.003038

52 N. Roohani, R. Hurrell, R. Kelishadi & R. Schulin (2013). Zinc and its importance for human health: an integrative review. *Journal of Research in Medical Sciences: The Official Journal of Isfahan University of Medical Sciences*, 18(2), 144–57.

53 H. H. Sandstead, A. S. Prasad, A. R. Schulert, Z. Farid, A. Miale Jr, S. Bassilly & W. J. Darby (1967). Human zinc deficiency, endocrine manifestations and response to treatment. *American Journal of Clinical Nutrition*, 20(5), 422–42.

54 H. W. Lopez, F. Leenhardt, C. Coudray & C. Remesy (2002). Minerals and phytic acid interactions: is it a real problem for human nutrition? *International Journal of Food Science & Technology*, 37(7), 727–39. doi:10.1046/j.1365-2621.2002.00618.x

55 R. S. Gibson, L. Perlas & C. Hotz (2006). Improving the bioavailability of nutrients in plant foods at the household level. *Proceedings of the Nutrition Society*, 65(2), 160–8. doi:10.1079/PNS2006489

56 National Health and Medical Research Council (2011). *A Modelling System to Inform the Revision of the Australian Guide to Healthy Eating*. Canberra: NHMRC.

57 M. Foster, A. Chu, P. Petocz & S. Samman (2013). Effect of vegetarian diets on zinc status: a systematic review and meta-analysis of studies in humans. *Journal of the Science of Food and Agriculture*, 93(10), 2362–71. doi:10.1002/jsfa.6179

58 Australian Government Department of Health and New Zealand Ministry of Health. Australian and New Zealand Nutrient Reference Values for Fluoride. Commonwealth of Australia as represented by the Department of Health. Available from www.nrv.gov.au/sites/default/files/content/resources/2017%20 NRV%20Fluoride%20Report.pdf.

PART 2

NUTRITION, SOCIETY AND THE HUMAN LIFECYCLE

2

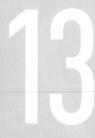

CHAPTER 13

NUTRITION FOR EXERCISE AND SPORT

MICHAEL LEVERITT

CHAPTER OBJECTIVES

This chapter will enable the reader to:

- briefly describe the role of physical activity and exercise in improving health
- describe the current recommendations for the intake of specific nutrients for exercising individuals and athletes
- identify how exercise performance and adaptations to training can be enhanced through carefully developed nutrition strategies
- discuss the influence of fluid intake, hydration status and ergogenic aids on sport and exercise performance.

KEY TERMS

Ergogenic aids	Hydration	Sports foods
Exercise	Physical activity	Training adaptation

KEY POINTS

- Exercise training and competition can increase the requirement for specific nutrients in order to promote optimal training adaptation, recovery, body composition and performance.
- Carbohydrate is the predominant fuel for high-intensity exercise and the consumption of carbohydrate during exercise is likely to enhance performance due to a variety of mechanisms; however, training with reduced carbohydrate availability can enhance the changes in the muscle in response to training.
- The amount, type and timing of protein intake can influence muscle protein synthesis after exercise. Immediate ingestion of 20–25 g of protein that is rapidly absorbed, contains all essential amino acids and is high in the amino acid leucine is best for stimulating protein synthesis after exercise.
- Adaptation to several weeks of a very high-fat diet enables individuals to use more fat as a fuel during exercise and this may benefit athletes involved in long duration events lasting several hours.
- Nutrient requirements for athletes and exercising individuals change frequently and sports nutrition strategies should be personalised to meet the specific training and performance goals of each athlete at any given point in time.

INTRODUCTION

Physical activity and exercise are important components of a healthy lifestyle. This chapter will briefly explore the relationship between physical activity and health, then discuss how exercise can increase the requirements for certain nutrients, in addition to providing recommendations about specific nutrition strategies that can enhance exercise performance. When reading this chapter, it is important to keep in mind that the amount of physical activity, exercise and sport undertaken by different individuals can vary significantly. Relatively modest amounts of physical activity can confer significant health benefits, whereas a large amount of exercise training might be required to achieve optimal performance in a sport. Therefore, the nutrition requirements for individuals involved in exercise and sport will vary considerably and are likely to be different depending on their goals. It is becoming increasingly clear that there is no one-size-fits-all approach to nutrition for exercise and sport. Instead, there are now broad guidelines developed for the intake of different nutrients, but these guidelines can be adapted to suit the specific needs of an individual depending on their level of physical activity and fitness, and the goals of their exercise training program. Given that athletes tend to be highly talented, trained and motivated individuals, understanding nutrition for exercise and sport may provide the vital ingredients for success.

STOP AND THINK

- What is the difference between physical activity and sport?
- How might physical activity influence requirements for nutrients?
- Why would sports nutrition be a specialty area in nutrition?

HOW DO PHYSICAL ACTIVITY AND EXERCISE INFLUENCE HEALTH?

Increasing physical activity and reducing sedentary behaviour can result in significant health benefits [1]. Individuals who are physically active have a reduced risk of developing cardiovascular disease (Figure 13.1), diabetes and cancer; and physically active people have a significantly reduced risk of early death from all causes. Physical activity can also benefit mental health and assist in reducing the progression of many chronic diseases in individuals who have already been diagnosed with disease.

While the health benefits of physical activity are universally acknowledged, it is important to recognise the subtle differences between physical activity, exercise and physical fitness. **Physical activity** refers to any bodily movement produced by skeletal muscles that requires energy expenditure. Physical activity can therefore be undertaken in many different domains or contexts, including: occupational physical activity; activities of daily living such as domestic activities and active commuting; and leisure time activity that includes recreational activities, exercise and sport. **Exercise** refers to physical activity that is planned, structured, repetitive and usually designed to enhance physical fitness. **Physical fitness** refers to the capacity to function effectively in activities of daily living, work, leisure or sport without undue fatigue. These definitions highlight that physical activity is a much broader term, encompassing many more activities than just exercise, whereas physical fitness refers to a capacity to perform certain tasks rather than describing a specific behaviour or activity. Interestingly, somewhat independent associations have been found

Physical activity
movement of skeletal muscles requiring energy expenditure.

Exercise
planned, structured repetitive actions designed to enhance physical fitness.

Physical fitness
capacity to undertake daily activity without undue fatigue.

FIGURE 13.1   MECHANISMS FOR INFLUENCE OF PHYSICAL ACTIVITY ON CARDIOVASCULAR DISEASES RISK

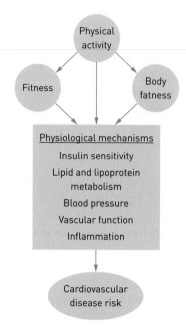

Source: J. M. R. Gill & D. Malkova (2006). Physical activity, fitness and cardiovascular disease risk in adults: interactions with insulin resistance and obesity. *Clinical Science*, 110(4), 409–25. doi:10.1042/cs20050207 (Figure 2)

between health and each of physical activity, vigorous exercise, physical fitness and also time spent in sedentary activities such as prolonged sitting [2]. Therefore, it is possible that physical activity, exercise and physical fitness each contribute to enhanced health in slightly different ways and it is important to be physically active, increase physical fitness through more vigorous exercise and reduce time spent in sedentary activities for the best overall improvements in health.

Increased physical activity and increased physical fitness are associated with health benefits that are also independent from overweight and obesity [3]. This means that overweight and obese individuals can significantly improve their health by increasing physical activity and physical fitness even if their weight does not change. This might be due to the effect of physical activity, particularly higher-intensity exercise on many metabolic pathways in the body that benefit health, but do not necessarily result in creating a sustained energy deficit that is required to reduce body weight over a long period of time. For example, exercise training causes a reduction in visceral fat, which is the fat around major organs that is capable of provoking inflammatory responses that initiate disease processes (Figure 13.2). However, overall body weight change after exercise training is usually modest, unless there is concurrent dietary energy restriction. Therefore, it is important to promote and encourage physical activity for improved health in all individuals, regardless of body weight.

Determining the exact amount of physical activity to recommend for optimal health benefits is difficult and complex. It is clear that the health benefits of physical activity occur over long periods of time and much of our understanding of these benefits comes from cohort studies in which it is difficult to specifically control variables like the intensity and duration of exercise (Table 13.1). Nevertheless, it appears that there is a dose–response relationship between the amount of physical activity and the

FIGURE 13.2 PHYSICAL INACTIVITY AND ABDOMINAL ADIPOSITY

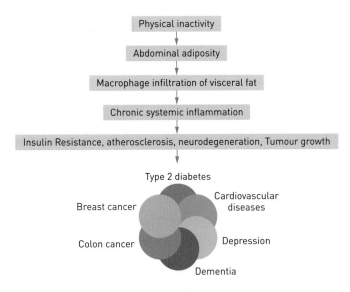

Source: B. Pedersen (2009). The diseasome of physical inactivity—and the role of myokines in muscle—fat cross talk. *Journal of Physiology*, 587(23), 5559–68. doi:10.1113/jphysiol.2009.179515

TABLE 13.1 RECOMMENDED COMPONENTS OF WEEKLY EXERCISE AND ACTIVITY FOR HEALTH

Component	Recommendation
Physical activity	150–300 minutes moderate intensity or 75–50 minutes vigorous intensity
Muscle strengthening	Undertaken on at least 2 days
Sedentariness (e.g. prolonged sitting)	Minimise time spent and break up as often as possible

Source: Department of Health (2017). *Australia's Physical Activity & Sedentary Behaviour Guidelines for Adults (18–64 Years)*. Canberra: Department of Health

reduction in the risk of disease and early death. More physical activity results in a greater reduction in the risk of disease and early death. However, this relationship is not linear and the biggest risk reductions occur when people shift from being sedentary to undertaking around 150 minutes of moderate intensity physical activity per week. Increasing physical activity above this level causes further health benefits, but the benefits progressively diminish as amount of activity is increased [4].

» CASE 13.1

AUSTRALIAN LEVELS OF PHYSICAL ACTIVITY

The most recent health survey in Australia suggests that only 55% of adults participated in sufficient physical activity [5]. This suggests that large-scale interventions that support people to be more physically active are urgently required. The amount of physical activity undertaken by Australian adults is likely to be influenced by a range of individual, social and environmental factors or determinants. It is important to fully understand these determinants in order to develop physical activity promotion interventions that are likely to have a significant impact on physical activity levels in the population.

- From the perspective of health research, why would it be useful to consider 'periods of physical activity' and 'states of sedentariness' separately?
- How does referring to physical activity as a 'lifestyle factor' help to view its role in the prevention of chronic disease?
- What contextual factors should be considered in research on physical activity levels in Australia?

See Chapter 3 for more on energy and adenosine triphosphate.

Energy systems
pathways in the body that produce energy, in the form of the molecule adenosine triphosphate (ATP), which fuels activity in the cells.

From a nutritional health perspective, the benefit of physical activity and exercise is the utilisation of energy in the body. The energy utilised for physical activity and exercise ultimately comes from food; however, the energy from food must be converted to a molecule called adenosine triphosphate (ATP) before it can be used by muscles to produce movement. There are limited stores of ATP in the body so it must be constantly produced to fuel activity. There are three **energy systems**, or pathways in the body that can produce ATP (Table 13.2).

The immediate energy system uses a molecule called creatine phosphate to rapidly generate ATP during very high-intensity, short-duration exercise. A fast energy system, anaerobic glycolysis, operates in the absence of oxygen to generate energy from glucose molecules at the start of high-intensity activities. A third energy system, oxidative phosphorylation or the aerobic energy system, generates ATP by breaking down carbohydrate and fat in the presence of oxygen. This energy system generates much more ATP than the other two systems, but the rate of ATP production is much slower and oxidative phosphorylation is the predominant energy system for endurance exercise that may last anywhere from a few minutes to several hours.

TABLE 13.2   ENERGY SYSTEMS IN OPERATION DURING ACTIVITY AND EXERCISE

Speed	Energy system	Molecular target	Relevant activity
Immediate	Phosphagen system	Creatine phosphate generates ATP	Very high-intensity, short-duration exercise
Fast	Anaerobic glycolysis	Generates ATP from glucose in the absence of oxygen	High-intensity activities lasting approximately 30–60 seconds
Slow	Aerobic system or oxidative phosphorylation	Generates ATP from carbohydrate and fat in the presence of oxygen	Endurance exercise (minutes to hours)

›› RESEARCH AT WORK

COMPENDIUM OF PHYSICAL ACTIVITIES

Energy expenditure during exercise is influenced by the intensity, duration and mode of activity. The compendium of physical activities provides a comprehensive list of the energy cost of several different activities [6]. The compendium is now published online to allow for updating as new data becomes available. The energy cost of activities is listed in metabolic equivalents (METs).

A MET is the ratio of energy expended during the exercise task compared with the amount of energy expended during rest. Therefore, the MET is a unit that represents the energy cost of an activity in multiples of the resting metabolic rate. For example, walking at a moderate pace is 3.5 METs, which means that this activity uses energy at a rate that is 3.5 times the energy expended at rest. The compendium provides a convenient tool to estimate energy expended during an exercise training program.

This is useful for a variety of reasons. The health benefits of physical activity appear to be most closely related to the amount of energy expended during physical activity. Therefore, an individual wanting to undertake an exercise training program to improve health might want to select activities that result in the greatest energy expenditure. However, an athlete training to improve performance might want estimate their energy expenditure and match this with energy intake from food in order to provide adequate fuel for training and avoid any adverse effects on body composition.

STOP AND THINK

- What is the relationship between physical activity, exercise and physical fitness?
- How would foods consumed be an important consideration for different types of exercise?

WHICH SPECIFIC NUTRIENTS ARE PARTICULARLY IMPORTANT FOR EXERCISING INDIVIDUALS AND ATHLETES?

Energy requirements of athletes and exercising individuals have traditionally been studied in the context of energy balance. Energy balance is simply the balance between energy intake and energy expenditure. Energy intake is provided through macronutrients in foods. However, adjusting energy intake to achieve a desired energy balance for an athlete or exercising individual can be problematic in sports nutrition practice. Energy intake is difficult to measure accurately by using methods that are inexpensive and realistic in practice, and there is also large variation in the estimation of energy expenditure in individuals undertaking large volumes of exercise training. In fact, the errors in the measurement of both energy intake and energy expenditure are often greater than any desired change in energy balance. A more useful concept in sports nutrition practice is **energy availability** [7]. Energy availability is defined as the difference between dietary energy intake and the energy expended during exercise. This is usually expressed in kilojoules or calories relative to an individual's fat free mass and it provides an indication of the amount of energy remaining for normal physiological function after the demands of exercise have been met. This is a more useful concept for sports nutrition practice because it enables a determination of whether energy intake is likely to be insufficient to sustain normal function.

Chronically low levels of energy availability have been associated with impaired menstrual function for women, reduced bone density, and disruptions in the endocrine and immune systems. Although low energy availability is more common in female athletes, it can also occur in men. As with many concepts in sports nutrition, there may not be critical values or thresholds of low energy availability that result in adverse consequences. It is generally considered that impaired function and performance may occur across a continuum of reductions in energy availability and that low energy availability may not necessarily occur at the same time as weight loss due to the body's ability to down-regulate

Energy requirement
The estimated dietary energy intake that is predicted to maintain energy balance.

Energy availability
the difference between dietary energy intake and the energy expended during exercise; indicates energy available for normal physiological function after the demands of exercise have been met.

See Chapter 7 for more on energy balance and body weight.

MICHAEL LEVERITT

TABLE 13.3   ENERGY AND MACRONUTRIENT CONSIDERATIONS FOR EXERCISE AND ATHLETIC ACTIVITY

Nutritional variable	Consideration	Implications
Energy	Energy availability: the difference between energy intake and the energy expended during exercise (expressed in kilojoules or calories relative to fat-free mass)	Maintaining normal physiological function and performance
Carbohydrate	Variable requirements: should be manipulated to suit the goals of individual athletes at any given point in their training schedule	Carbohydrate loading for enhanced performance Training with low carbohydrate availability for enhanced adaptation
Fat	Ability to use fat during exercise can be manipulated through both exercise training and dietary interventions	Keto-adaptation for endurance sports
Protein	Requirements increased in both endurance and strength/power athletes	The amount, type and timing of protein intake can influence muscle protein synthesis after exercise

resting metabolic rate when energy intake is reduced. While the consequences of low energy availability can be of significant concern for athletes, there is evidence that dietary interventions that increase energy availability can also result in the restoration of normal physiological function and performance (Table 13.3).

Carbohydrate

The introduction of the muscle biopsy technique in the 1960s enabled researchers to discover that carbohydrate is an important muscle fuel during exercise. Early studies demonstrated an association between the amount of glycogen stored in the muscle and the ability to exercise for long periods at a fixed intensity [8]. Both endogenous (stored in the body) and exogenous (consumed in foods and beverages) carbohydrate can be used as fuels during exercise. The contribution of carbohydrate breakdown to total energy expenditure increases as the intensity of exercise increases. Carbohydrate is also used by the central nervous system and may influence pacing strategies, concentration and perceptions of fatigue during exercise. Given these important roles of carbohydrate during exercise, it was once thought that all athletes and exercising individuals should consume a high-carbohydrate diet in order to maximise their performance, recovery and adaption to training. However, most athletes undertake periodised training programs in which the intensity, duration and frequency of training is manipulated at different times of the season or year in order to develop different characteristics that underpin successful performance. Consequently, carbohydrate requirements are not static and more recent guidelines suggest that carbohydrate intake should be manipulated to suit the goals of individual athletes at any given point in their training schedule [9].

See Chapter 4 for more on carbohydrates.

Carbohydrate stores in the muscle are unlikely to limit performance in a single bout of short-duration, high-intensity exercise such as sprinting or weightlifting. However, fatigue during repeated high-intensity exercise or multiple sets of resistance exercise may occur earlier if individuals have not consumed adequate carbohydrate in the days before exercising [10]. A moderate daily carbohydrate intake of 4–7 g/kg body mass has been recommended for athletes involved in strength and power sports [11], but it is likely that this requirement may vary during different phases of the training cycle, particularly if other training goals such as changes in body composition are desired.

Muscle glycogen depletion and reduced blood glucose concentration is associated with fatigue during long-duration endurance exercise. A high-carbohydrate diet in the days before a single bout of endurance exercise is associated with increased muscle glycogen storage and enhanced performance during exercise compared with the consumption of a low-carbohydrate diet [8]. Since these early discoveries in the 1960s, much research has been conducted on strategies to augment muscle glycogen stores before endurance events. Current recommendations suggest that a reduced training volume and a high carbohydrate intake of approximately 8–10 g/kg body mass for three to four days before the event is likely to result in optimal muscle glycogen storage. This form of 'carbohydrate loading' has been used for many decades by athletes competing in endurance and ultra-endurance sports.

» RESEARCH AT WORK

GLYCOGEN AVAILABILITY AND METABOLIC ADAPTATIONS

Hansen and colleagues conducted a study to determine if performing some endurance training sessions with low glycogen availability could enhance the metabolic adaptations to training [12]. Participants in this study completed 10 weeks of training involving knee extension exercise. Training with low glycogen availability was achieved by training one leg twice every second day, so that the second training bout was conducted without any opportunity to replenish the muscle glycogen used in the first training bout. The other leg trained once every day, which allowed the glycogen used from each training session to be fully replenished in the 24-hour period between training sessions. Results showed that the leg trained with low glycogen availability had a higher activity of metabolic enzymes involved in energy production and could exercise for longer at a fixed exercise intensity than the other leg. This was one of the first studies to show that training with low carbohydrate availability can enhance muscle adaptation and this nutrition strategy is now regularly used by athletes during specific phases of their training cycle.

Consuming carbohydrate during exercise is also associated with improved endurance performance [13]. Carbohydrate ingestion is likely to provide additional fuel for exercise and delay the depletion of muscle glycogen stores. Interestingly, improved performance occurs even when carbohydrate is consumed during exercise tasks lasting approximately one hour, which would not be long enough to fully deplete muscle glycogen stores. Some studies have shown that rinsing a carbohydrate solution in the mouth without ingestion can enhance performance during exercise lasting approximately one hour [14]. This suggests that carbohydrate consumption during exercise may have the capacity to improve performance through multiple mechanisms. The presence of carbohydrate in the mouth induces a signalling response to the central nervous system, which stimulates brain regions related to reward and motor control [15]. Carbohydrate consumption during these shorter-duration endurance exercise tasks is more likely to improve performance in studies where participants begin exercise after an overnight fast. Other studies that have provided carbohydrate-rich meals or periods of carbohydrate loading before exercise have typically not shown that carbohydrate can enhance performance during exercise tasks lasting approximately one hour [16]. These findings have practical applications for endurance athletes competing in events lasting approximately one hour or less, because many athletes find it uncomfortable to consume foods and beverages before and/or during exercise. If an athlete prefers to train or compete on an empty stomach, they may still be able to have enhanced performance where a small amount of carbohydrate is consumed during exercise. Other athletes might prefer to load up on carbohydrate before the event and not be distracted during the event by the need to consume foods or beverages.

While it is clear that very small amounts of carbohydrate, even without ingestion, can improve performance during events lasting approximately one hour, the potential of carbohydrate to enhance performance during longer events is likely to be determined by the amount and type of carbohydrate ingested [13] (Figure 13.3).

FIGURE 13.3 CARBOHYDRATE INTAKE RECOMMENDATIONS DURING EXERCISE BASED ON THE DURATION OF EXERCISE

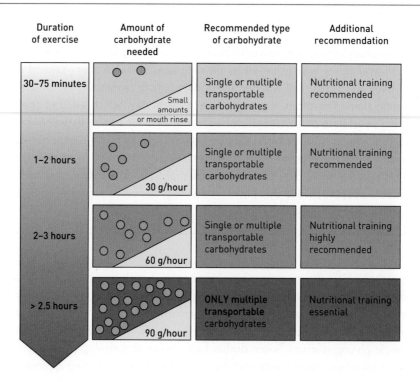

Source: A. Jeukendrup (2014). A step towards personalized sports nutrition: carbohydrate intake during exercise. *Sports Medicine*, 44(suppl. 1), S25–33. doi:10.1007/s40279-014-0148-z

≫ RESEARCH AT WORK

CARBOHYDRATE UTILISATION DURING EXERCISE

Studies using **metabolic isotope tracers** have enabled the determination of the rate at which ingested carbohydrate is used to produce energy during exercise. These studies have shown that maximal rates of exogenous glucose oxidation occur at approximately 1 g/min, which is much higher than other types of carbohydrate such as fructose and galactose, which are oxidised at a rate of 0.6 g/min [17]. These findings have led to recommendations that 30–60 g per hour of carbohydrate should be ingested during exercise lasting longer than one hour. Interestingly, studies using a mix of different types of carbohydrate during prolonged exercise lasting two to three hours have reported even higher exogenous carbohydrate oxidation rates of up to 1.8 g/min [18]. This is likely to occur because the rate-limiting step for exogenous carbohydrate oxidation appears to be the rate of absorption in the gut. Different types of carbohydrate are absorbed via different intestinal transport mechanisms and a mix of **multiple transportable carbohydrates** will produce a higher rate of exogenous carbohydrate oxidation compared with a single carbohydrate source. It is recommended that athletes consume 60–90 g/hour of multiple transportable carbohydrates (e.g. a mix of glucose and fructose) during exercise lasting two to three hours or longer.

Metabolic isotope tracer
a molecule functionally identical to the naturally occurring molecule, but labelled with a stable isotope to allow tracing of the path of the molecule through metabolic pathways during exercise.

Multiple transportable carbohydrates
carbohydrates containing a combination of monosaccharides that use different intestinal transporters for absorption.

The recommendations for carbohydrate intake during exercise are based on findings from laboratory studies usually conducted on stationary cycle ergometers. Exercise in this context is probably least likely to result in gastrointestinal discomfort compared with other modes of exercise, such as running, which are usually performed outdoors in variable environmental conditions. Therefore, it is possible that optimal intake of carbohydrate during long-duration exercise may be extremely difficult to achieve for endurance athletes in training or competition due to the potential for gastrointestinal discomfort associated with such a high intake of carbohydrate during exercise. Interestingly, some recent studies have suggested that it is possible to 'train' the gut to tolerate large carbohydrate intakes through repeated exposure during exercise [19]. Liquid, semi-liquid and solid forms of carbohydrate all appear to have similar benefits when consumed during exercise, which means that athletes should choose the form of carbohydrate they prefer and feel most comfortable consuming during exercise. It is important for athletes and exercising individuals to use carbohydrate recommendations as a guide or starting point, but they should be also encouraged to trial different carbohydrate intake strategies to identify which one best suits their individual requirements.

Despite the clear benefit of carbohydrate ingestion in enhancing performance during an acute bout of endurance exercise, it may also be possible for athletes to derive benefits from training with low carbohydrate availability [12]. Training after an overnight fast, or training while consuming a diet low in carbohydrate, or even just restricting carbohydrate intake after the previous training session all enable athletes to perform a training session with low carbohydrate availability. Training with low carbohydrate availability appears to result in a greater transcriptional activation of enzymes involved in carbohydrate metabolism and actually enhances the metabolic adaptations to training [20]. The disadvantage of this

MICHAEL LEVERITT

type of training is that performance during training may be reduced, which may compromise other non-metabolic training goals such as enhanced neuromuscular coordination. Many athletes now use a periodised approach to training where some training sessions are performed with low carbohydrate availability and some are performed with high carbohydrate availability, depending on the goals of the individual session and the specific phase of the training cycle. This is a good example of how athletes can use an understanding of sports nutrition to add value to their training programs and achieve the specific adaptations that maximise performance.

Fat

Fat is the largest source of stored energy in the body and is an important fuel for endurance exercise. One of the key metabolic adaptations to endurance training is an increase in the ability to oxidise fat to produce energy for movement. This has the potential to enhance performance by sparing more carbohydrate, which delays fatigue and enables athletes to exercise at a higher intensity towards the end of an event. The maximal rate of fat oxidation typically occurs at an exercise intensity of approximately 50% VO_2max. However, there is significant individual variation in the ability to oxidise fat during exercise. A large study of over 1000 athletes has reported that some athletes can oxidise around 75 g of fat per hour, whereas the maximal rate of fat oxidation in other athletes was only 10 g per hour [21]. Fat oxidation during exercise may be further enhanced when individuals adapt to several weeks of a very high-fat diet, and fat oxidation rates of over 100 g per hour have been reported after adapting to such a diet [22]. This shows that the ability to use fat during exercise can be manipulated through both exercise training and dietary interventions.

See Chapter 5 for more on fat.

Interest in the benefit of high-fat diets for endurance athletes has experienced a resurgence in recent years after these diets were previously discounted by many sports nutrition researchers and practitioners. Early studies on high-fat diets may have been limited by the duration of the dietary intervention, low participant numbers, the degree of carbohydrate restriction achieved during these studies and/or the duration of the exercise performance test used to assess the benefits of the intervention. A very high-fat diet providing >80% of energy from fat with very little carbohydrate (<50 g/day) is required to be consumed for several weeks in order to achieve a state of keto-adaptation. **Keto-adaptation** is when the body is adapted to use predominantly fat for activities requiring energy and is also able to tolerate relatively low levels of blood glucose due to the availability of ketones for the central nervous system. This state of keto-adaptation facilitates very high rates of fat oxidation during exercise, which can be an advantage to performance in events lasting several hours, such as ironman triathlons. Athletes in these events who are not in a state of keto-adaptation need to rely more on carbohydrate for energy, but this may be unavailable in the latter stages of the event due to muscle glycogen depletion and/or an inability to tolerate very high intakes of carbohydrate in foods and beverages during exercise.

Keto-adaptation

where the body is adapted to use predominantly fat for activities requiring energy and is also able to tolerate relatively low levels of blood glucose due to the availability of ketones for the central nervous system.

Keto-adaptation essentially provides athletes with an internal motor with a far greater capacity to produce energy for very long periods than their non-keto-adapted counterparts [23] (Figure 13.4). While the benefits of high-fat diets for endurance athletes are theoretically plausible, the evidence for benefit is provided mostly through anecdotal reports, and only a few studies with small participant numbers and limited measures of exercise performance have been conducted. This may be due to the difficulty in conducting these types of studies rather than due to an absence of any benefit. Another potential downside for athletes wanting to consume a very high-fat diet for long periods is that the dietary patterns required to achieve this are not typical of usual dietary patterns in most societies. This presents challenges for athletes if

FIGURE 13.4 THEORETICAL PARADIGM BY WHICH KETOGENIC DIETS MAY BENEFIT ATHLETES

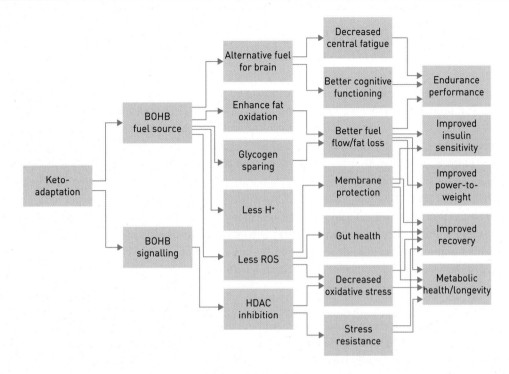

Abbreviations: BOHB: beta-hydroxybutyrate; ROS: reactive oxygen species; HDAC: histone deacetylase

Source: J. S. Volek, T. Noakes & S. D. Phinney (2015). Rethinking fat as a fuel for endurance exercise. *European Journal of Sport Science*, 15(1), 13–20. doi:10.1080/17461391.2014.959564

they regularly consume food that is prepared by others, train and compete away from home or are simply unwilling to undertake such a restriction in their food choices. Given the large individual variability in fat oxidation rates during exercise, there may also be some individuals who are more likely to benefit from a high-fat diet than others. Further research is required before high-fat diets can be universally recommended for endurance athletes involved in events lasting several hours. However, this is definitely an area worthy of further exploration for sports nutrition researchers and practitioners.

Protein

Protein is an important nutrient that plays a role in tissue growth, repair and regeneration. Protein is often considered in the context of strength- and power-based sports because high levels of muscle mass can often predict success in these sports. However, protein requirements of endurance athletes are also increased due to the high energy expenditure during endurance exercise. Although protein contributes only about 5% of total energy used during endurance exercise, the amount of protein required can be significant when exercise intensity is high and exercise duration is prolonged. Protein consumption during endurance exercise may actually enhance performance and improve recovery after exercise, although these effects are not always observed when adequate carbohydrate is provided during and after exercise. Daily protein recommendations for endurance athletes range from 1.0–1.6 g/kg body mass depending on exercise intensity and duration [24].

See Chapter 6 for more on protein.

> **» RESEARCH AT WORK**

PROTEIN INTAKE AND EXERCISE

Areta and colleagues conducted a study investigating the effects of manipulating the timing and distribution of protein intake on muscle protein synthesis after a single bout of resistance exercise [25]. They compared three different patterns of ingestion of 80 g of whey protein for 12 hours after resistance exercise. The protein was ingested in a pulsed (8 × 10g every 1.5 hours), intermediate (4 × 20g every 3 hours) or bolus (2 × 40g every 6 hours) pattern. All ingestion patterns resulted in enhanced protein synthesis; however, the intermediate pattern elicited significantly greater protein synthesis than the other two patterns of intake. This study clearly showed that the timing of protein intake after exercise can impact on muscle protein synthesis even when the total amount ingested is the same. The authors suggested it appears a minimum threshold of blood amino acid concentration is required to optimally stimulate muscle protein synthesis and that the intermediate pattern of protein intake was able to exceed this threshold on more occasions than the other two intake patterns. The data from this study suggest that athletes and exercising individuals wanting the greatest gains in muscle mass from a resistance training program should ingest protein in an intermediate pattern after each training session.

Resistance training
a form of exercise training requiring muscles to exert force against a resistance that might be provided by an external weight, band, object or an individual's own body weight; used to develop greater strength and lean body mass.

Protein recommendations for strength and power athletes have been based on studies investigating acute muscle protein synthesis after a bout of **resistance training** and studies investigating the effect of different amounts of dietary protein intake on changes in muscle mass and strength during a prolonged period of resistance training. Acute studies show that consuming protein after a bout of resistance exercise can enhance subsequent muscle protein synthesis [26]. The degree to which protein synthesis is augmented is determined by the amount, type and timing of protein intake. Approximately 20–25 g of protein appears to stimulate optimal muscle protein synthesis after an acute bout of resistance exercise, with very little further increases observed when greater amounts of protein are consumed [27]. Proteins that are rapidly absorbed, contain all essential amino acids and are high in the amino acid leucine, which is a trigger for protein synthesis in the muscle, appear to stimulate greater muscle protein synthesis than other proteins [28]. Higher rates of muscle protein synthesis are observed when whey protein is consumed after resistance exercise compared with the same amount of casein and soy protein. This is because whey protein is high in leucine and also causes a rapid rise in blood amino acids soon after it is consumed. An intermediate pattern of protein distribution in which 20–25 g of protein is consumed immediately following resistance exercise and then every three to four hours afterwards appears to result in greater muscle protein synthesis than larger amounts consumed less frequently or smaller amounts consumed more frequently [25]. Therefore, it is recommended that athletes undertaking resistance training aim to consume 20–25 g of rapidly absorbed, high-leucine protein such as whey protein immediately after and then every three to four hours subsequently in order to maximise protein synthesis after a bout of resistance training.

Although there is good evidence to support specific recommendations for the amount, type and timing of protein intake required to optimise muscle protein synthesis after a bout of resistance training, most of this evidence comes from acute studies investigating a single bout of resistance exercise. Longer-term studies that investigate the effects of consuming protein during a resistance training program suggest that the total amount of daily protein consumed, rather than the type or timing of protein intake, is the most important factor that contributes to gains in muscle mass and strength [29]. The subtle effects of the type and timing of protein in longer-term studies are possibly not always observed because many other factors contribute to changes in muscle mass and strength, and these factors are difficult to adequately control in longer-term training studies. Optimal gains in muscle mass and strength after a resistance training program are achieved when daily protein intake is approximately 1.6–2.0 g/kg body mass. This is over double the recommended amount for sedentary individuals, but is still relatively easy to achieve if an athlete consumes a typical Western-style dietary pattern in which high-protein foods such as meat, poultry, eggs and dairy foods are readily available. Some strength and power athletes consume protein in amounts that exceed current recommendations. While additional benefit is unlikely to result from exceeding protein recommendations, adverse effects of high protein intakes in fit and healthy individuals consuming a wide variety of foods are rarely observed.

Micronutrients

Exercise training results in an increased utilisation of many metabolic pathways that involve micronutrients. The requirements for most micronutrients can be achieved by athletes consuming a wide variety of nutrient-dense foods, particularly if the amount is increased to match the increased energy needs associated with training. However, there are some notable exceptions and the micronutrients of most concern for athletes are iron and vitamin D. The role of antioxidants during training adaptation is also worthy of consideration for athletes and exercising individuals.

See chapters 9-12 for more on micronutrients.

Exercise training can increase iron requirements above those of sedentary individuals. The exact amount of additional iron required by athletes is not known precisely and is likely to depend on the specific circumstances of individuals. Periods of rapid growth, training at high altitude, menstrual blood loss, haemolysis resulting from frequent foot strikes, or injury have the potential to negatively influence iron status in athletes. It has been observed that over one-third of active women have low iron status [30]. Iron consumption by athletes is often below recommended intakes for healthy individuals and low iron status can negatively impact on both health and exercise performance. Athletes with low iron status or deficiency may benefit from high-dose iron supplementation, but this is only recommended when close monitoring and the support of a health professional is available. It is prudent to recommend that athletes consume a variety of iron-rich foods in order to prevent low iron status. Also, regular monitoring of iron status in higher-risk groups such as female endurance athletes should be considered.

Vitamin D is an important nutrient for bone health, plays a role in immune function and is also involved in muscle growth and repair processes. Many athletes have poor vitamin D status, potentially due to long hours spent training indoors, increased use of sun protection and/or low dietary vitamin D intake [31]. Measuring vitamin D status is complex and there is currently much debate about exact serum concentrations that indicate insufficiency and deficiency. Low serum concentrations of vitamin D are associated with impaired muscle function; however, improved performance is not always observed when individuals with low vitamin D status receive vitamin D supplements. It is also unclear if any adverse effects result from long-term supplementation with high doses of vitamin D. Given the importance of vitamin D for many functions in the body and the impact low vitamin D status can have on performance, it is essential that research continues in this area in order to provide specific guidelines and recommendations for athletes.

Exercise causes a significant increase in the production of reactive oxygen species (ROS) due to an increase in the rates of many metabolic pathways. It is now recognised that ROS generation during exercise provides an important signalling process for many skeletal muscle adaptations. Supplementation with antioxidants during periods of moderate exercise training appears to blunt adaptations to training and is currently not recommended for exercising individuals [32]. However, antioxidants may offer some benefit during acute periods of very high training stress. Antioxidant systems in the body are complex and there is no simple test to measure an individual's antioxidant status at any given point in time, and this makes it difficult to provide specific recommendations for athletes. However, there appear to be no adverse effects on training adaptation associated with the consumption of vegetables and fruits that are high in antioxidants and these should be recommended for all athletes to promote overall health and well-being.

STOP AND THINK

- How does performing endurance training with low carbohydrate availability have the potential to enhance the metabolic adaptations to training?
- What food combinations (meals) might enable an athlete to have low carbohydrate availability during a training session?
- What are some disadvantages of training with low carbohydrate availability?

WHICH FOOD AND BEVERAGE CONSUMPTION PATTERNS MAY ENHANCE EXERCISE PERFORMANCE?

See Chapters 2–7 on food sources of macronutrients.

A great deal of emphasis in the research on diet and exercise/sports performance is conducted at the level of macronutrients, but food remains important as the staple source of everyday fuel. Manipulating the macronutrient composition of the diet by different food choices is covered in Part 1 of the book. This section will introduce two new areas specifically relevant to sports nutrition: fluids and sports supplements.

Fluids for hydration

See Chapter 8 for more on water, beverages and hydration.

The evaporation of sweat from the skin is the main mechanism used to regulate body temperature during exercise. Therefore, exercise that is high intensity, of prolonged duration and/or performed in hot environmental conditions can cause significant fluid loss. This fluid loss has the potential to impair both physical and cognitive performance by compromising cardiovascular and cellular function. The effects of dehydration on exercise performance are complex, with different amounts of dehydration potentially having different effects on specific performance tasks. For example, fluid losses equivalent to 2% of body mass appear to have negative effects on endurance capacity during exercise tasks performed at a fixed intensity. However, adverse effects on endurance time trial performance may not occur until fluid losses are greater than 4% of body mass [33]. Fluid loss during exercise can also vary significantly between individuals. This makes it difficult to develop universal recommendations for fluid intake. The amount of fluid consumed during exercise needs to be sufficient to prevent any negative effect of dehydration on performance and temperature regulation, but it is also important for athletes not to consume too much fluid during exercise. The consequences of excess fluid consumption range from the negative effects of carrying additional weight during exercise through to the severe consequences associated with the risk of **hyponatraemia**.

Hyponatraemia
a condition of low levels of sodium in the blood. Resulting symptoms can range in severity and include headache, nausea, confusion, seizures and coma.

Severe hyponatraemia is rare, but it can occur during prolonged exercise when the fluid ingested dilutes sodium in the blood, and this can result in severe consequences including death.

Current fluid intake guidelines are somewhat controversial and have been the subject of robust debate in recent years. A variety of hydration strategies may be effective for different athletes during exercise. Some studies show that simply drinking according to thirst may be just as effective as a planned fluid intake strategy designed to match fluid losses or restrict fluid losses to no more than 2% of body mass. Recommendations for athletes to drink to thirst during training and competition are problematic because there is not always an opportunity to consume fluid immediately when feeling thirsty in many sports; however, this recommendation may be the best way to avoid excess consumption of fluid. Recommendations to have a planned fluid intake strategy to restrict fluid loss to no more than 2% of body mass can also be problematic because body mass losses are not easy to measure in many sports. Athletes must rely on previous measures of fluid loss under similar conditions in order to implement this strategy. Therefore, there is no simple answer to the question of how much an athlete should drink during exercise. Nevertheless, it might be a good strategy for athletes to use thirst as an initial guide to fluid consumption, and then to regularly monitor fluid loss, fluid intake and performance to identify fluid consumption patterns that result in optimal performance in each individual.

TRY IT YOURSELF

Fluid loss during exercise can be estimated by measuring an individual's body weight before and after the exercise session. Calculate the fluid loss of a male rugby league player who weighs 95.3 kg at the beginning of a training session and then weighs 93.9 kg at the end of the training session. What percentage of his original body weight has been lost? What is the likely impact on performance from this level of dehydration?

Fluids containing sodium may enhance fluid retention and are generally recommended for individuals who lose a lot of sodium through sweat. However, water is the most appropriate beverage to consume during exercise for the vast majority of individuals. Some beverages promoted for use in sport contain additional ingredients such as carbohydrate and caffeine, which may benefit exercise performance. However, the requirement for these additional ingredients should be considered independently as they have similar benefits if provided in a beverage or in other forms.

Replacing fluid losses after exercise is important to ensure subsequent exercise is not commenced in a dehydrated state. It is generally recommended to consume around one and a half times the fluid lost during exercise because sweat losses continue after exercise and not all of the fluid consumed is retained in the body. The rate of fluid retention after exercise depends on the rate of fluid consumption and the composition of the rehydration beverage. Beverage components such as sodium, carbohydrate, protein and the overall amount of energy consumed can impact on fluid retention. Fluid from beverages high in kilojoules appears to be retained well after exercise because gastric emptying is slowed when energy is present. Slower gastric emptying allows the fluid to be absorbed more gradually. This prevents a rapid decline in plasma osmolality and sodium concentration and the stimulation of fluid excretion that might occur if the fluid was absorbed quickly. High-energy beverages such as milk and liquid meal replacement beverages have been shown to result in greater fluid retention compared with sports drinks and water [34]. However, the additional energy and sodium required to enhance fluid retention can also be consumed in the form of foods. Combining foods with plain water results in an equally effective rehydration strategy after exercise compared with a meal replacement beverage with similar nutrient composition [35].

Sports foods and ergogenic aids

Sports foods

specially formulated foods designed to help athletes or exercising individuals achieve specific nutritional or performance goals.

Understanding how different nutrients can enhance exercise performance has led to the development of specific **sports foods**, where nutrients are packaged in convenient forms. Sports drinks, gels, bars and dietary supplements in liquid, powder or capsule form are frequently used by athletes and exercising individuals. The vast majority of these specialised sports foods are simply convenient packages of nutrients, but athletes can often receive the same benefits from consuming the same nutrients in regular foods, which may also provide a cheaper alternative. Nevertheless, sports foods can have a role to play in an athlete's diet. For example, consuming protein after resistance exercise may enhance muscle protein synthesis. Most foods that are high in protein such as meat, poultry, eggs and dairy foods require refrigeration and are not always easy to access after a training session. A sports food such as a protein powder that can be mixed with water may be more convenient for an athlete to take to training and consume immediately after they finish exercise.

See Chapter 21 for more on functional foods.

» CASE 13.2

SPORTS SUPPLEMENTS AND ERGOGENIC AIDS

Placebo or belief effects are often associated with many sports nutrition supplements and ergogenic aids. There have even been well-controlled studies conducted with known ergogenic aids such as caffeine and carbohydrate that show that exercise performance is enhanced when participants are told they are receiving the ergogenic aid despite only being given a placebo [36; 37]. This has implications for ethical practice in sports nutrition, as it could be considered unethical to deceive an athlete by advising them to consume a supplement that is not likely to enhance performance.

For public health safety, sports foods are regulated under Standard 2.9.4 of the Food Standards Code. It is a requirement that labels on sports foods must:

1   state 'supplemented formulated sports food'
2   indicate the context of use—that is, in conjunction with a nutritious diet and appropriate exercise program
3   provide recommendations on quantity and frequency of intake (include amount for one day)
4   state 'not suitable for children under 15 years of age or pregnant women
5   should only be used under medical or dietetic supervision [38].
•   Do you think it is ethical for sports nutrition practitioners to promote placebo and belief effects in the athletes they work with?
•   What is the best advice to provide to an athlete who wants to use a supplement that has not been shown to be effective in enhancing performance?

Nutritional ergogenic aids

dietary supplements that enhance performance above levels anticipated under normal conditions.

Nutritional ergogenic aids are dietary supplements that enhance performance above levels anticipated under normal conditions. Ergogenic aids typically contain unusual amounts of nutrients or other components of foods that would not normally be consumed through food alone. There are many products available today that are marketed as being able to enhance exercise performance, but there is rarely strong scientific evidence to support the proposed

TABLE 13.4   COMMON ERGOGENIC AIDS IN SPORTS NUTRITION

Compound	Proposed physiological effects	Considerations
Caffeine	Effects on central nervous system, increasing arousal and reducing perception of effort	Dose will vary depending on source Available through common foods and beverages such as coffee
Nitrate-rich foods	Effect of nitric oxide on improving muscle function and consequently exercise performance	Nitrate content varies between foods and from food preparation
Bicarbonate	Enhanced capacity to buffer acid produced from exercise	Side effects of gastrointestinal discomfort
Beta-alanine (carnosine)	Increased levels of carnosine that may act as a buffer to acid produced in short-intensity exercise	Skin side effects Compliance with recommended protocol is difficult
Creatine	Increased creatine pool in muscle for enhanced ATP regeneration; increased lean muscle mass	Various protocols for use

benefits. Nevertheless, studies on some ergogenic aids such as caffeine, nitrates, bicarbonate, beta-alanine and creatine have shown a degree of effectiveness in enhancing performance under certain conditions (Table 13.4). More research is required to build the evidence base and ensure safe and ethical practice.

Caffeine is one of the most widely used pharmacologically active substances in the world and it has been shown to improve performance in a range of exercise tasks. The benefits of caffeine for athletes and exercising individuals are most likely related to its effects on the central nervous system: it increases arousal and reduces the perception of effort during exercise. The dose required to achieve optimal performance gains appears to be 3 mg/kg body mass [39]. This dose is equivalent to approximately 600 mL of a standard energy drink or two cups of coffee and is similar to the usual daily consumption of caffeine for many adults. The intake of caffeine at these relatively low doses is unlikely to result in any negative side effects, which is perhaps one reason why caffeine use in sport has not been restricted since 2004. Caffeine can improve performance when consumed in tablet form, coffee or energy drinks. However, the amount of caffeine in coffee and some energy drinks can vary significantly. Therefore, athletes may wish to consume caffeine in tablet form to be more certain of the exact dose that is being delivered. Caffeine is most effective when consumed approximately one hour before exercise [40], although studies have shown that small amounts of caffeine consumed in cola beverages can enhance performance when consumed in the concluding stages of an endurance exercise task [41]. Caffeine consumption during exercise does not cause dehydration and it has even been shown to enhance performance when consumed before exercise performed in hot conditions [42]. Athletes who normally consume large amounts of caffeine in their diet still receive similar benefits when consuming caffeine before exercise compared with athletes who do not consume much caffeine on a regular basis.

TRY IT YOURSELF

Caffeine has been shown to consistently enhance endurance exercise performance. The recommended dose is 3 mg/kg body mass consumed approximately 60 minutes before exercise. The average caffeine content of a cup of coffee is 100 mg, but this can range from 25 mg to over 200 mg depending on how it is prepared. An energy drink contains 80 mg of caffeine in a 250 mL can. Caffeine tablets, which are available at most pharmacies, contain exactly 100 mg of caffeine.

Which source of caffeine would you recommend for a 60 kg endurance athlete in order to achieve the recommended dose? Discuss the benefits and limitations of each caffeine source.

Nitrate-rich foods are becoming increasingly popular as an ergogenic aid given a potential capacity to enhance endurance exercise performance [43]. Many green leafy vegetables and beetroot are examples of foods with a high nitrate content. The nitrate content of foods can vary significantly due to growing conditions and loss of nitrate during cooking and preparation, which makes it difficult to predict how much dietary nitrate is being consumed through different foods. There are now many sports foods and beverages available that are usually made with concentrated beetroot juice and contain a known amount of nitrate. Once ingested, dietary nitrate can be converted to nitrite by bacteria in the mouth. Circulating nitrite is then converted into nitric oxide in blood and other tissues. It is thought that enhancing nitric oxide availability may improve muscle function and, consequently, exercise performance. Nitrate supplementation is thought to specifically enhance the efficiency of oxygen use during exercise and allows individuals to perform greater work for the same energy cost, improving their capacity to exercise at a fixed intensity for a longer duration before exhaustion. Daily intake of 400–500 mg of nitrate for approximately one week has been argued as the most effective at enhancing performance; however, benefits have also been shown after a single dose consumed two to three hours before exercise [44]. Importantly, the benefits of dietary nitrate supplementation are less evident in highly trained athletes, particularly when exercise performance is measured via a time-trial test rather than time to exhaustion tests. Thus, athletes may wish to monitor their individual response to nitrate supplementation to determine whether this is likely to be an effective nutrition strategy that contributes to their performance goals.

It has also been argued that performance in short-duration, high-intensity exercise can be improved after the ingestion of *sodium bicarbonate* [45]. The physiological principle is that increasing bicarbonate in the blood enhances the capacity to buffer acid produced by the muscle during exercise. Theoretically, this would have the potential to delay fatigue during high-intensity exercise. In practice, however, even with a clear mechanistic rationale, not all studies show a performance benefit. There also can be side effects associated with gastrointestinal discomfort and this may offset any potential benefits of an improved buffer capacity. Similar to nitrate supplementation, the benefits of bicarbonate ingestion appear to be less evident in highly trained individuals, possibly due to the already high buffer capacity developed through training in this population. Doses of 200–400 mg/kg body mass consumed 60 to 90 minutes before exercise appear to be optimal. However, athletes would need to trial the use of this supplement on several occasions during training to ensure that no adverse gastrointestinal side effects are likely to occur in competition.

Beta-alanine is a component of the dipeptide carnosine, which plays a role in buffering acid produced in the muscle during high-intensity exercise. Beta-alanine supplementation for several weeks may result in increased muscle carnosine and improved performance in short-duration (1–4 minutes), high-intensity exercise [46]. A daily dose of 6.4 g is used in most studies and it appears that at least four weeks of beta-alanine supplementation is required to elevate muscle carnosine concentration. Further increases in muscle carnosine concentration are observed after 10 weeks of supplementation. The daily dose is usually consumed on three to four occasions spread throughout the day in order to reduce the acute side effects associated with consumption of large doses of beta-alanine. Side effects can include tingling, flushing and a prickly sensation on the skin, and peak around 30 to 60 minutes after ingestion.

However, the protocol for beta-alanine supplementation is much more difficult for athletes to adhere to than protocols for other supplements as it involves several daily doses taken for several weeks.

Creatine has been used by athletes as an ergogenic aid for several decades. Supplementation with creatine monohydrate increases the creatine pool in muscles, which allows for more rapid ATP regeneration during repeated bouts of high-intensity exercise. Theoretically, this mechanism may enable a higher training intensity and improved adaptation to training, particularly resistance training, which involves repeated, high-force muscle contractions. Creatine supplementation also appears to positively influence anabolic processes in muscles that results in an increase in lean muscle mass after supplementation [47]. Studies have shown that creatine supplementation during a period of resistance training enhances gains in muscle strength and lean body mass [48]. Typical creatine supplementation protocols involve a short loading phase lasting five to seven days in which 20 g/day of creatine monohydrate is consumed in four daily intakes of 5 g each, evenly spaced throughout the day. This is then followed by a maintenance phase in which 3–5 g/day is consumed. The maintenance phase typically lasts for the duration of the training cycle in which improvements in maximal muscle strength and lean body mass are the primary goals.

STOP AND THINK

- Which characteristics of whey protein may contribute to enhancing muscle protein synthesis more than other protein sources? How much is recommended?
- What other dietary factors associated with overall protein intake need to be considered by athletes and exercising individuals wanting to gain lean body mass during a period of resistance training?
- How should the evidence be fully evaluated to support the use of sports supplements in training?

SUMMARY

- Physical activity and exercise are important components of a healthy lifestyle and being physically active reduces the risk of developing cardiovascular disease, diabetes and cancer.
- Energy availability is defined as the difference between dietary energy intake and the energy expended during exercise. This provides an indication of the amount of energy available for normal physiological function after the demands of exercise have been met. Low energy availability is associated with disrupted physiological function and can impair the overall health and well-being of athletes.
- The consumption of carbohydrate during exercise is likely to enhance endurance exercise performance. Performance is enhanced in events lasting approximately one hour even when carbohydrate is rinsed in the mouth and not ingested. Longer events require the ingestion of carbohydrate and events lasting two to three hours or longer are best enhanced when multiple transportable carbohydrate sources are ingested.
- Fat oxidation during exercise varies considerably across individuals. Adapting to a very high-fat diet has the potential to benefit some athletes competing in events lasting several hours; however, further research is warranted in this area.
- Protein requirements for athletes and exercising individuals are increased compared with sedentary individuals. The amount, type and timing of protein intake has the potential to influence muscle protein synthesis after resistance training, but having high daily protein intake appears to be the most important factor contributing to gains in strength and lean body mass after a period of resistance training.

- The requirements for most micronutrients can be achieved by athletes consuming a wide variety of foods, particularly if the amount of nutrient-dense foods is increased to match the increased energy needs associated with training. However, there are some notable exceptions and the micronutrients of most concern for athletes are iron and vitamin D.
- The influence of hydration status on exercise performance is variable and athletes are likely to benefit from a range of fluid intake strategies, including drinking to thirst, to enable optimal performance and reduce the risk of adverse events associated with excess fluid consumption.
- Ergogenic aids such as caffeine, nitrates, sodium bicarbonate, beta-alanine and creatine have the potential to enhance specific aspects of exercise performance, but scientific research is required to provide a strong evidence base of effects.

PATHWAYS TO PRACTICE

- Identifying key issues in nutrition for exercise and sport, in particular the significance of food choices, provides opportunities in the community health context where both physical activity and healthy eating are promoted at a community and population level.

- Understanding nutrition for exercise and sport provides opportunities in the food industry context where new product formulations are being developed and tested for specific sports foods.

- Understanding nutrition for exercise and sport is important for exercise and sports scientists who work with a range of different disciplines, including sports dietitians, to best support coaches and athletes to perform at their peak.

DISCUSSION QUESTIONS

1   How can physical activity and exercise improve health without necessarily causing weight loss?
2   What are the mechanisms by which carbohydrate improves performance when provided during endurance exercise?
3   What are the recommended amounts, types and timing of protein intake that result in optimal muscle protein synthesis after resistance training?
4   What are the advantages and disadvantages of different strategies of fluid intake during endurance exercise?
5   What is the position of a healthy eating pattern in providing the background to optimal sports performance and overall health?

USEFUL WEBLINKS

Australia's Physical Activity and Sedentary Behaviour Guidelines:
    www.health.gov.au/internet/main/publishing.nsf/content/health-pubhlth-strateg-phys-act-guidelines

Australian Bureau of Statistics—Australian Health Survey 2011–12—Physical activity:
    www.abs.gov.au/ausstats/abs@.nsf/Lookup/4364.0.55.004Chapter1002011-12

Australian Sports Commission—Sports nutrition:
    www.ausport.gov.au/ais/nutrition

Heart Foundation—Australian Physical Activity Network:
  www.heartfoundation.org.au/for-professionals/physical-activity/australian-physical-activity-network

Nutrition Australia—Sports Nutrition:
  www.nutritionaustralia.org/national/resources/sports-nutrition

Sports Dietitians Australia:
  www.sportsdietitians.com.au

FURTHER READING

Aragon, A. A., Schoenfeld, B. J., Wildman, R., Kleiner, S., VanDusseldorp, T., Taylor, L., … Antonio, J. (2017). International society of sports nutrition position stand: diets and body composition. *Journal of the International Society of Sports Nutrition*, 14, 16. doi:10.1186/s12970-017-0174-y

Beaulieu, K., Hopkins, M., Blundell, J. & Finlayson, G. (2016). Does habitual physical activity increase the sensitivity of the appetite control system? A systematic review. *Sports Medicine*, 46(12), 1897–919. doi:10.1007/s40279-016-0518-9

Benton, D., Braun, H., Cobo, J. C., Edmonds, C., Elmadfa, I., El-Sharkawy, A., … Watson, P. (2015). Executive summary and conclusions from the European Hydration Institute expert conference on human hydration, health, and performance. *Nutrition Reviews*, 73(suppl. 2), 148–50. doi:10.1093/nutrit/nuv056

Birkenhead, K. L. & Slater, G. (2015). A review of factors influencing athletes' food choices. *Sports Medicine*, 45(11), 1511–22. doi:10.1007/s40279-015-0372-1

Burdon, C. A., Spronk, I., Cheng, H. L. & O'Connor, H. T. (2017). Effect of glycemic index of a pre-exercise meal on endurance exercise performance: a systematic review and meta-analysis. *Sports Medicine*, 47(6), 1087–101. doi:10.1007/s40279-016-0632-8

Burke, L. M., Ross, M. L., Garvican-Lewis, L. A., Welvaert, M., Heikura, I. A., Forbes, S. G., … Hawley, J. A. (2017). Low carbohydrate, high fat diet impairs exercise economy and negates the performance benefit from intensified training in elite race walkers. *Journal of Physiology*, 595(9), 2785–807. doi:10.1113/JP273230

Heung-Sang Wong, S., Sun, F.-H., Chen, Y.-J., Li, C., Zhang, Y.-J. & Ya-Jun Huang, W. (2017). Effect of pre-exercise carbohydrate diets with high vs low glycemic index on exercise performance: a meta-analysis. *Nutrition Reviews*, 75(5), 327–38. doi:10.1093/nutrit/nux003

Jäger, R., Kerksick, C. M., Campbell, B. I., Cribb, P. J., Wells, S. D., Skwiat, T. M., … Antonio, J. (2017). International Society of Sports Nutrition Position Stand: protein and exercise. *Journal of the International Society of Sports Nutrition*, 14(1), 20. doi:10.1186/s12970-017-0177-8

Jeukendrup, A. E. (2017). Periodized nutrition for athletes. *Sports Medicine*, 47(1), 51–63. doi:10.1007/s40279-017-0694-2

Jeukendrup, A. E. (2017). Training the gut for athletes. *Sports Medicine*, 47(1), 101–10. doi:10.1007/s40279-017-0690-6

Kerksick, C. M., Arent, S., Schoenfeld, B. J., Stout, J. R., Campbell, B., Wilborn, C. D., ... Antonio, J. (2017). International Society of Sports Nutrition Position Stand: nutrient timing. *Journal of the International Society of Sports Nutrition*, 14(1), 33. doi:10.1186/s12970-017-0189-4

Kreider, R. B., Kalman, D. S., Antonio, J., Ziegenfuss, T. N., Wildman, R., Collins, R., ... Lopez, H. L. (2017). International Society of Sports Nutrition Position Stand: safety and efficacy of creatine supplementation in exercise, sport, and medicine. *Journal of the International Society of Sports Nutrition*, 14(1), 18. doi:10.1186/s12970-017-0173-z

Liao, C. D., Tsauo, J. Y., Wu, Y. T., Cheng, C. P., Chen, H. C., Huang, Y. C., ... Liou, T. H. (2017). Effects of protein supplementation combined with resistance exercise on body composition and physical function in older adults: a systematic review and meta-analysis. *American Journal of Clinical Nutrition*, 106(4), 1078–91. doi:10.3945/ajcn.116.143594

Lynch, H., Wharton, C. & Johnston, C. (2016). Cardiorespiratory fitness and peak torque differences between vegetarian and omnivore endurance athletes: a cross-sectional study. *Nutrients*, 8(11), 726.

Maughan, R. J., Watson, P., Cordery, P. A., Walsh, N. P., Oliver, S. J., Dolci, A., ... Galloway, S. D. (2016). A randomized trial to assess the potential of different beverages to affect hydration status: development of a beverage hydration index. *American Journal of Clinical Nutrition*, 103(3), 717–23. doi:10.3945/ajcn.115.114769

Maughan, R. J., Watson, P. & Shirreffs, S. M. (2015). Implications of active lifestyles and environmental factors for water needs and consequences of failure to meet those needs. *Nutrition Reviews*, 73(suppl. 2), 130–40. doi:10.1093/nutrit/nuv051

Somerville, V., Bringans, C. & Braakhuis, A. (2017). Polyphenols and performance: a systematic review and meta-analysis. *Sports Medicine*, 47(8), 1589–99. doi:10.1007/s40279-017-0675-5

Thomas, D. T., Erdman, K. A. & Burke, L. M. (2016). Position of the Academy of Nutrition and Dietetics, Dietitians of Canada, and the American College of Sports Medicine: nutrition and athletic performance. *Journal of the Academy of Nutrition and Dietetics*, 116(3), 501–28. doi:https://doi.org/10.1016/j.jand.2015.12.006

van Vliet, S., Burd, N. A. & van Loon, L. J. (2015). The skeletal muscle anabolic response to plant- versus animal-based protein consumption. *Journal of Nutrition*, 145(9), 1981–91. doi:10.3945/jn.114.204305

REFERENCES

1   M. Reiner, C. Niermann, D. Jekauc & A. Woll (2013). Long-term health benefits of physical activity—a systematic review of longitudinal studies. *BMC Public Health*, 13, 813. doi:10.1186/1471-2458-13-813

2   C. Bouchard, S. N. Blair & P. T. Katzmarzyk (2015). Less sitting, more physical activity, or higher fitness? *Mayo Clinic Proceedings*, 90(11), 1533–40. doi:10.1016/j.mayocp.2015.08.005

3   V. W. Barry, M. Baruth, M. W. Beets, J. L. Durstine, J. Liu & S. N. Blair (2014). Fitness vs. fatness on all-cause mortality: a meta-analysis. *Progress in Cardiovascular Diseases*, 56(4), 382–90. doi:10.1016/j.pcad.2013.09.002

4   P. Kelly, S. Kahlmeier, T. Goetschi, N. Orsini, J. Richards, N. Roberts, ... C. Foster (2014). Systematic review and meta-analysis of reduction in all-cause mortality from walking and cycling and shape of dose response relationship. *International Journal of Behavioral Nutrition and Physical Activity*, 11, 132. doi:10.1186/s12966-014-0132-x

5   Australian Bureau of Statistics (2015). *National Health Survey: First results, 2014–15—Exercise*. Retrieved from: www.abs.gov.au/ausstats/abs@.nsf/Lookup/by%20Subject/4364.0.55.001~2014-15~Main%20 Features~Exercise~29.

6   B. E. Ainsworth, W. L. Haskell, M. C. Whitt, M. L. Irwin, A. M. Swartz, S. J. Strath, ... A. S. Leon (2000). Compendium of physical activities: an update of activity codes and MET intensities. *Medicine & Science in Sports & Exercise*, 32(9 Suppl.), S498–504.

7   A. B. Loucks, B. Kiens & H. H. Wright (2011). Energy availability in athletes. *Journal of Sports Science*, 29 Suppl.1, S7–15. doi:10.1080/02640414.2011.588958

8   J. Bergstrom, L. Hermansen, E. Hultman & B. Saltin (1967). Diet, muscle glycogen and physical performance. *Acta Physiologica Scandinavica*, 71(2), 140–50. doi:10.1111/j.1748-1716.1967.tb03720.x

9   A. Jeukendrup (2014). A step towards personalized sports nutrition: carbohydrate intake during exercise. *Sports Medicine*, 44(Suppl.1), S25–33. doi:10.1007/s40279-014-0148-z

10 M. Leveritt & P. J. Abernethy (1999). Effects of carbohydrate restriction on strength performance. *Journal of Strength and Conditioning Research*, 13(1), 52–7.

11 G. Slater & S. M. Phillips (2011). Nutrition guidelines for strength sports: sprinting, weightlifting, throwing events, and bodybuilding. *Journal of Sports Science*, 29 Suppl.1, S67–77. doi:10.1080/02640414.2011.574722

12 A. K. Hansen, C. P. Fischer, P. Plomgaard, J. L. Andersen, B. Saltin & B. K. Pedersen (2005). Skeletal muscle adaptation: training twice every second day vs. training once daily. *Journal of Applied Physiology*, 98(1), 93–9. doi:10.1152/japplphysiol.00163.2004

13 N. M. Cermak & L. J. van Loon (2013). The use of carbohydrates during exercise as an ergogenic aid. *Sports Medicine*, 43(11), 1139–55. doi:10.1007/s40279-013-0079-0

14 J. M. Carter, A. E. Jeukendrup & D. A. Jones (2004). The effect of carbohydrate mouth rinse on 1-h cycle time trial performance. *Medicine & Science in Sports & Exercise*, 2107–11. doi:10.1249/01.mss.0000147585.65709.6f

15 E. S. Chambers, M. W. Bridge & D. A. Jones (2009). Carbohydrate sensing in the human mouth: effects on exercise performance and brain activity. *Journal of Physiology*, 587(Pt 8), 1779–94. doi:10.1113/jphysiol.2008.164285

16 B. Desbrow, S. Anderson, J. Barrett, E. Rao & M. Hargreaves (2004). Carbohydrate-electrolyte feedings and 1 h time trial cycling performance. *International Journal of Sport Nutrition and Exercise Metabolism*, 14(5), 541–9.

17 A. E. Jeukendrup (2010). Carbohydrate and exercise performance: the role of multiple transportable carbohydrates. *Current Opinion in Clinical Nutrition and Metabolic Care*, 13(4), 452–7. doi:10.1097/MCO.0b013e328339de9f

18 R. L. Jentjens & A. E. Jeukendrup (2005). High rates of exogenous carbohydrate oxidation from a mixture of glucose and fructose ingested during prolonged cycling exercise. *British Journal of Nutrition*, 93(4), 485–92.

19 R. J. S. Costa, A. Miall, A. Khoo, C. Rauch, R. Snipe, V. Camoes-Costa & P. Gibson (2017). Gut-training: the impact of two weeks repetitive gut-challenge during exercise on gastrointestinal status, glucose availability, fuel kinetics, and running performance. *Applied Physiology, Nutrition, and Metabolism*, 42(5), 547–57. doi:10.1139/apnm-2016-0453

20 J. A. Hawley & J. P. Morton (2014). Ramping up the signal: promoting endurance training adaptation in skeletal muscle by nutritional manipulation. *Clinical and Experimental Pharmacology and Physiology*, 41(8), 608–13. doi:10.1111/1440-1681.12246

21 R. K. Randell, I. Rollo, T. J. Roberts, K. J. Dalrymple, A. E. Jeukendrup & J. M. Carter (2017). Maximal fat oxidation rates in an athletic population. *Medicine & Science in Sports & Exercise*, 49(1), 133–40. doi:10.1249/MSS.0000000000001084

22 S. D. Phinney, B. R. Bistrian, W. J. Evans, E. Gervino & G. L. Blackburn (1983). The human metabolic response to chronic ketosis without caloric restriction: preservation of submaximal exercise capability with reduced carbohydrate oxidation. *Metabolism*, 32(8), 769–76.

23 J. S. Volek, T. Noakes & S. D. Phinney (2015). Rethinking fat as a fuel for endurance exercise. *European Journal of Sport Science*, 15(1), 13–20. doi:10.1080/17461391.2014.959564

24 M. Tarnopolsky (2004). Protein requirements for endurance athletes. *Nutrition*, 20(7–8), 662–8. doi:10.1016/j.nut.2004.04.008

25 J. L. Areta, L. M. Burke, M. L. Ross, D. M. Camera, D. W. West, E. M. Broad, ...V. G. Coffey (2013). Timing and distribution of protein ingestion during prolonged recovery from resistance exercise alters myofibrillar protein synthesis. *Journal of Physiology*, 591(9), 2319–31. doi:10.1113/jphysiol.2012.244897

26 K. D. Tipton & R. R. Wolfe (2004). Protein and amino acids for athletes. *Journal of Sports Science*, 22(1), 65–79. doi:10.1080/0264041031000140554

27 O. C. Witard, S. R. Jackman, L. Breen, K. Smith, A. Selby & K. D. Tipton (2014). Myofibrillar muscle protein synthesis rates subsequent to a meal in response to increasing doses of whey protein at rest and after resistance exercise. *American Journal of Clinical Nutrition*, 99(1), 86–95. doi:10.3945/ajcn.112.055517

28 J. E. Tang, D. R. Moore, G. W. Kujbida, M. A. Tarnopolsky & S. M. Phillips (2009). Ingestion of whey hydrolysate, casein, or soy protein isolate: effects on mixed muscle protein synthesis at rest and following resistance exercise in young men. *Journal of Applied Physiology*, 107(3), 987–92. doi:10.1152/japplphysiol.00076.2009

29 B. J. Schoenfeld, A. A. Aragon & J. W. Krieger (2013). The effect of protein timing on muscle strength and hypertrophy: a meta-analysis. *Journal of the International Society of Sports Nutrition*, 10(1), 53. doi:10.1186/1550-2783-10-53

30 L. M. Sinclair & P. S. Hinton (2005). Prevalence of iron deficiency with and without anemia in recreationally active men and women. *Journal of the American Dietetic Association*, 105(6), 975–8. doi:10.1016/j.jada.2005.03.005

31 G. L. Close, J. Russell, J. N. Cobley, D. J. Owens, G. Wilson, W. Gregson, ... J. P. Morton (2013). Assessment of vitamin D concentration in non-supplemented professional athletes and healthy adults during the winter months in the UK: implications for skeletal muscle function. *Journal of Sports Science*, 31(4), 344–53. doi:10.1080/02640414.2012.733822

32 D. Morrison, J. Hughes, P. A. Della Gatta, S. Mason, S. Lamon, A. P. Russell & G. D. Wadley (2015). Vitamin C and E supplementation prevents some of the cellular adaptations to endurance-training in humans. *Free Radical Biology and Medicine*, 89, 852–62. doi:10.1016/j.freeradbiomed.2015.10.412

33 E. D. Goulet (2013). Effect of exercise-induced dehydration on endurance performance: evaluating the impact of exercise protocols on outcomes using a meta-analytic procedure. *British Journal of Sports Medicine*, 47(11), 679–86. doi:10.1136/bjsports-2012-090958

34 B. Desbrow, S. Jansen, A. Barrett, M. D. Leveritt & C. Irwin (2014). Comparing the rehydration potential of different milk-based drinks to a carbohydrate-electrolyte beverage. *Applied Physiology, Nutrition, and Metabolism*, 39(12), 1366–72. doi:10.1139/apnm-2014-0174

35 N. Campagnolo, E. Iudakhina, C. Irwin, M. Schubert, G. R. Cox, M. Leveritt & B. Desbrow (2017). Fluid, energy and nutrient recovery via ad libitum intake of different fluids and food. *Physiology and Behavior*, 171, 228–35. doi:10.1016/j.physbeh.2017.01.009

36 V. R. Clark, W. G. Hopkins, J. A. Hawley & L. M. Burke (2000). Placebo effect of carbohydrate feedings during a 40-km cycling time trial. *Medicine and Science in Sports and Exercise*, 32(9), 1642–7.

37 C. J. Beedie, E. M. Stuart, D. A. Coleman & A. J. Foad (2006). Placebo effects of caffeine on cycling performance. *Medicine and Science in Sports and Exercise*, 38(12), 2159–64.

38 Food Standards Australia New Zealand (2016). Sports foods. Standard 2.9.4 Formulated supplementary sports foods. Retrieved from: www.foodstandards.gov.au/consumer/nutrition/sportfood/Pages/default.aspx.

39 B. Desbrow, C. Biddulph, B. Devlin, G. D. Grant, S. Anoopkumar-Dukie & M. D. Leveritt (2012). The effects of different doses of caffeine on endurance cycling time trial performance. *Journal of Sports Science*, 30(2), 115–20. doi:10.1080/02640414.2011.632431

40 T. L. Skinner, D. G. Jenkins, D. R. Taaffe, M. D. Leveritt & J. S. Coombes (2013). Coinciding exercise with peak serum caffeine does not improve cycling performance. *Journal of Science and Medicine in Sport*, 16(1), 54–9. doi:10.1016/j.jsams.2012.04.004

41 G. R. Cox, B. Desbrow, P. G. Montgomery, M. E. Anderson, C. R. Bruce, T. A. Macrides, ... L. M. Burke (2002). Effect of different protocols of caffeine intake on metabolism and endurance performance. *Journal of Applied Physiology*, 93(3), 990–9. doi:10.1152/japplphysiol.00249.2002

42 N. W. Pitchford, J. W. Fell, M. D. Leveritt, B. Desbrow & C. M. Shing (2014). Effect of caffeine on cycling time-trial performance in the heat. *Journal of Science and Medicine in Sport*, 17(4), 445–9. doi:10.1016/j.jsams.2013.07.004

43 N. F. McMahon, M. D. Leveritt & T. G. Pavey (2017). The effect of dietary nitrate supplementation on endurance exercise performance in healthy adults: a systematic review and meta-analysis. *Sports Medicine*, 47(4), 735–56. doi:10.1007/s40279-016-0617-7

44 R. K. Boorsma, J. Whitfield & L. L. Spriet (2014). Beetroot juice supplementation does not improve performance of elite 1500-m runners. *Medicine and Science in Sports and Exercise*, 46(12), 2326–34. doi:10.1249/MSS.0000000000000364

45 D. J. Peart, J. C. Siegler & R. V. Vince (2012). Practical recommendations for coaches and athletes: a meta-analysis of sodium bicarbonate use for athletic performance. *Journal of Strength and Conditioning Research*, 26(7), 1975–83. doi:10.1519/JSC.0b013e3182576f3d

46 B. Saunders, K. Elliott-Sale, G. G. Artioli, P. A. Swinton, E. Dolan, H. Roschel, ... B. Gualano (2017). Beta-alanine supplementation to improve exercise capacity and performance: a systematic review and meta-analysis. *British Journal of Sports Medicine*, 51(8), 658–69. doi:10.1136/bjsports-2016-096396

47 R. Cooper, F. Naclerio, J. Allgrove & A. Jimenez (2012). Creatine supplementation with specific view to exercise/sports performance: an update. *Journal of the International Society of Sports Nutrition*, 9(1), 33. doi:10.1186/1550-2783-9-33

48 J. D. Branch (2003). Effect of creatine supplementation on body composition and performance: a meta-analysis. *International Journal of Sport Nutrition and Exercise Metabolism*, 13(2), 198–226.

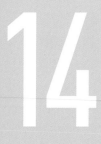

CHAPTER 14

NUTRITION DURING PREGNANCY AND LACTATION

SARA GRAFENAUER

CHAPTER OBJECTIVES

This chapter will enable the reader to:

- describe the impact of nutrition on early development in the foetus
- identify requirements for energy, nutrients and key foods during pregnancy and lactation
- outline the processes involved in breastfeeding and describe the benefits of breastfeeding for mother and their infants.

KEY TERMS

Breastfeeding   Lactation

Colostrum   Pregnancy

Gestation

KEY POINTS

- The peri-conceptual period, during pregnancy and the post-natal period are critical time points for nutrition where nutrient consumption has a major influence on future health.
- Nutrition provides a major environmental exposure for genetic expression in the child, and the mother's bodyweight and the maintenance of nutritional reserves are important considerations.

INTRODUCTION

This chapter addresses the significance of nutrition at the start of life, and this begins with the nutritional status of the parent. As a pregnancy provides the environment in which new life begins, the mother's body in particular needs to be adequately nourished prior to conception. This needs to continue throughout the pregnancy and then through the period of lactation, with breast milk providing the primary food for the newborn and the early periods of infancy. Understanding the nutritional needs of the mother requires an appreciation of the physiological changes that are occurring during these times and how this relates to nutrient requirements and food choices.

STOP AND THINK

- Why are food choices so important when planning a pregnancy and during the pregnancy itself?
- How might nutritional requirements change during pregnancy and lactation, and why?
- What are the benefits of breastfeeding an infant from birth?

HOW DOES NUTRITION HAVE AN IMPACT ON EARLY DEVELOPMENT IN THE FOETUS?

Identifying the nutritional requirements in pregnancy first requires an understanding of **pregnancy** itself. Pregnancy involves the rapid growth and development of the foetus, and as such makes significant demands on physiological and metabolic processes, and thereby nutrients and foods. Adequately nourishing the mother and foetus during this period is important for future physical and mental health. Foetal nutrition is now understood to influence the future health of the adult and even future generations [1].

Pregnancy
the period from embryonic implantation in the uterus to birth.

Pregnancy has been likened to a looking glass to the future. Health issues arising during this time can be an indication of diseases to come later in life. This is especially true for glycaemic control and hypertension. The unique nutritional requirements of pregnancy promote foetal growth while preserving the nutrition and energy stores of the mother.

For the individual, the peri-conceptual period may easily be overlooked as an important period for preparing the body for pregnancy, and many women are unaware that inadequate nutrient intakes can reduce their chance of conceiving. Nutrition affects oocyte development, which can impact on the ability to establish pregnancy in the first instance [2] and undernutrition can influence foetal development. Many pregnancies are unplanned [3] but peri-conceptual blood tests can be performed to check for disease immunity and any possible nutrient deficiencies [4]. Polycystic ovarian syndrome (PCOS) is a condition associated with increased weight, metabolic, hormonal and reproductive alterations that can affect fertility, but through weight loss and dietary modification pregnancy is made possible [2].

>> RESEARCH AT WORK

RESEARCH ON FOETAL PROGRAMMING

David Barker and colleagues proposed the 'early origins of adult disease' hypothesis. Infants born at the extreme ends of the birth weight distribution (very low or very high birth weight) were observed to have a higher prevalence of cardiovascular disease [5, 6]. 'Foetal programming', as this original hypothesis was known, is about more than just birth weight, and research is now focused on the role of the placenta. Early conception is the period of time from when the female egg (ova) is penetrated by the male sperm (spermatozoid), up to about eight weeks thereafter, when the embryo is considered a foetus. During this time, the foetal cells are nourished by the yolk sac within the egg since in this early phase there is no established nutrient supply from the mother. Nutrition during this time frame is key to establishing a well-developed placenta in terms of size, function and metabolism [2]. The placenta is the organ that provides nutrients and oxygen to the foetus and returns carbon dioxide and other waste products to be excreted. It is the weight of the placenta and the size and shape of its surface that affect nutrient transfer [6]. This phase of pregnancy is now thought to be central to the future health of the offspring, including implantation of the zygote, growth and compensatory expansion of the placenta and, in turn, delivery of nutrients to the foetus once this is required [5; 6]. Maternal energy needs are not increased at this stage, but diet quality is important in terms of the nutrients that reach the foetus via the complex 'supply line' [2; 7] once it is in place. Until such time, it is the mother's body weight and body composition, a result of much earlier nutritional intake, that influences nutrient availability from the blastocyst stage onward [6]. Undernutrition at this stage is the focus of research around postnatal health outcomes.

Despite the common belief that pregnancy involves eating for two, maternal energy needs are not increased until the second and third trimester of pregnancy. While a normal pregnancy lasts for about 40 weeks, this is broken into three trimesters of approximately 13 weeks each. By the second and third trimester, energy requirements do increase to incorporate the needs of the growing foetus. During the third trimester, especially towards the end of this period, the foetus is laying down fatty tissue (brown fat) in preparation for early life when energy is devoted to the birthing process, and thereafter to thermoregulation.

The additional energy requirements in pregnancy are relatively small compared with the mother's basal metabolic rate (BMR). The additional energy needs are to compensate for the expanded blood volume, the work performed by the heart, lungs and kidneys, the metabolic needs of the foetus and the additional needs required for physical activity with weight gain. Dietary guidance needs to emphasise nutrient rather than energy requirements [8].

Energy requirements are related to meeting nutrient needs and weight gain for a normal pregnancy. For a normal, singleton (one baby) full-term pregnancy, weight gain is normally between 11.5 and 16 kg and multiple births are associated with a 17–25 kg gain for healthy weight mothers [9]. There are International Guidelines for weight gain based on pre-pregnancy body mass index (BMI) [10] (Tables 14.1 and 14.2). Excess weight gain alone or combined with higher pre-pregnancy BMI places the mother and child at increased risk [11], although weight-loss diets are not recommended at any time during pregnancy [10] and conception may need to be delayed following rapid weight loss or bariatric surgery [12].

TABLE 14.1   RECOMMENDATIONS FOR TOTAL WEIGHT GAIN DURING PREGNANCY BASED ON PRE-PREGNANCY BMI

Pre-pregnancy BMI	Total weight gain (kg)*
Underweight: <8.5 kg/m²	12.7–18.2
Normal weight: 18.5–24.9 kg/m²	11.4–15.9
Overweight: 25.0–29.9 kg/m²	6.8–11.4
Obese: >30 kg/m²	5–9.1

*Calculated from Institute of Medicine & National Research Council (2009). *Weight Gain During Pregnancy: Reexamining the guidelines*. Washington, DC: National Academies Press.

TABLE 14.2   RECOMMENDED WEIGHT GAIN GUIDELINES FOR WOMEN CARRYING TWINS

Week of gestation	Maternal pre-gravid BMI weight status			
	Underweight (BMI<19.9)	Normal weight (BMI 20-24.9)	Overweight (BMI 25-29.9)	Obese (BMI>30)
	Kg/wk weight gain			
<20	0.57–0.79	0.45–0.68	0.45–0.57	0.34–0.45
20–28	0.68–0.79	0.57–0.79	0.45–0.68	0.34–0.57
>28	0.57	0.45	0.45	0.34

Source: B Luke, M.L. Hedger, C. Nugent, R.B. Newman, J.G. Mauldin, F.R Witter,& M.J. O'Sullivan (2003) Body mass index-specific sweight gains associated with optimal birth weights in twin pregnancies. *Journal of Reproductive Medicine*, 48(4), 217–24.

The duration of a full-term pregnancy is between 37 to 40 weeks **gestation**, although babies can be safely born before 37 weeks. For multiple births, 35 to 38 weeks is considered full term as the placenta ages faster [13], possibly undergoing calcification, and intrauterine growth of twins usually stops after 39 weeks [13].

Gestation
the period of pregnancy (usually around 40 weeks).

For singleton infants, 22 to 37 weeks is considered preterm. In Australia, preterm infants comprise between 7 and 12% of all births, but also account for two-thirds of perinatal deaths [14; 15]. Under 35 weeks, infants may not have a developed suck reflex and may require 'assisted' or tube feeding. Preterm infants are functionally immature, have low levels of brown fat and poor thermoregulatory mechanisms—lack of surfactant in the lungs affects respiratory functioning and increases risk of respiratory distress [9].

The principle of energy balance is important in managing weight and ensuring adequate nutrition during pregnancy. Overweight needs to be avoided. In Australia, for example, one-third of pregnant women are overweight or obese [16] and this is one of the key modifiable risk factors for poor pregnancy outcomes. Malnutrition can exist with obesity [17; 18], and despite excessive energy intake, micronutrient deficiencies have been noted. There needs to be a focus on correcting any nutrient issues early in a pregnancy, emphasising nutrient-rich foods and dietary patterns with limited 'extra' foods [19; 20]. When a woman is overweight or obese prior to becoming pregnant, weight gain expectations are lower; 7–11.5 kg and 5–9 kg respectively as per Institute of Medicine (IOM) guidelines [21]. Overweight women can be at increased risk during pregnancy of complications affecting their health, including gestational diabetes mellitus, pregnancy induced hypertension and pre-eclampsia, venous thrombo-embolism, labour induction and caesarean section [22; 23]. Overweight is linked with greater risks of depressive symptoms following delivery [24], and greater difficulties in breastfeeding, particularly in positioning the infant. Adverse effects of excess weight are closely aligned with BMI classification [25].

STOP AND THINK

- Why do nutrients play such an important role in the early development of the foetus?
- Why might pregnancy provide a mirror to the future of a woman's health?
- What factors need to be considered when determining energy requirements from food during pregnancy?

WHICH NUTRIENTS AND FOODS NEED SPECIAL ATTENTION IN PREGNANCY AND LACTATION?

It is known that many women in Australia have nutrient intakes below nationally recommended levels during pregnancy [26–28]. The nutritional requirements for pregnancy are defined within Australia's Nutrient Reference Values (NRVs; Table 14.3). Given their significance in the physiological changes that occur during pregnancy, iron, folate, iodine, vitamin D and long chain polyunsaturated fatty acids (LCPUFA) are key nutrients for consideration.

See Chapter 12 for more on iron.

Iron is found in red meats, fish, poultry, eggs and wholegrain cereals. Iron deficiency and iron deficiency anaemia (IDA) during pregnancy are risk factors for preterm delivery, prematurity and small for gestational age birth weight [29; 30]. Iron deficiency also has a negative effect on behavioural development and on intelligence, which may not be reversible [31]. Preventing iron deficiency in the foetus can be addressed by preventing iron deficiency in the pregnant woman. It has been shown that these issues can be reduced with iron supplementation [32]; however, iron-rich foods and using high vitamin C food choices to improve iron absorption are always preferred. The requirements for absorbed iron increase during pregnancy range from ~1.0 mg/day in the first trimester to 7.5 mg/day in the third trimester.

See Chapter 10 for more on folate.

Folate is a B group vitamin found in cereals, bread, vegetables and legumes. Deficiency in pregnant women is associated with neural tube defects in infants if folate is insufficient prior to conception. 400 μg of folic acid daily is recommended in addition to foods that are rich in folate or fortified with folic acid [33] for up to three months prior to conception and during pregnancy. The critical period for neural tube development is 17–30 days of gestation, a time when most women would not realise they are pregnant. A history of neural tube defect is an indication for a significantly higher dose of folate [4]. Interestingly, additional folate may be linked to increased twinning, and monitoring of multiple births now that fortification of the food supply (bread) is in place [34] will become important. Adequate folate and maintaining homocysteine levels are also thought to be important in prevention of pre-eclampsia (discussed later in this section).

See Chapter 12 for more on iodine.

Iodine is found in seafood, iodised table salt, bread and in low amounts in vegetables depending on the soil. Iodine is rapidly absorbed via the stomach and duodenum and is taken up by the thyroid depending on supply and the functional state of the thyroid. As maternal thyroid production increases in early gestation, there is increased demand and increased

TABLE 14.3 NRVs FOR NORMAL SINGLETON PREGNANCIES

Pregnant women	14–18 years	19–30 years	31–50 years
Macronutrients			
Protein (RDI*—g/day)	58	60	60
Dietary fats (AI**—g/day) Linoleic acid A-linolenic acid LC n-3 (DHA/EPA/DPA)	10 1.0 110	10 1.0 115	10 1.0 115
Dietary fibre (AI—g/day)	25	28	28
Water (AI—L/day)	2.4 (1.8—fluid only)	3.1 (2.3—fluid only)	3.1 (2.3—fluid only)
Micronutrients			
Vitamin A (retinol equivalents) (AI—µg/day)	700	800	800
Thiamin (RDI—mg/day)	1.4	1.4	1.4
Riboflavin (RDI—mg/day)	1.4	1.4	1.4
Niacin (niacin equivalents) (RDI—mg/day)	18	18	18
Vitamin B6 (RDI—mg/day)	1.9	1.9	1.9
Vitamin B12 (RDI—µg/day)	2.6	2.6	2.6
Folate (folate equivalents) (RDI—µg/day)	600	600	600
Pantothenic acid (AI—mg/day)	5.0	5.0	5.0
Biotin (AI—µg/day)	30	30	30
Vitamin C (RDI—mg/day)	55	60	60
Vitamin D (RDI—mg/day)	5	5	5
Vitamin E (α-tocopherol equivalents) (AI—mg/day)	8	7	7
Calcium (RDI—mg/day)	1300	1000	1000
Zinc (RDI—mg/day)	10	11	11
Iron (RDI—mg/day)	27	27	27

*RDI: recommended dietary intake
**AI: adequate intake

Source: National Health and Medical Research Council (2006). *Nutrient Reference Values for Australia and New Zealand, Including Recommended Dietary Intakes*. Canberra: NHMRC. © Commonwealth of Australia

iodine clearance as glomerular filtration via the kidneys increases [35]. Iodine readily crosses the placenta, facilitating the transfer of iodine to the foetus [36]. It is important to note that the most severe effects of deficiency are seen as a result of inadequate nutrition in pregnancy, ranging from reduced auditory capacity and loss of intelligence quotient (IQ) points, to mild retardation and, in extreme cases, cretinism [36]. Mild forms of iodine deficiency result in an average reduction in IQ of 10–13.5 points and it is unknown if adequate intakes later in childhood can reverse the neurocognitive damage caused by even mild maternal iodine deficiency in pregnancy [12].

See Chapter 9 for more on vitamin D.

Vitamin D is a fat-soluble vitamin made from exposure to adequate sunlight. Vitamin D presents at low levels in the Australian population [37] with >60% of women in the reproductive age group considered vitamin D deficient [12]. During pregnancy, the foetus is reliant on maternal supply for skeletal formation and cell differentiation [38]. Hypovitaminosis D during gestation may also result in rickets in infancy or childhood, and there are also respiratory connections with asthma [39]. While the key source for vitamin D is sunlight, care needs to be taken to avoid overt sun exposure that may encourage skin cancers. The food supply contains some natural sources of vitamin D (such as fatty fish) and fortified products (margarine, some dairy products) are also available. However, the level defined as 'adequate' for maternal vitamin D remains controversial [38] and some groups within the population may be considered at higher risk than others.

n-3 long chain polyunsaturated fatty acids (LCPUFA) are found in fish. Significant findings have emerged on the benefits of maternal n-3 LCPUFA, in particular docosahexaenoic acid (DHA) [40]. Fatty fish consumption during pregnancy and breastfeeding is associated with increased DHA levels in breast milk [41] and improved infant health outcomes, such as visual acuity and cognitive development [42]. Consumption of omega n-3 during pregnancy and breastfeeding is supported by a Cochrane Database Systematic Review [43] and a European Union Perinatal Lipid Intake Working Group assessment [44]. Recent key studies have identified that pre-term infants benefit most, as they essentially miss the rapid *in utero* growth characteristic of the last trimester, and the opportunity to accrue adequate fat reserves [45–47]; however, recent research suggests caution in this area [48].

Eating well is an important part of promoting health during pregnancy. Pregnant women can enjoy a wide variety of healthy nutritious foods throughout the full term. The Australian Guide to Healthy Eating (AGHE) is designed to meet the nutrient and energy requirements for all groups within the population with foods from each of the core food groups (Table 14.4).

Poor maternal nutrition needs to be avoided. The impacts are present, for example, in women who deliver preterm. Signs include a low pre-gravid body weight and BMI, poor weight gain for stage of pregnancy and poor foetal growth [32], resulting in low birth weight (<2500 g) or small for gestational age (<10th percentile for gestational age). Famine in the third trimester particularly influences circulating glucose, resulting in slower foetal growth and influencing birth size. The Dutch Famine of 1944–45 has been well documented for its effects on foetal growth [49]. Earlier in pregnancy, micronutrient deficits, particularly iron and folate, have been shown to influence pregnancy outcomes with consistency [32].

TABLE 14.4   AVERAGE RECOMMENDED FOOD INTAKE SERVES PER DAY FOR PREGNANCY (AGHE)

	Age	Vegetables and legumes/beans	Fruit	Grain	Lean meat, poultry, fish eggs, nuts, seeds and legumes/beans	Milk, yoghurt, cheese and/or alternatives
Women	19–50	5	2	6	2.5	2.5
	51–70	5	2	4	2	4
	70+	5	2	3	2	4
Pregnant		5	2	8.5	3.5	2.5
Lactating		7.5	2	9	2.5	2.5

Source: National Health and Medical Research Council (2013). *Australian Dietary Guidelines*. Canberra: NHMRC. © Commonwealth of Australia

Some women experience some nausea and vomiting in the early part of the pregnancy. However, if vomiting is severe and protracted and/or affects weight gain of the mother or the foetus (measured during ultrasound examinations), problems may arise. The term **hyperemesis gravidarum** refers to a condition where there may be a need for hospitalisation for correction of dehydration and electrolyte disturbance [50] and artificial feeding (into the duodenum) may be required. The cause of hyperemesis is largely unknown, although there is some research investigating the diet prior to pregnancy, particularly consumption of a healthy diet including vegetables, fish and moderate water intake as a possible link [51].

Other women may show clinical signs of glucose intolerance during pregnancy. **Gestational diabetes mellitus** (GDM), which literally means 'diabetes in pregnancy', is one of the most common metabolic disorders encountered by pregnant women, affecting approximately 10–13% of pregnant women in Australia [52]. It is commonly defined as 'any degree of glucose intolerance with onset or first recognition during pregnancy' [53]. Pregnant women with GDM have an impaired ability to metabolise carbohydrate foods they consume, resulting in higher post-meal blood glucose levels (BGLs). A high post-meal BGL was found to be associated with a range of adverse pregnancy outcomes, including giving birth to a baby with a high birth weight [54; 55]. However, if properly treated, pregnant women with GDM may achieve similar pregnancy outcomes as those with a healthy pregnancy. Recent studies suggest that a carbohydrate-controlled, low glycaemic index (GI) eating pattern may be an effective dietary strategy to manage post-meal BGLs [56; 57]. If dietary management fails, insulin injections is the preferred treatment due to the uncertain effects of oral hypoglycaemic agents commonly used in type 2 diabetes on the growing foetus [58].

Food safety is particularly important during all stages of pregnancy, as a severe bacterial infection can affect the mother and the foetus, possibly resulting in stillbirth. Some foods need to be avoided—for example, soft cheese, luncheon meats, raw and smoked fish and seafood, pre-prepared salads, sprouts and pâté [59; 60]—as these foods are more likely to be a risk for contamination with the food-borne bacterium *Listeria monocytogenes*. It is important to check that foods are properly cooked and stored. For example, cold food must be kept cold, below 4°C, and cooked food must be hot, such that the temperature of the food is above 60°C. Buffet-style foods are discouraged as there is risk of contamination and foods not being held at the correct temperature. 'Left-over' food should also be treated with care and discarded if not eaten within two days, even if it has been stored correctly. Raw or undercooked eggs should also not be consumed as these are a risk for *Salmonella* [61]. Although the messages about listeriosis may rank lower than others in pregnancy, prevention is simple and it is an important public health message.

Although fish is encouraged in the diet as a source of protein and because fatty fish (salmon, tuna, sardines and mackerel) contain a source of omega-3 fatty acids, heavy metals may be a source of concern in certain types of fish. Pregnant women are advised to consume no more than one serve per fortnight of shark, marlin or swordfish and no other fish that fortnight, or one serve of orange roughly (deep sea perch) and no other fish that week [62].

For most people, moderate caffeine consumption (~3 cups instant or espresso style) can be part of a healthy diet. The Australian Dietary Guidelines recommend a maximum of 300 mg/day for pregnant women [63] (Table 14.5).

Alcohol consumed by a breastfeeding mother is concentrated in breast milk within 30–60 minutes of ingestion [64]. The blood alcohol concentration of the mother is influenced by body weight,

Hyperemesis gravidarum
excessive vomiting associated with pregnancy and requiring hospitalisation.

Gestational diabetes mellitus
glucose intolerance during pregnancy.

See Chapter 23 for more on food safety.

TABLE 14.5   CAFFEINE CONTENT OF BEVERAGES, 2018

Beverage	Serving size	mg of caffeine per serve
Espresso coffee (short black)	50 mL	145
Formulated caffeinated beverages	250 mL can	80
Instant coffee	1 tsp/250 mL cup	80
Coca-Cola	375 mL can	48.75
Black tea	250 mL cup	50
Energy drink (soft drink)	250 mL can	80
Milk chocolate	50 g	10

Source: www.foodstandards.gov.au/consumer/generalissues/Pages?Caffeine.aspx

proportion of adipose tissue to lean muscle tissue, the stomach contents at the time of alcohol ingestion, rate of alcohol consumption, and the amount and the strength of alcohol. However, even small amounts of alcohol, if passed to an infant, could have a negative effect as newborns have very limited ability to metabolise alcohol [64].

Breastfeeding
suckling and nourishing an infant via the breast.

Lactation
production of milk from the breast.

During **breastfeeding** the nutrient and energy needs of the mother are increased and are in proportion to the volume of milk produced (**lactation**) [65]. The nutrient requirements are higher than when the infant was in utero, especially if exclusively breastfeeding (Table 14.6).

While breast milk is the sole food of the infant, the mother's energy requirements will be higher compared with when complementary foods are introduced. Over time, some of the additional requirements of breastfeeding can be derived from body stores, but advice regarding the dietary pattern and balancing food intake is important as breastfeeding has no sustained impact on maternal weight gain or loss [8]. Mothers will often feel very thirsty while breastfeeding and it is important to replace fluids regularly with water, and also energy-dense, nutrient-rich fluids like milk. Caffeine can pass into breast milk, possibly disturbing sleep patterns of the infant, so an awareness of the caffeine content of foods and fluids is necessary.

It is suggested that women who return to their pre-pregnancy weight by about six months have a lower risk of being overweight 10 years later [66]. Either diet and exercise or diet alone are effective in assisting with post-partum weight loss, although there is insufficient data for breastfeeding women [66]. While low-intensity activity should not affect breast milk supply, higher levels of activity may need to be adjusted according to how both mother and baby respond. Weight loss can influence breast milk supply and the composition, as components of protein breakdown can be detected in breast milk. Infants may exhibit signs of fussiness following exercise if the session was heavy.

STOP AND THINK

- Why are certain nutrients important during pregnancy and lactation?
- Which particular nutritional problems can emerge during pregnancy?
- Which foods may require special attention during pregnancy and lactation?

TABLE 14.6 NRVs FOR LACTATION

Requirements for breastfeeding women	14–18 years	19–30 years	31–50 years
Macronutrients			
Protein (RDI*—g/day)	63	67	67
Dietary fats (AI**—g/day) Linoleic acid A-linolenic acid LC n-3 (DHA/EPA/DPA)	12 1.2 140	12 1.2 145	12 1.2 145
Dietary fibre (AI—g/day)	27	30	30
Water (AI—L/day)	2.9 (2.3—fluid only)	3.5 (2.6—fluid only)	3.5 (2.6—fluid only)
Micronutrients			
Vitamin A (retinol equivalents) (AI—µg/day)	1100	1100	1100
Thiamin (RDI—mg/day)	1.4	1.4	1.4
Riboflavin (RDI—mg/day)	1.6	1.6	1.6
Niacin (niacin equivalents) (RDI—mg/day)	17	17	17
Vitamin B6 (RDI—mg/day)	2.0	2.0	2.0
Vitamin B12 (RDI—µg/day)	2.8	2.8	2.8
Folate (folate equivalents) (RDI—µg/day)	500	500	500
Pantothenic acid (AI—mg/day)	6.0	6.0	6.0
Biotin (AI—µg/day)	35	35	35
Vitamin C (RDI—mg/day)	80	85	85
Vitamin D (RDI—mg/day)	5	5	5
Vitamin E (α-tocopherol equivalents) (AI—mg/day)	12	11	11
Calcium (RDI—mg/day)	1300	1000	1000
Zinc (RDI—mg/day)	11	12	12
Iron (RDI—mg/day)	10	9	9

*RDI: recommended dietary intake
**AI: adequate intake

Source: National Health and Medical Research Council (2006). *Nutrient Reference Values for Australia and New Zealand, Including Recommended Dietary Intakes.* Canberra: NHMRC. © Commonwealth of Australia

HOW DOES BREASTFEEDING WORK?

Breastfeeding is provided by the mother to her baby from the time immediately after birth. The physiological processes are part of the sequence of events so, by nature, breast milk is the best food for infants. In 2003 the World Health Organization (WHO) recommended that all infants be exclusively breastfed for at least six months after birth [67]. That said, it is important that infants be managed individually as they move towards the introduction of solid foods to ensure that growth is optimal. Arguably, there is a 'window of tolerance' for introducing solids from between four and seven months [68]. The WHO also recommends breastfeeding up to the age of two years as part of the infant's diet; however, from a social point of view, there may be little support for continuing breastfeeding for this extended period of time [69]. Breastfeeding should continue until 12 months and beyond for as long as the mother and child desire. In Australia there is now a high-level enduring strategy to support breastfeeding and to measure the progress on increasing the number of babies who are breastfed exclusively up to six months [70].

From the early stages of pregnancy, breast tissue develops, particularly ductal growth, and prepares for the arrival of the infant. Maternal blood supply increases to breast tissue and around the abdomen. During the course of pregnancy, a number of changes to the physiological structure of breast tissue occur, in response to rising levels of progesterone, prolactin and placental lactogen [71], collectively called stage I lactogenesis (Figure 14.1). At birth, the removal of placenta triggers hormonal changes, and there is an abrupt drop in progesterone, signalling stage II lactogenesis [71].

FIGURE 14.1 STRUCTURE OF THE BREAST TISSUE AND DEVELOPMENT OF THE MILK DUCTS—LOBULAR ALVEOLAR COMPLEXES

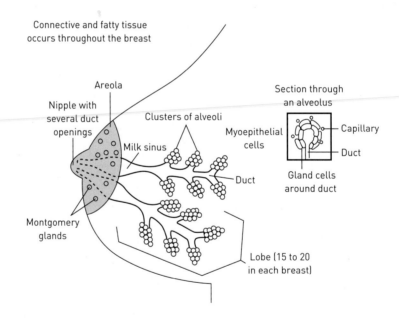

Initiating breastfeeding

Colostrum

initial secretion from breast before breast milk and contains immune factors.

The birthing process triggers hormones that prepare the body for breastfeeding and release of **colostrum**, the immunological forerunner to breast milk. Colostrum contains high levels of protein, but less fat than breast milk. It also contains vitamins A and B12, lactoferrin, immunoglobulin A, enzymes, maternal antibodies, living cells (leukocytes, neutrophils and macrophages) and probiotics providing some protection against illness

[63; 72]. Infants born via the birth canal acquire beneficial bacteria that is unique and protective for the period immediately following the birth, up until they are receiving adequate nutrition (from breast milk) to stimulate their own bacterial profile within their gut. Infants born via caesarean section do not obtain the same beneficial bacterial profile and tend to acquire a bacterial profile according to the environment in which they are delivered. Early breastfeeding following caesarean section is known to assist in the development of an improved profile in these infants.

Following delivery, there are hormonal changes within the body, such that all the processes required to initiate feeding are available (stage II lactogenesis). Early attachment and simulation of feeding encourages production. Nerve stimulation as the infant suckles stimulates release of prolactin and oxytocin. Prolactin is the hormone responsible for producing breast milk. In this early phase, the endocrine system is the major mechanism to control milk production and so what occurs is taken care of by the 'automatic' systems of the body. This changes to autocrine control as supply is stimulated as feeding continues within a supply–demand feedback mechanism [73].

Typically, milk comes in within 48–72 hours post-delivery [70]. This signals a change in volume and composition of the milk with transition milk being 90–100% whey, whereas mature milk (by eight months of age) is closer to 50% whey and 50% casein. This increase in volume has been found to be delayed following caesarean section [71] compared with a vaginal delivery, and delayed for primiparous (first delivery) versus multiparous women (subsequent delivery) [71], but not to the extent that feeding cannot be initiated. Women should be made aware that following a caesarean section, and/or if they are first-time mothers, onset of lactation may be delayed up to 72 hours. With the initiation of breastfeeding, engorgement may occur and ice-packs can be used to ease any related discomfort between feeds [74]. Trying different feeding positions can assist and this is a key time to support new parents.

As feeding continues, the key factors are related to the frequency of feeds, the spacing between feeds and the duration of feeds. The autocrine system takes the place of the previous endocrine control. The storage capacity of the breast, the amount of milk taken at each feed and the degree to which the breast is emptied determines the amount and rate of milk synthesised between feeds. Supply responds to demand.

Early skin-to-skin contact following delivery and in the weeks following delivery has been shown to impact positively on the mother–child bond, benefiting breastfeeding outcomes and cardiorespiratory stability and reducing infant crying [75]. Feeding must be learnt and it may take up to eight weeks for the mother to feel confident with the process, so the days and weeks following the birth are important in establishing a good supply and patterns of feeding (Figures 14.2 and 14.3). In Australia, 96% of women initiate breastfeeding [76]; however, a much smaller percentage reach six months with exclusive breastfeeding. This may represent acceptance that early colostrum is very important for the newborn infant, but lack of support is thought to be the main contributor to discontinued feeding.

TRY IT YOURSELF

Consider whether you have ever observed a woman breastfeeding her baby. How did the social conditions support the breastfeeding? Discuss the importance of social support structures and values that enable women to breastfeed in accordance with public health guidelines.

FIGURE 14.2 POSITIONING FOR BREASTFEEDING

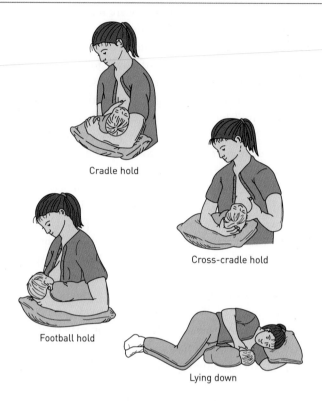

Cradle hold

Cross-cradle hold

Football hold

Lying down

FIGURE 14.3 SUCKLING INFANT POSITION

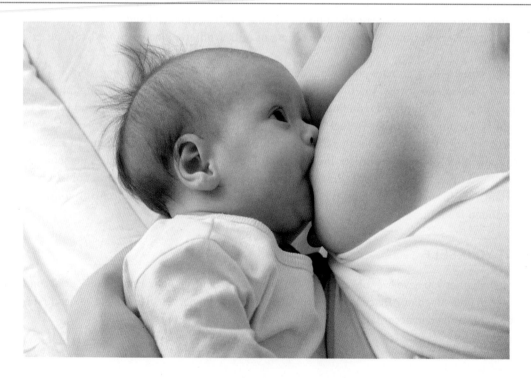

The 'let-down' is in response to prolactin: this is best described as pin-prickles or tingles followed by a rushing feeling as the breast milk is let down, although the sensation differs between women. Breast tissue needs to be checked throughout the day. Before a feed in the early weeks and months, breast tissue will feel swollen and hard. After a feed, breast tissue should feel smooth and as if the ducts are emptied. Some lumpiness is normal, but should be massaged out as blocked milk ducts can result in mastitis.

The infant is born with a sucking reflex when born at term, close to or around 40 weeks. This is an innate reflex and when attached to the breast (not the nipple but the areola area surrounding the nipple), the sucking response will stimulate the let-down. It is the periodic attachment of the infant that stimulates breast milk supply. If breast tissue is not stimulated at regular intervals in the early weeks and months of breastfeeding, supply can be affected. This is one reason why complementary feeding (with infant formula) is discouraged in this early time frame.

Establishing supply is key to the first 16 weeks post-delivery. Baby-led breastfeeding is encouraged such that there are no restrictions placed on the frequency or length of feeds [77] compared with scheduled feeding, where the frequency and length of feeds is predetermined [73]. As a general guide during the first weeks of life, most infants feed 8–12 times within a 24-hour period. It appears that breastfed infants have a greater degree of control of meal size and the intervals between feeds compared with infants who are formula fed [78] and this influences a slower rate of growth [72]. From birth to 12 months, breast milk or a commercial infant formula is the most important fluid. Any fluid supplementation while breastfeeding supply is being established may decrease milk removal and therefore affect milk production [79]. Additional water may be needed in hot weather after six months of age, and boiled, cooled tap water may be given [76].

The composition of breast milk changes within a day (higher lactose in the morning and a fattier composition at night) and within a single feed; again, the fore-milk is higher in carbohydrate-restoring glucose levels and the hind-milk, being higher in fat, provides satiety between feeds [80] (Figure 14.4). Consequently, the energy content of breast milk can vary, with a range of between 270 and 315 kJ per 100 mL identified [80; 81]. Ensuring the infant completes the feed, obtaining the more calorific hind-milk by fully emptying the breast, can be important for growth. Just getting the fore-milk can cause more gas production (due to the high lactose content), result in shorter periods of sleep (not enough fat to sustain the infant during sleep) and poorer growth.

FIGURE 14.4 VARIATION IN BREAST MILK COMPOSITION SHOWING EARLY- AND LATE-STAGE SECRETION

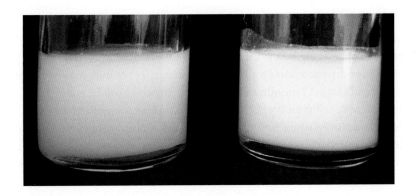

>> CASE 14.1

EXPLORING THE NUTRITIONAL PROPERTIES OF BREAST MILK

Although there is a great deal known to date about the composition of human breast milk, this knowledge will always be limited by the ability of the scientific techniques of the day to identify and measure components. Currently, we know that colostrum, the low-volume fluid released prior to milk secretion, is nutrient and energy dense, particularly high in protein and rich in immunoglobulins. This yellow-ish-coloured thick fluid is important in helping to colonise the gut with bifidus bacteria, a protective feature of breastfeeding. Within the first year of life, the whey and casein composition in breast milk changes to match the requirements of the infant. Whey is easily digestible and leaves the gut quickly, and as the first year of life progresses, the proportion of whey decreases and casein increases. Casein forms a distinct curd in the gut in response to gastric acid and remains there longer, providing greater satiety as the infant moves towards eight months of age. Mature milk continues to provide immune factors to the infant.

Breast milk is designed by nature to address the nutritional requirements of the infant, but has other protective effects. Research indicates that breastfeeding reduces the incidence of infectious diseases, including gastrointestinal and respiratory infections [82], and reduces the risk of otitis media, atopic eczema and, possibly, allergic rhinitis in childhood [82; 83]. Breastfed infants are thought to have lower rates of allergy, although breastfeeding is not a guarantee for avoiding allergy, as there is a large genetic component to susceptibility. The diet through infancy and childhood is more likely to affect the risk of allergy (asthma, eczema and other allergy) than the mother's diet during pregnancy as influences *in utero* are likely to be minimal [84–87]. Continued research in this area is developing greater clarity on this topic [88–90].

See Chapter 24 on nutrition and research.

- Typically a food is valued for its macro and micronutrient composition, and substitutes aim to mimic this composition. What other bioactive components do we now know that breast milk contains and how does this knowledge add to the evidence of its superiority as a first food for infants?
- Why might there be other health benefits from breast feeding (in addition to normal growth and development)?
- Why are dietary immune factors important for supporting infant health?

Ceasing breastfeeding

Ceasing breastfeeding may be voluntary or involuntary. In any case, it can be an emotional experience for the mother. When an infant is being weaned, it is ideal that it is done gradually. If this is not possible, and it is early in the lactation period, mastitis can be a risk. Self-expressing breast milk may be required to avoid this situation. Towards the end of the 12 months of breastfeeding, the child will be consuming a diverse range of foods and the nutrition obtained from breast milk will be secondary to meals. At this stage, it is much easier to decrease feeds and, eventually, when both mother and child are happy, they can wean completely. Some parents will decide to continue breastfeeding for longer periods, but it important to note that the dominant sucking reflex from birth will have changed, and by 12 months a child can sip and swallow from a normal cup, which is different from the action of sucking. Transitioning from a bottle at this stage is particularly important and a cup should be used by 12 months of age for complementary fluids like water and milk. It is generally not necessary to cease breast feeding during short-term illnesses as important anti-infective substances are passed via the breast milk to the infant, and this can be managed under proper medical supervision. Medications should be checked to confirm they are safe for the infant as some may pass into the breast milk.

Problems during breastfeeding

Mastitis is a condition whereby the breast becomes tender and swollen, usually due to infection (bacterial) via cracked nipples. Milk ducts may also become blocked and inflamed due to inadequate emptying of milk. Early signs of mastitis are flu-like symptoms, so a medical consultation and possible prescription of antibiotics may be needed to resolve the condition. During this time, it is usually recommended that feeding continues as ceasing breastfeeding may make the condition worse. Feeding from the breast that is worst affected first may help clear the blockage. Prevention of mastitis has not been adequately studied [91], although ensuring proper attachment, completely draining the breast at a feed and maintaining checks may be useful preventions.

≫ CASE 14.2

BREAST MILK SUBSTITUTES

In some cases, breastfeeding is not successful. If is it not possible to breastfeed, an appropriate infant formula needs to be selected [76]. Rather than approximate the nutritional makeup of breast milk, the composition of commercial infant formula aims to replicate the health outcomes observed for breastfed infants in terms of weight gain, gastrointestinal health and allergy. Breastfed infants may gain weight more slowly, particularly from three to 12 months of age, and this is thought to be an important feature in disease prevention later in life. Breastfed infants are better protected from a range of bacterial infections because of the natural bifidobacteria obtained from breastfeeding. Technological advances in infant formula now include tested, lower levels of protein to better match weight gain rates of breastfed infants [92–95]; the addition of probiotic bacteria for improved gastrointestinal health and recovery after infection [96–99]; and partially hydrolysed protein that has been clinically tested to reduce allergy in those infants that are not breastfed [100; 101].

The mean protein concentration of mature-term milk and preterm milk ranges from 0.8–1.2 g per 100 mL and 1.5–1.9 g per 100 mL. Fat is most variable and ranges from 3.7–4 g per 100 mL and 3.5–3.6 g per 100 mL. Lactose tends to fall between 6–7 g per 100 mL and is less variable [102]. Iron is reported between 0.1–1.6 mg/L and is diurnal, matching the changes in fat content within a day and is highest in transitional milk [103]. Cow's milk contains iron that is poorly absorbed, whereas full-term breast milk contains 0.3–0.5 µg/mL, and infant formula contains a median of 4–7 µg/mL as it is also not as well absorbed [104]. Regular cow's milk, goat's milk, soy or nut milks must not be used for infants in place of a commercial infant formula. Homemade (or DIY) formula should never be considered as it is not supported by scientific research and is unlikely to meet the precise needs of the infant or the food standards set by Food Standards Australia New Zealand (FSANZ).

Particular care should be taken to prepare formula to instructions and that equipment is sterile [76]. Formula feeding to a schedule has been found to be associated with rapid weight gain in infancy and parents who choose to use formula should be encouraged to feed on demand as is done with breastfeeding [105]. Simulating other features of breastfeeding are also recommended while formula feeding—for example, maintaining eye contact and swapping sides to assist with ocular development.

- What areas of particular care need to be taken when choosing and using breast milk substitutes?
- What additional research and support is needed to help address the issue of poor breastfeeding rates in Australia?

>> RESEARCH AT WORK

PROTEIN CONTENT OF INFANT FORMULA

The macronutrient composition of formula, in particular the protein content, has recently been shown to be important. In a large randomised controlled trial [106], babies born at term were fed infant formula and follow-on formula with either a lower protein content (1.77 g protein/100 Kcal and 2.2 g protein/100 Kcal) or a higher protein content (2.9 g protein/100 Kcal and 4.4 g protein/100 Kcal, respectively). It was found that weight-for-length Z score at two years of age was greater in the group of infants who received the formula with the higher protein content, translating into a higher BMI and 2.4-fold increased risk of obesity at six years of age [107]. The increased weight was in part related to a greater visceral fat mass, indicating that there may be metabolic consequences for these children as they grow older [108]. In contrast, the children who received the lower-protein formula showed no decrement in mental performance at eight years of age and performed similarly to children who were not randomised and who were breastfed [109].

STOP AND THINK

- What is colostrum and why is it an important component of breastfeeding newborn infants?
- How does the production of breast milk change over time and why?
- What actions help to support breast milk supply?

SUMMARY

- Pregnancy is a particular physiological state with implications for nutrition and food choice, and key nutrients have significant roles to play in supporting a healthy conception and pregnancy (iron, folate, LCPUFAs, iodine and vitamin D).
- Weight gain of the mother during pregnancy is an important parameter, adjusted according to pre-pregnancy weight and based on single or multiple foetuses.
- Pregnant women should enjoy a wide variety of nutritious foods throughout their term, although care should be taken with the safe preparation of food and the selection of seafood. Alcohol consumption should be avoided during pregnancy.
- Some nutrition-related conditions require health professional care during pregnancy such as diabetes, pre-eclampsia (high blood pressure) and severe vomiting.

- By nature, the national requirements for infants are met through breastfeeding. Breastfeeding on demand is the best choice for all infants. Infant formula is the only other acceptable choice if breastfeeding is not successful. If using formula, feeding on demand rather than by a schedule is advisable.
- Breast tissue changes from the beginning of pregnancy. The initiation of colostrum and then milk production is influenced by the mode of delivery of the infant, number of previous infants and stimulation of the nerves in breast tissue. Hormones and the endocrine system are responsible at first, changing to the autocrine system and a supply–demand scenario as feeding progresses.
- When breastfeeding, nutritional needs and requirements for fluids are greater, and dramatic weight loss is not recommended during lactation as this may affect breast milk supply.

PATHWAYS TO PRACTICE

- Parents will often take advice about parenting from family members. Skills in nutrition communications will help describe the nutritional needs for pregnancy and breastfeeding.
- Many areas in public health practice provide opportunities to contribute to reviews—for example, see <www.health.gov.au/breastfeeding> for updates to the *Australian National Breastfeeding Strategy: 2017 and beyond.*

DISCUSSION QUESTIONS

1. How would you approach a discussion with a mother-to-be about alcohol consumption?
2. If you have never experienced breastfeeding, how would you approach this topic in a group session with parents-to-be, considering that supporting breastfeeding is one of the Australian Dietary Guidelines?
3. How would a vegetarian mother-to-be ensure she met nutritional requirements for pregnancy? Which particular foods would be important?
4. What are the important considerations for weight gain during pregnancy and weight loss following delivery?
5. There are many reasons why breastfeeding is often not continued long term. What conditions may hinder breastfeeding within the first year of an infant's life?

USEFUL WEBLINKS

Australian Breastfeeding Association (ABA):
    www.breastfeeding.asn.au Promotes and protects breastfeeding. Counsellors can be contacted on the breastfeeding hotline (phone 1800 686 268).

Australian National Breastfeeding Strategy: 2017 and beyond:
    www.health.gov.au/breastfeeding

Community Health Centres:
    www.betterhealth.vic.gov.au/health/healthyliving/community-health-centres. Early childhood health service and community health centres are staffed by health professionals who specialise in child and family health throughout Australia.

Karitane:

www.karitane.com.au. Parent help centre Karitane provides support on a wide range of issues via consultation with child and family health nurses providing consultation (phone 1300 227 464). Residential services are available.

MotherSafe:

www.mothersafe.org.au. Provides a comprehensive counselling service for women and their healthcare providers concerned about exposures during pregnancy and breastfeeding in New South Wales.

Tresillian Parent's Help Line:

www.tresillian.org.au. NSW-based parent help centre, where people can speak to a registered nurse via phone (1800 272 736) or online. Residential services are available.

FURTHER READING

Bass, J. L., Gartley, T. & Kleinman, R. (2016). Unintended consequences of current breastfeeding initiatives. *JAMA Pediatrics*, 170(10), 923–4. doi:10.1001/jamapediatrics.2016.1529

Berti, C., Agostoni, C., Davanzo, R., Hyppönen, E., Isolauri, E., Meltzer, H. M., ... Cetin, I. (2017). Early-life nutritional exposures and lifelong health: immediate and long-lasting impacts of probiotics, vitamin D, and breastfeeding. *Nutrition Reviews*, 75(2), 83–97. doi:10.1093/nutrit/nuw056

Bravi, F., Wiens, F., Decarli, A., Dal Pont, A., Agostoni, C. & Ferraroni, M. (2016). Impact of maternal nutrition on breast-milk composition: a systematic review. *American Journal of Clinical Nutrition*, 104(3), 646–62. doi:10.3945/ajcn.115.120881

Emmett, P. M., Jones, L. R. & Golding, J. (2015). Pregnancy diet and associated outcomes in the Avon Longitudinal Study of Parents and Children. *Nutrition Reviews*, 73(Suppl.3), 154–74. doi:10.1093/nutrit/nuv053

Flynn, A. C., Dalrymple, K., Barr, S., Poston, L., Goff, L. M., Rogozińska, E., ... Thangaratinam, S. (2016). Dietary interventions in overweight and obese pregnant women: a systematic review of the content, delivery, and outcomes of randomized controlled trials. *Nutrition Reviews*, 74(5), 312–28. doi:10.1093/nutrit/nuw005

Garcia, A. H., Voortman, T., Baena, C. P., Chowdhurry, R., Muka, T., Jaspers, L., ... van den Hooven, E. H. (2016). Maternal weight status, diet, and supplement use as determinants of breastfeeding and complementary feeding: a systematic review and meta-analysis. *Nutrition Reviews*, 74(8), 490–516. doi:10.1093/nutrit/nuw016

Gould, J. F., Treyvaud, K., Yelland, L. N, et al. (2017). Seven-year follow-up of children born to women in a randomized trial of prenatal DHA supplementation. *JAMA—Journal of the American Medical Association*, 317(11), 1173–5. doi:10.1001/jama.2016.21303

Hughes, H. K., Landa, M. M. & Sharfstein, J. M. (2017). Marketing claims for infant formula: the need for evidence. *JAMA Pediatrics*, 171(2), 105–6. doi:10.1001/jamapediatrics.2016.3837

Martin, C. R., Ling, P. R. & Blackburn, G. L. (2016). Review of infant feeding: key features of breast milk and infant formula. *Nutrients*, 8(5), 279. doi:10.3390/nu8050279

McGuire, M. K. & McGuire, M. A. (2015). Human milk: mother nature's prototypical probiotic food? *Advances in Nutrition: An International Review Journal*, 6(1), 112–23. doi:10.3945/an.114.007435

Muktabhant, B., Lawrie, T. A., Lumbiganon, P. & Laopaiboon, M. (2015). Diet or exercise, or both, for preventing excessive weight gain in pregnancy. *The Cochrane Database of Systematic Reviews*, 6, CD007145. doi:10.1002/14651858.CD007145.pub3

Pannia, E., Cho, C. E., Kubant, R., Sánchez-Hernández, D., Huot, P. S. P. & Harvey Anderson, G. (2016). Role of maternal vitamins in programming health and chronic disease. *Nutrition Reviews*, 74(3), 166–80. doi:10.1093/nutrit/nuv103

Rollins, N. C., Bhandari, N., Hajeebhoy, N., Horton, S., Lutter, C. K., Martines, J. C., ...Victora, C. G. (2016). Why invest, and what it will take to improve breastfeeding practices? *The Lancet*, 387(10017), 491–504. doi:10.1016/S0140-6736(15)01044-2

Schoenaker, D. A. J. M., Mishra, G. D., Callaway, L. K. & Soedamah-Muthu, S. S. (2016). The role of energy, nutrients, foods, and dietary patterns in the development of gestational diabetes mellitus: a systematic review of observational studies. *Diabetes Care*, 39(1), 16–23. doi:10.2337/dc15-0540

Silva-Zolezzi, I., Samuel, T. M. & Spieldenner, J. (2017). Maternal nutrition: opportunities in the prevention of gestational diabetes. *Nutrition Reviews*, 75(Suppl.1), 32–50. doi:10.1093/nutrit/nuw033

The Lancet (2017). Editorial. Breastfeeding: a missed opportunity for global health. *The Lancet*, 390(10094), 532. doi:10.1016/S0140-6736(17)32163-3

Victora C. G., Bahl, R., Barros, A. J. D., França, G. V. A., Horton, S., Krasevec, J., ... Richter, L. (2016). Breastfeeding in the 21st century: epidemiology, mechanisms, and lifelong effect. *The Lancet*, 387(10017), 475–90. doi:10.1016/S0140-6736(15)01024-7

REFERENCES

1 A. A. Geraghty, K. L. Lindsay, G. Alberdi, F. M. McAuliffe & E. R. Gibney (2015). Nutrition during pregnancy impacts offspring's epigenetic status—evidence from human and animal studies. *Nutrition and Metabolic Insights*, 8(Suppl.1), 41–7. doi:10.4137/nmi.s29527

2 K. Kind (2006). Diet around conception and during pregnancy—effects on fetal and neonatal outcomes. *Reproductive BioMedicine Online*, 12(5), 532–41.

3 C. Read, D. Bateson, E. Weisberg & J. Estoesta (2009). Contraception and pregnancy then and now: examining the experiences of a cohort of mid-age Australian women. *Australian and New Zealand Journal of Obstetrics and Gynaecology*, 49, 429–33.

4 J. M. Harnisch, P. H. Harnisch & D. R. Harnisch (2012). Family medicine obstetrics: pregnancy and nutrition. *Primary Care: Clinics in Office Practice*, 39, 39–54.

5 K. L. Thornburg, P. F. O'Tierney & S. Louey (2010). Review: the placenta is a programming agent for cardiovascular disease. *Trophoblast Research*, 24, S54–S59.

6 D. J. P. Barker (2012). Developmental origins of chronic disease. *Public Health*, 126, 185–9.

7 J. Harding (2001). The nutritional basis of the fetal origins of adult disease. *International Journal of Epidemiology*, 30, 15–23.

8   Dietary Guidelines Advisory Committee (2010). *Report of the Dietary Guidelines Advisory Committee on the Dietary Guidelines for Americans.* Washington, DC: US Department of Agriculture, Agricultural Research Service. Retrieved from: www.cnpp.usda.gov/Publications/DietaryGuidelines/2010/DGAC/Report/2010DGACReport-camera-ready-Jan11-11.pdf.

9   C. K. Ballard, L. Bricker, K. Reed, L. Wood & J. P. Neilson (2011). Nutritional advice for improving outcomes in multiple pregnancies (review). *The Cochrane Library*, 6.

10 Institute of Medicine & National Research Council (2009). *Weight Gain During Pregnancy: Reexamining the guidelines.* Washington, DC: National Academies Press.

11 P. van der Pligt, K. Campbell, J. Willcox, J. Opie & E. Denney-Wilson (2011). Opportunities for primary and secondary prevention of excess gestational weight gain: general practitioners' perspectives. *BMC Family Practice*, 12(124).

12 A. Clark (2015). The role of nutrition in pregnancy. *Medicine Today*, 16(12), 16–22.

13 M. E. Rosello-Soberon, L. Fuentes-Chaparro & E. Casanueva (2005). Twin pregnancies: eating for three? Maternal nutrition update. *Nutrition Reviews*, 63(9), 295–302.

14 S. K. Tracy, M. B. Tracy, J. Dean, P. Laws & E. Sullivan (2007). Spontaneous preterm birth of liveborn infants in women at low risk in Australia over 10 years: a population-based study. *BJOG: An International Journal of Obstetrics and Gynecology*, 114, 731–5.

15 J. P. Newnham, D. S. Sahota, C. Y. Zhang, B. Xu, M. Zheng, D. A. Doherty, ... Y. Hu (2011). Preterm birthrates in Chinese women in China, Hong Kong and Australia—the price of westernisation. *Australian and New Zealand Journal of Obstetrics and Gynaecology*, 51, 426–31.

16 Australian Institute of Health and Welfare (2015). *Australia's Mothers and Babies 2013—in brief. Perinatal statistics series no. 31.* Cat. no. PER 72. Canberra: AIHW.

17 M. Via (2012). The malnutrition of obesity: micronutrient deficiencies that promote diabetes. *ISRN Endocrinology*, 2012, article 103472, 1–8.

18 C. H. S. Ruxton (2011). Nutritional implications of obesity and dieting. *Nutrition Bulletin*, 36, 199–211.

19 National Health and Medical Research Council (2013). *Healthy Eating During Your Pregnancy.* Canberra: NHMRC.

20 J. Josefson (2011). The impact of pregnancy nutrition on offspring obesity. *Journal of the American Dietetic Association*, 111(1), 50–2. doi:10.1016/j.jada.2010.10.015

21 K. Rasmussen & A. Yaktine (2009). *Weight Gain During Pregnancy: Reexamining the guidelines.* Washington, DC: National Academies Press.

22 I. Guelinckx, R. Devlieger, K. Beckers & G. Vansant (2008). Maternal obesity: pregnancy complications, gestational weight gain and nutrition. *Obesity Reviews*, 9, 140–50.

23 American Dietetic Association and American Society for Nutrition (2009). Position of the American Dietetic Association and American Society for Nutrition Obesity, Reproduction, and Pregnancy Outcomes. *Journal of the American Dietetic Association*, 109, 918–27.

24 S. Y. Han, A. A. Brewis & A. Wutich (2016). Body image mediates the depressive effects of weight gain in new mothers, particularly for women already obese: evidence from the Norwegian Mother and Child Cohort study. *BMC Public Health*, 16, 664.

25 The Royal Australian and New Zealand College of Obstetricians and Gynaecologists (2013). *Management of Obesity in Pregnancy.* Melbourne: RANZCOG.

26 A. Hure, A. Young, R. Smith & C. Collins (2009). Diet and pregnancy status in Australian women. *Public Health Nutrition*, 12(6), 853–61. doi:10.1017/S1368980008003212

27 L. Malek, W. Umberger, M. Makrides & S. J. Zhou (2015). Adherence to the Australian Dietary Guidelines during pregnancy: evidence from a national study. *Public Health Nutrition*, 19(7), 1155–63. doi:10.1017/S1368980015002232

28 K. Bookari, H. Yeatman & M. Williamson (2017). Falling short of dietary guidelines: what do Australian pregnant women really know? A cross-sectional study. *Women and Birth*, 30(1), 9–17. doi:http://dx.doi.org/10.1016/j.wombi.2016.05.010

29 T. O. Scholl (2011). Maternal iron status: relation to fetal growth, length of gestation, and iron endowment of the neonate. *Nutrition Reviews*, 69(suppl. 1), S23–S29. doi:10.1111/j.1753-4887.2011.00429.x

30 N. A. Alwan, J. E. Cade, H. J. McArdle, D. C. Greenwood, H. E. Hayes & N. A. B. Simpson (2015). Maternal iron status in early pregnancy and birth outcomes: insights from the Baby's Vascular Health and Iron in Pregnancy study. *British Journal of Nutrition*, 113(12), 1985–92. doi:10.1017/S0007114515001166

31 N. Hovdenak & K. Haram (2012). Influence of mineral and vitamin supplements on pregnancy outcome. *European Journal of Obstetrics Gynecology and Reproductive Biology*, 164(2), 127–32.

32 D. J. P. Barker, R. Bergmann & P. L. Ogra (eds). (2007). *The Window of Opportunity: Pre-pregnancy to 24 months of age*. Vevey, Switzerland: Nestec Ltd.

33 Food Standards Australia New Zealand (2016). Folic acid/folate and pregnancy. Retrieved from: www.foodstandards.gov.au/consumer/generalissues/pregnancy/folic/Pages/default.aspx.

34 E. E. Muggli & J. L. Halliday (2007). Folic acid and risk of twinning: a systematic review of the recent literature, July 1994–July 2006. *Medical Journal of Australia*, 186(5), 243–8.

35 A. M. Leung, E. N. Pearce & L. E. Braverman (2011). Iodine nutrition in pregnancy and lactation. *Endocrinology and Metabolism Clinics of North America*, 40, 765–77.

36 K. E. Charlton, L. Gemming, H. Yeatman & G. Ma (2010). Suboptimal iodine status of Australian pregnant women reflects poor knowledge and practices related to iodine nutrition. *Nutrition*, 26, 963–8.

37 C. A. Nowson, J. J. McGrath, P. R. Ebeling, A. Haikerwal, R. M. Daly, K. M. Sanders, ... R. S. Mason (2012). Vitamin D and health in adults in Australia and New Zealand: a position statement. *Medical Journal of Australia*, 196(11), 1–7.

38 D. K. Dror & L. H. Allen (2010). Vitamin D inadequacy in pregnancy: biology, outcomes, and interventions. *Nutrition Reviews*, 68(8), 465–77.

39 S. N. Karras, H. Fakhoury, G. Muscogiuri, W. B. Grant, J. M. van den Ouweland, A. M. Colao & K. Kotsa (2016). Maternal vitamin D levels during pregnancy and neonatal health: evidence to date and clinical implications. *Therapeutic Advances in Musculoskeletal Disease*, 8(4), 124–35. doi:10.1177/1759720X16656810

40 U. Ramakrishnan, I. Gonzalez-Casanova, L. Schnaas, A. DiGirolamo, A. D. Quezada, B. C. Pallo, ... R. Martorell (2016). Prenatal supplementation with DHA improves attention at 5 y of age: a randomized controlled trial. *American Journal of Clinical Nutrition*, 104(4), 1075–82. doi:10.3945/ajcn.114.101071

41 R. L. Duyff (2012). *American Dietetic Association Complete Food and Nutrition Guide*, 4th edn. Boston, MA: Houghton Mifflin Harcourt.

42 V. Leventakou, T. Roumeliotaki, D. Martinez, H. Barros, A.-L. Brantsaeter, M. Casas, ... L. Chatzi (2014). Fish intake during pregnancy, fetal growth, and gestational length in 19 European birth cohort studies. *American Journal of Clinical Nutrition*, 99(3), 506–16. doi:10.3945/ajcn.113.067421

43 M. Makrides, L. Duley & S. F. Olsen (2009). Marine oil, and other prostaglandin precursors, supplementation for pregnancy uncomplicated by pre-eclampsia or intrauterine growth restriction. *Cochrane Database of Systematic Reviews*, 3.

44 B. Koletzko, I. Cetin & J. T. Brenna (2007). Dietary fat intakes for pregnant and lactating women. *British Journal of Nutrition*, 98, 873–7.

45 D. J. Palmer, T. Sullivan, M. S. Gold, S. L. Prescott, R. Heddle, R. A. Gibson & M. Makrides (2012). Effect of n-3 long chain polyunsaturated fatty acid supplementation in pregnancy on infants' allergies in first year of life: randomised controlled trial. *British Medical Journal*, 344(7845), 1–11.

46 M. Makrides, R. A. Gibson, A. J. McPhee, L. Yelland, J. Quinlivan, P. Ryan & DOMInO Investigative Team (2010). Effect of DHA supplementation during pregnancy on maternal depression and neurodevelopment of young children: a randomized controlled trial. *JAMA—Journal of the American Medical Association*, 304(15), 1675–83.

47 M. Makrides (2012). DHA supplementation during the perinatal period and neurodevelopment: do some babies benefit more than others? *Prostaglandins, Leukotrienes and Essential Fatty Acids*, 88(1), 87–90.

48 C. T. Collins, M. Makrides, A. J. McPhee, T. R. Sullivan, P. G. Davis, M. Thio, … Robert A. Gibson (2017). Docosahexaenoic acid and bronchopulmonary dysplasia in preterm infants. *New England Journal of Medicine*, 376, 1245–55. doi:10.1056/NEJMoa1611942

49 Z. Stein, M. Susser, G. Saenger & F. Marolla (eds). (1975). *Famine and Human Development: The Dutch hunger winter of 1944/45*. New York: Oxford University Press.

50 S. Sonkusare (2011). The clinical management of hyperemesis gravidarum. *Archives of Gynecology and Obstetrics*, 283(6), 1183–92.

51 M. Haugena, Å. Vikanesa, A. L. Brantsætera, H. M. Meltzera, A. M. Grjibovskia & P. Magnus (2011). Diet before pregnancy and the risk of hyperemesis gravidarum. *British Journal of Nutrition*, 106, 596–602.

52 R. G. Moses, G. J. Morris, P. Petocz, F. San Gil & D. Garg (2011). The impact of potential new diagnostic criteria on the prevalence of gestational diabetes mellitus in Australia. *Medical Journal of Australia*, 194(7), 338–40.

53 American Diabetes Association (2009). Diagnosis and classification of diabetes mellitus. *Diabetes Care*, 32(suppl. 1), S62–S67. doi:10.2337/dc09-S062

54 C. M. Peterson & L. Jovanovic-Peterson (1991). Percentage of carbohydrate and glycemic response to breakfast, lunch, and dinner in women with gestational diabetes. *Diabetes*, 40(suppl. 2), 172–4. doi:10.2337/diab.40.2.S172

55 L. Jovanovic-Peterson, C. M. Peterson, G. F. Reed, B. E. Metzger, J. L. Mills, R. H. Knopp & J. H. Aarons (1991). Maternal postprandial glucose levels and infant birth weight: the Diabetes in Early Pregnancy study. *American Journal of Obstetrics and Gynecology*, 164(1), 103–11. doi:http://dx.doi.org/10.1016/0002-9378(91)90637-7

56 T. P. Markovic, R. Muirhead, S. Overs, G. P. Ross, J. C. Y. Louie, N. Kizirian, … J. C. Brand-Miller (2016). Randomized controlled trial investigating the effects of a low-glycemic index diet on pregnancy outcomes in women at high risk of gestational diabetes mellitus: the GI Baby 3 study. *Diabetes Care*, 39(1), 31–8. doi:10.2337/dc15-0572

57 J. C. Y. Louie, T. P. Markovic, N. Perera, D. Foote, P. Petocz, G. P. Ross & J. C. Brand-Miller (2011). A randomized controlled trial investigating the effects of a low–glycemic index diet on pregnancy outcomes in gestational diabetes mellitus. *Diabetes Care*, 34(11), 2341–6. doi:10.2337/dc11-0985

58 The Royal Australian College of General Practitioners (2016). *General Practice Management of Type 2 Diabetes: 2016–18—13.3 Gestational diabetes mellitus*. Melbourne: RACGP.

59 D. Bondarianzadeh, H. Yeatman & D. Condon-Paoloni (2011). A qualitative study of the Australian midwives' approaches to listeria education as a food-related risk during pregnancy. *Midwifery*, 27, 221–8.

60 Food Standards Australia New Zealand (2011). Listeria. Retrieved from: www.foodstandards.gov.au/consumerinformation/listeria.

61 New Zealand Ministry of Health (2006). *Food and Nutrition Guidelines for Healthy Pregnant and Breastfeeding Women: A background paper*. Revised 2008. Wellington: NZ Ministry of Health.

62 Food Standards Australia New Zealand (2011). Fish. Retrieved from: www.foodstandards.gov.au/consumerinformation/mercuryinfish.cfm.

63 National Health and Medical Research Council (2013). *Australian Dietary Guidelines*. Canberra: NHMRC.

64 T. M. Cassidy & R. C. Giglia (2012). Psychosocial and cultural interventions for reducing alcohol consumption during lactation. *The Cochrane Library*.

65 Food Standards Australia New Zealand (2012). *NUTTAB 2010*. Canberra: FSANZ.

66 A. R. Amorim Adegboye, Y. M. Linne & P. M. C. Lourenco (2012). Diet or exercise, or both, for weight reduction in women after childbirth (review). *The Cochrane Library*, 2.

67 M. S. Kramer & R. Kakuma (2009). Optimal duration of exclusive breastfeeding (review). *The Cochrane Library*, 1.

68 S. L. Prescott, P. Smith, M. Tang, D. J. Palmer, J. Sinn, S. J. Huntley, … M.. Makrides (2008). The importance of early complementary feeding in the development of oral tolerance: concerns and controversies. *Pediatric Allergy and Immunology*, 19(5), 375–80.

69 M. J. Renfrew, F. M. McCormick, A. Wade, B. Quinn & T. Dowswell (2012). Support of healthy breastfeeding mothers with healthy term babies (review). *The Cochrane Library*, 5.

70 The COAG Health Council (2016). *Australian National Breastfeeding Strategy 2010–2015: Final progress report*. Canberra: COAG Health Council. Retrieved from: www.health.gov.au/internet/main/publishing.nsf/Content/D94D40B034E00B29CA257BF0001CAB31/$File/ANBS-2010-2015-Final-Progress-Report%20.pdf.

71 J. A. Scott, C. W. Binns & W. H. Oddy (2007). Predictors of delayed onset of lactation. *Maternal and Child Nutrition*, 3, 186–93.

72 S. Ip, M. Chung, G. Raman, P. Chew, N. Magula, D. DeVine, T. Trikalinos & J. Lau (2007). Breastfeeding and maternal and infant health outcomes in developed countries. *Evidence Report Technology Assessment (Full Report)*, 153, 1–186.

73 A. Fallon, C. Engel, D. Devane, C. Dring, E. H. Moylett & G. Fealy (2011). Baby-led versus scheduled breastfeeding for healthy newborns (protocol). *The Cochrane Library*, 4.

74 L. Mangesi & T. Dowswell (2010). Treatments for breast engorgement during lactation (review). *The Cochrane Library*, 9.

75 E. R. Moore, G. C. Anderson, N. Bergman & T. Dowswell (2012). Early skin-to-skin contact for mothers and their healthy newborn infants (review). *The Cochrane Library*, 5.

76 National Health and Medical Research Council (2012). *Infant Feeding Guidelines for Health Workers*. Canberra: NHMRC.

77 Division of Child Health and Development World Health Organization (1998). *Evidence for the Ten Steps to Successful Breast Feeding*. Geneva: WHO.

78 H. Demmelmair, J. von Rosen & B. Koletzko (2006). Long-term consequences of early nutrition. *Early Human Development*, 82(8), 567–74.

79 G. E. Becker, S. Remmington & T. Remmington (2011). Early additional food and fluids for healthy breastfed full-term infants (review). *The Cochrane Library*, 12.

80 A. Prentice (1996). Constituents of human milk. *Food and Nutrition Bulletin*, 17, 305–12.

81 National Health and Medical Research Council (2011). *Draft Australian Dietary Guidelines Incorporating the Australian Guide to Healthy Eating*. Canberra: NHMRC.

82 M. S. Kramer, B. Chalmers, E. D. Hodnett, Z. Sevkovskaya, I Dzikovich, S. Shapiro, ... E. Helsing (2001). Promotion of breastfeeding intervention trial (PROBIT): a randomized trial in the Republic of Belarus. *JAMA—Journal of the American Medical Association*, 285, 413–21.

83 C. G. Victora, R. Bahl, A. J. Barros, G. V. França, S. Horton, J. Krasevec, ... Lancet Breastfeeding Series Group (2016). Breastfeeding in the 21st century: epidemiology, mechanisms, and lifelong effect. *The Lancet*, 387, 475–90.

84 L. Chatzi, M. Torrent, I. Romieu, R. Garcia-Esteban, C. Ferrer, J. Vioque, ... J. Sunyer (2008). Mediterranean diet in pregnancy is protective for wheeze and atopy in childhood. *Thorax*, 63(6), 507.

85 J. De Batlle, J. Garcia-Aymerich, A. Barraza-Villarreal, J. M. Antó & I. Romieu (2008). Mediterranean diet is associated with reduced asthma and rhinitis in Mexican children. *Allergy*, 63(10), 1310–16.

86 N. E. Lange, S. L. Rifas-Shiman, C. A. Camargo, Jr, D. R. Gold, M. W. Gillman & A. A. Litonjua (2010). Maternal dietary pattern during pregnancy is not associated with recurrent wheeze in children. *Journal of Allergy and Clinical Immunology*, 126(2), 250–5.

87 S. O. Shaheen, K. Northstone, R. B. Newson, P. M. Emmett, A. Sherriff & A. J. Henderson (2009). Dietary patterns in pregnancy and respiratory and atopic outcomes in childhood. *Thorax*, 64(5), 411–17.

88 B. I. Nwaru, H. M. Takkinen, O. Niemela, M. Kaila, M. Erkkola, S. Ahonen, ... S. M. Virtanen (2013). Introduction of complementary foods in infancy and atopic sensitization at the age of 5 years: timing and food diversity in a Finnish birth cohort. *Allergy*, 68(4), 507–16. doi:10.1111/all.12118

89 B. I. Nwaru, H. M. Takkinen, M. Kaila, M. Erkkola, S. Ahonen, J. Pekkanen, ... S. M. Virtanen (2014). Food diversity in infancy and the risk of childhood asthma and allergies. *Journal of Allergy and Clinical Immunology*, 133(4), 1084–91. doi:10.1016/j.jaci.2013.12.1069

90 D. Ierodiakonou, V. Garcia-Larsen, A. Logan, A. Groome, S. Cunha, J. Chivinge, ... R. J. Boyle (2016). Timing of allergenic food introduction to the infant diet and risk of allergic or autoimmune disease: a systematic review and meta-analysis. *JAMA—Journal of the American Medical Association*, 316(11), 1181–92. doi:10.1001/jama.2016.12623

91 M. A. Crepinsek, L. Crowe, K. Michener & N. A. Smart (2012). Interventions for preventing mastitis after childbirth (review). *The Cochrane Library*, 3.

92 B. Koletzko, R. von Kries, R. Closa, J. Escribano, S. Scaglioni, M. Giovannini, ... for the European Childhood Obesity Trial Study Group (2009). Lower protein in infant formula is associated with lower weight up to age 2 y: a randomized clinical trial. *American Journal of Clinical Nutrition*, 89, 1836–45.

93 B. Koletzko, R. von Kries, R. C. Monasterolo, J. Escribano Subías, S. Scaglioni, M. Giovannini, ... for the European Childhood Obesity Trial Study Group (2009). Can infant feeding choices modulate later obesity risk? *American Journal of Clinical Nutrition*, 89(suppl.), 1S–7S.

94 D. Turck, C. Grillon, E. Lachambre, P. Robiliard, L. Beck, J.-L. Maurin, ... L.-D. Van Egroo (2006). Adequacy and safety of an infant formula with a protein/energy ratio of 1.8 g/100 kcal and enhanced protein efficiency for term infants during the first 4 months of life. *Journal of Paediatric Gastroenterology and Nutrition*, 43, 364–71.

95 N. C. R. Raiha, A. Fazzolari-Nesci, C. Cajozzo, G. Puccio, A. Monestier, G. Moro, … F. Haschke (2002). Whey predominant, whey modified infant formula with protein/energy ratio of 1.8 g/100 kcal: adequate and safe for term infants from birth to four months. *Journal of Pediatric Gastroenterology and Nutrition*, 35, 275–81.

96 H. D. Holscher, L. A. Czerkies, P. Cekola, R. Litov, M. Benbow, S. Santema, … K. A. Tappenden (2012). Bifidobacterium lactis Bb12 enhances intestinal antibody response in formula-fed infants: a randomized, double-blind, controlled trial. *Journal of Parenteral and Enteral Nutrition*, 36(suppl. 1), 106S–117S.

97 J. Lee, D. Seto & L. Bielory (2008). Meta-analysis of clinical trials of probiotics for prevention and treatment of pediatric atopic dermatitis. *Journal of Allergy and Clinical Immunology*, 121, 116–21.

98 M. H. Floch, W. A. Walker, S. Guandalini, P. Hibberd, S. Gorbach, C. Surawicz, … L. A. Dielman (2008). Recommendations for probiotic use. *Journal of Clinical Gastroenterology*, 42, S104–S108.

99 C. Binns & M. K. Lee (2010). The use of probiotics to prevent diarrhea in young children attending child care centers: a review. *Journal of Experimental and Clinical Medicine*, 2(6), 269–73.

100 The Australasian Society of Clinical Immunology and Allergy (2008). *Infant Feeding Advice*. Balgowlah, NSW: ASCIA. Retrieved from: www.rch.org.au/uploadedFiles/Main/Content/allergy/ASCIA_Infant_Feeding_Advice_2010.pdf.

101 D. D. Alexander & M. D. Cabana (2010). Partially hydrolyzed 100% whey protein infant formula and reduced risk of atopic dermatitis: a meta-analysis. *Journal of Pediatric Gastroenterology and Nutrition*, 50(4), 422–30.

102 Y. S. Casadio, T. M. Williams, C. T. Lai, S. E. Olsson, A. R. Hepworth & P. E. Hartman (2010). Evaluation of a mid-infrared analyser for the determination of the macronutrient composition of human milk. *Journal of Human Lactation*, 26, 376–83.

103 A. Shashiraj, M. M. Faridi, O. Singh & U. Rusia (2006). Mother's iron status, breastmilk iron and lactoferrin: are they related? *European Journal of Clinical Nutrition*, 60(7), 903–8.

104 M. L. Fernández-Sánchez, et al. (2012). Iron content and its speciation in human milk from mothers of preterm and full-term infants at early stages of lactation: a comparison with commercial infant milk formulas. *Microchemical Journal*, 105, 108–14. doi:10.1016/j.microc.2012.03.016

105 S. Mihrshahi, D. Battistutta, A. Magarey & L. A. Daniels (2011). Determinants of rapid weight gain during infancy: baseline results from the NOURISH randomised controlled trial. *BMC Paediatrics*, 11(99), 1–8.

106 B. Koletzko, R. von Kries, R. Closa, J. Escribano, S. Scaglioni, M. Giovannini, … European Childhood Obesity Trial Study Group (2009). Lower protein in infant formula is associated with lower weight up to age 2 y: a randomized clinical trial. *American Journal of Clinical Nutrition*, 89, 1836–45.

107 M. Weber, V. Grote, R. Closa-Monasterolo, J. Escribano, J. P. Langhendries, E. Dain, … European Childhood Obesity Trial Study Group (2014). Lower protein content in infant formula reduces BMI and obesity risk at school age: follow-up of a randomized trial. *American Journal of Clinical Nutrition*, 99, 1041–51.

108 D. Gruszfeld, M. Weber, K. Gradowska, P. Socha, V. Grote, A. Xhonneux, … for the European Childhood Obesity Study Group (2016). Association of early protein intake and pre-peritoneal fat at five years of age: follow-up of a randomized clinical trial. *Nutrition, Metabolism and Cardiovascular Diseases*, 26, 824–32.

109 J. Escribano, V. Luque, J. Canals-Sans, N. Ferré, B. Koletzko, V. Grote, … R. Closa-Monasterolo (2016). Mental performance in 8-year-old children fed reduced protein content formula during the 1st year of life: safety analysis of a randomised clinical trial. *British Journal of Nutrition*, 22, 1–9.

CHAPTER 15

NUTRITION DURING INFANCY AND CHILDHOOD

SARA GRAFENAUER, KANITA KUNARATNAM AND VICKI FLOOD

CHAPTER OBJECTIVES

This chapter will enable the reader to:

- define the periods identified as infancy and childhood and the implications for nutritional requirements
- discuss the food requirements for infants and young children and the significance of the development of healthy eating habits
- identify key dietary problems that emerge during childhood and recognise effective approaches to developing healthy food habits, in particular for the prevention of childhood obesity.

KEY TERMS

Breast milk

Childhood obesity

Complementary feeding

Weaning

KEY POINTS

- Following breastfeeding, complementary foods are introduced to meet increased nutritional requirements at around six months of age in line with developmental milestones.
- Childhood obesity is a significant public health problem in various parts of the globe, including Australia. Monitoring growth of children enables awareness of this problem, which can occur without due care in food and beverage choices.
- Healthy eating habits are developed in the context of supportive environments, beginning with families and broadening to school and community contexts.

OXFORD UNIVERSITY PRESS

INTRODUCTION

The birth of a child marks the first stage of separate existence entering a pathway of growth, development, maturation and ageing. Nutritional intakes are particularly important to support the rapid growth and development that occurs during childhood. Infancy is the very early stage of childhood and adolescence marks the end of childhood.

Food choices in the early years not only influence body composition and growth rate, but also the establishment of eating patterns that continue throughout life. Dietary intakes during childhood are critical in setting the scene for health in the future. In this period, in particular, nutritional health is tied to the development of eating behaviours. Dietary intake is dependent on the foods made available to the growing child and the ways in which meals and snacking are managed. Breast milk provides the best first food, and feeding infants occurs in a close physical context. The weaning period, in which other foods are introduced, is a significant time for the development of the child's systems, including the gut, and it also introduces new feeding contexts that relate to meals and particular skills development. As the child grows older and more independent, the food environment again changes. In time, deeper considerations of the types and amounts of accessible foods must be considered as well as opportunities for physical activity and learning about the value of food.

In recent decades, childhood obesity has emerged as a particular health concern and excessive growth during infancy may be a risk factor for lifetime obesity. However, it appears that being at either end of the weight spectrum may be associated with health risks in later life. For example, one study found that infants in the highest size distribution for weight or body mass index (BMI) were at increased risk of adult and childhood obesity [1], while another study showed that thinness at birth was associated with increased risk of diabetes and chronic disease in later life [2]. The prenatal period may also have an impact. Indeed, the situation was different for pre-term infants in one study indicating early weight gain (0–3 months) had a more significant impact on BMI (+4.9 s.d. [standard deviation]), than later infancy weight gain from three months to one year (BMI +2.5 s.d.) ($p < 0.05$) at age 19 years [3]. In this case, the pre-term infants had a gestational age of <32 weeks and weighed about 1.5 kg at birth. It is interesting to note, however, that the time period of early catch-up growth can also be associated with detrimental metabolic effects. It has been suggested that improvements in linear growth in the first two years should be the focus, avoiding excessive weight gain relative to height gain (BMI) after the age of two years [4; 5]. With concerns about the prevalence of childhood obesity in the community, the monitoring of weight during childhood has become an issue, particularly in recognising and dealing with it before lifetime health concerns set in.

STOP AND THINK

- What are the main implications for nutrition during infancy and childhood?
- Why is the development of healthy eating habits so critical during infancy and childhood?
- What sectors in the community are responsible for supporting healthy eating habits during infancy and childhood?

WHAT ARE THE MAIN NUTRITION-RELATED ISSUES DURING INFANCY AND CHILDHOOD?

Nutritional gap
inadequate nutrient intakes—for example, when breast milk no longer meets all nutritional requirements of the growing infant.

As the infant grows in size and the nutritional composition of breast milk no longer provides all the additional needs, a **nutritional gap** emerges and complementary foods need to be introduced into the diet. With this stage comes tastes of a range of new foods and the development of eating behaviours that carry the individual throughout life. As such, there are particular implications for family food practices. At the same time, the development of the immune system and associated maturation of the gut impact on food tolerance may need to be taken into consideration. As the child grows, the main public health concern is over-feeding resulting in childhood obesity. For infants and children, in particular, nutritional needs go hand in hand with the development of healthy eating behaviours.

For the generally well population, the first major nutritional target alongside successful breastfeeding is the well-timed and appropriate introduction of solid foods in the first year of life (Table 15.1). The purpose is the delivery of energy and nutrients that meet requirements for adequate growth and development that can no longer be met with breast milk alone. Introducing solid foods should aim to eventually expose the child to the full range of usual family foods by two years of age.

The timing of introduction of solid foods is important, and should match nutritional and developmental requirements. Concerns regarding introduction of solid foods too early are based on the possibility that any food may reduce breast milk production, the key source of energy and fat in the infant's diet. It is also likely that the infant is not developmentally ready, either physically or physiologically. Lack of head and neck control is a risk for aspiration of food particles into the airway. Similarly, lack of tongue control and a persistent extrusion reflex mean that a properly formed bolus cannot be formed and passed to the back of the mouth in preparation for swallowing. The gastrointestinal tract needs to be fully matured to make use of the nutrients in digestive and absorptive processes and the kidneys must be prepared for the solute load [6]. Introducing solids is also risky due to exposure to possible pathogens and diarrhoeal disease. The younger infant is less

TABLE 15.1   KEY POINTS FOR CONSIDERATION WITH THE INTRODUCTION OF SOLID FOODS TO INFANTS

Developmental considerations	Nutritional considerations	Food considerations
Head and neck control	Increased energy requirements	Breast milk
Tongue control	Limiting nutrients, iron, zinc	Modified textures in food
Maturation of gut	Managing food tolerance	Iron-fortified cereals
Motor skills development	Development of immune system	Vegetables
Speech development	Acceptance of taste and textures	Fruit
Increased movement	Healthy snacks	Protein-rich foods
Growth rate	Portion sizes	Water and milk
	Suitable beverages Food hygiene and safety	Low sugar, low salt

well prepared for a gastrointestinal insult, dehydrates quickly and would recover more slowly from a bout of infection. In addition, providing solid food before 3–4 months may increase the risk of allergy [7].

On the other hand, delaying the introduction of solid food until after six months can impact on the health and development of the infant. Micronutrient deficiency, particularly iron and zinc status, are threatened when weaning practices are inappropriately delayed [8]. Growth rates usually will falter, leaving the infant in a position where their immune protection can be compromised. Growth includes weight and length gains, and development of the brain measured by head circumference is also a critical part of the normal monitoring of well babies. When iron is depleted at this early age, it is difficult to realise the extent of the damage to brain development, and whether it is reversible is not known [9]. The introduction of foods also influences the development of motor skills within the oral cavity, such as chewing and the general movement of food, which, in turn, impacts on speech development. Delaying the introduction of food decreases the acceptance of new tastes and textures, increasing feeding difficulties for the carer and reducing the overall adequacy of the diet. However, this can also occur if the texture of foods is not progressed appropriately within the 12-month time frame from purée to chunky food pieces [10]. Contrary to earlier beliefs, new research indicates that if 'the window of opportunity' is missed in introducing solid foods, especially in relation to the development of oral tolerance to foods, there may be an increased risk of allergy [11].

The National Health and Medical Research Council (NHMRC) Infant Feeding Guidelines (2012) state that 'around 6 months of age infants are physiologically and developmentally ready for new foods, textures and modes of feeding and need more nutrients than can be provided by breast milk or formula. Delaying the introduction of solid foods beyond this age may increase the risk of developing allergic syndromes' [11]. The European Society of Paediatric Gastroenterology (ESPGHAN) states that solid foods should not be introduced before 17 weeks [12]. The introduction of solid foods (also termed 'complementary foods' or 'weaning foods') is part of the weaning process, is aligned with the growth and development through the first 12 months of life, and follows certain guiding principles [13].

From a general development perspective, the infant needs to show signs of interest in food, be able to maintain head control for a period of time and be able to move food from the front of the mouth to the back of the mouth and swallow safely. The NHMRC Infant Feeding Guidelines [11] provide recommendations for continued breastfeeding while introducing complementary foods so that the infant benefits from the immunomodulatory potential of breast milk. Interestingly, Australian research has also found that infants who are breastfed for longer also tend to consume a wider variety of foods [14], possibly due to the flavours that pass through the milk, as described earlier [15].

TRY IT YOURSELF

Body weight is one of the best indicators that the infant is receiving adequate energy (calories/kilojoules) in their diet. Monitoring growth during the first 12 months of life and onwards is a regular part of a health check, as is monitoring developmental milestones.

Consider Aidan and Ella, twins born at 38 weeks (term for twins), breastfed for 13 months and given the same types of food. Using the WHO growth charts (see www.cdc.gov/growthcharts or www.who.int/childgrowth/standards/en), which were developed using data from breastfed infants, plot each twin's

    SARA GRAFENAUER, KANITA KUNARATNAM AND VICKI FLOOD

weight and length. Compare how their weight changed up to three years of age. Consider the similarities and differences, and the factors that might have influenced them.

Age	Aidan		Ella	
(months)	Weight (kg)	Height (cm)	Weight (kg)	Height (cm)
0	3.30	49.0	2.98	49.0
6	7.75	68.0	7.30	65.5
12	10.70	77.5	9.10	76.0
18	12.00	–	10.80	–
24	13.80	88.0	12.00	90.0
36	15.2	97.5	14.20	99.8

By around six months of age, there are important reasons for an infant to progress to a more complex diet. The infant's iron stores developed throughout the later part of pregnancy become depleted, so that the introduction of complementary foods becomes critically important from a nutritional point of view. Breast milk alone cannot fulfil the infant's requirements for iron, zinc or vitamin D [8]. Developmentally, the gastrointestinal and renal systems have reached an appropriate level of maturity to deal with a more complex diet. The infant is ready to master new oral motor skills as the suck reflex becomes less dominant at around 4–6 months, moving to the next stage of 'munching' [16]. Changes in the oral cavity related to speech development, particularly how the tongue moves, are also linked to timely introduction of a range of foods. Progression through various textures of food up to and even beyond 12 months of age helps to build the foundations for healthy eating habits in the longer term. By around one year of age, the energy provided by complementary foods has displaced much of the energy that had been derived earlier from breast milk or formula [17], and being breastfed is replaced by independent feeding of most food items [18].

Australian data from 1998–2001 showed the introduction of solid food and cow's milk occurs in a step-wise process, gradually flattening out [19] (Figure 15.1). The more recent 2010 Australian National Infant Feeding Survey showed that at six months of age 91.5(+1)% of infants had received solid foods within the past 24 hours [20].

The foods given during infancy need to meet the emerging nutritional gap and be at least as nutritious as breast milk, with the total diet contributing at a minimum 30–40% of energy from fat [14; 21]. Breast milk contains about 50% fat, but many foods normally given at the early stages of introducing complementary foods in Australia are low in fat and energy [12; 21]—for example, fruit, vegetables and cereals—so breast milk remains an important dietary component [11]. The foods also need to be adapted in terms of texture and would normally be offered as a purée. Importantly, foods should not contain added sodium or sugar and not be too high in fibre as this may affect nutrient absorption [10]. Within the first year, the texture of foods needs to change towards a more lumpy texture and then to whole, soft foods and, finally, to a diversity of normal family meals. Repeated exposure and the variety of foods offered helps determine acceptance [10] and, therefore, impacts on the nutritional adequacy of the diet.

FIGURE 15.1 TRENDS IN INTRODUCING SOLID FOODS TO INFANTS IN AUSTRALIA 1998–2001

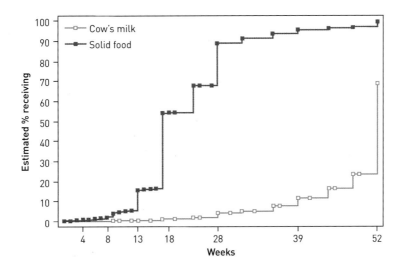

Source: S. M. Donath & L. H. Amir (2005). Breastfeeding and the introduction of solids in Australian infants: data from the 2001 National Health Survey. *Australian and New Zealand Journal of Public Health*, 29(2), 171–5. doi:10.1111/j.1467-842X.2005.tb00069.x

≫ CASE 15.1

INTRODUCING ALLERGENIC FOODS TO INFANTS

The timing of introduction of solid foods has been the subject of much debate—for example, since the 1980s delaying the introduction of potential allergenic foods to children at increased risk of allergy has been argued [22]. More recent research has indicated that delaying introduction of foods can lead to increased risk of allergic disease [7]. These studies reflect the ongoing need for research in this area and the influence that new research has on current debates and potential differences in recommendations around the world.

As many as 90% of all allergies relate to peanuts and egg [23]. These foods were traditionally avoided in infant diets; however, the position on this has recently changed. The NHMRC Infant Feeding Guidelines notes the literature, citing there is little evidence that delaying the introduction of solid foods reduces the risk of allergy, and there is insufficient evidence that avoiding allergenic foods is needed [11]. The immune system of the human gut needs to learn to differentiate between foreign proteins that are a problem, such as viral and bacterial particles, and those from foods such as peanut, fish and eggs. It is thought that the optimal timing of this opportunity is around the age of introduction of solid foods (>4 months) [7; 11; 24]. The results from the LEAP study [25] and the STEP trial [26], among others, suggest a benefit in including high-risk allergenic foods (particularly peanuts) and of the food remaining in an infant's diet. The NHMRC Infant Feeding Guidelines advise a variety of foods be introduced in those with a family history of allergies [11]. Breakdown of the cutaneous barrier of the skin early in life (due to dry skin caused potentially by beard rash or reactions to washing powders or soaps), together with abnormal immune reactivity, and possible environmental antigen exposure to food proteins on table tops, on hands and from dust, is thought to be the precursor to eczema and allergy [27]. It may be important that breast milk, containing immunomodulatory factors, be present in the gut together with newly introduced foods and possible allergens, so continued breastfeeding is an important part of the recommendations [27; 28].

- How does this case study exemplify the way in which new research informs practice?
- How would a family with a strong history of food allergy best approach food issues with new infants?
- Why does breastfeeding remain so significant in this scenario?

Food allergy
immune response to food allergen with production of antibodies leading to swelling, hives, vomiting.

Anaphylaxis
the most severe form of allergic reaction leading to difficulty breathing, swelling of tongue and throat and possible collapse

Food intolerance
non-immune adverse reaction to food such as migraine or irritable bowel

Food allergy is an immune-mediated response to ingestion and can result in swelling of the lips, face and eyes; hive or welts; eczema/rash; abdominal pain; vomiting or tingling in the mouth. It may or may not occur with **anaphylaxis**. Food allergies have increased over the past decades, with certain food allergies now 2–12 times as prevalent [23]. Non-immune-related responses can be referred to as **food intolerance**. The cause of the increase in food allergy is unknown and is not limited to known family history. Correct diagnosis of food allergy should be made under the professional guidance of a registered medical practitioner specialising in allergic disease or an immunologist. Usually this involves skin prick or RAST testing and oral food challenges. The NHMRC Infant Feeding Guidelines state that if food restrictions are required for medical reasons, the advice of a dietitian needs to be sought to ensure the nutritional adequacy of the modified diet [11]. In high-risk families (those with a family history of allergy), parents may wish to seek guidance from a paediatrician conjointly with a paediatric accredited practising dietitian (APD), particularly if feeding has already been a concern, including faltering growth.

STOP AND THINK

- Why do complementary foods need to be introduced to infants at around six months of age?
- What are the limiting nutritional factors in breast milk that need supplementation with food at this age?
- How might trends in complementary feeding in Australia change over time, and why?

WHICH FOODS NEED TO BE INTRODUCED DURING INFANCY, AND HOW?

Initially, solid foods are given after a feed so as not to displace the milk feed. Later, the food consumed is more important and the milk feed becomes secondary in terms of the nutritional value in driving growth and development. Feeding of solid foods is part of an important experiential learning process such that new foods are best given in the morning when the infant is alert. Infants are born with an ability to learn to like new foods [15; 29], having tasted many flavours from the mother's diet *in utero* via the amniotic fluids [15; 30] and via breast milk [15]. Due to declining iron levels, iron-fortified rice cereals made with breast milk or formula to a soft or 'sloppy' texture or finely puréed meat or poultry are often chosen as first foods. Rice cereal is inexpensive and so this is a good choice for the infant's first tastes, where a great deal of food may be extruded from the oral cavity as they become familiar with the new experience. Since there is an innate liking of sweet foods, vegetables, rather than fruits, can be introduced first, although the NHMRC Infant Feeding Guide does not specify the order [11].

To encourage the infant to acquire a taste for the flavour of the different vegetables, each vegetable is best served singly [30]. Vegetables can be easily introduced at the beginning of weaning. Neo-phobia (or fear of the new) is more common between 2 and 4 years of age, beginning at ~18 months [29], and it is more difficult to introduce 'bitter' tasting vegetables, which are normally rejected [10; 31]. Some sweeter vegetables (e.g. carrot) may be preferred over other vegetables that may contain bitter flavours (e.g. some green vegetables) [32]. Repeated exposure over this early time frame is the key to success, with as many as 8–10 exposures required before a food is accepted [31; 33; 34]. Caregivers need to repeatedly offer foods despite their perception that the infant dislikes the food item [35]. Encouraging 'taking a taste' increases liking of vegetables, in particular, and this strategy can be used by caregivers [36]. Research on competing tastes has shown that although foods differ greatly, such as green beans and puréed peach, acceptance of each food is learnt independently [35]. New foods can be offered every 4–5 days and the types of foods should be changed frequently to expand variety. For simplicity, this can involve choosing foods that have a suitable texture (raw) or can be prepared to a suitable texture when cooked and either mashed or chopped into small cubes. Teeth do not need to have emerged before progressing the texture of foods through to 'chunky' or to soft finger food-sized pieces.

>> CASE 15.2

FOOD SAFETY AND PREPARATION

Foods provided to infants should have minimal risk of contamination. Hygienic food preparation and storage of fresh and cooked foods needs to be observed. In addition, safe swallowing is a key concern. The infant needs to be able to form a bolus and move the food parcel to the back of the mouth and swallow without choking or risking inhalation. Certain foods, like nuts, are not advisable in the weaning diet due to choking risk [11]. Foods selected need to be texturally appropriate and served in appropriate amounts. If a wide variety of foods is offered, the infant is more likely to accept more novel foods and meals as weaning progresses [30]. There are many options of foods for feeding to an infant and it is important that they are given the best start nutritionally and not fed pre-prepared adult foods, many of which are too high in salt and sugar.

Most infants in Australia are initially fed home-prepared weaning foods; however, this changes with time [37]. Home-prepared weaning foods are an economical choice and bulk preparation can save a great deal of time. Foods can be served separated and the texture can be altered more readily according to the stage of development. While commercial options are available in different age range specifications, the texture cannot be varied beyond what is contained within the can, jar or pouch, and there may be wastage at mealtime, making them a more expensive option. Often, more than one flavour is combined together (e.g. pumpkin with corn). Some packaging relies on the infant sucking rather than clearing a spoon and this may influence an infant's desire to reject more challenging family foods.

When going out for the day, it is important that parents are prepared with foods for the young infant or child. Although foods such as soft-serve ice cream may have the right texture and appear to be like milk, they are not appropriate food choices given the sugar content.

- How can parents prepare safe and nutritious foods, available in small amounts, for their infant?
- How might food safety considerations influence food choices for infants when outside the home?
- How can parents ensure their infants are receiving quality safe foods at all times?

SARA GRAFENAUER, KANITA KUNARATNAM AND VICKI FLOOD

At about 4–7 months of age, signs of early chewing appear, coinciding with increased strength of suck, and the movement of the gag reflex from the mid to the posterior third of tongue. The developmental stage allows differing textures to be consumed. At about six months, feeding behaviour changes distinctly from sucking to biting and the infant learns when to use these new skills, particularly once teeth begin to emerge. The ability to 'sweep a spoon' with the top lip at around six months is a key developmental step [12].

At around six months of age, infants are able to grasp foods and bring them to their mouth, suggesting that some degree of baby-led weaning is possible once finger foods can be given [38]. This gives family members an opportunity to model eating behaviours. Importantly, no salt or sugar should be added to foods, and caregivers may need to be reminded of this if they are feeding normal family foods to the infant at an early stage [38]. Commercially prepared sauce and flavour bases are usually high in sodium and these should be exchanged for tastes and flavours such as garlic, herbs and mild spices.

At around eight months of age, solid foods can begin to be given before the usual milk feed and a greater range of foods can now be introduced. This is a transition point for the infant, and once the infant is taking a greater quantity of solid food, milk may be replaced as the main source of energy and nutrients. Tongue flexibility allows small lumps to be chewed and swallowed [12]. Finely minced meat (lamb, beef, pork), chicken or fish can be introduced. Dairy foods such as yoghurt, custard and cheese also help to add protein to the diet. Encouraging self-feeding using finger foods with soft fruit and toast fingers can help encourage progress with different textures. At the end of this period, the diet pattern should be moving towards three meals and some snack options. Snack options also need to contribute to the nutritional needs, as only small amounts of food can be consumed at any one time. Developmentally, the infant should be completely clearing the spoon with their lips and demonstrating both biting and chewing. They are also capable of lateral movements of the tongue, enabling movement of food towards the teeth for grinding foods. The presence of teeth is not necessary for this to occur, and infants are adept at using their gums to grind foods.

≫ RESEARCH AT WORK

IDENTIFYING PROBLEMS WITH DIETARY CHOICES FOR INFANTS

Problems with developing dietary habits have been identified in studies of Australian infants. Of particular concern to researchers is the balance between consumption of healthy food categories (e.g. vegetables, fruits) versus those that are energy dense and nutrient poor, defined as 'non-core' or 'discretionary' (e.g. cakes, biscuits, potato chips). In an analysis of the inFANT program in Melbourne, infants were found to double their consumption of sweetened beverages, savoury and sweet-energy dense snacks between 9 and 18 months of age [39] with up to 90% of children aged 12–36 months consuming at least one serve in the previous 24 hours [40]. In another report, half of the infants in a study of 16–24-month-old children exceeded the upper limits for sodium (62% >1000 mg/day) and this increased to 114% between the two time points examined [41]. Weaning diets low in iron have also been highlighted [14; 41].

At 8–12 months of age, finger foods and experimentation with self-feeding become important and children need to be offered the opportunity to explore and feed themselves; otherwise, this developmental milestone may be delayed. Lumpy textures need to be introduced by 10 months or these textures may be rejected and cause feeding difficulties [12]. By 12 months, infants will demonstrate rotary chewing movement and greater jaw stability. Children of this age are often tired by the night-time meal, so in many cases it is ideal that the main meal is served at lunch, when it is likely that a greater variety of the foods will be consumed. Meats can be finely chopped to encourage consumption, but they need to be moist, as dry textures are more difficult for the infant to consume. Meats can also be given as finger food in strips or attached to a finger food–sized bone (e.g. lamb cutlet). Sucking and chewing on meat will extract some of the important nutrition (iron), even if this is not swallowed by the infant.

TRY IT YOURSELF

Identify raw foods that would be an appropriate texture as a complementary food. Provide finger food ideas for an eight-month-old child.

Each meal may be carefully considered. By 12 months, breakfast can include an adult cereal choice such as oat porridge or a flaked wheat or breakfast biscuit option. Meat, vegetables and a starchy choice (potato/pasta, rice or bread) should be the basic structure of a meal at lunch and dinner. Any of the options listed can be given as mini-meals or as snacks in addition to high-calcium choices such as yoghurt or custard. Full-fat cow's milk can be given as a drink after 12 months of age, but this should not be given in a bottle. A two-handle 'sipper' cup is preferable to bottles with a teat since the child can now safely form a fluid bolus and should be preparing to drink from a normal cup. Reduced-fat milk is an option after two years of age, but this needs to be balanced against adequate weight gain and the adequacy and quality of the overall diet.

≫ CASE 15.3

BEVERAGES FOR INFANTS

Apart from the need for breast milk, the choice of beverages for infants may be a cause for concern in terms of creating balance in overall energy and nutrient intakes. While breast milk is both a beverage and a food, water is also provided to infants. Water is recommended through the Australian Dietary Guidelines [42] as the main drink for all family members. The case for water as a beverage lies in its ability to provide hydration and provide protective properties for dentition (neutralising acidity in the oral cavity and delivering fluoride). The NHMRC Infant Feeding Guidelines state that cow's milk (fresh, UHT or made up powdered milk) should not be used as the main drink before 12 months of age [11], but it is suitable for milk-based desserts (custards) and with cereal. After 12 months, pasteurised cow's milk is a good source of nutrients, but should be limited to 500 mL/day so as not to reduce diversity in the diet. Reduced-fat milks are not recommended in the first two years of life, and others argue that lower-fat varieties should not be given before 2–3 years of age [12] to ensure that the fat intake from this source is not limited.

The case for fruit juice is more contentious. The vitamin C delivered in fruit juice might be better provided by whole fruit cut into easy-to-eat portions. The NHMRC Infant Feeding Guidelines [11] referred to the position of the American Academy of Pediatrics [43] in arriving at its position that fruit juice is not necessary or recommended for infants under 12 months. The issues are related to dental health, nutritional displacement of better foods/beverages and bowel problems. If consumed, a limit of 120–180 mL/day was suggested [44].

- What is the best beverage for infants at various ages?
- What are the main nutritional issues for consideration in managing beverage consumption in infants?
- What areas of research on this topic would be informative?

    SARA GRAFENAUER, KANITA KUNARATNAM AND VICKI FLOOD

>> **RESEARCH AT WORK**

MEASURING FOOD INTAKES IN INFANTS

Understanding the fluctuations in food intake from meal-to-meal and day-to-day can help in developing guidelines for infant feeding. Infants have an innate ability to regulate food energy intake to match cues of hunger and satiety [40], so their appetite in addition to the milk feed may be small. Food refusal is also characteristic of the early weaning period; however, this is more likely to be due to unfamiliar textures and new experiences rather than a dislike of specific foods [17]. One study on intake variability in the weaning period found the amounts of food consumed averaged from 30 g per feed in the first weeks, to 80 g within one month and 120 g by about six weeks [17]. By one year of age, Young and Drewett reported a median of 146 g of food per meal [45]. In researching or monitoring this early phase of solid food introduction, a single measure of food intake is inappropriate and not representative of usual intake. A food record or diary is important in determining the adequacy of the diet and to capture the variability of intake and the range of foods being consumed. Thus, only small amounts of food need to be prepared, and experience with new foods appears critical to acceptance in the longer term.

Parents who set a good example by eating fruit and vegetables tend to have children who consume better food choices and are less fussy [31]. Exerting pressure on children to eat and restricting access to specific foods may focus the child's attention on the restricted food and their desire of those forbidden foods; however, this may depend on whether the food is kept at home or not [33]. Whether restrictions early in childhood lead to overeating of forbidden foods and a dislike of approved foods is yet to be fully understood. Either way, as the core social unit, the family serves as a role model for eating behaviours. The main areas of parental control on food consumption by infants relate to the type of food, as well as the timing [31] and the location. Providing planned mealtimes is one way to manage this scenario, as well as creating a suitable setting where appropriate attention can be given to building healthy eating behaviours. This may include, for example, discussing the meal with the child, highlighting foods they have eaten and enjoyed in the past. Previous exposure clearly plays a role in the type of food consumed. Research has demonstrated that exposure to fruit and vegetables before two years of age predicts food variety up to school age and beyond [40]. Serving size is another area that should be addressed. As a practical guide, a tablespoon (tbsp) can be used as a guide for serving sizes of individual foods for children up to five years. For example, a four year old would have 4 tbsp of fruit or vegetable per serve. The child's palm can be used as a guide for the meat serving size. Providing young children with a diet comprising healthy foods in reasonable-portion sizes is a good start for dealing with the later stages of childhood when they are exposed to a much broader food environment and a greater range in the quality of foods from which they can choose.

STOP AND THINK

- Which foods are good examples of first foods? Why?
- How does the significance of milk change as the child consumes a more diverse diet?
- How can parents achieve the best profile of foods offered to children within and outside the home?

HOW CAN NUTRITION-RELATED PROBLEMS EMERGING DURING CHILDHOOD BE ADDRESSED?

In Australia, moving from early childhood to the preschool and primary school years brings further variations in nutritional requirements and exposure to food. The school years are important milestones in development, with a characteristic acceleration in growth. This phase is usually accompanied by changes in food sources and influences, with peers eventually becoming an important factor over parental opinion. There is usually a combination of factors at play. These include changes in psychosocial patterns—for example, from dependence on parental authority to independent thought processes; and familial patterns and family functioning may change—for example, if both parents are working outside the home, choices may be made by other caregivers and children may be making decisions and choices about their own meals. Social patterns develop further—for example, increasing socialisation with friends, peer pressure, eating out, fast-food consumption and media influence. Finally, changing environmental patterns can occur with increasing sedentary lifestyles, increased screen time (from television, computer, video games and online social media) and a decline in sports-related physical activities [46].

This combination of physical, psychosocial and environmental factors may predispose the growing child to an obesogenic lifestyle. Obesity is the major nutrition-related problem during childhood in the Australian population. Based on the 2014–15 National Health Survey, 27.4% of children aged 5–17 years were classified as overweight or obese, with 20.2% overweight and 7.4% obese [47]. Among 2–4 year olds, 20% of children were already classified as overweight or obese, with a higher proportion among boys (21.2%) compared with girls (17.9%). By the age of 16–17 years, 32.9% of teenagers were classified as overweight or obese, again with a notably higher proportion among boys (38.7%) than girls (26.7%) [48]. According to the National Nutrition and Physical Activity Survey (NNPAS), 84% of 2–4 year olds averaged at least six or more hours of physical activity per day from both outdoor and indoor play [49]. But also, they spent close to 1.5 hours (83 minutes) per day on sedentary screen time watching TV/DVD or playing electronic games. By the age of 5–17 years, children only spent 91 minutes per day on physical activity, with over two and quarter hours (136 minutes) spent on screen-based leisure activity [49]. Dietary problems can emerge from this environmental context that relate to energy imbalance.

Energy balance and nutritional adequacy

Challenges in this age group are the need to improve diet quality and physical activity, and to ensure optimal nutrition for growth, especially with the sudden growth spurts before puberty, while emphasising the need for healthy food choices both at home and outside the home (Table 15.2). Dietary problems typically emerge with excess consumption of total dietary energy, saturated fatty acids (SFA) and added sugars, along with insufficient consumption of micronutrients such as calcium, magnesium, iron, folate, zinc, vitamin B and n-3 fatty acids [50].

In a recent study among two-year-old Australian children [50], it was found that the dietary intake of this age group was characterised by low vegetable consumption and high discretionary food intake. Most children (92%) reported consuming the Australian Dietary Guidelines (ADG) recommendations of one serve of fruit per day, but only 20% reported consuming the recommended 2.5 serves of vegetables per day, with mean serves of fruit of 2.2 (s.d. 1.2) and vegetables 1.7 (s.d. 1.2) [42]. Importantly, this study also investigated the association of the child's diet compared with the mother's food habits, and

SARA GRAFENAUER, KANITA KUNARATNAM AND VICKI FLOOD

TABLE 15.2   RECOMMENDED SERVINGS OF FOODS FOR AUSTRALIAN CHILDREN AGED 2–11 YEARS

Food group (single serve size)	Gender	2–3 years	4–8 years	9–11 years
Vegetables and legumes (75 g/0.5cup)	Boy	2.5	4.5	5
	Girl	2.5	4.5	5
Fruit (150 g/1medium piece)	Boy	1	1.5	2
	Girl	1	1.5	2
Grains (bread, cereal, rice, pasta) (1 slice bread/0.5 cup cereal, rice, pasta)	Boy	4	4	5
	Girl	4	4	5
Lean meat, fish, eggs, nuts, legumes (65 g meat/100 g fish/1 cup legumes/30 g nuts/2 eggs)	Boy	1	1.5	2.5
	Girl	1.5	1.5	2.5
Milk, cheese, yoghurt (1 cup/40 g cheese/200 g yoghurt)	Boy	1.5	2	2.5
	Girl	1.5	1.5	3

Source: National Health and Medical Research Council (2013). *Healthy Eating for Children—Brochure*. Canberra: NHMRC. © Commonwealth of Australia

found the two were highly correlated, indicating the importance of modelling healthy food behaviours by parents [51].

According to the ADG [42], one serve of discretionary foods contributes approximately 550 kJ of energy. Discretionary foods include items such as sweet biscuits, cakes, desserts and pastries; processed meats and sausages; ice creams and other ice confections, confectionary and chocolate; savoury pastries and pies; commercial burgers, fried foods, potato chips, crisps and other fatty or salty snacks; cream, butter and spreads; sugar-sweetened drinks, energy drinks and cordials. In 2011–12, the Australian Health Survey reported that children aged 2–3 years were consuming an average of 5–6 serves of discretionary foods daily, while children aged 4–8 years were consuming close to 6–7 serves of discretionary foods per day [52]. Discretionary foods accounted for 30.2% of energy intake among 2–3 year olds, 37.5% among 4–8 year olds and almost 40.1% of energy intake among 14–18 year olds. The largest discretionary food contributor to 2–3 year olds' energy was sweet and savoury biscuits (3.9%), while for 4–8 year olds it was cakes, muffins, scones and cake-type desserts (5%). Among 14–18 year olds, confectionary and cereal/nut/fruit/seed bars and soft drinks and flavoured mineral water contributed 3.7% and 3.6%, respectively [52].

In an Australian study involving children below two years of age, it was found that consumption of discretionary foods was inversely associated with consumption of core foods. As the intake of most micronutrients was notably lower among children in the highest quintile of discretionary food consumption, the main foods consumed were high in energy but nutrient poor [53].

The fatty acid profile of the diets of Australian children is also of concern, as it is high in SFAs but low in n-3 polyunsaturated fatty acids (PUFA) [54], suggesting a low fish intake. The NHMRC recommends replacing energy-dense low-nutrient foods with marine n-3 PUFA-rich foods, such as oily fish, to prevent chronic disease [55]. One concern, however, is the high methylmercury content of some fish, which may impede child development, with associated neurological effects [56]. According to the Heart Foundation, although the absolute risk of seafood-borne illness is extremely low in the type of fish commonly consumed in Australia [57], it would be prudent to recommend two or three servings of fish per week (150–225 g/week; where one serve of fish ~75 g for young children) for children up to six years, and up to 300–450 g/week, where one serve of fish is ~150 g for older children [46].

» CASE 15.4

WATER—THE PREFERRED BEVERAGE FOR CHILDREN

In an Australian study, 63–68% of 2–8-year-old Australian children were found to drink sugar-sweetened beverages [58]. Excessive fruit juice consumption has also been associated with several health issues in young children, including toddler 'diarrhoea', short stature and the risk of obesity [59]. Water is necessary for metabolism and for non-human physiological functions, including provision of essential minerals such as calcium, magnesium and fluoride. It is especially important in children, as young children may not be able to indicate when they are thirsty and they rely on caregivers to offer them water frequently. Using data from the Third National Health and Nutrition Examination Survey (NHANES III), the US Dietary Reference Intake committee [60] recommended that children aged 1–3 years consume a total of 1.3 L (~0.9 L from beverages/day or ~4 cups/day); children aged 4–8 years are recommended to take a total of 1.7 L (~1.2 L from beverages/day or ~5 cups/day). For older children and adolescents, for boys 9–13 years the recommendation is 2.4 L of total water per day (~1.8 L from beverages/day or 8 cups); for girls 9–13 years it is 2.1 L of total water per day (~1.6 L from beverages or 7 cups).

- How often should young children be offered a drink of water?
- What are the risks associated with providing sugar-sweetened beverages to children instead of water?
- What other components in the diet provide water in addition to beverages?

Childhood obesity

Childhood obesity has emerged as a major public health concern in Australia and globally. In the 2014–15 National Health Survey [48], about one in four children (27.4%) aged 5–17 years were overweight or obese, comprising 20.2% overweight and 7.4% obese. In the same survey, among 2–4-year-old children 20% of children were classified as overweight or obese, with 21.2% of boys (14.2% overweight and 6.7% obese) and 17.9% of girls (8.7% overweight and 9.0% obese) classified as overweight/obese. According to the Australian Aboriginal and Torres Strait Islander Health Survey (2012–13), 22.4% of Indigenous children aged 2–4 years old were classified as overweight/obese (15.6% overweight and 6.5% obese) [61]. Interestingly, among this population the proportion of overweight/obese 2–4-year-old children was higher among girls (27.1%) (19.9% overweight and 7.2% obese) than boys (17.8%) (11.8% overweight and 5.9% obese). High rates of overweight and obesity were also notable among older children aged 5–14 years, with 37.7% classified as overweight or obese, comprised of 24.4% overweight and 13.5% obese [61]. The prevalence of overweight and obesity among preschoolers in developed countries in 2010 was 11.7%, and this is set to rise to 14.1% in 2020 [62]. Australian preschoolers are already far exceeding the estimated international

Childhood obesity
excess body fat that occurs during childhood, where obesity is defined as a BMI greater than 30 kg/m².

benchmarks for overweight/obesity. Despite reported stabilisation in prevalence rates of overweight and obesity in children over the past few years, these rates remain high and still represent a significant health issue [63]. Monitoring weight is hence an important part of managing childhood obesity in the population.

>> CASE 15.5

MEASURING WEIGHT STATUS IN CHILDREN

Body mass index (BMI) is used as a measure of obesity within populations. When the US NHANES III data was used to determine predictive ability of BMI-for-age in determining body fatness, it was found that both BMI-for-age and weight-for-stature performed equally well in screening for underweight and overweight among children 3–5 years of age. For school-aged children (six years and above), BMI-for-age had higher validity than weight-for-stature in predicting underweight and overweight status [64]. The BMI is the most common means for defining a healthy body weight for adults and children. Although BMI for children and adults is calculated the same way, it is interpreted differently. This is because, as children grow, the amount of body fat changes with age, so BMI for children needs to be interpreted in relation to a child's age, and there are gender differences. As BMI for children and adolescents is age- and gender-specific, the age and gender of a child must be considered when interpreting their BMI.

Two main approaches have been developed to identify children with high body weight based on BMI. One is based on the US Centers for Disease Control and Prevention (CDC) growth reference charts [65], which are used to classify children aged two years and older as 'overweight' or 'at risk of overweight', respectively, and the other is based on the International Obesity Taskforce (IOTF) recommendations. The IOTF links childhood BMI cut-off points with adult overweight (BMI = 25 kg/m²) and obesity (BMI = 30 kg/m²) thresholds [66] and is used primarily for obesity surveillance in research settings [67]. As no local BMI-for-age reference charts exist, Australian experts have endorsed the IOTF classification system charts proposed by Cole and colleagues as the most appropriate measurement of adiposity in children and adolescents for research and population-monitoring purposes [68]. However, in clinical situations where growth monitoring is an important evaluation tool and greater measurement precision is necessary, exact percentiles tend to be preferred by clinicians [65]. The NHMRC recommends the use of BMI scores plotted on the BMI-for-age percentile charts (for boys or girls) as an initial (first level) assessment to assist in identifying children who *may* be overweight or obese. For children aged 2–18 years, either the CDC or WHO BMI percentile charts may be used, with the same chart used over time to allow for consistent monitoring of growth [11] (Table 15.3 and Figure 15.2).

TABLE 15.3   RECOMMENDED BMI-FOR-AGE CUT-OFFS FOR CHILDREN TWO YEARS AND OLDER

BMI category	Percentile standard (CDC cut-offs)[1]	Percentile standard (WHO cut-offs)[2]
Obese	⩾95th percentile	⩾99th percentile
At risk of overweight/overweight	85th to <95th percentile	85th to 97th percentile
Healthy weight	>5th to <85th percentile	15th to 50th percentile
Underweight	⩽5th percentile	<3rd percentile

Source: [1]V. Khadilkar & A. Khadilkar (2011). Growth charts: a diagnostic tool. *Indian Journal of Endocrinology and Metabolism*, 15(suppl. 3), S166–S171; [2]National Health and Medical Research Council (2013). *Clinical Practice Guidelines for the Management of Overweight and Obesity in Adults, Adolescents and Children in Australia*. Melbourne: NHMRC. © Commonwealth of Australia

FIGURE 15.2 TIMELINE OF GROWTH CHARTS IN AUSTRALIA

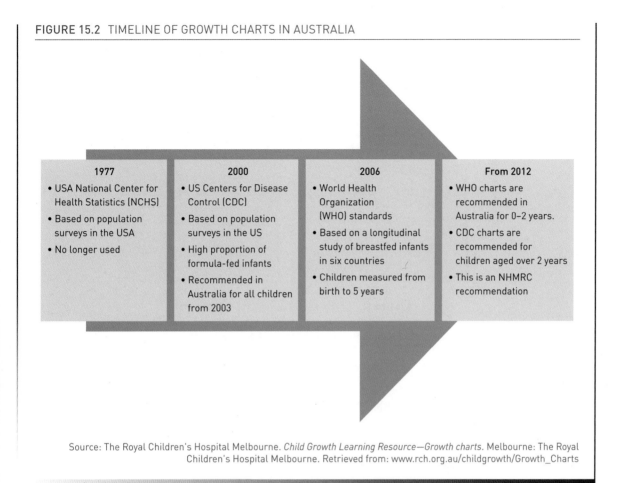

1977	2000	2006	From 2012
• USA National Center for Health Statistics (NCHS) • Based on population surveys in the USA • No longer used	• US Centers for Disease Control (CDC) • Based on population surveys in the US • High proportion of formula-fed infants • Recommended in Australia for all children from 2003	• World Health Organization (WHO) standards • Based on a longitudinal study of breastfed infants in six countries • Children measured from birth to 5 years	• WHO charts are recommended in Australia for 0–2 years. • CDC charts are recommended for children aged over 2 years • This is an NHMRC recommendation

Source: The Royal Children's Hospital Melbourne. *Child Growth Learning Resource—Growth charts*. Melbourne: The Royal Children's Hospital Melbourne. Retrieved from: www.rch.org.au/childgrowth/Growth_Charts

In clinical assessments, BMI percentiles are used for assessing individual size and growth patterns. In this context, transition from weight-for-length (for 2–5 years) to the BMI-for-age charts from 24 to 36 months occurs when a child can stand unassisted and is able to adequately follow directions for correct posture and stature measurement [65]. Once BMI is calculated and plotted on the BMI-for-age growth charts, a percentile ranking can be obtained. Percentiles indicate the relative position of the child's BMI number among children of the same sex and age [68] (Figure 15.3).

In population settings, BMI z-scores are used for assessing growth patterns. Body mass index z-scores (or BMI s.d. scores) correspond to growth chart percentiles, and are measures of relative weight adjusted for child age and sex. Given a child's age, sex, BMI and an appropriate reference standard, a BMI z-score (or its equivalent BMI-for-age percentile) can be determined [68]. According to Armitage and Berry [69], z-score = (observed value)−(median reference value of a population)/standard deviation of reference population (Figures 15.4 and 15.5).

Previous reports have implicated individual factors in causing rising levels of obesity among children and adolescents [70]. These include increased energy intake, sedentary lifestyles, decreased walking and cycling, decreased physical activity, and changes in family structure and dynamics. However, recent findings have alluded to multifactorial contributors and combined cumulative effect of genetic, biological, psychological, cultural and environmental factors occurring at crucial points of time, which have culminated in the rise in childhood obesity [71].

FIGURE 15.3 BMI PERCENTILES FOR AGE

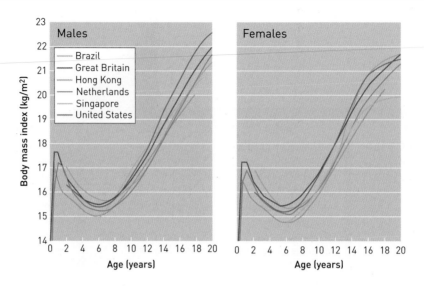

Source: R. J. Kuczmarski, C. L. Ogden, S. S. Guo, L. M. Grummer-Strawn, K. M. Flegal, Z. Mei, ... C. L. Johnson (2002). 2000 CDC growth charts for the United States: methods and development. *Vital and Health Statistics*, 11(246), 1–190

FIGURE 15.4 MEDIAN CHILDREN'S BMI BY AGE AND SEX IN SIX NATIONALLY REPRESENTATIVE DATABASES

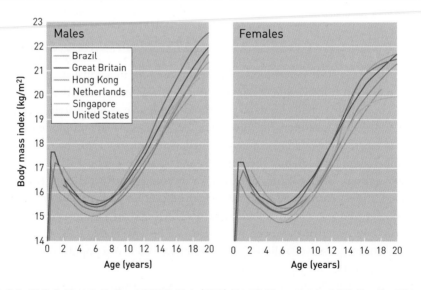

Source: T. J. Cole, M. C. Bellizzi, K. M. Flegal & W. H. Dietz (2000). Establishing a standard definition for child overweight and obesity worldwide: international survey. *British Medical Journal*, 320(7244), 1240

FIGURE 15.5 INTERNATIONAL CUT-OFF POINTS FOR BMI BY SEX FOR OVERWEIGHT AND OBESE CHILDREN PASSING THROUGH BMI 25 AND 30 KG/M² AT AGE 18

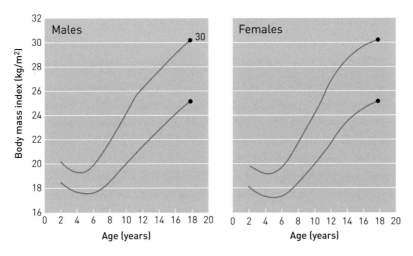

Source: T. J. Cole, M. C. Bellizzi, K. M. Flegal & W. H. Dietz (2000). Establishing a standard definition for child overweight and obesity worldwide: international survey. *British Medical Journal*, 320(7244), 1240

>> RESEARCH AT WORK

AN ECOLOGICAL MODEL OF CHILDHOOD OBESITY

Gebel and colleagues [72] proposed an ecological model that explains the complex factors associated with obesity in a fairly concise manner (Figure 15.6). The framework shows how the physical environment influences nutrition and physical activity behaviour, either directly or mediated by the social environment

FIGURE 15.6 ECOLOGICAL FRAMEWORK OF FACTORS INFLUENCING WEIGHT

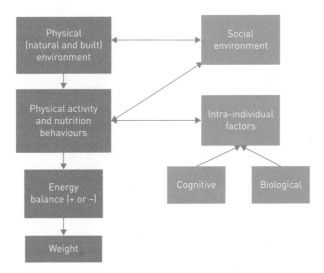

Source: K. Gebel, L. King, A. Bauman, P. Vita, T. Gill, A. Rigby & A. Capon (2005). *Creating Healthy Environments: A review of links between the physical environment, physical activity and obesity*. Sydney: NSW Health Department and NSW Centre for Overweight and Obesity

 SARA GRAFENAUER, KANITA KUNARATNAM AND VICKI FLOOD

(i.e. social, economic, cultural and political factors) that affect physical activity and nutrition behaviour. It also includes the interplay at the individual level (i.e. cognitive factors such as knowledge, attitudes and beliefs, and biological factors such as age, sex, race, individual physiological responsiveness and genetic makeup) that contributes to the development of overweight and obesity.

For children, there has also been a consistent body of evidence that obesity that manifests in childhood is likely to persist into adulthood, with its associated health risks [73]. Besides the physiological impacts, individuals who are overweight or obese may tend to experience stigmatisation and emotional disturbances. Psychosocial consequences among obese children and adolescents include social isolation and discrimination [74]. These children are also likely to have poor self-esteem and to adopt high-risk behaviours such as smoking and binge drinking in later life [75] (Table 15.4).

It has been noted that by school age, most childhood lifestyle behaviours such as feeding practices, satiety cues and sedentary behaviours may have already been learnt, and hence are difficult to change. Intrauterine, infancy and preschool periods have been identified as critical periods for programming long-term regulation of energy balance [5; 62; 76]. A review of interventions has argued that although there is a range of interventions for use in reducing the risk of childhood obesity, there is still a lack of knowledge of the specific interventions that are the most effective and cost-effective [77]. The authors also highlighted the need for interventions to be focused on a population level for implementation, rather than short-term individually based interventions, and that there are research gaps among younger children aged 0–3 years, and 0–5 years in particular. Overall, it has

TABLE 15.4   HEALTH CONSEQUENCES OF OVERWEIGHT IN CHILDREN

Short-term consequences[1]	Long-term consequences[2, 3]
Low self-esteem Teasing, bullying or even rejection by peers Joint pain Chronic inflammation Asthma Impaired glucose tolerance (IGT), type 2 diabetes, metabolic syndrome and high blood pressure	Chronic diseases—e.g. obesity, insulin resistance, type 2 diabetes mellitus, hypertension, hyperlipidaemia, atherosclerosis, left ventricular hypertrophy and cardiovascular disease Fatty liver (non-alcoholic)/steatohepatitis Asthma (exacerbation) Renal (proteinuria) Depression Stroke and certain types of cancers Bone and joint issues, e.g. slipped capital femoral epiphysis, Blount's disease Obstructive sleep apnoea Pseudomotor cerebri Poor quality of life

Sources: [1] J. J. Reilly, E. Methven, Z. C. McDowell, B. Hacking, D. Alexander, L. Stewart & C. J. H. Kelnar (2003). Health consequences of obesity. *Archives of Disease in Childhood*, 88, 748–52; [2] S. R. Daniels, D. K. Arnett, R. H. Eckel, S. S. Gidding, L. L. Hayman, S. Kumanyika, … C. L. Williams (2005). Overweight in children and adolescents: pathophysiology, consequences, prevention, and treatment. *Circulation*, 111(15),1999–2012. [3] A. S. Singh, C. Mulder, J. W. R. Twisk, W. van Mechelen & M. J. M. Chinapaw (2008). Tracking of childhood overweight into adulthood: a systematic review of the literature. *Obesity Reviews*, 9(5), 474–88.

been increasingly recognised that strategies to prevent obesity onset should commence as early as possible, with an inherent focus on early interventions before the age of five years. These should include nutrition and lifestyle interventions that would improve linear growth in the first two years of life and avoid excess weight gain relative to height (BMI) after that age [4]. Parents should be equipped with the skills to inculcate healthy lifestyle behaviours in their children from birth, such as exclusive breastfeeding (for at least the first six months of life); increasing consumption of fruits, vegetables and whole grains; reducing saturated fat intake and discretionary foods, and sugary foods and beverages; limiting screen time; and encouraging physical activity and outdoor play. This will help lay the foundations for healthy lifestyle habits that have a continuing impact across the lifespan.

STOP AND THINK

- Why has childhood obesity emerged as a major nutrition-related problem?
- Why is it necessary to differentiate between measuring obesity in children individually at the clinical level and as a group at the population level?
- What approaches can be taken to address the problem of childhood obesity at the public health level? What research is needed to help make this more effective?

SUMMARY

- As infants grow, their nutritional requirements increase and solid foods need to be introduced. The timing needs to match changed physiological needs and developmental stage.
- The development of healthy eating habits is very important in all stages of child development. This should align with national dietary guidelines, with a focus on consuming recommended servings of vegetables, fruit, cereals, lean meats and milk/cheese/yoghurt.
- Childhood obesity can be prevented through judicious choice of foods and beverages throughout this stage of development.

PATHWAYS TO PRACTICE

- Early childhood services and baby health clinics have significant opportunities to provide nutrition education and support for parents of infants and young children to develop healthy dietary practices.
- As part of the external environmental influences on children's eating habits, child care services, preschools, schools and sporting organisations can ensure that nutritious foods and beverages are strongly promoted and made available as primary, if not exclusive, choices for infants and children.
- Skills development in preparing suitable meals for infants and children can be provided via a number of different means, from cooking classes to providing online recipes and chat rooms.
- In industry, food standards apply for the development of infant foods. These relate to important nutrients and guidelines appropriate for infant products.

DISCUSSION QUESTIONS

1   Which aspects of child development are particularly relevant to the timing of the introduction of solid foods to infants?

2   How might the choice of foods and texture during the introduction of solid foods relate to the above?

3   What are some of the controversies surrounding the exact timing of the introduction of solid foods to infants?

4   Why is the early establishment of healthy eating habits in children important?

5   What are some of the issues concerning the measurement of weight status in children?

6   How is an ecological framework helpful for understanding the development of childhood obesity?

USEFUL WEBLINKS

Australian Breastfeeding Association—
www.breastfeeding.asn.au/bfinfo/index.html

Department of Health—Breastfeeding:
www.health.gov.au/internet/main/Publishing.nsf/Content/health-pubhlth-strateg-brfeed-index.htm

Department of Health—Get up and grow caring for our kids:
www.health.gov.au/internet/main/publishing.nsf/Content/gug-resource-order-guide

Eat for Health—Healthy eating for children brochure:
www.eatforhealth.gov.au/sites/default/files/content/The%20Guidelines/n55f_children_brochure.pdf

Eat for Health—Infant Feeding Guidelines:
www.eatforhealth.gov.au/guidelines

Pregnancy, Birth and Baby:
www.pregnancybirthbaby.org.au

The Royal Children's Hospital Melbourne—Child growth learning:
resource www.rch.org.au/childgrowth

The Royal Children's Hospital Melbourne—Growth charts:
www.rch.org.au/childgrowth/Growth_Charts

The WHO Child Growth Standards:
www.who.int/childgrowth/standards/en

US Centers for Disease Control and Prevention Growth Chart:
www.cdc.gov/growthcharts

US Department of Agriculture—Infant Nutrition:
www.nal.usda.gov/fnic/infant-nutrition

World Health Organization—Complementary feeding:
www.who.int/nutrition/topics/complementary_feeding/en

World Health Organization—Infant nutrition:
www.who.int/topics/infant_nutrition/en

FURTHER READING

Abrams, E. M., Greenhawt, M., Fleischer, D. M. & Chan, E. S. (2017). Early solid food introduction: role in food allergy prevention and implications for breastfeeding. *Journal of Pediatrics*, 184, 13–18. doi:10.1016/j.jpeds.2017.01.053

Bell, K. A., Wagner, C. L., Feldman, H. A., Shypailo, R. J. & Belfort, M. B. (2017). Associations of infant feeding with trajectories of body composition and growth. *American Journal of Clinical Nutrition*, 106(2), 491–8. doi:10.3945/ajcn.116.151126

Berti, C., Agostoni, C., Davanzo, R., Hyppönen, E., Isolauri, E., Meltzer, H. M., ... Cetin, I. (2017). Early-life nutritional exposures and lifelong health: immediate and long-lasting impacts of probiotics, vitamin D, and breastfeeding. *Nutrition Reviews*, 75(2), 83–97. doi:10.1093/nutrit/nuw056

Brown, A. & Lee, M. D. (2015). Early influences on child satiety-responsiveness: the role of weaning style. *Pediatric Obesity*, 10(1), 57–66. doi:10.1111/j.2047-6310.2013.00207.x

Buvinger, E., Rosenblum, K., Miller, A. L., Kaciroti, N. A. & Lumeng, J. C. (2017). Observed infant food cue responsivity: associations with maternal report of infant eating behavior, breastfeeding, and infant weight gain. *Appetite*, 112, 219–26. doi:10.1016/j.appet.2017.02.002

Cole, N. C., An, R., Lee, S.-Y. & Donovan, S. M. (2017). Correlates of picky eating and food neophobia in young children: a systematic review and meta-analysis. *Nutrition Reviews*, 75(7), 516–32. doi:10.1093/nutrit/nux024

de Barse, L. M., Jansen, P. W., Edelson-Fries, L. R., Jaddoe, V. W. V., Franco, O. H., Tiemeier, H. & Steenweg-de Graaff, J. (2017). Infant feeding and child fussy eating: the Generation R Study. *Appetite*, 114, 374–81. doi:10.1016/j.appet.2017.04.006

De Beer, M., Vrijkotte, T. G. M., Fall, C. H. D., Van Eijsden, M., Osmond, C. & Gemke, R. J. B. J. (2015). Associations of infant feeding and timing of linear growth and relative weight gain during early life with childhood body composition. *International Journal of Obesity*, 39(4), 586–92. doi:10.1038/ijo.2014.200

Emmett, P. M. & Jones, L. R. (2015). Diet, growth, and obesity development throughout childhood in the Avon Longitudinal Study of Parents and Children. *Nutrition Reviews*, 73(suppl. 3), 175–206. doi:10.1093/nutrit/nuv054

Fangupo, L. J., Heath, A. L. M., Williams, S. M., Somerville, M. R., Lawrence, J. A., Gray, A. R., ... Taylor, R. W.. (2015). Impact of an early-life intervention on the nutrition behaviors of 2-y-old children: a randomized controlled trial. *American Journal of Clinical Nutrition*, 102(3), 704–12. doi:10.3945/ajcn.115.111823

Fangupo, L. J., Heath, A. L. M., Williams, S. M., Williams, L. W. E., Morison, B. J., Fleming, E. A., ... Taylor, R. W. (2016). A baby-led approach to eating solids and risk of choking. *Pediatrics*, 138(4). doi:10.1542/peds.2016-0772

Fewtrell, M., Bronsky, J., Campoy, C., Domellöf, M., Embleton, N., Mis, N. F., ... Molgaard, C. (2017). Complementary feeding: a position paper by the European Society for Paediatric Gastroenterology, Hepatology, and Nutrition (ESPGHAN) committee on nutrition. *Journal of Pediatric Gastroenterology and Nutrition*, 64(1), 119–32. doi:10.1097/MPG.0000000000001454

Foterek, K., Buyken, A. E., Bolzenius, K., Hilbig, A., Nöthlings, U. & Alexy, U. (2016). Commercial complementary food consumption is prospectively associated with added sugar intake in childhood. *British Journal of Nutrition*, 115(11), 2067–74. doi:10.1017/S0007114516001367

Foterek, K., Hilbig, A. & Alexy, U. (2015). Associations between commercial complementary food consumption and fruit and vegetable intake in children. Results of the DONALD study. *Appetite*, 85, 84–90. doi:10.1016/j.appet.2014.11.015

Garza, C. (2015). Fetal, neonatal, infant, and child international growth standards: an unprecedented opportunity for an integrated approach to assess growth and development. *Advances in Nutrition: An International Review Journal*, 6(4), 383–90. doi:10.3945/an.114.008128

Hetherington, M. M., Schwartz, C., Madrelle, J., Croden, F., Nekitsing, C., Vereijken, C. M. J. L. & Weenen, H. (2015). A step-by-step introduction to vegetables at the beginning of complementary feeding. The effects of early and repeated exposure. *Appetite*, 84, 280–90. doi:10.1016/j.appet.2014.10.014

Jensen, S. M., Ritz, C., Ejlerskov, K. T., Mølgaard, C. & Michaelsen, K. F. (2015). Infant BMI peak, breastfeeding, and body composition at age 3 y. *American Journal of Clinical Nutrition*, 101(2), 319–25. doi:10.3945/ajcn.114.092957

Johnson, S. L. (2016). Developmental and environmental influences on young children's vegetable preferences and consumption. *Advances in Nutrition: An International Review Journal*, 7(1), 220S–231S. doi:10.3945/an.115.008706

Kamran, A., Sharifirad, G., Nasiri, K., Soleymanifard, P., Savadpour, M. T. & Akbarhaghighat, M. (2017). Determinants of complementary feeding practices among children aged 6–23: a community based study. *International Journal of Pediatrics*, 5(3), 4551–60. doi:10.22038/ijp.2016.7811

Keller, K. L. & Adise, S. (2016). Variation in the ability to taste bitter thiourea compounds: implications for food acceptance, dietary intake, and obesity risk in children. *Annual Review of Nutrition*, 36(1), 157–82. doi:10.1146/annurev-nutr-071715-050916

Lobstein, T., Jackson-Leach, R., Moodie, M. L., Hall, K. D., Gortmaker, S. L., Swinburn, B. A., ... McPherson, K. (2015). Child and adolescent obesity: part of a bigger picture. *The Lancet*, 385(9986), 2510–20. doi:10.1016/S0140-6736(14)61746-3

Martin, R. M., Kramer, M. S., Patel, R., et al. (2017). Effects of promoting long-term, exclusive breastfeeding on adolescent adiposity, blood pressure, and growth trajectories: a secondary analysis of a randomized clinical trial. *JAMA Pediatrics*, 171(7), e170698. doi:10.1001/jamapediatrics.2017.0698

Maslin, K. & Venter, C. (2017). Nutritional aspects of commercially prepared infant foods in developed countries: a narrative review. *Nutrition Research Reviews*, 30(1), 138–48. doi:10.1017/S0954422417000038

Mennella, J. A., Daniels, L. M. & Reiter, A. R. (2017). Learning to like vegetables during breastfeeding: a randomized clinical trial of lactating mothers and infants. *American Journal of Clinical Nutrition*, 106(1), 67–76. doi:10.3945/ajcn.116.143982

Mennella, J. A., Reiter, A. R. & Daniels, L. M. (2016). Vegetable and fruit acceptance during infancy: impact of ontogeny, genetics, and early experiences. *Advances in Nutrition: An International Review Journal*, 7(1), 211S–219S. doi:10.3945/an.115.008649

Moghaddam, H. T., Khademi, G., Abbasi, M. A. & Saeidi, M. (2015). Infant and young child feeding: a key area to improve child health. *International Journal of Pediatrics*, 3(6), 1083–92. doi:10.22038/ijp.2015.5603

Mok, E., Vanstone, C. A., Gallo, S., Li, P., Constantin, E. & Weiler, H. A. (2017). Diet diversity, growth and adiposity in healthy breastfed infants fed homemade complementary foods. *International Journal of Obesity*, 41(5), 776–82. doi:10.1038/ijo.2017.37

Nicklaus, S. (2015). The role of food experiences during early childhood in food pleasure learning. *Appetite*, 104, 3–9. doi:10.1016/j.appet.2015.08.022

Patro-Gołąb, B., Zalewski, B. M., Kołodziej, M., Kouwenhoven, S., Poston, L., Godfrey, K. M., ... Szajewska, H. (2016). Nutritional interventions or exposures in infants and children aged up to 3 years and their effects on subsequent risk of overweight, obesity and body fat: a systematic review of systematic reviews. *Obesity Reviews*, 17(12), 1245–57. doi:10.1111/obr.12476

Robinson, S. M., Crozier, S. R., Harvey, N. C., Barton, B. D., Law, C. M., Godfrey, K. M., ... Inskip, H. M. (2015). Modifiable early-life risk factors for childhood adiposity and overweight: an analysis of their combined impact and potential for prevention. *American Journal of Clinical Nutrition*, 101(2), 368–75. doi:10.3945/ajcn.114.094268

Scheepers, L. E. J. M., Penders, J., Mbakwa, C. A., Thijs, C., Mommers, M. & Arts, I. C. W. (2015). The intestinal microbiota composition and weight development in children: the KOALA Birth Cohort study. *International Journal of Obesity*, 39(1), 16–25. doi:10.1038/ijo.2014.178

Turati, F., Bertuccio, P., Galeone, C., Pelucchi, C., Naldi, L., Bach, J. F., ... Peroni, D. (2016). Early weaning is beneficial to prevent atopic dermatitis occurrence in young children. *Allergy: European Journal of Allergy and Clinical Immunology*, 71(6), 878–88. doi:10.1111/all.12864

Woo, J. G., Herbers, P. M., McMahon, R. J., Davidson, B. S., Ruiz-Palacios, G. M., Peng, Y. M. & Morrow, A. L. (2015). Longitudinal development of infant complementary diet diversity in 3 international cohorts. *Journal of Pediatrics*, 167(5), 969–74. doi:10.1016/j.jpeds.2015.06.063

Woo Baidal, J. A., Locks, L. M., Cheng, E. R., Blake-Lamb, T. L., Perkins, M. E. & Taveras, E. M. (2016). Risk factors for childhood obesity in the first 1,000 days: a systematic review. *American Journal of Preventive Medicine*, 50(6), 761–79. doi:10.1016/j.amepre.2015.11.012

REFERENCES

1   J. Baird, D. Fisher, P. Lucas, J. Kleijnen, H. Roberts & C. Law (2005). Being big or growing fast: systematic review of size and growth in infancy and later obesity. *British Medical Journal*, 331(7522), 929. doi:10.1136/bmj.38586.411273.E0

2   J. G. Eriksson, T. Forsén, J. Tuomilehto, C. Osmond & D. J. P. Barker (2003). Early adiposity rebound in childhood and risk of type 2 diabetes in adult life. *Diabetologia*, 46(2), 190–4. doi:10.1007/s00125-002-1012-5

SARA GRAFENAUER, KANITA KUNARATNAM AND VICKI FLOOD

3   A. M. Euser, M. J. Finken, M. G. Keijzer-Veen, E. T. Hille, J. M. Wit, F. W. Dekker & Dutch POPS-19 Collaborative Study Group (2005). Associations between prenatal and infancy weight gain and BMI, fat mass, and fat distribution in young adulthood: a prospective cohort study in males and females born very preterm. *American Journal of Clinical Nutrition*, 81(2), 480–7.

4   R. Uauy, J. Kain, V. Mericq, J. Rojas & C. Corvalan (2008). Nutrition, child growth, and chronic disease prevention. *Annals of Medicine*, 40(1), 11–20. doi:10.1080/07853890701704683

5   D. J. Barker (2004). The developmental origins of chronic adult disease. *Acta Paediatrica Supplement*, 93(446), 26–33.

6   D. Davies & B. O'Hare (2004). Weaning: a worry as old as time. *Current Paediatrics*, 14(2), 83–96.

7   S. L. Prescott, P. Smith, M. Tang, D. J. Palmer, J. Sinn, S. J. Huntley, ... M. Makrides (2008). The importance of early complementary feeding in the development of oral tolerance: concerns and controversies. *Pediatric Allergy and Immunology*, 19(5), 375–80. doi:10.1111/j.1399-3038.2008.00718.x

8   H. Przyrembel (2012). Timing of introduction of complementary food: short- and long-term health consequences. *Annals of Nutrition and Metabolism*, 60(suppl. 2), 8–20.

9   M. K. Georgieff (2011). Long-term brain and behavioral consequences of early iron deficiency. *Nutrition Reviews*, 69(suppl. 1), S43–S48.

10 S. Nicklaus (2011). Children's acceptance of new foods at weaning. Role of practices of weaning and of food sensory properties. *Appetite*, 57(3), 812–15.

11 National Health and Medical Research Council (2012). *Infant Feeding Guidelines*. Canberra: NHMRC.

12 C. Agostoni, T. Decsi, M. Fewtrell, O. Goulet, S. Kolacek, B. Koletzko, ... J. Rigo (2008). Complementary feeding: a commentary by the ESPGHAN Committee on Nutrition. *Journal of Pediatric Gastroenterology and Nutrition*, 46(1), 99–110.

13 K. Hamilton, L. Daniels, N. Murray, K. M. White & A. Walsh (2012). Mothers' perceptions of introducing solids to their infant at six months of age: identifying critical belief-based targets to promote adherence to current infant feeding guidelines. *Journal of Health Psychology*, 17(1), 121–31. doi:10.1177/1359105311409786

14 J. A. Conn, M. J. Davies, R. B. Walker & V. M. Moore (2009). Food and nutrient intakes of 9-month-old infants in Adelaide, Australia. *Public Health Nutrition*, 12(12), 2448–56.

15 L. Cooke & A. Fildes (2011). The impact of flavour exposure in utero and during milk feeding on food acceptance at weaning and beyond. *Appetite*, 57(3), 808–11. doi:10.1016/j.appet.2011.05.317

16 H. Törölä, M. Lehtihalmes, A. Yliherva & P. Olsén (2012). Feeding skill milestones of preterm infants born with extremely low birth weight (ELBW). *Infant Behavior and Development*, 35(2), 187–94.

17 M. van Dijk, S. Hunnius & P. van Geert (2009). Variability in eating behavior throughout the weaning period. *Appetite*, 52(3), 766–70.

18 M. van Dijk, S. Hunnius & P. van Geert (2012). The dynamics of feeding during the introduction to solid food. *Infant Behavior and Development*, 35(2), 226–39.

19 S. M. Donath & L. H. Amir (2005). Breastfeeding and the introduction of solids in Australian infants: data from the 2001 National Health Survey. *Australian and New Zealand Journal of Public Health*, 29(2), 171–5. doi:10.1111/j.1467-842X.2005.tb00069.x

20 Australian Institute of Health and Welfare (2011). *2010 Australian National Infant Feeding Survey: Indicator results*. Canberra: AIHW.

21 R. Uauy & A. D. Dangour (2009). Fat and fatty acid requirements and recommendations for infants of 0–2 years and children of 2–18 years. *Annals of Nutrition and Metabolism*, 55(1–3), 76–96.

22 J. F. Soothill (1980). Dietary antigen avoidance: postponement or prevention? *The Lancet*, 315(8168), 604. doi:10.1016/s0140-6736(80)91098-3

23 B. Symon & M. Bammann (2012). Feeding in the first year of life: emerging benefits of introducing complementary solids from 4 months. *Australian Family Physician*, 41(4), 226.

24 Australian Society of Clinical Immunology and Allergy (2016). *Infant Feeding Advice*. Retrieved from: www. allergy.org.au/images/pcc/ASCIA_PCC_Infant_Feeding_Advice_2016.pdf.

25 G. Du Toit, G. Roberts, P. H. Sayre, H. T. Bahnson, S. Radulovic, A. F. Santos, … M. Feeney (2015). Randomized trial of peanut consumption in infants at risk for peanut allergy. *New England Journal of Medicine*, 372(9), 803–13.

26 D. J. Palmer, J. Metcalfe, M. Makrides, M. S. Gold, P. Quinn, C. E. West, … S. L. Prescott (2013). Early regular egg exposure in infants with eczema: a randomized controlled trial. *Journal of Allergy and Clinical Immunology*, 132(2), 387–92, e381.

27 G. Lack (2012). Update on risk factors for food allergy. *Journal of Allergy and Clinical Immunology*, 129, 1187–97.

28 A. Ivarsson, O. Hernell, H. Stenlund & L. A. Persson (2002). Breast-feeding protects against celiac disease. *American Journal of Clinical Nutrition*, 75, 914–21.

29 S. D. Brown & G. Harris (2012). Disliked food acting as a contaminant during infancy. A disgust based motivation for rejection. *Appetite*, 58(2), 535–8. doi:10.1016/j.appet.2012.01.010

30 S. J. Caton, S. M. Ahern & M. M. Hetherington (2011). Vegetables by stealth. An exploratory study investigating the introduction of vegetables in the weaning period. *Appetite*, 57(3), 816–25.

31 L. L. Birch & J. O. Fisher (1998). Development of eating behaviors among children and adolescents. *Pediatrics*, 101(3), 539–49.

32 C. A. Forestell & J. A. Mennella (2012). More than just a pretty face. The relationship between infant's temperament, food acceptance, and mothers' perceptions of their enjoyment of food. *Appetite*, 58(3), 1136–42. doi:10.1016/j.appet.2012.03.005

33 J. O. Fisher & L. L. Birch (1999). Restricting access to palatable foods affects children's behavioral response, food selection, and intake. *American Journal of Clinical Nutrition*, 69(6), 1264–72.

34 S. A. Sullivan & L. Birch (1994). Infant dietary experience and acceptance of solid foods. *Paediatrics*, 93(2), 271–7.

35 C. A. Forestell & J. A. Mennella (2007). Early determinants of fruit and vegetable acceptance. *Pediatrics*, 120(6), 1247–54. doi:10.1542/peds.2007-0858

36 S. Anzman-Frasca, J. S. Savage, M. E. Marini, J. O. Fisher & L. L. Birch (2012). Repeated exposure and associative conditioning promote preschool children's liking of vegetables. *Appetite*, 58(2), 543–53. doi:10.1016/j.appet.2011.11.012

37 A. Arora, M. Gay & D. Thirukumar (2012). Parental choice of infant feeding behaviours in South West Sydney: a preliminary investigation. *Health Education Journal*, 71(4), 461–73. doi:10.1177/0017896912444180

38 H. Rowan & C. Harris (2012). Baby-led weaning and the family diet. A pilot study. *Appetite*, 58(3), 1046–9.

39 S. Lioret, S. A. McNaughton, A. C. Spence, D. Crawford & K. J. Campbell (2013). Tracking of dietary intakes in early childhood: the Melbourne InFANT Program. *European Journal of Clinical Nutrition*, 67(3), 275–81. doi:http://www.nature.com/ejcn/journal/v67/n3/suppinfo/ejcn2012218s1.html

40 L. Chan, A. Magarey & L. Daniels (2011). Maternal feeding practices and feeding behaviors of Australian children aged 12–36 months. *Maternal & Child Health Journal*, 15(8), 1363–71. doi:10.1007/s10995-010-0686-4

41 K. Webb, I. Rutishauser & N. Knezevic (2008). Foods, nutrients and portions consumed by a sample of Australian children aged 16–24 months. *Nutrition & Dietetics*, 65(1), 56–65. doi:10.1111/j.1747-0080.2007.00224.x

42 National Health and Medical Research Council (2013). *Australian Dietary Guidelines*. Canberra: NHMRC.

43 American Academy of Pediatrics (2001). The use and misuse of fruit juice in pediatrics. *Pediatrics*, 107(5), 1210–13. doi:10.1542/peds.107.5.1210

44 M. B. Heyman & S. A. Abrams (2017). Fruit juice in infants, children, and adolescents: current recommendations. *Pediatrics*, 139(6). doi:10.1542/peds.2017-0967

45 B. Young & R. Drewett (2000). Eating behaviour and its variability in 1-year-old children. *Appetite*, 35(2), 171–7. doi:10.1006/appe.2000.0346

46 S. S. Gidding, B. A. Dennison, L. L. Birch, S. R. Daniels, M. W. Gilman, A. H. Lichtenstein, … L. Van Horn (2006). Dietary recommendations for children and adolescents: a guide for practitioners. *Pediatrics*, 117(2), 544–59.

47 Australian Bureau of Statistics (2014). *National Health Survey: First results, 2014–15—Children's risk factors*. ABS: Canberra. Retrieved from: www.abs.gov.au/ausstats/abs@.nsf/Lookup/by%20Subject/4364.0.55.001~2014-15~Main%20Features~Children's%20risk%20factors~31.

48 Australian Bureau of Statistics (2014). *National Health Survey: First results, 2014–15—Australia*. Table 16.3 Children's Body Mass Index, waist circumference, height and weight(a)(b), Proportion of persons. ABS: Canberra. Retrieved from: www.abs.gov.au/AUSSTATS/abs@.nsf/DetailsPage/4364.0.55.0012014-15?OpenDocument.

49 Australian Bureau of Statistics (2013). *Australian Health Survey: Physical activity, 2011–12. National Nutrition and Physical Activity Survey*. ABS: Canberra. Retrieved from: www.abs.gov.au/ausstats/abs@.nsf/Lookup/4364.0.55.004Chapter1002011-12.

50 S. J. Osendarp, K. I. Baghurst, J. Bryan, E. Calvaresi, D. Hughes, M. Hussaini, … NEMO Study Group (2007). Effect of a 12-mo micronutrient intervention on learning and memory in well-nourished and marginally nourished school-aged children: 2 parallel, randomized, placebo-controlled studies in Australia and Indonesia. *American Journal of Clinical Nutrition*, 86(4), 1082–93.

51 K. Kunaratnam, M. Halaki, L. M. Wen, L. A. Baur & V. M. Flood (2018). Mother–child dietary behaviours and their observed associations with socio-demographic factors: findings from the Healthy Beginnings Trial. *British Journal of Nutrition*, 119(4), 464–71.

52 Australian Bureau of Statistics (2014). *Australian Health Survey: Nutrition First results—Foods and nutrients, 2011–12—Discretionary foods*. ABS: Canberra. Retrieved from: www.abs.gov.au/ausstats/abs@.nsf/Lookup/by%20Subject/4364.0.55.007~2011-12~Main%20Features~Discretionary%20foods~700.

53 K. L. Webb, M. Lahti-Koski, I. Rutishauser, D. J. Hector, N. Knezevic, T. Gill, … S. R. Leeder (2006). Consumption of 'extra' foods (energy-dense, nutrient-poor) among children aged 16–24 months from western Sydney, Australia. *Public Health Nutrition*, 9(8), 1035–44.

54 S. J. Zhou, R. A. Gibson, R. S. Gibson & M. Makrides (2012). Nutrient intakes and status of preschool children in Adelaide, South Australia. *Medical Journal of Australia*, 196(11), 696–700.

55 National Health and Medical Research Council (2006). *Nutrient Reference Values for Australia and New Zealand, Including Recommended Dietary Intakes.* Canberra: NHMRC.

56 E. Oken & D. C. Bellinger (2008). Fish consumption, methylmercury and child neurodevelopment. *Current Opinion in Pediatrics*, 20(2), 178–83. doi:10.1097/MOP.0b013e3282f5614c

57 D. Colquhoun, A. Ferreira-Jardim, T. Udell & B. Eden (2008). *Review of Evidence: Fish, fish oils, n-3 polyunsaturated fatty acids and cardiovascular health.* Canberra: National Heart Foundation of Australia.

58 A. M. Rangan, J. Kwan, V. M. Flood, J. C.Y. Louie & T. P. Gill (2011). Changes in 'extra' food intake among Australian children between 1995 and 2007. *Obesity Research & Clinical Practice*, 5(1), e55–e63. doi:http://dx.doi.org/10.1016/j.orcp.2010.12.001

59 B. A. Dennison (1996). Fruit juice consumption by infants and children: a review. *Journal of the American College of Nutrition*, 15(Suppl.5), 4s–11s.

60 Panel on Dietary Intake for Electrolytes and Water Standing Committee on the Scientific Evaluation of Dietary Reference Intakes (2005). *Dietary Reference Intakes for Water, Potassium, Sodium, Chloride, and Sulfate.* Washington, DC: National Academies Press.

61 Australian Bureau of Statistics (2014). *Australian Aboriginal and Torres Strait Islander Health Survey—First results, 2012–13—Australia.* ABS: Canberra. Retrieved from: www.abs.gov.au/ausstats/abs@.nsf/Lookup/A07BD 8674C37D838CA257C2F001459FA?opendocument.

62 M. de Onis, M. Blössner & E. Borghi (2010). Global prevalence and trends of overweight and obesity among preschool children. *American Journal of Clinical Nutrition*, 92(5), 1257–64. doi:10.3945/ajcn.2010.29786

63 M. Wabitsch, A. Moss & K. Kromeyer-Hauschild (2014). Unexpected plateauing of childhood obesity rates in developed countries. *BMC Medicine*, 12, 17.

64 Z. Mei, L. M. Grummer-Strawn, A. Pietrobelli, A. Goulding, M. I. Goran & W. H. Dietz (2002). Validity of body mass index compared with other body-composition screening indexes for the assessment of body fatness in children and adolescents. *American Journal of Clinical Nutrition*, 75(6), 978–85.

65 R. J. Kuczmarski, C. L. Ogden, S. S. Guo, L. M. Grummer-Strawn, K. M. Flegal, Z. Mei, … C. L. Johnson (2002). 2000 CDC growth charts for the United States: methods and development. *Vital and Health Statistics*, 11(246), 1–190.

66 T. J. Cole, M. C. Bellizzi, K. M. Flegal & W. H. Dietz (2000). Establishing a standard definition for child overweight and obesity worldwide: international survey. *British Medical Journal*, 320(7244), 1240. doi:10.1136/bmj.320.7244.1240

67 P. T. Katzmarzyk, C. L. Craig & L. Gauvin (2007). Adiposity, physical fitness and incident diabetes: the physical activity longitudinal study. *Diabetologia*, 50(3), 538–44. doi:10.1007/s00125-006-0554-3

68 P. T. Espinel & L. King (2009). *A Framework for Monitoring Overweight and Obesity in NSW.* Sydney: NSW Department of Health and the Physical Activity Nutrition Obesity Research Group.

69 P. Armitage, G. Berry & J.N.S. Matthews (2002). *Statistical Methods in Medical Research*, 4th edn. Oxford: Blackwell.

70 Australian Institute of Health and Welfare (2004). *A Rising Epidemic: Obesity in Australian children and adolescents.* Canberra: AIHW.

71 S. Caprio, S. R. Daniels, A. Drewnowski, F. R. Kaufman, L. A. Palinkas, A. L. Rosenbloom & J. B. Schwimmer (2008). Influence of race, ethnicity, and culture on childhood obesity: implications for prevention and treatment: a consensus statement of Shaping America's Health and the Obesity Society. *Diabetes Care*, 31(11), 2211–21. doi:10.2337/dc08-9024

72 L. K. K. Gebel, A. Bauman, P. Vita, T. Gill, A. Rigby & A. Capon (2005). *Creating Healthy Environments: A review of links between the physical environment, physical activity and obesity.* Sydney: NSW Health Department and NSW Centre for Overweight and Obesity.

73 American Academy of Pediatrics Committee on Nutrition (2003). Prevention of pediatric overweight and obesity. *Pediatrics*, 112(2), 424–30.

74 R. S. Strauss & H. A. Pollack (2003). Social marginalization of overweight children. *Archives of Pediatrics & Adolescent Medicine*, 157(8), 746–52. doi:10.1001/archpedi.157.8.746

75 R. S. Strauss (2000). Childhood obesity and self-esteem. *Pediatrics*, 105(1), e15–e15.

76 D. J. Barker, J. G. Eriksson, T. Forsen & C. Osmond (2002). Fetal origins of adult disease: strength of effects and biological basis. *International Journal of Epidemiology*, 31(6), 1235–9.

77 E. Waters, A. de Silva-Sanigorski, B. J. Burford, T. Brown, K. J. Campbell, Y. Gao, ... C. D. Summerbell (2011). Interventions for preventing obesity in children. *Cochrane Database of Systematic Reviews*, 12. doi:10.1002/14651858.CD001871.pub3

CHAPTER 16

NUTRITION DURING ADOLESCENCE

CLARE COLLINS, REBECCA HASLAM, ANNETTE MURPHY,
KRISTINE PEZDIRC AND LEE ASHTON

CHAPTER OBJECTIVES

This chapter will enable the reader to:

- define adolescence and the key changes that occur within this life stage
- describe the nutritional requirements of adolescence and the concerns for nutrition during this life stage
- recognise effective approaches to developing healthy food habits and adequate nutritional intakes for adolescents.

KEY TERMS

Adolescence   Social modelling

Nutritional requirements

KEY POINTS

- Adolescence is a period of rapid human growth and development following childhood and preceding adulthood.
- Requirements for energy and nutrients vary between individuals, so recommendations should account for factors such as physical activity level and body size. If negative habits are formed, they can result in obesity and predispose adolescents for diseases such as cardiovascular disease and diabetes.
- It is important to provide modelling and education for adolescents on the preparation and consumption of healthy meals. Adolescents' dietary habits are influenced by their family and peers as well as settings such as the school canteen. Long-term health relies on positive influences during the period of adolescence.

INTRODUCTION

This chapter will cover the definition of adolescence, the factors that influence an adolescent's food intake and the critical nutrition-related concerns for adolescents including overweight and obesity, diabetes, nutrition for active adolescents and vegetarianism. The chapter will also cover nutrient and food group recommendations and also current dietary intakes for adolescents.

WHAT IS ADOLESCENCE?

Adolescence
a transitional period of growth and development between childhood and adulthood (ages 10–19).

Puberty
the onset of sexual maturation in humans.

The World Health Organization (WHO) defines **adolescence** as the ages from 10 to 19 years where rapid human growth and development occurs, after childhood and before adulthood [1]. Timing of the key physiological changes during adolescence can vary from person to person, although the order of changes is the same.

The age of onset of **puberty** can vary from 8–15 years of age. Menarche is a female's first menstruation and indicates ovulation has begun. Spermarche, a male's first ejaculation, indicates sperm production has begun. During puberty, there are a number of changes that occur. The testicles and ovaries mature and hormone changes occur with increases in testosterone for males and estradiol for females [2]. These hormonal changes commonly lead to moodiness and sexual urges; however, physical changes may also play a role [3].

Physical changes include body hair growth and distribution, changes to voice, and the development of breasts and acne. There is usually a sudden period of growth where muscle mass increases in males and fat mass increases in females [4]. Changing circadian rhythms cause adolescents to stay up later and sleep later into the morning, which can lead to inadequate sleep relative to needs. Adolescent brain regions develop at different rates, and the rate varies between individuals and sexes. The brain regions related to emotions and impulse mature first, followed by rationality and logic [5].

Adolescence should be a healthy period of life with a low prevalence of risk factors and chronic disease and where individuals perform at an optimal level. However, as adolescents seek the development of independence, they are also exposed to and can engage in risky health behaviours, which increase their likelihood of accidents and adverse health outcomes [6]. They may also be prone to developing psychological conditions such as depression and eating disorders [7]. Thus, adolescence can be a time marked by key changes in lifestyle and the formation of new eating behaviours. During this time, healthy eating habits are of critical importance, as high rates in physical growth are associated with higher requirements for some nutrients [8]. Adherence to healthy food patterns during adolescence increases the chance of these patterns continuing into adulthood and helps to delay or prevent chronic disease risk such as cardiovascular disease in later life [9].

STOP AND THINK

- How has the concept of adolescence emerged in modern society?
- What are some of the health risks that are particular to this age group?
- What are the implications of these changes for maintaining nutritional health?

WHAT ARE THE NUTRITIONAL REQUIREMENTS DURING ADOLESCENCE?

The major growth spurt that occurs during adolescence requires sufficient energy and nutrient requirements to support growth and development [10; 11]. Bone health, including teeth, is an important consideration in all life stages, but as peak bone mass is reached by the age of 30, adequate nutrition is particularly important in adolescents. Insufficient intake of calcium and excessive intake of discretionary foods such as sugar-sweetened beverages can have an impact on bone health.

Recall from previous chapters that *energy* is required by the body for metabolic and physiological functions, including breaking down of food into nutrients, muscle activity, growth and development. Sources of energy predominately come from carbohydrates, fats and protein [11]. During adolescence, energy requirements are influenced by basal metabolic rate (BMR), physical activity levels (PAL) and increased requirements to support pubertal growth and development. BMR is the amount of energy required to maintain basic life functions and contributes to approximately 45–70% of daily energy expenditure. During adolescence, BMR is higher compared to adulthood, to accommodate for the increased rates of growth and development during this life stage [11]. Physical activity levels also play a role in an individual's energy requirements: the more physically active a person is the higher their energy requirements are [11; 12].

Table 16.1 provides guidance for calculating energy requirements (megajoules[MJ]/ day) for adolescents based on selecting the most appropriate PAL. The PAL includes relevant growth factors for age and corresponds to the following activities: 1.2: best rest; 1.4: very sedentary; 1.6: light activity;1.8: moderate activity ; 2.0: heavy activity; 2.2: vigorous activity [11].

See Chapters 1, 3 and 7 on food consumption and energy.

TABLE 16.1   ESTIMATED ENERGY REQUIREMENTS FOR ADOLESCENTS (MJ/DAY)

	BMR (MJ/day)	PAL 1.2	PAL 1.4	PAL 1.6	PAL 1.8	PAL 2.0	PAL 2.2
Boys							
10 years	5.1	6.3	7.3	8.3	9.3	10.4	11.4
14 years	6.6	8.0	9.3	10.6	11.9	13.2	14.6
18 years	7.7	9.4	10.9	12.5	14.0	15.6	17.1
Girls							
10 years	4.7	5.7	6.7	7.6	8.5	9.5	10.4
14 years	5.7	6.9	8.1	9.2	10.3	11.5	12.6
18 years	6.0	7.3	8.5	9.7	10.9	12.1	13.3

Abbreviations: BMR: basal metabolic rate; PAL: physical activity level

Source: National Health and Medical Research Council (2006). *Nutrient Reference Values for Australia and New Zealand, Including Recommended Dietary Intakes.* Canberra: NHMRC. © Commonwealth of Australia

TRY IT YOURSELF

Calculate the energy requirements (kJ/day) for a 14-year-old male who plays representative soccer for his school plus trains two times (60 minutes) per week.

CLARE COLLINS, REBECCA HASLAM, ANNETTE MURPHY, KRISTINE PEZDIRC AND LEE ASHTON

Carbohydrate is a macronutrient used for energy production in the body and includes sugars and starch [11; 13]. Carbohydrates are found naturally occurring in fruits, dairy foods and grains as well as processed foods [12; 13]. Total carbohydrate intake should contribute to 45–65% of total energy intake [14].

Protein is a macronutrient which is required by the body for growth, repair and maintenance. Requirements for protein are higher in adolescence and are higher again in males than females [11; 12]. Protein can be obtained from the diet through animal products including meat, poultry, fish and dairy foods, as well as non-meat products such as legumes, eggs, tofu and seeds [12; 13]. Protein intake is recommended to contribute to 5–20% of total energy intake. Protein requirements can be calculated using adolescent weight in kilograms (kg) [11] (Table 16.2).

Fat is the most energy-dense macronutrient and is required in the body for the absorption of fat-soluble vitamins. Dietary sources of fat may be saturated, monounsaturated or polyunsaturated depending on their chemical structure [13]. Saturated fats are found predominately in animal products—for example, the fat in meat—while monounsaturated and polyunsaturated fats are found in plant-based foods such as olive oil [12]. Fat intake is recommended to contribute 20–35% of total energy intake, with no more than 10% of energy coming from saturated fat sources [14]. In adolescence, total fat requirements for ages 9–13 years are 70 mg/day, while the fat requirements at ages 14–18 years are greater, with males requiring 125 mg/day and females 85 mg/day [11].

Fibre is a component of all plant materials that resists digestion in the small intestine and ferments at least partially in the large intestine. Physiological effects from fibre include increased laxation, reduction in blood cholesterol and modulation of blood glucose levels [11]. Sources of fibre include fruits, vegetables, breads and cereals [14]. Requirements for adequate fibre intake for males at ages 9–13 years is 24 g/day and for ages 14–18 years is 28 g/day. For females, requirements are 20 g/day for ages 9–13 years and 22 g/day for 14–18 year olds [11].

Calcium is required for the development and maintenance of bones as well as muscle and cardiac function [11]. Dairy foods such as milk, cheese and yoghurt are the major sources of calcium. The estimated average requirement (EAR) for calcium for boys and girls aged 12–18 years is 1050 mg/day and this can be obtained by consuming 3½ serves of dairy and dairy alternatives per day [11; 12].

Iron in the body is predominantly found in haemoglobin, which is used to transport oxygen around the body, and it is also required for immune system, muscle and cognitive functioning [11; 13]. From the diet, iron is obtained from red meat, poultry, fish and wholegrain cereals. The EAR for children aged 9–13 years is 6 mg/day and for ages 14–18 years is 8 mg/day [11].

TABLE 16.2   PROTEIN REQUIREMENTS FOR ADOLESCENTS (G/DAY)

	EAR	RDI
Boys		
9–13 years	31 g/day (0.78 g/kg)	40 g/day (0.94 g/kg)
14–18 years	49 g/day (0.76 g/kg)	65 g/day (0.99 g/kg)
Girls		
9–13 years	24 g/day (0.61 g/kg)	35 g/day (0.87 g/kg)
14–18 years	35 g/day (0.62 g/kg)	45 g/day (0.77 g/kg)

Abbreviations: EAR: estimated average requirement; RDI: recommended dietary intake

Source: National Health and Medical Research Council (2006). *Nutrient Reference Values for Australia and New Zealand, including Recommended Dietary Intakes*. Canberra: NHMRC. © Commonwealth of Australia

Folate is essential for DNA synthesis and is required to prevent neural tube defects during foetal development in pregnancy. Since 2009, Food Standards Australia New Zealand (FSANZ) has mandated the fortification of folate in wheat flour. Naturally occurring sources of folate include fruit and vegetables, especially green leafy vegetables [11; 18]. For males and females aged 9–13 years, the EAR is 250 µg/day. Males and females aged 14–18 years have increased folate requirements of 330 µg/day [11].

Sodium is found most commonly in foods as salt and is required by the body for extracellular fluid and to maintain cell membrane potential. Adequate intake (AI) of sodium is 400–800 mg/day for ages 9–13 years and 460–920 mg/day for ages 14–18 years (both males and females) [11]. The upper level (UL) of intake for ages 9–13 years is 2000 mg/day and for 14–18 year olds it is 2300 mg/day [11].

Zinc is required in the body to help maintain the structural integrity of proteins and regulate gene expression. A variety of food groups contain zinc, including, meat, fish, grains and dairy foods. The zinc EAR for ages 9–13 years (males and females) is 5 mg/day [11]. For ages 14–18 years, the EAR is 11 mg/day for males and 6 mg/day for females [11].

≫ RESEARCH AT WORK

ALCOHOL CONSUMPTION IN ADOLESCENTS

Alcohol is widely consumed by adolescents. Research has shown that 28% of adolescents aged 12–17 years report drinking alcohol and 3.4% drink alcohol on a weekly basis [15; 16]. Abstinence from alcohol is recommended during adolescence, especially before the age of 14 years, when it increases the risk of alcohol-related harm or injury. Increased risks associated with binge drinking, including impaired brain development, injury, death and drink driving, are reported for adolescents who consume alcohol compared with older age groups [16; 17]. Abstaining from alcohol is the best option for adolescents.

≫ CASE 16.1

INADEQUATE NUTRIENT INTAKES AND IMPROVING DIETARY CHOICES BY AUSTRALIAN ADOLESCENTS

According to results from the Australian Health Survey 2011–13 comparing usual adolescent intakes to the Australian Nutrient Reference Values (NRVs), inadequate intakes of calcium, iron, folate and zinc are common in these age groups (Table 16.3) [13].

TABLE 16.3   PROPORTION OF ADOLESCENTS NOT MEETING EAR FOR MICRONUTRIENTS

Nutrient	Males		Females	
	12–13 years	14–18 years	12–13 years	14–18 years
Inadequate calcium (%)	67	71	84	90.3
	9–13 years			
Inadequate iron (%)	3.3	8.3	10.5	40.1
Inadequate folate (%)	0.4	1.2	1.2	7.9
Inadequate zinc	0.3	27.4	2.3	10.0

Source: Australian Bureau of Statistics (2015). *Australian Health Survey: Usual nutrient intakes, 2011–2012.* Cat. no. 4364.0.55.008. Canberra: ABS

CLARE COLLINS, REBECCA HASLAM, ANNETTE MURPHY, KRISTINE PEZDIRC AND LEE ASHTON

The Australian Health Survey indicated that an inadequate intake of calcium was common in adolescent males and females when compared with their age/sex-specific EARs [13]. For males aged 12–13 years, 67% had inadequate intake, while at the age of 14–18 years 71% did not meet their EAR for calcium. For females aged 12–13 years and 14–18 years, 84% and 90.3% had inadequate intake of calcium, respectively. Inadequate iron intake is more prevalent in females than males. In ages 9–13 years, only 3.3% of males had inadequate intake compared with 10.5% of females of the same age. Higher rates of inadequate iron intake were reported in ages 14–18 years, with 8.3% of males and 40.1% of females not meeting the EAR. In ages 9–13 years, inadequate folate intake based on the EAR was seen in 0.4% of males and 1.2% of females, while in ages 14–18 years, 1.2% of males and 7.9% of females had an inadequate intake of folate. Inadequate intake of zinc was more prevalent in older males than females when based on the EAR. Only 0.3% of males aged 9–13 years had inadequate intake while 2.1% of females of the same age had inadequate intake of zinc. In the older age group (14–18 years old), the proportion of males with an inadequate zinc intake was 27.4%, and for females it was 10.0%. A large proportion of the population was shown to have an excess intake of sodium: in males aged 9–13 years and males aged 14–18 years, 83.2% and 86.4% exceeded the UL, respectively. For females aged 9–13 years, 68.7% reached the UL, while 50.6% of 14–18-year-old females exceeded the UL.

In terms of foods consumed, the recommended vegetables and fruit intakes for adolescent males are 5 to 5½ serves of vegetables and 2 serves of fruit per day, while females between 9–18 years of age require 5 serves of vegetables and 2 serves of fruit [12]. The results from the National Health Survey 2014–15 reported on average 68.1% of 2–18 year olds are meeting the target for fruit intakes and only 5.4% meet their recommended serves of vegetables [19]. Per day, on average, children aged 2–18 years of age consumed 2 serves of fruit and 1.9 serves of vegetables. Girls were also more likely to meet the recommended serves of fruit than boys (71.8% compared to 65.0%). Adolescents aged 12–18 years are recommended to have at least 3½ serves of milk, cheese, yoghurt and dairy alternatives per day [20]. However, the Australian Health Survey indicates that less than 2% of adolescents are meeting the recommended serves [20]. A higher proportion of males (68%) and females (83%) participating in the survey had less than 2 serves per day. The recommended amount of lean meats and alternatives for males and females aged 12–18 years is 2½ serves. The Australian Health Survey indicated that approximately 9.5% of males were most likely to meet these recommendations while less than 1% females were able to reach this target [20]. For adolescents aged 12–13 years, where 6 serves of grains and cereals for males and 5 serves for females are recommended, 35% of males and 27% females were meeting their targets. Only 14% of adolescents aged 14–18 years were meeting the recommended 7 serves of grains and cereals per day.

Excessive consumption of discretionary foods

According to the Australian Health Survey, adolescents and young adults consume more soft drinks, burgers and chips than any other age group. Children and adolescents aged 9–11 and 12–13 years were the second-highest group in this category, with 39% of total energy consumption coming from discretionary foods [20]. Around 41% of total energy consumption from adolescents aged 14–18 years came from discretionary foods, the highest compared to other age groups.

- How might the findings from the Australian Health Survey inform the development of public health initiatives to improve the nutrient intakes of adolescents?

- What does the pattern of food intakes by adolescents tell us about their food choices?

- Do adolescents need further guidance and encouragement in making healthy food choices?

STOP AND THINK
....

- Why are certain key nutrients critical during adolescent growth?
- Which nutrients are likely to be at risk of insufficient intake, and why?
- How does inadequate nutritional intake relate to food and beverages choices?
- What kinds of approaches might be needed to improve the nutritional intake of Australian adolescents?

WHAT ARE THE HEALTH CONCERNS RELATING TO NUTRITION DURING ADOLESCENCE?

Adolescence is a critical stage of development, and therefore poor nutritional intake can have a substantial impact on health during adulthood. From a preventive health perspective, the development of chronic disease risk is a major concern for nutrition during this period of maturation. Other health conditions that may be implicated during adolescence include eating disorders, distorted body image and the development of acne (Table 16.4). As nutrition underpins both the structure and function of the human body, there are additional considerations for academic and sporting performance, and the special needs of adolescent pregnancy.

TABLE 16.4   NUTRITION-RELATED PROBLEMS/ISSUES SEEN DURING ADOLESCENCE

Chronic disease risk	Functional issues
Overweight/obesity	Acne
Heart disease risk	Cognitive performance
Diabetes	Sports performance
Pregnancy	Eating disorders

Overweight/obesity

Overweight and obesity is a significant health problem across all age groups, with over a quarter of Australian children and adolescents overweight or obese [19]. Excess weight in adolescence increases the risk of overweight and obesity in adulthood [21] and also increases the lifetime risk of developing chronic diseases such as diabetes, cardiovascular disease and specific cancers [22]. Adolescent obesity is also linked with psychosocial issues, including body dissatisfaction, overeating and depression [22]. Excessive consumption of energy-dense, nutrient-poor foods (e.g. confectionary, soft drinks, takeaway foods), and low intake of fruits and vegetable serves and being physically inactive are all contributors to overweight and obesity [22]. Australian adolescents have one of the highest intakes of energy-dense, nutrient-poor foods and lowest intakes of fruit and vegetable serves [13].

Adolescent food intake is influenced by parental eating behaviours , convenience, cost and a lack of concern about healthy eating [23]. Adolescents are reaching an age where increased independence also impacts on their food choices. Increasing the knowledge of healthy eating in adolescents is an important strategy for reducing overweight and obesity. The development of skills such as selecting, preparing and cooking healthy meals will support the sustainability of these behaviours over the longer term.

CLARE COLLINS, REBECCA HASLAM, ANNETTE MURPHY, KRISTINE PEZDIRC AND LEE ASHTON

The National Health and Medical Research Council (MHMRC) uses the 5As framework to manage body weight in adolescents: ask and assess, advise, assist and arrange follow-up [24]. A family approach to weight management is the goal of these guidelines, promoting involvement by the family as a whole in modifying the family food environment, physical activity habits and long-term monitoring and assessment of these behaviours. Support and modelling of a healthy food habits and participation in regular physical activity with family and friends have been shown to increase the likelihood of adolescents mimicking these behaviours [25; 26].

Dietary modifications such as increasing intake of fruit and vegetables, increasing the consumption of fibre-rich foods, decreasing consumption of sugar-sweetened beverages and also eating breakfast have been shown to reduce adiposity in adolescents [25]. Therefore, by following the dietary guidelines and including a variety of fruits, vegetables, wholegrains, lean meats and alternatives, fat-reduced dairy foods and alternatives and limiting the consumption of energy-dense, nutrient-poor foods, as well as encouraging family members to model healthy eating, can help to minimise overweight and obesity in adolescents [12; 26]. School-based interventions are also another area where behaviour change in adolescents can be successful [27].

Cardiovascular disease

Cardiovascular disease is a primary cause of morbidity and mortality in developed countries. Risk factors that contribute to cardiovascular disease include obesity, high blood pressure, dyslipidaemia (abnormal blood fats and/or elevated total blood cholesterol), impaired glucose tolerance (high blood sugars) and vascular (vein) abnormalities. Dietary intake can play a significant role in the development of these risk factors.

Research conducted in the Young Finns study, one of the largest follow-up studies into cardiovascular risk from childhood to adulthood tracking over 30 years, has shown that the atherogenic process begins in childhood [28]. The study shows that childhood risk factors measured at or after age nine years (moving into adolescence) have the strongest associations with later atherosclerosis and subsequent heart disease.

The Bogalusa study also identifies that risk factors for cardiovascular disease are present at an early age [29]. Fibrous-plaque lesions were detected in coronary arteries in over 30% of adolescents aged 16–20 years and a high body mass index (BMI) and blood pressure and abnormal lipid profiles were associated with cardiovascular risk. A traditional dietary pattern characterised by low intakes of fruits and vegetables was associated with increased arterial wall thickness, with an associated increased risk of cardiovascular disease, especially in males, whereas a high intake of vegetables was independently associated with increased arterial elasticity (cardioprotective) in both genders [29]. Consuming a diet that is energy dense, high in total fat and low in fibre is positively associated with cardiometabolic risk factors. This process begins in childhood and tracks in adolescence [30]. Dietary intake is a modifiable factor that can reduce the risk of cardiovascular disease. Foods that can decrease the risk of cardiovascular disease are listed in Table 16.5.

Type 1 diabetes
an auto-immune condition where the immune system destroys the beta-cells in the pancreas that produce insulin, thus requiring insulin therapy.

Diabetes

There are a number of types of diabetes, all of which have nutritional implications. **Type 1 diabetes** is an auto-immune disease in which the immune system destroys the beta-cells in the pancreas that produce insulin, thus requiring insulin therapy. The exact cause of the condition is not known, but it is not linked to modifiable lifestyle factors. Type 1 diabetes

TABLE 16.5 FOODS CONSIDERED PROTECTIVE AGAINST THE RISK OF CARDIOVASCULAR DISEASE AND TYPE 2 DIABETES

Food	Value
Fruit and vegetables	High fibre content, antioxidant compounds that may protect vessel walls, high source of folate, which may help lower blood levels of homocysteine (linked to an increased risk of heart disease)
Oily fish	Such as sardines, tuna and salmon: contain omega-3 fatty acids
Vegetable oils	Corn, soy and safflower, which contain omega-6 fatty acids, and those containing omega-3 fatty acids such as canola and olive oil. All of these may help to lower LDL cholesterol
Whole grains	Unrefined grains, bread and breakfast cereals, legumes, certain types of rice and pasta, with low glycaemic index, can help keep blood sugar levels within a narrower range
Legumes	Soy protein has been shown to lower LDL cholesterol levels, especially if blood cholesterol levels are high

is one of the most common chronic diseases in adolescence, with approximately 2400 Australians diagnosed with type 1 diabetes every year. The peak time of diagnosis in Australia is between the ages of 10 and 14 years, with around 95% of the diabetes found in children being type 1 [31]. Having a healthy dietary pattern does not reduce the risk of being diagnosed with the disease, but it will help with management and insulin therapy. Following a healthy diet is vital during this growth period, and accredited practising dietitians (APDs) play a key role in supporting families with dietary guidance.

Unlike type 1 diabetes, *type 2 diabetes* is linked to body weight, and insulin is still produced by the body but is less effective. In the past two decades, a rise in the prevalence of type 2 diabetes has been reported in children and adolescents. Modifiable risk factors include a nutrient inadequate diet and physical inactivity, both of which lead to overweight and obesity, which is a high risk factor for developing the disease. People diagnosed with diabetes at an earlier age have a greater risk of complications due to longer exposure to the disease. Other evidence indicates that adolescents with type 2 diabetes have a higher rate of comorbidities at diagnosis, such as high blood pressure [32].

One of the biggest issues with adolescents and diabetes is adherence to an appropriate healthy dietary pattern. This is due to a number of factors, including increased concerns about social setting and body image, a change in responsibility for diabetes management from parents to teens, increased risk-taking behaviours, incomplete knowledge and understanding of treatment and future health risks, burnout from constant care of a chronic illness and physiological changes that lead to greater insulin resistance during puberty [33]. Foods that can decrease the risk of type 2 diabetes are listed in Table 16.5.

>> CASE 16.2

A HYPOTHETICAL CASE OF AN ADOLESCENT WITH A FAMILY HISTORY OF DIABETES AND CARDIOVASCULAR DISEASE

Jackson is a 14-year-old teenager attending the local high school and living with his mother, father and 12-year-old sister. His mother and father both have a family history of diabetes and cardiovascular disease, and they work full-time outside the home. Jackson cares for his younger sister after school until his parents get home, usually after 6.30 p.m. Jackson has been bullied at school for being a bit 'chubby'

CLARE COLLINS, REBECCA HASLAM, ANNETTE MURPHY, KRISTINE PEZDIRC AND LEE ASHTON

but his mum calls it 'puppy fat'. Jackson does not play organised sport but enjoys time 'gaming' and chatting with other gamers online. Jackson's current weight is 88 kg and he is 160 cm tall.

- What are Jackson's key concerns (social, physical and medical) in relation to his health?
- What diseases is Jackson at risk of developing?
- What approaches could be taken by Jackson's family, school and health workers to reduce his risk of chronic diseases?

Eating disorders and body image

Eating disorder
a preoccupation with eating, exercising, weight or body shape.

Eating disorders and distorted body image may also be affect health during adolescence. **Eating disorders** are classified as a mental illness and include preoccupation with eating, exercising, weight or body shape [34]. The *Diagnostic and Statistical Manual of Mental Disorders (DSM-5)* specifies the diagnostic criteria for eating disorders [35]. Eating disorders are the third most common chronic illness for young females [36] and can affect any age group, but the average age of onset is during adolescence [37].

There is a variety of different types of eating disorders, including anorexia nervosa, bulimia nervosa, binge eating disorder and other specified feeding and eating disorders (OSFED) [34]. Anorexia nervosa can be restrictive, involve binge-eating or purging and is characterised by low body weight, obsessive fear of weight gain and body image distortion; it affects 0.3% of people aged 13–18 years [34; 38]. Bulimia nervosa is characterised by recurrent binge-eating followed with compensatory behaviours such as overexercising, vomiting, use of laxatives or fasting; it affects 0.9% of adolescents. Binge-eating disorders are characterised by extreme intakes of food, even when not hungry, and affect 1.6% of adolescents. OSFED includes atypical anorexia nervosa, low frequency/duration binge-eating or bulimia nervosa, as well as those that are not classified but cause distress or impaired functioning [34; 38].

Adolescence is a period of intense change, which can result in increased stress, confusion and anxiety. Physical changes occur interlinked with increased feelings of self-consciousness, body image concerns, changes in self-esteem and comparisons with peers. Additionally, there are many hormonal and brain changes that can influence an adolescent's development, both physically and psychologically. Adolescents start to explore their sexuality and evaluate and change their peer groups. Eating disorders may present themselves as a way of coping with this large flux and as an attempt by adolescents to control some aspects of their life when they feel powerless in other areas [37]. Prevention or early detection is the best management technique for dealing with eating disorders. It is important that the person experiencing an eating disorder is supported by a multidisciplinary team including a general practitioner (or other medical professionals), mental health professional and an Accredited Practicing Dietitian (APD).

Acne

Adolescents are more prone to acne because of the hormonal changes that they experience during puberty, and around 85% of adolescents have at least mild acne. However, there may be some dietary factors that worsen acne and limiting the intake of these foods may lead to some improvements. Most recently, the focus has been on moderating dairy foods, with the exception of cheese, and lowering the glycaemic index (GI) of foods usually consumed [39–42]. The whey and casein proteins in dairy products, except for cheese (which does not seem to have the same effect), promote growth by stimulating an increase in insulin and insulin-like growth factor (IGF). Foods with a high GI or glycaemic load (GL) also trigger a higher insulin response, which in turn increases IGF. While the biochemical mechanisms are complex, high intakes of dairy or high GI/GL foods potentially exacerbate acne. Therefore, limiting excessive intake of dairy and consuming a low-GI/GL diet may help improve the condition of acne.

Academic performance

Nutritional status can play an important role in contributing to adolescent cognitive performance and potentially help optimise academic success. Studies of nutrition and academic performance have typically focused on the impact of breakfast [43; 44]. Evidence from two systematic reviews shows positive associations between habitual breakfast consumption and academic achievement [43–45]. Generally, these positive associations have been attributed to improvements in working memory and attention [46–48]. Specifically, breakfast consumption has been linked with an increased ability to remember information during lessons and the ability to remain on-task and sustain attention during learning activities [43]. However, breakfast is the most frequently skipped meal, with 20–30% of children and adolescents reported to regularly skip breakfast in developed countries [49; 50].

Studies looking more at diet intake holistically have found positive associations between overall healthier eating patterns (i.e. higher intakes of fruit and vegetables and lower intakes of energy-dense, nutrient-poor foods) and academic performance among adolescents [45; 51–54]. In studies that have explored the association with dietary patterns overall, the consumption of specific foods has also been related to positive academic performance. Intake of omega-3 fatty acids, specifically from fish, has been associated with higher school grades in Swedish adolescents [55], while in a sample of American adolescents, school grades were inversely associated with daily intake of sugar-sweetened beverages [56]. Energy-dense nutrient poor foods (i.e. junk foods) have also been negatively associated with academic performance [45].

Despite the associations between diet patterns and academic performance, many studies are cross-sectional; therefore, the potential effect of confounding factors cannot be excluded. For example, socioeconomic status (SES) is known to be a central determinant of academic performance [57; 58]; however, some studies have failed to adequately adjust for SES in analyses. Future research should consider the relationship between SES and academic performance.

Sports performance

Adolescents who participate in sport, whether recreationally or at an elite level, have higher nutritional demands compared to less active adolescents and adult athletes. Increased nutritional requirements are necessary to support growth and repair, athletic performance and also general wellness and academic performance [59]. A whole-food approach to nutrition for sporting performance should be emphasised and supplement use discouraged under most circumstances [60]. Encouraging adolescent athletes to take interest in food and nutrition and up-skill in meal planning and preparation is important. Many adolescents are still attending school, so planning meals and snacks is important to ensure adequate food and nutrient intake throughout the day.

See Chapter 13 for more on sports performance.

Active adolescents can be exposed to misinformation about nutrition for sporting performance, and food intake can be adversely influenced by incorrect nutrition messages. The development of unhealthy eating behaviours in adolescent athletes can be a concern, particularly if restrictive eating patterns develop, as these can have detrimental impacts on growth and performance. Eating behaviours can be influenced by peers, team mates, celebrities and even coaching staff, who may pressure adolescents to lose weight to improve sporting performance. For females, this can develop into a more severe health condition known as the female athlete triad, which consists of disordered eating, menstrual dysfunction and low bone mineral density. Therefore, it is important that the athlete develops a healthy relationship with food that has a focus on intuitive and mindful eating and meets their nutritional requirements [61; 62].

Active adolescents have higher energy and protein requirements, as well as greater needs for fluid, iron, calcium and vitamin D [60; 63]. *Energy* requirements are difficult to estimate due to the variability in intensity, duration and frequency of participation in sport or physical activity. The use of predictive energy equations specific to the adolescent age group is recommended, with adjustment for different physical activity levels [64]. However, these equations should be used as a guide only, as it is not uncommon to see reported intakes lower than estimated requirements in weight-stable adolescents. Growth should be measured over time to determine if energy intake is appropriate. The use of 'energy availability' (Energy intake − Exercise energy expenditure) in this age group may be beneficial, and gives an estimation of the energy remaining after exercise for optimal growth and development [60]. *Protein* intake recommendations for adolescents are currently based on the same data that informs adult requirements. The recommended dietary intake (RDI) for protein in adolescents is 0.8 g/kg/day; however, this guideline does not account for participation in heavy exercise. Protein intakes between 1.35−1.6 g/kg/day appear sufficient for positive nitrogen balance in active adolescents. Adult athletes are recommended 1.3−1.8 g/kg/day and as high as 2.5 g/kg/day during heavy periods of exercise with a regular spread of protein across the day (~20 g of high-quality protein at main meals). Therefore, the current consensus is that adolescents should follow protein guidelines of adult athletes, including a regular intake of protein across the day [60]. *Carbohydrate* intake should be tailored to the individual adolescent, based on current body weight and ensuring enough carbohydrate is consumed to fuel their training and competition energy demands. There is insufficient evidence for the development of adolescent-specific guidelines for carbohydrate intake, and little research exists to suggest that requirements should differ from those of adults. There are carbohydrate recommendations related during exercise (30−60 g/hour), immediate post-exercise recovery (1−1.2 g/kg/hour) and daily recovery (3−10 g/kg/day), and these vary greatly depending on intensity and duration (<1 hour/day to 4−5 hours/day). Recommendations for dietary fat intake reflect those of the general population, which are to choose lean meats, include sources of unsaturated fat including plant-based sources and limit intake of foods high in saturated fat, such as fried takeaway foods and baked products. There is currently insufficient evidence to suggest that adolescent athletes have higher requirements for *iron*, *calcium* and *vitamin D* compared to non-athletes. However, these nutrients are important for sporting performance, growth and development. Intakes of these nutrients in adolescent athletes still fall below the recommendations, so encouragement and education around the importance and appropriate intakes of these nutrients is needed. *Water* is the most appropriate fluid replacement during routine exercise, as sports drinks may contribute to excess energy intake and electrolyte losses are generally lower in adolescents than adults. Sports drinks may have a place in the hydration strategies of competitive adolescent athletes. Adolescents need to be educated about the best fluids for hydration, the importance of commencing exercise hydrated, taking opportunities to hydrate during sessions and monitoring fluid losses to ensure replacement during recovery is adequate [60].

See Chapter 13 for more on sports nutrition.

>> CASE 16.3

VEGETARIAN EATING HABITS

In general terms, a vegetarian is someone who abstains from eating meat. However, there are a number of variations to the term, with different categories of vegetarians. For example, lacto-ovo vegetarians consume dairy and eggs, pesco-vegetarians eat fish and seafood, while a flexitarian has been defined as a person who consciously reduces their meat intake on three or more days per week. Vegans abstain from eating animals and their by-products altogether. Few studies report the prevalence of vegetarianism, particularly in adolescents. However, an estimate of 6% of the adolescent population has been suggested, inclusive of all types of vegetarians [65].

Because vegetarians do not consume meat, it means they must have a diverse diet to ensure they obtain adequate nutrients, particularly protein, iron, zinc, calcium and vitamin B12 [65; 66]. Plant proteins have a lower digestibility than animal-based sources, meaning an increased intake is required. However, requirements should not be hard to meet if a variety of sources are included across the day [66; 67]. The absorption of non-animal sources of iron and zinc, such as green leafy vegetables, legumes and nuts and seeds, is affected by fibre, phytates and tannins generally found in grains, legumes, tea and coffee. Therefore, higher intakes of these minerals may be required [66]. Non-dairy consuming vegetarians are at risk of a calcium deficiency, so options such as calcium-fortified products may provide adequate calcium. Vitamin B12 is found solely in animal products, and vegans are at risk of a deficiency in this nutrient. To prevent deficiency, supplementation and consumption of fortified foods will be necessary for vegans [66].

- Given the results of the Australian Health Survey on the dietary intake of adolescents, which nutrients would need particular attention if this group also chose to limit their diet by vegetarianism or veganism?
- Which plant-based foods would be of particular importance in vegetarian diets consumed by adolescents?
- What areas of additional focus would be required for those also engaging in competitive sports?

Pregnancy during adolescence

Being pregnant during adolescence can create extreme nutritional risk [68; 69]. Many adolescents have unhealthy eating habits and their intakes are often high in fat, sugar and energy, and low in micronutrients such as iron, folate, zinc and calcium. Lifestyle factors and lack of nutrition knowledge contribute to these eating habits. Furthermore, adolescents often find it difficult to foresee potential future outcomes of their current behaviour and may not see themselves as at risk. Pregnant adolescents are at risk of preterm delivery, low birth weight (LBW), infant mortality, anaemia and gestational weight gain. The prenatal environment has implications on developing future obesity, cardiovascular disease and diabetes in both the mother and her offspring [70]. To achieve positive health outcomes for both mother and infant, the focus should be on appropriate gestational weight gain and adequate nutrition [68; 69].

See Chapter 14 for more on pregnancy in adolescence.

STOP AND THINK

- What particular areas of future health as an adult are likely to be affected by nutritional status and habits during adolescence?
- Why is it important to consider each adolescent on an individual basis when assessing nutritional issues?
- What are some of the significant public health issues relating to adolescent health and nutrition, and what health promotion strategies could be put in place?

WHAT MIGHT BE EFFECTIVE APPROACHES TO DEVELOPING HEALTHY FOOD HABITS AND ADEQUATE NUTRITIONAL INTAKES FOR ADOLESCENTS?

Factors that influence adolescent eating patterns are complex and include the social environmental (e.g. peer influences, social norms), physical environment (e.g. proximity of school, fast-food outlets, food availability at home) and policy factors (e.g. school canteen policies) [71]. Understanding these influences may assist in helping to form healthy eating practices during this important life stage (Table 16.6).

See Chapter 20 for more on the social and behavioral aspects of eating.

TABLE 16.6   ENVIRONMENTAL/SOCIAL FACTORS INFLUENCING NUTRITIONAL INTAKES DURING ADOLESCENCE

Influencer	Nature of influence
Social norms of behaviour	Influence and imitation
Family circumstances	Food provision
Peer group inclusion	Selection of foods
School environment	Nutrition education

Social norms (or what is considered typical) are likely to influence the initiation and maintenance of eating behaviours [72]. If adolescents are surrounded by others who regularly eat unhealthy foods, this can influence what is perceived as normal or appropriate behaviour [73]. Therefore, adolescents may perceive the consumption of unhealthy foods to be acceptable, or even desirable. This process is also called **social modelling** [74] in that individuals form beliefs and attitudes about the behaviours they observe in others, which in turn shape their own behaviour [72]. As a result, adolescents are likely to mimic the eating behaviours of those with whom they interact closely and regularly [75]. The most influential interaction partners for adolescents include family, friends and peer groups.

Social modelling

learning to imitate others by observing their behaviour.

Although parents are still considered the main influence, there is growing evidence that adolescent eating behaviours are also heavily influenced by *friends and peers* as adolescents broaden their social networks and assume greater independence [82]. Similarities in eating patterns are observed between adolescent friends, particularly for total energy intakes and consumption of wholegrains, dairy products and vegetables [82]. Peer influence affects the sexes differently. Research has shown that boys are more likely to consume unhealthy foods when in the presence of their peers [83], while girls tended to choose healthier foods in the presence of peers [78]. For both sexes, higher kilojoule intakes have been reported in friendship groups that include peers who are overweight [83; 84]. The relationships between peers and dietary habits are further impacted by issues of perceived body image, peer approval and popularity [85; 86]. Studies have reported that 'popular' adolescents consume more high-kilojoule foods [87; 88]. This could be due to 'healthy eating' conflicting with the desired image they wish to portray among friends and this can affect their social image and standing among peers [89].

>> RESEARCH AT WORK

FAMILY INFLUENCES ON ADOLESCENT EATING HABITS

Parents are the main influencers of adolescent dietary intake [76] and are usually the main providers of food that adolescents can easily access. When it comes to healthy eating, descriptive norms (i.e. what parents do) have been found to be more important than injunctive norms (i.e. what parents say). The family mediates adolescents' eating habits through provision of food, shaping food attitudes and preferences, and influencing values that impact on development of lifelong eating habits [77]. Family meals are an opportunity for parents to model, influence or reinforce healthy eating behaviours and the selection of more nutritious foods by their adolescents [78]. Family breakfasts can influence weight status, with lower rates of excess weight associated with consumption of more regular family breakfasts [79]. More frequent consumption of family meals has also been found to be linked with higher intakes of fruit, vegetables and dairy foods, as well as lower intakes of sugar-sweetened beverages [80; 81].

The *school environment* also can have a powerful influence on adolescent eating behaviours, as adolescents can spend a third of their waking day at school. Adolescents can consume a large proportion of their total daily energy at school with foods eaten at lunch comprising around 35–40% of their total daily energy intake [90]. In schools, adolescents are offered a variety of eating options and opportunities—for example, there may be government-regulated nutrition programs such as Breakfast Clubs, as well as school canteens, vending machines and food outlets encountered on the way to and from school; in some cases, students may be allowed to leave school to buy food [91]. Links have been found between unhealthy school food environments (i.e. those offering energy-dense, nutrient-poor snacks beverages to students) and poorer dietary behaviours among young adolescents [91]. A systematic review has shown that school nutrition programs that increase availability of healthy foods can improve dietary behaviours among adolescents [92].

>> RESEARCH AT WORK

PACE+ INTERVENTION FOR ADOLESCENTS

As many adolescents fail to meet national dietary guidelines, this study looked to evaluate the long-term effects (12 months) of a home-based intervention designed to improve physical activity and nutrition behaviours among 878 adolescent girls and boys aged 11 to 15 years in the United States [93]. Specifically, the nutrition intervention components consisted of computer-assisted dietary assessment (for total intake of fat and servings per day of fruits and vegetables) and stage-based goal setting followed by brief health care provider counselling and 12 months of monthly mail and telephone counselling. Results showed that the percentage of adolescent girls meeting recommended dietary guidelines was significantly improved for consumption of saturated fat. All other changes in meeting dietary guidelines did not differ between groups for either boys or girls. Findings also showed that when compared to control, there was a trend for girls in the intervention group to improve the number of serves of fruit and vegetables, but this was not significant (intervention vs control change, 3.5 to 4.2 servings/day vs 3.5 to 3.9 servings/day, respectively). No intervention effects were seen with percentage of calories from fat for either boys or girls. This intervention demonstrated some positive improvements for diet in girls, but highlights the difficulties in making sustained dietary changes in this population group, particularly in boys.

≫ CASE 16.4

TECHNOLOGICAL OPPORTUNITIES FOR NUTRITION EDUCATION FOR ADOLESCENTS

Recent advances in technology provide opportunities to use interactive and engaging delivery modes to assist in the promotion of healthy eating habits among adolescents. Internationally, adolescents are actively engaged in the technological environment. Between 2014 to 2015, in the United Kingdom, United States and Australia, ≥69% of adolescents owned a smartphone, while ≥65% used this smartphone to access the internet and ≥74% of adolescents used a computer to access the internet [94–97].

A systematic review of seven web-based weight management programs in adolescents found that most studies (75%) had clinically and statistically significant changes to outcomes such as reducing dietary total fat intake and BMI, and facilitating weight loss [98]. Also, a smartphone obesity prevention trial for adolescent boys in low-income communities (the ATLAS RCT) showed long-term (one year) significant reductions in sugar-sweetened beverage consumption [99]. Although further research is required to determine the effectiveness of technology-based interventions and in determining which types of technology are most effective, initial studies have highlighted the potential for innovative, technology interventions in improving adolescent dietary and physical activity behaviours.

- What types of technology-based applications might be useful for nutrition education involving Australian adolescents?
- Which kinds of information might have the best influence on improving nutritional intakes?
- What might be the limitations of relying on applications for nutrition promotion in this group?

STOP AND THINK

- Which organisations significant in the lives of adolescents may be able to provide effective guidance and support for healthy eating habits during this life stage?
- How can social norms be influenced to encourage healthy eating habits among adolescents?
- Why does family remain so important in supporting healthy eating habits in adolescents?

SUMMARY

- Adolescence is a period of rapid growth and increased nutrient requirements. It is a stage where adolescents can be influenced by peers, family and social media.
- It is important that adolescents have role models who positively influence their dietary choices and that efforts are made to educate and up-skill adolescents in nutrition.
- The current food and nutrient intake of adolescents is generally inadequate and this can increase the risk of developing chronic diseases, particularly in later years.
- Factors such as physical activity level and body size can influence nutrient requirements, so recommendations should be tailored to the individual.
- Nutrition intervention in adolescents needs to include technology as a mode of delivery to ensure maximum engagement.

PATHWAYS TO PRACTICE

- Schools and community organisations play a large part in influencing the nutritional intake of adolescents. There are many roles for teachers and sports managers to promote nutrition and ensure a healthy food environment for the adolescents under their care and supervision.

- Adolescents with health conditions who use primary health care and related community health services (including pharmacies) would benefit from high-quality nutrition guidance and access to healthy foods and relevant products.

- Food budgeting, cooking and shopping skills can all be developed in the home during adolescence to support current and future food choices that protect health and prepare well for adulthood.

DISCUSSION QUESTIONS

1 What would be the place, if any, of nutritional and dietary supplements for adolescents?
2 What are the health implications for adolescent females who decide to follow a vegan diet?
3 What are ways that families can help with providing a healthy environment in order to help with healthy eating habits for their adolescent children?
4 What strategies can schools implement in order to provide a healthy environment for their students?
5 Discuss the role/influence of social media in adolescent nutrition.

USEFUL WEBLINKS

Australian Dietary Guidelines:
>   www.eatforhealth.gov.au/guidelines/australian-guide-healthy-eating

Find Your Ideal Figure:
>   www.8700.com.au. A great way to learn about the energy requirements and kilojoule content of foods and what is required to burn these off. With other useful tools, tips and links to support healthy eating habits.

Healthy Eating Quiz:
>   http://healthyeatingquiz.com.au. A short quiz that asks about a person's eating habits. At the end of the quiz, personalised feedback on the person's food consumption patterns is provided, identifying any areas for improvement and providing suggestions for ways to increase the variety of foods in their diet.

Sports Dietitians Australia:
>   www.sportsdietitians.com.au/factsheets/children/nutrition-for-the-adolescent-athlete. Provides recommendations on sports nutrition for adolescent athletes.

Resources to support health professionals working with eating disorders

Centre for Eating and Dieting Disorders:
>   http://cedd.org.au

Centre of Excellence in Eating Disorders:
>   www.ceed.org.au

CLARE COLLINS, REBECCA HASLAM, ANNETTE MURPHY, KRISTINE PEZDIRC AND LEE ASHTON

Journal of Adolescent Health:

    www.jahonline.org

National Eating Disorders Collaboration:

    www.nedc.com.au

The Butterfly Foundation:

    https://thebutterflyfoundation.org.au

FURTHER READING

Desbrow, B., McCormack, J., Burke, L. M., Cox, G. R., Fallon, K., Hislop, M., … Leveritt, M. (2014). Sports Dietitians Australia position statement: sports nutrition for the adolescent athlete. *International Journal of Sport Nutrition and Exercise Metabolism*, 24(5), 570–84. doi: http://dx.doi.org/10.1123/ijsnem.2014-0031

National Health and Medical Research Council (2013). *Clinical Practice Guidelines for the Management of Overweight and Obesity in Adults, Adolescents and Children in Australia*. Canberra: NHMRC.

National Health and Medical Research Council. (2006). *Nutrient Reference Values for Australia and New Zealand, Including Recommended Dietary Intakes*. Canberra: NHMRC.

REFERENCES

1   World Health Organization (2016). *Maternal, Newborn, Child and Adolescent Health: Adolescent development*. Retrieved from: www.who.int/maternal_child_adolescent/topics/adolescence/dev/en.

2   E.A. Shirtcliff, R. E. Dahl & S. D. Pollak (2009). Pubertal development: correspondence between hormonal and physical development. *Child Development*, 80(2), 327–37.

3   C. L. Sisk & J. L. Zehr (2005). Pubertal hormones organize the adolescent brain and behavior. *Frontiers in Neuroendocrinology*, 26(3), 163–74.

4   J. M. Tanner (1981). Growth and maturation during adolescence. *Nutrition Reviews*, 39(2), 43–55.

5   B. Casey, R. M. Jones & T. A. Hare (2008). The adolescent brain. *Annals of the New York Academy of Sciences*, 1124(1), 111–26.

6   N. R. Council (2007). *Preventing Teen Motor Crashes: Contributions from the behavioral and social sciences: Workshop report, Chapter 3*. Washington, DC: National Academies Press.

7   J. M. Cyranowski, E. Frank, E. Young & M. K. Shear (2000). Adolescent onset of the gender difference in lifetime rates of major depression: a theoretical model. *Archives of General Psychiatry*, 57(1), 21–7.

8   D. C. Cusatis & B. M. Shannon (1996). Influences on adolescent eating behavior. *Journal of Adolescent Health*, 18(1), 27–34.

9   C. C. Dahm, A. K. Chomistek, M. U. Jakobsen, K. J. Mukamal, A. H. Eliassen, H. D. Sesso, … S. E. Chiuve (2016). Adolescent diet quality and cardiovascular disease risk factors and incident cardiovascular disease in middle-aged women. *Journal of the American Heart Association*, 5(12), e003583.

10 Better Health Channel (2012). *Food and Your Life Stages*. Retrieved from: www.betterhealth.vic.gov.au/health/healthyliving/food-and-your-life-stages.

11 National Health and Medical Research Council (2006). *Nutrient Reference Values for Australia and New Zealand, Including Recommended Dietary Intakes*. Canberra: NHMRC.

12 National Health and Medical Research Council (2013). *Educator Guide*. Canberra: NHMRC.

13 Australian Bureau of Statistics (2015). *Australian Health Survey: Usual nutrient intakes, 2011–2012*. Cat. no. 4364.0.55.008. Retrieved from: www.ausstats.abs.gov.au/Ausstats/subscriber.nsf/0/31EEAEBF2A09 D051CA257DFF000CA865/$File/australian%20health%20survey,%20usual%20nutrient%20intakes%20 2011-12.pdf.

14 National Health and Medical Research Council (2014). *Summary. Recommendations to Reduce Chronic Disease Risk*. Retrieved from: www.nrv.gov.au/chronic-disease/summary.

15 Australian Institute of Health and Welfare (2013). *National Drug Strategy Household Survey (NDSHS)*. Retrieved from: www.aihw.gov.au/alcohol-and-other-drugs/ndshs.

16 Better Health Channel (2016). *Alcohol and Teenagers*. Retrieved from: www.betterhealth.vic.gov.au/health/ healthyliving/alcohol-teenagers.

17 World Health Organization (2014). *Global Status Report on Alcohol and Health*. Geneva: WHO.

18 Food Standards Australia New Zealand (2016). *Folic Acid Fortification*. Retrieved from: www.foodstandards. gov.au/consumer/nutrition/folicmandatory/Pages/default.aspx.

19 Australian Bureau of Statistics (2015). *National Health Survey: First results, 2014–15*. Cat. no. 4364.0.55.001. Retrieved from: www.ausstats.abs.gov.au/Ausstats/subscriber.nsf/0/CDA852A349B4CEE6CA257F15000 9FC53/$File/national%20health%20survey%20first%20results,%202014-15.pdf.

20 Australian Bureau of Statistics (2016). *Australian Health Survey: Consumption of food groups from the Australian Dietary Guidelines, 2011–12: Australia*. Cat. no. 4364.0.55.012. Retrieved from: www.abs.gov.au/ausstats/ abs@.nsf/Lookup/4364.0.55.012main+features12011-12.

21 F. M. Biro & M. Wien (2010). Childhood obesity and adult morbidities. *American Journal of Clinical Nutrition*, 91(5), 1499S–1505S.

22 N. K. Güngör1 (2014). Overweight and obesity in children and adolescents. *Journal of Clinical Research in Pediatric Endocrinology*, 6(3), 129–43. doi:10.4274/jcrpe.1471

23 S. Jenkins & S. D. Horner (2005). Barriers that influence eating behaviors in adolescents. *Journal of Pediatric Nursing*, 20(4), 258–67.

24 National Health and Medical Research Council (2013). *Clinical Practice Guidelines for the Management of Overweight and Obesity in Adults, Adolescents and Children in Australia*. Retrieved from: www.nhmrc.gov.au/_ files_nhmrc/publications/attachments/n57_obesity_guidelines_140630.pdf.

25 B. A. Spear, S. E. Barlow, C. Ervin, D. S. Ludwig, B. E. Saelens, K. E. Schetzina & E. M. Taveras (2007). Recommendations for treatment of child and adolescent overweight and obesity. *Pediatrics*, 120(suppl. 4). doi:10.1542/peds.2007-2329F

26 D. L. Thomason, N. Lukkahatai, J. Kawi, K. Connelly & J. Inouye (2016). A systematic review of adolescent self-management and weight loss. *Journal of Pediatric Health Care*, 30(6), 569–82. doi:10.1016/ j.pedhc.2015.11.016

27 E. M. Van Sluijs, A. M. McMinn & S. J. Griffin (2007). Effectiveness of interventions to promote physical activity in children and adolescents: systematic review of controlled trials. *British Medical Journal*, 335(7622), 703.

28 J. E. Kaikkonen, V. Mikkilä, C. G. Magnussen, M. Juonala, J. S. Viikari & O. T. Raitakari (2013). Does childhood nutrition influence adult cardiovascular disease risk? Insights from the Young Finns Study. *Annals of Medicine*, 45(2), 120–8.

29 G. S. Berenson, S. R. Srinivasan, W. Bao, W. P. Newman, R. E. Tracy & W. A. Wattigney (1998). Association between multiple cardiovascular risk factors and atherosclerosis in children and young adults. *New England Journal of Medicine*, 338(23), 1650–6. doi:10.1056/nejm199806043382302

30 G. Appannah, G. K. Pot, R. C. Huang, W. H. Oddy, L. J. Beilin, T. A. Mori, ... G. L. Ambrosini (2015). Identification of a dietary pattern associated with greater cardiometabolic risk in adolescence. *Nutrition, Metabolism and Cardiovascular Diseases*, 25(7), 643–50.

31 Juvenile Diabetes Research Foundation (2015). What is type 1 diabetes? Retrieved from: www.jdrf.org.au/what-is-type-1-diabetes.

32 Australian Institute of Health and Welfare (2014). *Type 2 Diabetes in Australia's Children and Young People: A working paper.* Canberra: AIHW.

33 J. S. Borus & L. Laffel (2010). Adherence challenges in the management of type 1 diabetes in adolescents: prevention and intervention. *Current Opinion in Pediatrics*, 22(4), 405.

34 Eating Disorders Victoria (2016). Eating disorders explained. Retrieved from: www.eatingdisorders.org.au/eating-disorders/what-is-an-eating-disorder.

35 American Psychiatric Association (2013). *Diagnostic and Statistical Manual of Mental Disorders (DSM-5®).* Washington, DC: American Psychiatric Association Publishing.

36 National Eating Disorders Collaboration (2016). Eating disorders in Australia. Retrieved from: www.nedc.com.au/eating-disorders-in-australia.

37 Eating Disorders Victoria (2017). Eating disorders and adolescents. Retrieved from: www.eatingdisorders.org.au/eating-disorders/eating-disorders-children-teens-and-older-adults/eating-disorders-a-adolescents.

38 Headspace (2016). Understanding eating disorders—for health professionals. Retrieved from: www.headspace.org.au/health-professionals/understanding-eating-disorders-for-health-professionals.

39 F. W. Danby (2010). Nutrition and acne. *Clinics in Dermatology*, 28(6), 598–604.

40 B. C. Melnik (2011). Evidence for acne-promoting effects of milk and other insulinotropic dairy products. *Milk and Milk Products in Human Nutrition*, 67, 131–45. Basel: Karger Publishers.

41 J. Burris, W. Rietkerk & K. Woolf (2013). Acne: the role of medical nutrition therapy. *Journal of the Academy of Nutrition and Dietetics*, 113(3), 416–30.

42 R. N. Smith, N. J. Mann, A. Braue, H. Mäkeläinen & G. A. Varigos (2007). The effect of a high-protein, low glycemic–load diet versus a conventional, high glycemic–load diet on biochemical parameters associated with acne vulgaris: a randomized, investigator-masked, controlled trial. *Journal of the American Academy of Dermatology*, 57(2), 247–56.

43 K. Adolphus, C. L. Lawton & L. Dye (2013). The effects of breakfast on behaviour and academic performance in children and adolescents. *Frontiers in Human Neuroscience*, 7.

44 A. Hoyland, L. Dye & C. L. Lawton (2009). A systematic review of the effect of breakfast on the cognitive performance of children and adolescents. *Nutrition Research Reviews*, 22(2), 220–43.

45 T. Burrows, S. Goldman, K. Pursey & R. Lim (2017). Is there an association between dietary intake and academic achievement: a systematic review. *Journal of Human Nutrition and Dietetics*, 30(2), 117–40.

46 K. A. Wesnes, C. Pincock & A. Scholey (2012). Breakfast is associated with enhanced cognitive function in schoolchildren. An internet based study. *Appetite*, 59(3), 646–9.

47 S. B. Cooper, S. Bandelow, M. L. Nute, J. G. Morris & M. E. Nevill (2012). Breakfast glycaemic index and cognitive function in adolescent school children. *British Journal of Nutrition*, 107(12), 1823–32.

48 K. Widenhorn-Müller, K. Hille, J. Klenk & U. Weiland (2008). Influence of having breakfast on cognitive performance and mood in 13-to 20-year-old high school students: results of a crossover trial. *Pediatrics*, 122(2), 279–84.

49 P. R. Deshmukh-Taskar, T. A. Nicklas, C. E. O'Neil, D. R. Keast, J. D. Radcliffe & S. Cho (2010). The relationship of breakfast skipping and type of breakfast consumption with nutrient intake and weight status in children and adolescents: the National Health and Nutrition Examination Survey 1999–2006. *Journal of the American Dietetic Association*, 110(6), 869–78.

50 K. Corder, E. van Sluijs, R. Steele, A. Stephen, V. Dunn, D. Bamber, ... U. Ekelund (2011). Breakfast consumption and physical activity in British adolescents. *British Journal of Nutrition*, 105(02), 316–21.

51 D. MacLellan, J. Taylor & K. Wood (2008). Food intake and academic performance among adolescents. *Canadian Journal of Dietetic Practice and Research*, 69(3), 141–4.

52 P. Correa-Burrows, R. Burrows, Y. Orellana & D. Ivanovic (2015). The relationship between unhealthy snacking at school and academic outcomes: a population study in Chilean schoolchildren. *Public Health Nutrition*, 18(11), 2022–30.

53 Á. Logi Kristjánsson, I. Dóra Sigfúsdóttir & J. P. Allegrante (2010). Health behavior and academic achievement among adolescents: the relative contribution of dietary habits, physical activity, body mass index, and self-esteem. *Health Education & Behavior*, 37(1), 51–64.

54 N. C. Øverby, E. Lüdemann & R. Høigaard (2013). Self-reported learning difficulties and dietary intake in Norwegian adolescents. *Scandinavian Journal of Public Health*, 41(7), 754–60.

55 M. A. Åberg, N. Åberg, J. Brisman, R. Sundberg, A. Winkvist & K. Torén (2009). Fish intake of Swedish male adolescents is a predictor of cognitive performance. *Acta Paediatrica*, 98(3), 555–60.

56 S. Park, B. Sherry, K. Foti & H. M. Blanck (2012). Self-reported academic grades and other correlates of sugar-sweetened soda intake among US adolescents. *Journal of the Academy of Nutrition and Dietetics*, 112(1), 125–31.

57 S. Machin & A. Vignoles (2004). Educational inequality: the widening socio-economic gap. *Fiscal Studies*, 25(2), 107–28.

58 A. McCulloch & H. E. Joshi (2001). Neighbourhood and family influences on the cognitive ability of children in the British National Child Development Study. *Social Science & Medicine*, 53(5), 579–91.

59 A. Jeukendrup & L. Cronin (2011). Nutrition and elite young athletes. *The Elite Young Athlete*, 56, 47–58. Basel: Karger Publishers.

60 B. Desbrow, J. McCormack, L. M. Burke, G. R. Cox, K. Fallon, M. Hislop, ... M. Leveritt (2014). Sports Dietitians Australia position statement: sports nutrition for the adolescent athlete. *International Journal of Sport Nutrition and Exercise Metabolism*, 24(5), 570–84. doi: http://dx.doi.org/10.1123/ijsnem.2014-0031

61 M. E. Bingham, M. E. Borkan & P. A. Quatromoni (2015). Sports nutrition advice for adolescent athletes: a time to focus on food. *American Journal of Lifestyle Medicine*, 9(6), 398–402.

62 D. Clifford, A. Ozier, J. Bundros, J. Moore, A. Kreiser & M. N. Morris (2015). Impact of non-diet approaches on attitudes, behaviors, and health outcomes: a systematic review. *Journal of Nutrition Education and Behavior*, 47(2), 143–55.

63 Sports Dietitians Australia (n.d.). Nutrition for the adolescent athlete. Retrieved from: www.sportsdietitians. com.au/factsheets/children/nutrition-for-the-adolescent-athlete.

64 R. J. Maughan (2008). *The Encyclopedia of Sports Medicine: An IOC Medical Commission Publication, Nutrition in Sport* (vol. 7). Chichester: John Wiley & Sons.

65 C. L. Perry, M. T. McGuire & D. Neumark-Sztainer (2002). Adolescent vegetarians: how well do their dietary patterns meet the healthy people 2010 objectives? *Archives of Pediatrics and Adolescent Medicine*, 156(5), 431–7. doi:10.1001/archpedi.156.5.431

66 M. Amit (2010). Vegetarian diets in children and adolescents. *Paediatric Child Health*, 15(5), 303–8.

67 K. A. Marsh, E. A. Munn & S. K. Baines (2013). Protein and vegetarian diets. *Medical Journal of Australia*, 199(4 Suppl), S7–S10. doi:10.5694/mjao11.11492

68 K. Montgomery (2003). Improving nutrition in pregnant adolescents: recommendations for clinical practitioners. *Journal of Perinatal Education*, 12(2), 2230.

69 J. N. Nielsen, J. Gittelsohn, J. Anliker & K. O'Brien (2006). Interventions to improve diet and weight gain among pregnant adolescents and recommendations for future research. *Journal of the American Dietetic Association*, 106(11), 1825–40.

70 C. Lenders, T. McElrath & T. Scholl (2000). Nutrition in adolescent pregnancy. *Current Opinion in Pediatrics*, 12(3), 291–6.

71 K. J. Sawka, G. R. McCormack, A. Nettel-Aguirre & K. Swanson (2015). Associations between aspects of friendship networks and dietary behavior in youth: findings from a systematized review. *Eating Behaviors*, 18, 7–15.

72 S.-J. Salvy, K. De La Haye, J. C. Bowker & R. C. Hermans (2012). Influence of peers and friends on children's and adolescents' eating and activity behaviors. *Physiology & Behavior*, 106(3), 369–78.

73 S. Higgs (2015). Social norms and their influence on eating behaviours. *Appetite*, 86, 38–44.

74 A. Bandura & R. H. Walters (1977). *Social Learning Theory*. Englewood Cliffs, NJ: Prentice Hall.

75 R. C. Hermans, A. Lichtwarck-Aschoff, K. E. Bevelander, C. P. Herman, J. K. Larsen & R. C. Engels (2012). Mimicry of food intake: the dynamic interplay between eating companions. *PLOS ONE*, 7(2), e31027.

76 S. Pedersen, A. Grønhøj & J. Thøgersen (2015). Following family or friends. Social norms in adolescent healthy eating. *Appetite*, 86, 54–60.

77 M. Story, D. Neumark-Sztainer & S. French (2002). Individual and environmental influences on adolescent eating behaviors. *Journal of the American Dietetic Association*, 102(3), S40–S51.

78 S.-J. Salvy, A. Elmo, L. A. Nitecki, M. A. Kluczynski & J. N. Roemmich (2010). Influence of parents and friends on children's and adolescents' food intake and food selection. *American Journal of Clinical Nutrition*, 93(1), 87–92. doi: 10.3945/ajcn.110.002097

79 F. N. Vika, S. J. T. Veldea, W. V. Lippevelded, Y. Maniose, E. Kovacsf, N. Janh, ... E. Berea (2016). Regular family breakfast was associated with children's overweight and parental education: results from the ENERGY cross-sectional study. *Preventative Medicine*, 91, 197–203. doi:http://dx.doi.org/10.1016/j.ypmed.2016.08.013

80 T. M. Videon & C. K. Manning (2003). Influences on adolescent eating patterns: the importance of family meals. *Journal of Adolescent Health*, 32(5), 365–73.

81 N. I. Larson, D. Neumark-Sztainer, P. J. Hannan & M. Story (2007). Family meals during adolescence are associated with higher diet quality and healthful meal patterns during young adulthood. *Journal of the American Dietetic Association*, 107(9), 1502–10. doi:http://dx.doi.org/10.1016/j.jada.2007.06.012

82 M. Bruening, M. Eisenberg, R. MacLehose, M. S. Nanney, M. Story & D. Neumark-Sztainer (2012). Relationship between adolescents' and their friends' eating behaviors: breakfast, fruit, vegetable, whole-grain, and dairy intake. *Journal of the Academy of Nutrition and Dietetics*, 112(10), 1608–13. doi:10.1016/j.jand.2012.07.008

83 K. Sawka, G. McCormack, A. Nettel-Aguirre & K. Swanson (2015). Associations between aspects of friendship networks and dietary behavior in youth: findings from a systematized review. *Eating Behaviours*, 18, 7–15. doi:10.1016/j.eatbeh.2015.03.002.

84 S.-J. Salvy, K. De la Haye, J. C. Bowker & R. C. J. Hermans (2012). Influence of peers and friends on children's and adolescents' eating and activity behaviors. *Physiology & Behavior*, 106(3), 369–78. doi:10.1016/j.physbeh.2012.03.022

85 M. Lieberman, L. Gauvin, W. M. Bukowski & D. R. White (2001). Interpersonal influence and disordered eating behaviors in adolescent girls: the role of peer modeling, social reinforcement, and body-related teasing. *Eating Behaviors*, 2(3), 215–36.

86 H. Shroff & J. K. Thompson (2006). Peer influences, body-image dissatisfaction, eating dysfunction and self-esteem in adolescent girls. *Journal of Health Psychology*, 11(4), 533–51.

87 K. De la Haye, G. Robins, P. Mohr & C. Wilson (2010). Obesity-related behaviors in adolescent friendship networks. *Social Networks*, 32(3), 161–7.

88 K. De la Haye, G. Robins, P. Mohr & C. Wilson (2013). Adolescents' intake of junk food: processes and mechanisms driving consumption similarities among friends. *Journal of Research on Adolescence*, 23(3), 524–36.

89 M. Stead, L. McDermott, A. M. MacKintosh & A. Adamson (2011). Why healthy eating is bad for young people's health: identity, belonging and food. *Social Science & Medicine*, 72(7), 1131–9.

90 J. Burghardt, A. Gordon, N. Chapman, P. Gleason & T. Fraker (1993). *The School Nutrition Dietary Assessment Study: School food service, meals offered, and dietary intakes*. Alexandria, VA: USDA, Food & Nutrition Service.

91 M.Y. Kubik, L. A. Lytle, P. J. Hannan, C. L. Perry & M. Story (2003). The association of the school food environment with dietary behaviors of young adolescents. *American Journal of Public Health*, 93(7), 1168–73.

92 E. Van Cauwenberghe, L. Maes, H. Spittaels, F. J. van Lenthe, J. Brug, J.-M. Oppert & I. De Bourdeaudhuij (2010). Effectiveness of school-based interventions in Europe to promote healthy nutrition in children and adolescents: systematic review of published and 'grey' literature. *British Journal of Nutrition*, 103(06), 781–97.

93 K. Patrick, K. J. Calfas, G. J. Norman, et al. (2006). Randomized controlled trial of a primary care and home-based intervention for physical activity and nutrition behaviors: Pace+ for adolescents. *Archives of Pediatric and Adolescent Medicine*, 160(2), 128–36. doi:10.1001/archpedi.160.2.128

94 A. Lenhart (2015). Teens, social media & technology overview 2015. *Pew Research Center*, 9.

95 A. Lenhart (2014). Teens and technology: understanding the digital landscape. Retrieved from: www.pewinternet.org/2014/02/25/teens-technology-understanding-the-digitallandscape.

96 Ofcom (2015). *Children and Parents: Media Use and Attitudes Report*. Retrieved from: www.ofcom.org.uk/research-and-data/media-literacy-research/childrens/children-parents-nov-15.

97 Australian Communications and Media Authority (2016). Aussie teens and kids online. Retrieved from: www.acma.gov.au/theACMA/engage-blogs/engage-blogs/Research-snapshots/Aussie-teens-and-kids-online.

98 J.-Y. An, L. L. Hayman, Y.-S. Park, T. K. Dusaj & C. G. Ayres (2009). Web-based weight management programs for children and adolescents: a systematic review of randomized controlled trial studies. *Advances in Nursing Science*, 32(3), 222–40.

99 J. J. Smith, P. J. Morgan, R. C. Plotnikoff, K. A. Dally, J. Salmon, A. D. Okely, … D. R. Lubans (2014). Smartphone obesity prevention trial for adolescent boys in low-income communities: the ATLAS RCT. *Pediatrics*, 134(3), e723–31.

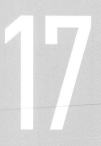

CHAPTER 17

NUTRITION DURING ADULTHOOD AND THE PREVENTION OF CHRONIC DISEASE

LINDA TAPSELL

CHAPTER OBJECTIVES

This chapter will enable the reader to:

- outline the main nutritional issues during adulthood
- describe the evidence on relationships between diet and the development of chronic disease
- identify key foods and dietary patterns that are associated with reduced chronic disease risk.

KEY TERMS

Cardiovascular disease

Hypertension

Obesity

Type 2 diabetes

KEY POINTS

- Nutritional requirements for sustaining health during adulthood need to be met with judicious choices of nutrient-dense foods while keeping within energy requirements.
- Research on the relationship between dietary characteristics and disease end points (or biomarkers of disease) exposes the potency of food in the prevention of chronic diseases.
- Both protective and detrimental effects of foods can be demonstrated by scientific means, enabling clear differentiation among foods and dietary patterns.

OXFORD UNIVERSITY PRESS

INTRODUCTION

Adulthood is the period where the body reaches maturation. There will be variation in size and shape, and in genetic profiles, as well as levels of physical activity, all of which will influence nutritional requirements. For women, there may be the additional demands of pregnancy and lactation. The consumption of food remains fundamental to the maintenance of the human system. The multiple bioactive compounds delivered by food have effects on processes that can influence future health, including hormone regulation, inflammatory responses, cell differentiation and growth, and DNA repair (Figure 17.1). Compounds in food may also affect metabolic processes associated with the development of cancer cells [1]. See Chapter 14 on nutrition during pregnancy and lactation.

Metabolomic research shows that diets delivering different nutrient profiles will lead to different blood profiles of metabolic products such as triglycerides and amino acids. Thus, consuming a diet produces a coordinated metabolic change. This means differential effects of diet composition can be observed through a range of cardiometabolic disease indicators [2]. Likewise, measuring changes in cardiometabolic and endocrine biomarkers such as total cholesterol, triglycerides,

FIGURE 17.1 BIOACTIVE FOOD COMPONENTS CAN INFLUENCE GENETIC AND EPIGENETIC EVENTS ASSOCIATED WITH A HOST OF DISEASE PROCESSES

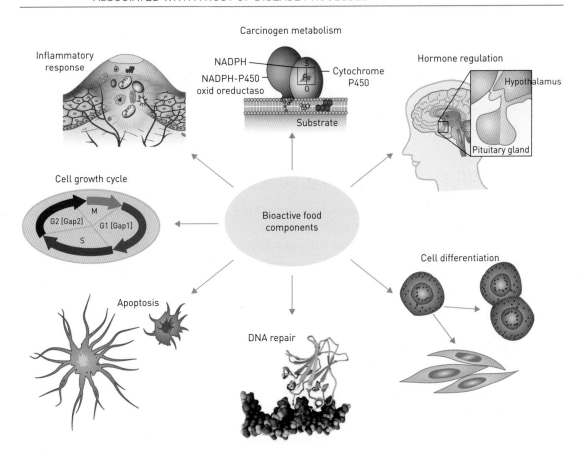

Source: E. Trujillo, C. Davis & J. Milner (2006). Nutrigenomics, proteomics, metabolomics, and the practice of dietetics. *Journal of the American Dietetic Association*, 106(3), 406

See Chapter 7 on energy intake and weight management.

Type 2 diabetes
disease associated with insulin resistance (high blood sugar and high blood insulin levels) and/or some degree of insulin insufficiency (high blood sugar only).

Cardiovascular disease
disease, likely to be inflammatory, that affects the circulation of blood around the body through the cardiovascular system.

insulin, adiponectin and leptin can help assess the value of different dietary patterns [3]. As the sophistication of this research develops, the potency of effects of food on health become more apparent.

At the whole body level, simply consuming too much food itself creates problems. For many adults, overweight or obesity is already present. With overweight and obesity comes the risk of metabolic decline, which may in turn lead to **type 2 diabetes** and **cardiovascular disease**. It remains important to consume foods that are less likely to lead to overweight, by making sure foods that deliver essential nutrients are included in the diet and that the overall quantity of food and beverages does not lead to overconsumption of energy. A higher dietary energy density (kJ energy/kg food) can be associated with more weight gain [4]. Considering the energy density (kJ energy/g food) and nutrient density (amount nutrients/100 g food) of individual foods will help assure that multiple nutrients are consumed while staying within energy needs [5; 6]. These are fundamental principles in diet and nutrition.

Even if a state of energy balance is achieved, nutrient intakes can be under-consumed or over-consumed. A spectrum of dietary influences occurs, from the level of individual nutrients through to single foods and whole dietary patterns. Research helps to identify which foods need to be included to support health, and those that need to be limited within the current food supply. Studies of dietary patterns, particularly those associated with traditional cuisines, help to shape this research in terms of acceptable food forms and culinary practices.

STOP AND THINK

- How do the characteristics of an individual influence adult nutrient and energy needs?
- Why is entering adulthood as overweight or obese a health risk?
- Which categories of foods are likely to be more protective of health during adulthood and why?

WHAT ARE THE MAIN NUTRITIONAL CONCERNS IN ADULTHOOD?

Once maturation has been achieved (and excluding pregnancy and lactation), the main nutritional goal is to maintain health and functionality. Adequate nutrition is achieved by providing essential nutrients in keeping with the guidance provided by the Nutrient Reference Values (NRVs; www.nrv.gov.au). These values cover macronutrients: protein to support tissue maintenance and growth and prevent malnutrition; carbohydrates as the major source of energy, in particular for delivering glucose to the brain; and fat for its various functions in the body, including as an energy source. Essential nutrients include vitamin A for vision, normal immune function and reproduction and those central to metabolic processes, such as thiamin (involved in energy conversion), riboflavin, vitamin B6 (involved in metabolism of amino acids), magnesium (involved in biochemical activity), selenium (with antioxidant potential and involvement in thyroid metabolism, alongside iodine) and zinc (with various regulatory roles). Calcium and phosphorus are required to maintain bones, along with vitamin C to maintain healthy connective tissues. Iron and vitamin B12 are required for carrying oxygen in the blood and the formation of blood, respectively. Recall that these nutrients are best consumed in foods. Nutritional imbalance can occur when consumption of nutrients from foods is inadequate and this can occur with both over- and under-consumption of energy.

See Chapter 2 on dietary guidelines.

>> CASE 17.1

NUTRIENT INTAKES OF AUSTRALIANS, 2011–12

The Australian Health Survey 2011–12 provided the most recent overview of nutrient and food intakes in the Australian population [7]. Key general results included:

- Low calcium intakes are very likely in females (73%), but also in males (51%).
- Low iron intakes are most likely in females (24% not meeting requirements compared with 3% in males).
- About one in 12 (9%) adult females (>19 years) were not meeting folate requirements from foods.
- Throughout adulthood females were less likely to meet thiamin requirements than males.
- Nutrient intakes less likely to be inadequately consumed were protein, vitamin C, vitamin B12, phosphorus and selenium (and folate, iodine and iron in males).
- Older adults (>71 years) were less likely to meet requirements for a number of nutrients, including protein, compared with their younger counterparts.
- Compared with the recommended five servings of vegetables/legumes/beans per day, adults (>19 years) consumed on average three servings, and only 4% consumed the minimum recommended amount.
- Thirty-five per cent of total dietary energy came from discretional foods, defined in the Australian Dietary Guidelines (ADG; www.eatforhealth.gov.au) as nutrient-poor and not included in the recommended food groups.

In Australia and New Zealand, some foods are fortified (enriched) with nutrients in keeping with Food Standards (www.foodstandards.gov.au). Mandatory fortification requires certain vitamins and minerals to be added to certain foods. For example, most wheat flour for making bread is required to be fortified with thiamin and folic acid. Iodised salt should also be used if required in the bread (Standard 2.1.1), and vitamin D should be added to margarines and spreads (Australia only, Standard 2.4.2).

Voluntary fortification occurs when food manufacturers have the choice to add these nutrients, provided they meet the permissions code (Standard 1.3.2). The term 'enrichment' can mean the same as fortification, although it can also relate to the practice of adding nutrients back into a food after they have been processed out (e.g. in the case of cereal products and B group vitamins and iron).

See Case 21.2 in Chapter 21 on functional foods.

- What are the implications of these nutritional intakes for the health of adult Australians?
- Which foods are implicated, and where does dietary change need to occur?
- Why are nutritional concerns for older adults different from those of younger adults?

While lack of food (dietary energy) results in malnutrition, protein-energy malnutrition is of particular concern as protein is such a critical component of the body's structure and function. In Australia, malnutrition of all forms is a major concern for elderly adults, particularly those living in institutions. Malnutrition can also occur with excess energy intake, where the quality of the diet is very poor. This can occur when foods consumed are predominantly energy rich and nutrient poor, and when food preparation does not protect the labile nutrient content of the food.

See Chapter 6 on protein.
See Chapter 18 on nutrition in older age.

>> **CASE 17.2**

HIDDEN CASE OF VITAMIN C DEFICIENCY

Clinical cases of vitamin C deficiency have now been reported among people with diabetes mellitus. In a recent publication of seven cases in Sydney (four males, three females), the mean weight was 107 + 30 kg and all reported a low intake of fruit and vegetables [8]. The primary symptom was ulcers that failed to heal, but low levels of vitamin C were measured and bleeding gums were also reported. The authors noted the importance of considering micronutrient deficiencies even in the presence of overweight and obesity [8]. One case reported in the local media [9] indicated she ate very little fruit and significantly overcooked vegetables.

- How could an abundant food supply put people at risk of micronutrient deficiency?
- What does this case reveal for nutrition education needs in the community?
- What is the role of vitamin supplements and food in this scenario?

Identifying nutritional concerns in adults can involve an assessment of energy and nutrient intakes in relation to physiological requirements. It also involves profiling of food intakes and their energy and nutrient density, and examining overall health profiles such as weight and chronic disease status.

STOP AND THINK

- How do nutrients continue to support the functioning of the body throughout adulthood?
- Why do food choices remain important during this stage of life, and what are the challenges for ensuring a healthy diet?
- What are some of the at-risk groups in the adult community for nutritional inadequacy?

HOW IS DIET RELATED TO THE DEVELOPMENT OF CHRONIC DISEASE IN ADULTHOOD?

Chronic lifestyle-related diseases are diseases that result from the breakdown of fundamental systems within the body, such as the cardiovascular system, leading to disability and death. In general, they are associated with lifestyle choices, including smoking, the type of food regularly consumed and the type and level of activity (including sleep). The most common chronic diseases (cardiovascular disease, type 2 diabetes and obesity) have shared aspects of pathophysiology. While from a treatment perspective obesity itself is a chronic disease, being overweight is also associated with the development of CVD and diabetes. It is now known that rather than being an inert substance, body fat (namely, visceral fat) is actively engaged in a cascade of events that can lead to chronic disease linked with basal inflammatory processes [10].

See Chapter 7 on obesity and chronic disease.

Gut microbiota
populations of microbes living in the gastrointestinal tract, estimated in the trillions.

The role of the gastrointestinal tract in body fat production and distribution is also being increasingly appreciated [11]. The **gut microbiota** can influence the development of obesity and metabolic diseases through molecular interactions with human host systems (Figure 17.2). These can relate to the laying down of fat, the development of basal

FIGURE 17.2 SYSTEMS INFLUENCED BY NUTRITION

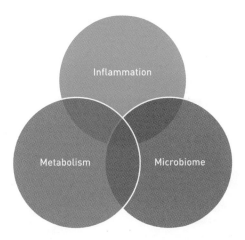

inflammation and the emergence of insulin resistance [12]. Research on the impact of dietary factors on gut microbiota is an exciting new area for nutrition scientists. For example, faecal metabolic profiling has now emerged as an important tool in understanding how what we eat has an impact on how our body stores and processes fat via interactions with bacteria in the gut, effects that appear stronger than the genetic profile [13].

CVD is the leading cause of death for Australians [14]. The disease presents with damage to blood vessels, so that the blood supply becomes limited, restricting the supply of oxygen to the cells. This can result in cell death, leading to myocardial infarction, commonly referred to as a heart attack. Research on CVD can have a number of '**end points**', from sudden death to 'events' such as myocardial infarction, or the presence of disease risk factors, such as high blood cholesterol, which are modifiable through diet. Dietary studies can use various measures of CVD end points to establish effects and associations with disease prevention.

End point
measureable condition or marker used in trials and observational studies to indicate presence of a disease.

Vascular disease can also contribute to death from stroke, where the cells in the brain, rather than the heart, die from lack of oxygen, this time as a result of a 'cerebrovascular accident'. Hypertension is a major risk factor for stroke and CVD. In a 2015 report, it contributed 42% of the CVD burden for Australians [15]. A significant proportion of the Australian adult population has high blood pressure [16].

» RESEARCH AT WORK

REDUCING RISK OF CVD: EVIDENCE FOR DIETARY PATTERNS AND FOODS

Research on dietary patterns and CVD risk has been substantial in past decades [17]. The PREDIMED randomised controlled trial involved a five-year dietary intervention, testing the effect of a Mediterranean diet (MedDiet) supplemented with extra virgin olive oil (EVOO) or mixed nuts on CVD in 7447 adults (aged 55–80 years) from across Spain [18]. The control group were advised on a low-fat diet. The primary end points were major cardiovascular events (myocardial infarction, stroke, death from cardiovascular disease). At the end of the trial, 288 events were found, 109 in the control, 96 in the Med-EVOO group and 83 in the

Med-Nut group. Rigorous statistical analysis, including adjustments for potential confounders, found the MedDiet groups had about a 30% reduction in risk of cardiovascular events compared with the controls. This seminal study provides direct evidence of the effect of a Mediterranean dietary pattern on reducing cardiovascular risk.

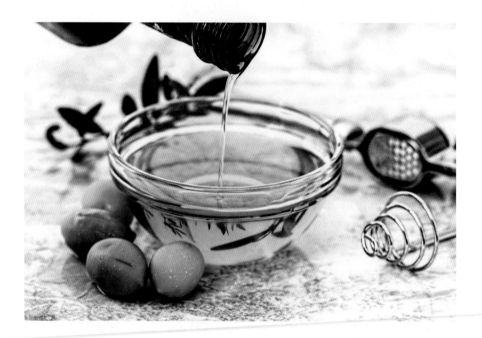

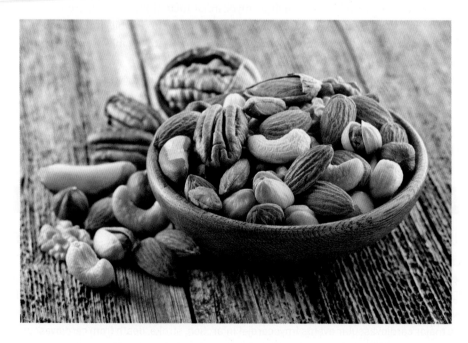

Since the PREDIMED trial, meta-analyses of cohort studies and clinical trials involving the Mediterranean diet have confirmed the beneficial effects, although there is some inconsistency in results (measured as CVD risk or other health outcomes). More high-quality studies are required to increase the confidence of estimates of the size of the effect [19]. The components of the diet linked to mechanisms behind effects are proposed as plant polyphenols, unsaturated fatty acids, fibre, vitamins and minerals, affecting pathways related to reduced oxidation, inflammation, body weight, blood pressure, LDL cholesterol and fasting glucose [19].

In a similar vein, the Portfolio dietary pattern was constructed by researchers in Canada to include four cholesterol-lowering foods with approved health claims from the United States, Canada or Europe (Table 17.1). A recent systematic review and meta-analysis of clinical trials examined effects of this approach on blood lipids, blood pressure, markers of inflammation, body weight and 10-year risk of coronary heart disease [20]. The analysis indicated the dietary pattern produced clinically meaningful improvements in LDL-cholesterol (high certainty) and moderate evidence of effects in other outcomes.

TABLE 17.1   CORE FOOD COMPONENTS OF PORTFOLIO DIETARY PATTERN

Diet component	Amount	Food sources
Nuts	42 g	Tree nuts and peanuts
Plant protein	50 g	Soy, pulses, beans, lentils
Viscous soluble fibre	20 g	Oats, barley, psyllium, eggplant, okra, apples, oranges, berries
Plant sterols	2 g	Enriched margarines

Source: Adapted from L. Chiavaroli, S. K. Nishi, T. A. Khan, C. R. Braunstein, A. J. Glenn, S. B. Mejia, … J. L. Sievenpiper (2018). Portfolio dietary pattern and cardiovascular disease: a systematic review and meta-analysis of controlled trials. *Progress in Cardiovascular Diseases*. doi:https://doi.org/10.1016/j.pcad.2018.05.004

Cardiovascular disease is often a cause of mortality in people with type 2 diabetes mellitus. The disease is associated with high blood glucose levels (hyperglycaemia) that have emerged after periods of 'insulin resistance'. The condition of insulin resistance occurs when high levels of insulin secreted by the pancreas fail to assist in the transport of glucose from the blood vessels to cells, with subsequent metabolic consequences. Eventually, insulin insufficiency is seen as the β-cells in the pancreas slowly fail to produce adequate insulin. Given the central position of fuel utilisation in diabetes, diet plays an important role across the spectrum of disease risk, development and management.

The development of chronic disease occurs throughout life, but it generally emerges clinically during adulthood. Understanding the disease development process is important in establishing preventive health strategies. **Biomarkers** of disease have been identified from studies of the pathophysiology of the disease, along with the relationships between factors associated with pathology and disease events, including mortality. In general, biomarkers reflect and locate the area of physiologic or metabolic dysfunction—for example, blood pressure indicates the risk to the cardiovascular system, while glucose and insulin levels are indicative of problems with fuel delivery that is manifest in diabetes.

Biomarkers

biological measurements that are indicative of the risk or presence of chronic disease or the consumption of a food.

» RESEARCH AT WORK

THE MEDITERRANEAN DIET AND CHRONIC DISEASE PREVENTION

Subsequent publications on the PREDIMED study have addressed components of the diet, as well as the effect of the MedDiet on secondary outcomes, such as biomarkers of disease. A review of the teachings of the PREDIMED study concluded that the dietary pattern, rich in unsaturated fat and compounds with antioxidant activity, was useful for CVD prevention. In addition to reducing CVD events, the incidence of diabetes was reduced in the MedDiet groups compared with controls, and beneficial effects on lipid profiles, blood pressure, inflammation and the influence on genetic expression were reported [21]. A more recent pre-specified secondary analysis further demonstrated favourable long-term effects on central adiposity and weight maintenance [22]. Given the size of the study population and the duration of the intervention, the PREDIMED trial was a landmark study of the effects of diet on chronic disease prevention. The body of publications on the trial also provides a broad understanding of the relationship between disease end points/biomarkers and dietary parameters, including the total diet, individual foods and significant components within key foods characteristics of the MedDiet pattern (see www.predimed.es).

One of the earliest biomarkers of CVD taken up into preventive health practice was blood cholesterol levels. The recognition of circulating cholesterol as a risk factor has been maintained given its presence in atherosclerotic plaque, associations with CVD exposed through observational epidemiology, and the reduced risk of coronary heart disease and total mortality seen with the use of the cholesterol-lowering drugs known as statins [17]. Cholesterol is transported via lipoprotein fractions: low-density lipoprotein (LDL) cholesterol refers to the fraction that delivers cholesterol away from the liver to the cells, whereas high-density lipoprotein (HDL) cholesterol is involved in reverse cholesterol transport back to the liver. Other lipoprotein fractions (e.g. very-low-density lipoprotein and intermediate-density lipoprotein), known as remnants, have also been implicated with atherogenic properties, as have pathways associated with the HDL fraction [23], so in time measures additional to total cholesterol and LDL/HDL fractions may become common. This may include measures of the oxidised LDL fraction that gets closer to the understanding the inflammatory process that underlies the development of CVD [24]. The role of dietary factors in manipulating lipid fractions, including reduced oxidised LDL fractions, remains a major component of the study of the diet–health relationship.

High blood pressure, or hypertension, is another well-established biomarker of CVD. Blood pressure is a function of the volume of blood pumped out by the heart (cardiac output) and resistance felt through the blood vessels (peripheral vascular resistance). On the other hand, the kidneys are responsible for managing fluid volume (water and electrolyte content), excreting ingested electrolytes and water daily. Volume content is tightly controlled by the regulation of sodium excretion, which means sodium plays a key role in the maintenance of blood pressure [25]. The relationship between blood pressure and salt and water excretion originally gained attention in the discipline of physiology [26]. Thus, studies of hypertension and diet have traditionally focused on dietary sodium, a single nutrient. The interpretation of evidence indicating sodium intakes are too high has been challenged from a physiological perspective with due consideration given to homeostatic mechanisms, such as the renin-angiotenson-aldosterone system (RAAS) [25]; however, these concerns have been addressed when the totality of evidence is considered for policy development [27].

Alongside the more traditional biomarkers of chronic disease, innovative biomarkers have emerged as the understanding of dysfunction in the system becomes more exposed. Biomarkers of inflammation are studied extensively given the association with the pathology of obesity and CVD [28]. Various **inflammatory biomarkers** have been found to expose the risk of cardiovascular events [29]. Examples of these biomarkers include C-reactive protein (CRP), tumour necrosis factor-alpha (TNF-α), interleukin-6 (IL-6), and many more. There are complex interactions between these biomarkers, however, and they have varying functions. Measures of multiple biomarkers are likely required to better understand risk [29]. In addition, the vascular dysfunction that occurs with inflammation can be studied using brachial flow mediated dilation (FMD), a non-invasive measure of endothelial function associated with risk of cardiovascular events [30]. Inflammatory biomarkers and measures of endothelial function now appear as end points in studies of the diet–disease relationship.

> **Inflammatory biomarkers**
> molecular components of pathways associated with inflammation.

» CASE 17.3

OBESITY AND HEART DISEASE RISK IN PRACTICE

The nature of the association between obesity and cardiovascular disease creates a great deal of discussion, in research, health policy and practice, and the media. With the gradual breakdown of the cardiovascular system, heart disease could be seen as a consequence of ageing, but substantial scientific research has shown this is preventable, at least in the earlier stages of life. The impact of overweight on individuals may vary, but at a population level the relationships can be clearly seen. These relationships are examined through the assessment of risk factors, and the distribution of these risk factors may give an indication of when and how best to intervene.

In a cross sectional study of 1,294,174 adults across a broad geographical area, researchers from the US Centers for Disease Control examined data on cardiometabolic risk factors (CMRF) for over 1 million adults who had attended for primary health care between 1 January 2012 and 31 December 2013 as part of the PORTAL weight cohort study [31]. The distribution of risk factors varied with age, degree of overweight and ethnicity. Researchers found that high blood pressure was the most common CMRF (59.9%), followed by prediabetes/high blood glucose levels (47.2%), low HDL cholesterol (33.7%) and high triglycerides (32.2%) [32]. Among overweight individuals, 18.6% had none of the CMRF and the proportion was less for obese individuals, which may reflect early medical management. Increasing age was strongly and independently associated with CMRF. The authors noted that factors that explain any differences observed could be body fat distribution, cardiometabolic fitness, weight-loss interventions with diet and exercise, cigarette smoking, family history and the presence or absence of systemic inflammation, but the distribution remained informative. Importantly, the analysis provided insights into when cardiovascular disease emerges in the population, which CMRF appear first and in which groups, and the impact of medical and lifestyle interventions at various life stages. Future research was suggested to examine the order in which CMRF develop during the life stages and the characteristics of individuals who do not have CMRF.

- When dealing with obesity and CMRF, what is the difference between population statistics and the test results for an individual?
- How might disease risk be managed at the population and individual levels?
- What does this study of CMRF profiles tell us about diet and the development of chronic disease?

Cardiometabolic risk factors (CMRF)
clinical measurements that have been shown to be associated with the development of cardiovascular disease and type 2 diabetes.

Metabolic syndrome
a cluster of CMRF (raised blood pressure, dyslipidaemia, raised fasting glucose, central adiposity) that occur together more often than by chance alone.

While research seeks to find new and better assessments of disease risk, their integration into practice requires substantive review of the overall evidence before being taken up. In practice, standard measures of CVD risk, such as total and LDL cholesterol levels, are referred to in both determining the need for dietary change and assessing dietary change effects. Chronic diseases develop over long periods of time and need sustained management. Poor diet quality over a lifetime can lead to chronic disease—for example, where the vascular and glucose homeostasis systems begin to break down. In practice, reference to **cardiometabolic risk factors (CMRF)** provides an indication of the degree of breakdown (Figure 17.3). Dietary factors can be implicated in chronic disease development by direct association with disease end points or through their association with biomarkers of the disease. Where relevant, preventive health strategies are built around driving dietary change based on evidence of relationships between dietary factors and CMRF. Where certain CMRF have been seen to cluster, the term **metabolic syndrome** has some utility in identifying people at risk and promoting appropriate changes in lifestyle behaviours.

FIGURE 17.3 FACTORS CONTRIBUTING TO CARDIOMETABOLIC RISK

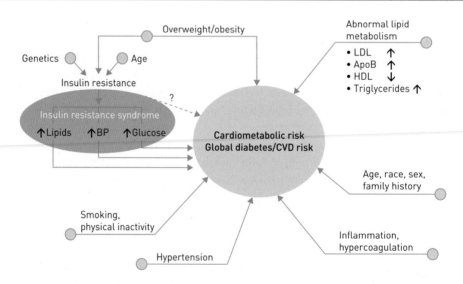

Source: J. D. Brunzell, M. Davidson, C. D. Furberg, R. B. Goldberg, B. V. Howard, J. H. Stein & J. L. Witztum (2008). Lipoprotein management in patients with cardiometabolic risk. *Consensus Conference Report from the American Diabetes Association and the American College of Cardiology Foundation*, 51(15), 1512–24. doi:10.1016/j.jacc.2008.02.034 (Figure 1: Factors contributing to cardiometabolic risk)

≫ CASE 17.4

THE CLINICAL UTILITY OF 'METABOLIC SYNDROME' AS A CONCEPT

Poor diet can lead to metabolic disturbances that can be observed through biomarkers that reflect risk of type 2 diabetes or cardiovascular disease. 'Metabolic syndrome' (MetS) reflects the presence of a number of these risk factors, including high waist circumference, high levels of blood triglycerides, high blood pressure, high blood glucose and low levels of blood HDL (good) cholesterol. Whether metabolic syndrome actually exists is debated in the literature, but the concept has emerged from observations that these risk factors tend to occur together, and the connections have been confirmed in analyses of population data [33]. The clinical descriptions are based on the presence of a pre-diabetic state that is linked to visceral adiposity (seen with high waist circumference) and the presence of an inflammatory condition induced by the presence of obesity [34]. While many definitions of metabolic syndrome have emerged over time, a consensus definition was published in 2009 [35]. Further analyses of data from large population studies have demonstrated that the cut-off points for clinical measures defining the condition are sufficient for clinical practice and research [36].

To examine the clinical utility of the MetS equation developed in the consensus statement [35], researchers examined data on 374 participants volunteering for a weight-loss trial in Wollongong, Australia. Among these, 137 participants (34%) were estimated as having MetS. Compared with those without MetS, they were older, more overweight and had a 4.5% increased risk of cardiovascular disease. They were also eight times more likely to develop coronary heart disease and 12 times more likely to develop insulin resistance (a pre-diabetic state). This study showed that the equation developed by a group of experts from a range of medical disciplines proved useful in identifying people at risk for future cardiovascular disease. In practice, the analysis underlined the need to lose weight to reduce chronic disease risk [37].

- How might the concept of MetS be useful for identifying dietary patterns that might protect against chronic disease?
- Which dietary factors might be significant in relation to risk factors identified in MetS?
- How does the concept of MetS align with that of food synergy?

STOP AND THINK

- How are the developments of obesity, cardiovascular disease and type 2 diabetes connected?
- What is the value of biomarkers of disease in managing the risk of chronic disease through dietary change?
- How is the evidence for relationships between diet and chronic disease established?

WHICH ARE THE BEST FOODS TO INCLUDE IN THE DIET TO PREVENT CHRONIC DISEASE IN ADULTHOOD?

Understanding the processes that are involved in the development of chronic disease and the associations with dietary factors exposes the principles of diets for preventing chronic disease. While the research is uneven, a number of dietary factors have been identified in the literature as associated with cardiometabolic risk [38]. These factors have been shown to influence the pathways outlined, producing varying degrees of evidence of dietary effects. The evidence for these relationships is positive, mixed or negative, with the top list of foods appearing positive and the bottom list increasingly negative (Figure 17.4).

FIGURE 17.4 IDENTIFIED EFFECTS BETWEEN DIETARY AND CARDIOMETABOLIC RISK FACTORS

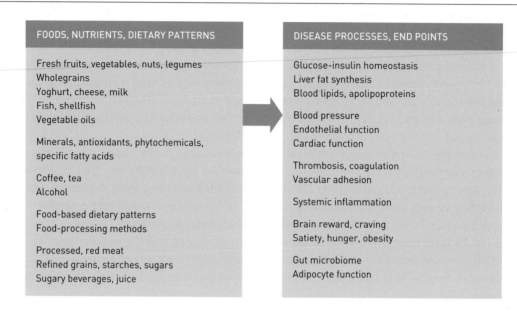

Source: Adapted from D. Mozaffarian (2016). Dietary and policy priorities for cardiovascular disease, diabetes, and obesity. a comprehensive review. *Circulation*, 133(2),187–225. doi:10.1161/circulationaha.115.018585

TRY IT YOURSELF

Which of the foods in your diet would be defined as refined grains, sugary beverages or processed meats? How does the amount and frequency of consumption of these foods in your diet compare with the amount of fruit, vegetables, nuts, yoghurt, wholegrains and fish you eat?

See Chapters 1 and 2 on research into dietary patterns and dietary guidelines.

Nutritious foods

foods delivering substantial amounts of nutrients and with evidence of protective effects on health.

Discretionary foods

foods of poor nutritional value, containing high amounts of saturated fat, salt and added sugar and potentially having detrimental effects on health.

The dietary factors in Figure 17.4 include foods, food components, dietary patterns, food processing and preparation methods and beverages. These relationships are studied in many ways, from laboratory experiments to epidemiological studies and clinical trials. Even though the dietary factor researched may be a nutrient, food or dietary pattern, they are all interrelated. A low-fat diet, for example, is characterised by its nutrient composition and the foods that together form this particular profile. Research on food-based dietary patterns provides evidence of effects of diets and cuisines, and also helps to identify key foods that may be delivering components that have an impact on effects [39]. The evidence-based review for Australian Dietary Guidelines (www.eatforhealth.gov.au) addressed the effects of different foods, nutrients and dietary patterns on the risk of chronic disease [40]. The categories of foods are given as either **nutritious foods** or foods to limit. Nutritious foods were listed as vegetables, legumes, beans, fruit, cereals—mostly wholegrain/high fibre—lean meat, poultry, fish, eggs, tofu, nuts, seeds, legumes, beans, and milk, yoghurt, cheese or alternatives. Foods to limit were described as containing high amounts of saturated fat, salt and added sugar. The latter group are referred to as **discretionary foods**, with examples being cakes, pastries, processed meats, confectionary, many commercial fried foods and sugar-sweetened beverages. The term 'discretionary' is used because they do not form the basis of the diet that meets the nutritional requirements.

When dietary guidelines are developed and updated, evidence for the relationship between consumption of individual foods and health outcomes is systematically reviewed (Table 17.2). The extent to which any food group may be identified and included in recommendations is dependent on the volume and quality of research on that food at that time. Research is ongoing, however, so the evidence base is constantly expanding. Shifts in guidance can be expected as new data is taken on board, but in the main, the increasing volume of research also means the confidence with which statements are made tends to improve with time.

See Chapter 2 on dietary guidelines.

TABLE 17.2 SUMMARY OF QUALIFIED EVIDENCE STATEMENTS REGARDING FOOD GROUP CONSUMPTION AND DISEASE RISK

Food group	Overweight/obesity	Type 2 diabetes	Cardiovascular disease	Hypertension/stroke
Vegetables			Reduced risk	Reduced risk stroke
Fruit			Reduced risk	Reduced risk stroke
Cereals	Reduced risk weight gain (wholegrain)	Reduced risk (wholegrain)	Reduced risk (oats, barley)	
Milk/cheese/yoghurt			Reduced risk	Reduced risk stroke/ hypertension

Source: Adapted from National Health and Medical Research Council (2011). *A Review of the Evidence to Address Targeted Questions to Inform the Revision of the Australian Dietary Guidelines.* Canberra: NHMRC. © Commonwealth of Australia

Reviewing research requires a working knowledge of quality reviews and independent searching from high-quality scientific journals. Meta-analyses provide stronger forms of evidence because they combine the data from a number of human studies, bearing in mind that these studies can be in the form of observations from large population groups (determining associations between the dietary factor and disease) and randomised controlled trials (providing direct evidence of effects). All research designs have inherent limitations, but it is important to keep up to date as the evidence continues to evolve.

» RESEARCH AT WORK

IDENTIFYING FOODS ASSOCIATED WITH DECREASED OR INCREASED CHRONIC DISEASE RISK

Identifying the relationship between food consumption patterns and changes in weight has been studied in large observational studies of human populations (prospective cohort) and in randomised controlled trials (RCTs) where the food of interest is the main dietary variable. Recognising that weight gain in US adults occurs at the rate of about half a kilogram a year, researchers from Harvard University examined the association between intakes of food categories and changes in weight. They analysed data from 120,877 healthy non-obese adults enrolled in the Nurse Health and Health Professional Cohort Studies. They measured consumption of foods and changes in weight over a four-year period. The cohort gained on average 0.83 kg (3.35 lb). The weight gain was inversely associated with consumption of vegetables (-0.22 lb), wholegrains (-0.37 lb), fruits (-0.49 lb), nuts (-0.57 lb) and yoghurt (-0.82 lb), but positively associated with intake of potato chips (1.69 lb), potatoes (1.28 lb), sugar-sweetened beverages (1.00 lb), unprocessed red meat (0.95 lb) and processed red meats (0.93 lb) [41].

This was one of the first observational studies that began to differentiate between types of foods and weight gain. While the total diet is the ultimate dietary factor influencing body weight, the implication of this research is that some foods are associated with patterns of food choice that protect against weight gain, while others are part of a deleterious set of food choices. A focus on individual foods helps to provide more detailed dietary guidance for more effective lifestyle behaviours.

A more recent report using a set of meta-analyses examined the effects of different foods on chronic disease [38]. Study end points were coronary heart disease (CHD), stroke and diabetes mellitus. The analyses showed fruits (each serving/day 100 g), vegetables (each serving/day 100 g), green leafy vegetables (each serving/day 100 g), legumes (each 4 servings per week/400g), wholegrains (high vs low) and nuts and seeds (each 4 servings/week 113g) to be associated with reduced risk. Compared with the first study discussed here [41], which was based on two prospective studies conducted from a single centre, this report [38] brought together data from a wide range of studies, both prospective cohort and RCTs, to compile the evidence separately on each food. Research will be ongoing, reflecting the types of research that are amenable to different foods. Where results are consistent, confidence builds in the direction of the effect of consuming that food. For example, in this second analysis [38], the results for nuts were obtained from RCTs and showed effects on the reduction of CHD death, non-fatal CHD and diabetes. A more recent meta-analysis [42] found that 28 g/day increase in nut intake produced reductions in CHD, stroke and diabetes. Note the evidence was consistent in two different studies conducted by different groups and published in different journals. When this consistency begins to emerge in the evidence base, confidence in the direction of results increases. The corollary, of course, is that single studies are of limited value and should not be taken as strong evidence of effects.

The pattern of evidence is also highly varied for each food group, including the degree of specificity for protective effects with disease end points [38]. In some cases, the food category itself is very broad. For example, there are many different types of dairy food [43], but there is also a large amount of research available. Because a number of products are also high in saturated fat, this group is implicated in concerns for dietary saturated fat. At the same time, the evidence for cardiovascular risk with high consumption of saturated fat remains a subject of scientific debate [44], and particularly in the case of dairy food [45]. In these cases, the extent of the scientific literature available and the use of meta-analyses [46] and systematic reviews [47–50] are valuable in informing the debates.

Across the globe, the need to discriminate between foods that promote or impede health has become part of efforts to reduce the risk of cardiometabolic disorders. Overall, and with food supply issues considered, the group of foods defined as wholegrains, fruit, vegetables, fish, nuts, seeds, beans, legumes and milk, and key nutrients (dietary fibre, polyunsaturated fat, seafood and plant omega-3 fatty acids and calcium) appear to provide protection against the development of cardiovascular disease and diabetes. On the other hand, other foods including sugary beverages and unprocessed meat, along with dietary levels of nutrients such as saturated fatty acids, trans-fatty acids, cholesterol and sodium, have emerged as detrimental to health [51]. Although there are variations across global regions, the consumption of unhealthy food items has increased despite the availability of healthy foods. In Australia, there appears to be no major decline in overall diet quality, but Australia remains among the worst countries for having unhealthy items in the diet [51].

Consuming too many deleterious foods impedes the prevention of chronic disease in adulthood. Recall that nutritious foods formed the basis for the dietary modelling underpinning the Australian

Dietary Guidelines. This was translated into the Australian Guide to Healthy Eating (AGHE), which outlines the relative amounts and types of foods in a healthy diet [40]. The dietary modelling produced Foundation diets, which were calculated to deliver adequate intakes of essential nutrients within dietary energy constraints for any given age and size [52]. As discussed above, because the dietary modelling included relatively unprocessed foods (with minimal amounts of added salt and sugar), and constrained the amounts of foods high in saturated fat, a distinction was created between 'core' foods (nutrient-dense foods) and 'discretionary' foods.

See Chapter 2 on dietary guidelines.

Problems with dietary behaviour in the Australian population are apparent in analyses of the recent Australian Health Survey, which suggests that 35% of energy consumed comes from discretionary food categories [7]. This analysis also showed that the major culprits are 'cereal foods and cereal food products' and 'vegetable products and dishes'. These represent alternative versions of the recommended categories of 'cereal foods (mostly wholegrains)' and 'vegetables' respectively, but prepared and processed in such a way as to reduce nutritional quality. In developing a healthy diet for chronic disease prevention, it becomes apparent that choice of cuisine and food preparation techniques play important roles.

It is arguable that cuisine factors underpinned the success of the PREDIMED trial [18], which demonstrated the effect of Mediterranean diet on cardiovascular disease risk reduction in regions across Spain. While the foods involved in this diet were consistent with known protective foods, the trial also demonstrated the effect of a culturally recognised cuisine that participants were able to develop and maintain. In the United States, the well-researched DASH diet plan displays a similar pattern of food choices, but there is more emphasis on the combination of foods and less on cuisine (Table 17.3). There is also an emphasis on restricting sodium in the diet, an element highly prevalent in processed and takeaway foods, so home-prepared cuisine may be implied.

See Chapter 11 for further discussion on the DASH diet.

TABLE 17.3   DESCRIPTION OF THE DASH EATING PLAN

Recommendations	Eat vegetables, fruits, wholegrains Include low-fat dairy products, fish, poultry, beans, nuts, vegetable oils Limit foods high in saturated fats Limit sugar-sweetened beverages and sweets	
Food group	**Servings/day ***	**Serving size**
Grains	6–8	1 slice bread, ½ cup cereal
Vegetables	4–5	½–1 cup
Fruit	4–5	1 medium or ½ cup
Fish, poultry, meat	<6	30 g or 1 egg
Low-fat dairy products	2–3	1 cup or 45 g (cheese)
Fats and oils	2–3	1 tsp
Sodium	2300 mg or less	(in food)
Nuts, seeds, dried peas, beans	4–5/week	45 g nuts, ½ cup beans, 2 tbsp peanut butter or seeds
Sweets	No more than 5/week	1 tbsp sugar or jam

*based on 2000 calories (8386 kJ)/day

Source: www.nhlbi.nih.gov/health-topics/dash-eating-plan

» CASE 17.5

VEGETARIAN DIETS

Minimally refined plant foods form the main category of foods aligned with preventive health goals. Fresh vegetables, fruits, nuts and legumes form the basis of the DASH and Mediterranean dietary patterns, and studies show that these foods are associated with reduced risk of chronic disease [38; 42; 53–56]. The case for including vegetables in weight management rests with effects on satiety and satiation [57], but new study designs need to be developed to show that this is the case [58; 59].

There are many definitions of vegetarian diets and they often involve food exclusions, so there may be concern for nutritional adequacy. Plant-based dietary patterns, including vegetarian diets, are an example of an alternative cuisine that can also meet nutritional needs. A slightly different set of foods is identified as providing some of the key nutrients, and the way in which the foods are prepared will also vary in a culinary sense [60–62]. A review of plant-based foods has shown that these dietary patterns can be adequate [63]. The approach to demonstrating adequacy is based on recognising the food groups that deliver key nutrients to achieve this balance (Table 17.4).

TABLE 17.4   FEATURES OF A HEALTHY VEGETARIAN DIET

Food group	Includes	Descriptive use
Vegetables	Legumes and salads	Mostly
Cereals	Rice, pasta, bread	Moderate
Protein-rich plant foods	Nuts, seeds, eggs, tofu, tempeh	Moderate smaller
Calcium-rich plant foods	Soy, milk, yoghurt	Inclusive
Fruit	Fresh whole fruits	Inclusive
Oil	Canola	Culinary

Source: A. Saunders, K. Marsh, C. Zeuschner & M. E. Reid (2012). Is a vegetarian diet adequate? Concepts and controversies in plant-based nutrition. *Medical Journal of Australia Open*, 1(suppl. 2), 1–48

- Why might it be difficult to meet nutritional requirements in a vegetarian diet?
- Which food groups require particular attention, and why?
- How might nutritional inadequacies be addressed if food is not available?

From observations of eating patterns and prevalence of disease, there is a growing body of evidence in the scientific literature about the relationship between food and health, but the details of this relationship are often debated. The studies that produce this evidence could focus on individual nutrients (e.g. amount and type of fat in the diet), or on whole foods (e.g. vegetables) and on whole diets (e.g. Mediterranean versus cholesterol-lowering diet patterns). While the early observations of the relationship between dietary saturated fat and cholesterol levels and coronary heart disease were made some 60 years ago [64], there is now some dispute as to whether all dietary saturated fats have the same effect [65]. It is argued that the foods that deliver saturated fat are important [45], and the cuisine effect needs to be considered more than a single nutrient [66]. The situation reflects the way in which much of the early research was conducted, where it was common practice to convert data on reported foods to that of nutrients, based on the nutrient composition of foods.

Other nutrients such as sodium and carbohydrate (specifically added sugar) have also been part of the debate, but while nutrient-based approaches to healthy dietary patterns leave the food choices more open, dietary modelling tends to return to the same group of foods. The only difference between dietary patterns then becomes emphasis, and some possible shifts around certain foods—for example, oils, dairy foods, meats and legumes. A Mediterranean diet is not a low-fat diet, but the origins of low-fat dietary advice have generally been in other Western cultures with high intakes of saturated fats reflected in local dietary patterns with different types of foods (Table 17.5). These patterns often include other poor dietary qualities such as a low intake of vegetables.

TABLE 17.5   FEATURES OF THE MEDITERRANEAN DIET AND AUSTRALIAN DIETARY GUIDELINES

Food group	Includes	Descriptive use
Mediterranean diet		
Oil	Extra virgin olive oil	Culinary fat
Plant products	Fresh vegetables and fruit, cereal foods (bread, pasta, rice), legumes, tree nuts, aromatic herbs and spices	Abundant
Seafood and fish	Fish and shellfish	Frequent
Alcohol	Wine	Moderate with meals
Animal products and sugar	Meat, milk, sugar	Low
Australian Dietary Guidelines		
Vegetables	Legumes, vegetables in range of colours	Mostly
Fruit	Fresh	Include
Grain foods	Mostly wholegrain cereals	Include
Dairy foods/alternatives	Milk, cheese, yoghurt, mostly reduced fat	Include
Protein-rich foods	Meats, fish, eggs, nuts, legumes, tofu, seeds	Smaller amounts
Unsaturated oils and spreads	Olive oil, canola oil	Culinary use

Source: J. Salas-Salvado, J. Fernandez-Ballart, E. Ros, M. A. Martínez-González, M. Fito, R. Estruch, ... M. I. Covas (2008). Effect of a Mediterranean diet supplemented with nuts on metabolic syndrome status: one-year results of the PREDIMED randomized trial. *Archives of Internal Medicine*, 168(22), 2449–58. doi:10.1001/archinte.168.22.2449; National Health and Medical Research Council (2013). *Australian Dietary Guidelines*. Canberra: NHMRC. © Commonwealth of Australia

TRY IT YOURSELF

The PREDIMED study [67] characterised the Mediterranean diet, and a healthy diet is implied in the Australian Dietary Guidelines statement.

- What are the similarities and differences between these food lists?
- How might they translate to ideas for meals?
- How could your usual eating pattern incorporate these characteristics and still reflect a set of meals that could feasibly be consumed throughout the week?

Poor dietary quality may indeed lie within the case against high dietary sodium intakes. Reviews suggest that reducing sodium intake can reduce blood pressure [68], with estimations that reducing sodium intake 100 mmol/day could reduce diastolic blood pressure by 1.4 to 2.5 mm Hg and subsequently reduce risk of stroke [69]. Stronger evidence was provided of long-term effects (around 19 years) in the follow-up of two landmark Trials of Hypertension Prevention (TOHP I and II). Here, reducing dietary salt in adults with untreated pre-hypertension (BP = <140/80–89 mm Hg) resulted in significant reductions in cardiovascular disease [70]. Also, the potassium content of the diet appears to have an inverse association with blood pressure, meaning the sodium-to-potassium ratio (Na:K) of the diet is also implicated in blood pressure regulation [71], and likely reflects the quality food choices, with fresh fruit and vegetables delivering potassium. The evidence supporting the inclusion of any single food in a healthy dietary pattern is gradually expanding, with increasing numbers of studies focusing on health outcomes in the context of improved methodologies and study designs for examining dietary effects. There is an increasing emphasis on the effects of the whole food as opposed to just the individual nutrients it is known to deliver [72]. There is also a focus on how consuming these foods may influence weight management, cardiovascular risk factors such as cholesterol levels and blood pressure, and pre-diabetic factors such as glucose and insulin responses. Observational studies highlight the associations between consumption of particular foods and the risks of developing cardiovascular disease, type 2 diabetes and cancer.

See Chapter 11 on sodium-to-potassium ratio and blood pressure.

STOP AND THINK

- Why is the nutrient profile of a food significant in the prevention of chronic disease?
- How can consumers distinguish between foods that are 'naturally nutrient rich' and those that may have an inadequate nutrient value, or too much of certain nutrients, such as sodium, fat and carbohydrate?
- How are nutrients, foods and whole diets connected in delivering prevention from chronic disease risk?

SUMMARY

- The best food choices for the prevention of chronic disease centre on nutrient-rich foods such as vegetables, fruit and wholegrains, then lean meat, poultry, fish, eggs, tofu, nuts, seeds, legumes and beans, and low-fat milk, cheese and yoghurt.
- Fats (spreads) and oils that contain mostly unsaturated fats are suggested for culinary use and to ensure a balance in the quality of fats in the diet.
- The combination of specific foods chosen on a daily basis constitutes a healthy diet pattern.
- There are a number of healthy diet patterns based on nutrient-rich foods for which there is evidence of reduced risk of chronic disease. Examples include the Mediterranean diet pattern, the DASH diet pattern and a plant-based dietary pattern. In each case, an understanding of how the foods contained in those diet patterns come to form a cuisine is important, with special attention being paid to meeting overall nutritional adequacy.
- Not all foods have a place in a healthy diet pattern, and certain categories of foods should be routinely limited. These include foods with a high saturated fat content (such as pies, fried foods, chips and cakes), a high sugar content (including sugar-sweetened drinks) and salty foods.
- Choosing the best foods for chronic disease prevention is just part of an overall healthy lifestyle. Physical activity is an important adjunct to achieving the benefits of a healthy dietary pattern.

PATHWAYS TO PRACTICE

- Promoting food choices that may be of benefit in the prevention of chronic disease requires a deep knowledge of food composition, the ability to distinguish between foods and the value of targeting specific foods.

- Generally, foods that are relatively unprocessed tend to be identifiable as protective; however, the types and amounts of foods in the total diet will influence overall health. While some minimally processed foods will naturally deliver sodium, saturated fat and sugar, it is the addition of these nutrients to foods that likely creates the imbalance that causes problems for health.

- Nutrition research continues to develop new knowledge and understanding of the effects of nutrients, foods and whole diets on health, which constantly translates to practice.

DISCUSSION QUESTIONS

1. Why does managing body weight appear to be the most important factor to consider in managing chronic lifestyle-related disease?
2. Which dietary factor is the most significant in managing body weight?
3. Which foods may be the best choices for managing body weight and chronic disease risk, and why?
4. Which food components, foods and dietary patterns are implicated in managing risk for chronic lifestyle-related disease?
5. How can we discriminate between foods and beverages so that we can make the best choices in preventing lifestyle-related disease?

USEFUL WEBLINKS

A review of the evidence to address targeted questions to inform the revision of the Australian Dietary Guidelines:

www.eatforhealth.gov.au/sites/default/files/files/the_guidelines/n55d_dietary_guidelines_evidence_report.pdf

Australian Dietary Guidelines:

www.eatforhealth.gov.au

Australian Health Survey:

www.abs.gov.au/australianhealthsurvey

Food Standards Australia New Zealand:

www.foodstandards.gov.au

Heart Foundation—Heart disease in Australia:

www.heartfoundation.org.au/about-us/what-we-do/heart-disease-in-australia

Nutrient Reference Values for Australia and New Zealand:

www.nrv.gov.au

PREDIMED study:

www.predimed.es

FURTHER READING

OBESITY PREVALENCE

Apovian, C. M. (2016). The obesity epidemic: understanding the disease and the treatment. *New England Journal of Medicine*, 374, 177–9.

Bastien, M., Poirier, P., Lemieux, I. & Després, J. P. (2014). Overview of epidemiology and contribution of obesity to cardiovascular disease. *Progress in Cardiovascular Diseases*, 56, 369–81.

Berrigan, D., Troiano, R. P. & Graubard, B. I. (2016). BMI and mortality: the limits of epidemiological evidence. *The Lancet*, 388, 734–6.

Bhupathiraju, S. N., Willett, W. C. & Hu, F. B. (2016). Body mass index and all-cause mortality. *JAMA—Journal of the American Medical Association*, 316, 991.

Casazza, K., Fontaine, K. R., Astrup, A., Birch, L. L., Brown, A. W., Bohan Brown, M. M., ... Allison, D. B. (2013). Myths, presumptions, and facts about obesity. *New England Journal of Medicine*, 368, 446–54.

Danaei, G. (2014). Metabolic mediators of the effects of body-mass index, overweight, and obesity on coronary heart disease and stroke: a pooled analysis of 97 prospective cohorts with 1.8 million participants. *The Lancet*, 383, 970–83.

Di Cesare, M., Bentham, J., Stevens, G. A., Zhou, B., Danaei, G., Lu, Y., et al. (2016). Trends in adult body-mass index in 200 countries from 1975 to 2014: a pooled analysis of 1698 population-based measurement studies with 19.2 million participants. *The Lancet*, 387, 1377–96.

Flegal, K. M., Kruszon-Moran, D., Carroll, M. D., Fryar, C. D. & Ogden, C. L. (2016). Trends in obesity among adults in the United States, 2005 to 2014. *JAMA—Journal of the American Medical Association*, 315, 2284–91.

Malik, V. S., Willett, W. C. & Hu, F. B. (2013). Global obesity: trends, risk factors and policy implications. *Nature Reviews Endocrinology*, 9, 13–27.

Mariscalco, G., Wozniak, M. J., Dawson, A. G., Serraino, G. F., Porter, R., Nath, M., ... Murphy, G. J. (2017). Body mass index and mortality among adults undergoing cardiac surgery: a nationwide study with a systematic review and meta-analysis. *Circulation*, 135, 850–63.

WEIGHT MANAGEMENT

Vadiveloo, M. K. & Parekh, N. (2015). Dietary variety: an overlooked strategy for obesity and chronic disease control. *American Journal of Preventive Medicine*, 49, 974–9.

INFLAMMATION AND OBESITY

Calder, P. C., Ahluwalia, N., Brouns, F., Buetler, T., Clement, K., Cunningham, K., ... Winklhofer-Roob, B. M. (2011). Dietary factors and low-grade inflammation in relation to overweight and obesity. *British Journal of Nutrition*, 106, S5–S78.

Esser, N., Legrand-Poels, S., Piette, J., Scheen, A. J. & Paquot, N. (2014). Inflammation as a link between obesity, metabolic syndrome and type 2 diabetes. *Diabetes Research and Clinical Practice*, 105, 141–50.

Gregor, M. F. & Hotamisligil, G. S. (2011). Inflammatory mechanisms in obesity. *Annual Review of Immunology*, 29, 415–45.

Jung, U. J. & Choi, M. S. (2014). Obesity and its metabolic complications: the role of adipokines and the relationship between obesity, inflammation, insulin resistance, dyslipidemia and nonalcoholic fatty liver disease. *International Journal of Molecular Sciences*, 15, 6184–223.

Lumeng, C. N. & Saltiel, A. R. (2011). Inflammatory links between obesity and metabolic disease. *Journal of Clinical Investigation*, 121, 2111–17.

Ye, J. & McGuinness, O. P. (2013). Inflammation during obesity is not all bad: evidence from animal and human studies. *American Journal of Physiology—Endocrinology and Metabolism*, 304, E466–E477.

MICROBIOTA AND OBESITY

Aron-Wisnewsky, J. & Clément, K. (2016). The gut microbiome, diet, and links to cardiometabolic and chronic disorders. *Nature Reviews Nephrology*, 12, 169–81.

Baghurst, K. (2012). Nutritional recommendations for the general population. In J. Mann & A.S. Truswell (eds). *Essentials of Human Nutrition*, 4th edn. New York: Oxford University Press.

Barlow, G. M., Yu, A. & Mathur, R. (2015). Role of the gut microbiome in obesity and diabetes mellitus. *Nutrition in Clinical Practice*, 30, 787–97.

Blaut, M. (2015). Gut microbiota and energy balance: role in obesity. *Proceedings of the Nutrition Society*, 74, 227–34.

Boulangé, C. L., Neves, A. L., Chilloux, J., Nicholson, J. K. & Dumas, M. E. (2016). Impact of the gut microbiota on inflammation, obesity, and metabolic disease. *Genome Medicine*, 8.

Cho, I. & Blaser, M. J. (2012). The human microbiome: at the interface of health and disease. *Nature Reviews Genetics*, 13, 260–70.

Corfe, B. M., Harden, C. J., Bull, M. & Garaiova, I. (2015). The multifactorial interplay of diet, the microbiome and appetite control: current knowledge and future challenges. *Proceedings of the Nutrition Society*, 74, 235–44.

Cotillard, A., Kennedy, S. P., Kong, L. C., Prifti, E., Pons, N., Le Chatelier, E., … Layec, S. (2013). Dietary intervention impact on gut microbial gene richness. *Nature*, 500, 585–8.

Cox, A. J., West, N. P. & Cripps, A. W. (2015). Obesity, inflammation, and the gut microbiota. *The Lancet Diabetes and Endocrinology*, 3, 207–15.

Delzenne, N. M., Neyrinck, A. M. & Cani, P. D. (2013). Gut microbiota and metabolic disorders: how prebiotic can work? *British Journal of Nutrition*, 109, S81–S85.

Delzenne, N. M., Neyrinck, A. M., Bäckhed, F. & Cani, P. D. (2011). Targeting gut microbiota in obesity: effects of prebiotics and probiotics. *Nature Reviews Endocrinology*, 7, 639–46.

Flint, H. J., Scott, K. P., Louis, P. & Duncan, S. H. (2012). The role of the gut microbiota in nutrition and health. *Nature Reviews Gastroenterology and Hepatology*, 9, 577–89.

Gérard, P. (2016). Gut microbiota and obesity. *Cellular and Molecular Life Sciences*, 73, 147–62.

Hersoug, L. G., Mÿller, P. & Loft, S. (2016). Gut microbiota-derived lipopolysaccharide uptake and trafficking to adipose tissue: implications for inflammation and obesity. *Obesity Reviews*, 17, 297–312.

Kau, A. L., Ahern, P. P., Griffin, N. W., Goodman, A. L. & Gordon, J. I. (2011). Human nutrition, the gut microbiome and the immune system. *Nature*, 474, 327–36.

Komaroff, A. L. (2017). The microbiome and risk for obesity and diabetes. *JAMA—Journal of the American Medical Association*, 317, 355–6.

Kong, L. C., Holmes, B. A., Cotillard, A., Habi-Rachedi, F., Brazeilles, R., Gougis, S., … Clément, K. (2014). Dietary patterns differently associate with inflammation and gut microbiota in overweight and obese subjects. *PLOS ONE*, 9(10), e109434.

Kumari, M. & Kozyrskyj, A. L. (2017). Gut microbial metabolism defines host metabolism: an emerging perspective in obesity and allergic inflammation. *Obesity Reviews*, 18, 18–31.

Lean, M. E. J. & Malkova, D. (2016). Altered gut and adipose tissue hormones in overweight and obese individuals: cause or consequence. *International Journal of Obesity*, 40, 622–32.

Murphy, E. A., Velazquez, K. T. & Herbert, K. M. (2015). Influence of high-fat diet on gut microbiota: a driving force for chronic disease risk. *Current Opinion in Clinical Nutrition and Metabolic Care*, 18, 515–20.

National Health and Medical Research Council (2012). *Infant Feeding Guidelines: Information for Health Workers*. Canberra: NHMRC.

National Health and Medical Research Council (2012). *Management of Overweight and Obesity in Adults, Adolescents and Children: Clinical practice guidelines for primary care health professionals*. Draft for public consultation. Canberra: NHMRC.

National Health and Medical Research Council (2013). *Australian Dietary Guidelines*. Canberra: NHMRC.

Neyrinck, A. M., Schüppel, V. L., Lockett, T., Haller, D. & Delzenne, N. M. (2016). Microbiome and metabolic disorders related to obesity: which lessons to learn from experimental models? *Trends in Food Science and Technology*, 57, 256–64.

Pei, R., Martin, D. A., Dimarco, D. M. & Bolling, B. W. (2017). Evidence for the effects of yogurt on gut health and obesity. *Critical Reviews in Food Science and Nutrition*, 57, 1569–83.

Portune, K. J., Benítez-Páez, A., Del Pulgar, E. M. G., Cerrudo, V. & Sanz, Y. (2017). Gut microbiota, diet, and obesity-related disorders—the good, the bad, and the future challenges. *Molecular Nutrition and Food Research*, 61(1).

Rosenbaum, M., Knight, R. & Leibel, R. L. (2015). The gut microbiota in human energy homeostasis and obesity. *Trends in Endocrinology and Metabolism*, 26, 493–501.

Salonen, A., Lahti, L., Salojärvi, J., Holtrop, G., Korpela, K., Duncan, S. H., … De Vos, W. M. (2014). Impact of diet and individual variation on intestinal microbiota composition and fermentation products in obese men. *ISME Journal*, 8, 2218–30.

Sen, T., Cawthon, C. R., Ihde, B. T., Hajnal, A., Dilorenzo, P. M., De La Serre, C. B. & Czaja, K. (2017). Diet-driven microbiota dysbiosis is associated with vagal remodeling and obesity. *Physiology and Behavior*, 173, 305–17.

Sonnenburg, J. L. & Bäckhed, F. (2016). Diet-microbiota interactions as moderators of human metabolism. *Nature*, 535, 56–64.

Valsecchi, C., Carlotta Tagliacarne, S. & Castellazzi, A. (2016). Gut microbiota and obesity. *Journal of Clinical Gastroenterology*, 50, S157–S158.

Vitaglione, P., Mennella, I., Ferracane, R., Rivellese, A. A., Giacco, R., Ercolini, D., ... Fogliano, V. (2015). Whole-grain wheat consumption reduces inflammation in a randomized controlled trial on overweight and obese subjects with unhealthy dietary and lifestyle behaviors: role of polyphenols bound to cereal dietary fiber. *American Journal of Clinical Nutrition*, 101, 251–61.

REFERENCES

1   E. Trujillo, C. Davis & J. Milner (2006). Nutrigenomics, proteomics, metabolomics, and the practice of dietetics. *Journal of the American Dietetic Association*, 106(3), 403–13. doi:10.1016/j.jada.2005.12.002

2   T. Esko, J. N. Hirschhorn, H. A. Feldman, Y.-H. H. Hsu, A. A. Deik, C. B. Clish, ... D. S. Ludwig (2017). Metabolomic profiles as reliable biomarkers of dietary composition. *American Journal of Clinical Nutrition*, 105(3), 547–54. doi:10.3945/ajcn.116.144428

3   H. B. AlEssa, V. S. Malik, C. Yuan, W. C. Willett, T. Huang, F. B. Hu & D. K. Tobias. (2017). Dietary patterns and cardiometabolic and endocrine plasma biomarkers in US women. *American Journal of Clinical Nutrition*, 105(2), 432–41. doi:10.3945/ajcn.116.143016

4   H. Du & E. Feskens (2010). Dietary determinants of obesity. *Acta Cardiology*, 65(4), 377–86. doi:10.2143/ac.65.4.2053895

5   B. J. Rolls, A. Drewnowski & J. H. Ledikwe (2005). Changing the energy density of the diet as a strategy for weight management. *Journal of the American Dietetic Association*, 105(5 Suppl.1), S98–103. doi:10.1016/j.jada.2005.02.033

6   A. Drewnowski (2003). The role of energy density. *Lipids*, 38(2), 109–15. doi:10.1007/s11745-003-1039-3

7   Australian Bureau of Statistics (2015). *Australian Health Survey: First results, 2011–12*. Canberra: ABS.

8   D. J. Christie-David & J. E. Gunton (2017). Vitamin C deficiency and diabetes mellitus—easily missed? *Diabetic Medicine*, 34(2), 294–6. doi:10.1111/dme.13287

9   K. Aubusson (2016). Scurvy surprise: archaic sickness that struck down sailors resurfaces in Sydney. *Sydney Morning Herald*, 29 November. Retrieved from: www.smh.com.au/national/health/scurvy-surprise-archaic-sickness-that-struck-down-sailors-resurfaces-in-sydney-20161129-gszrhx.html.

10 V. D. Dixit (2008). Adipose-immune interactions during obesity and caloric restriction: reciprocal mechanisms regulating immunity and health span. *Journal of Leukocyte Biology*, 84(4), 882–92. doi:10.1189/jlb.0108028

11 Y. Y. Lam, A. J. Mitchell, A. J. Holmes, G. S. Denyer, A. Gummesson, I. D. Caterson, ... L. H. Storlien (2011). Role of the gut in visceral fat inflammation and metabolic disorders. *Obesity*, 19(11), 2113–20. doi:10.1038/oby.2011.68

12 C. L. Boulangé, A. L. Neves, J. Chilloux, J. K. Nicholson & M.-E. Dumas (2016). Impact of the gut microbiota on inflammation, obesity, and metabolic disease. *Genome Medicine*, 8(1), 42. doi:10.1186/s13073-016-0303-2

13 J. Zierer, M. A. Jackson, G. Kastenmüller, M. Mangino, T. Long, A. Telenti, ... C. Menni (2018). The fecal metabolome as a functional readout of the gut microbiome. *Nature Genetics*, 50(6), 790–5. doi:10.1038/s41588-018-0135-7

14 Australian Bureau of Statistics (2016). *Causes of Death, Australia, 2015*. Canberra: ABS.

15 Australian Institute of Health and Welfare (2015). *Cardiovascular Disease, Diabetes and Chronic Kidney Disease—Australian facts—Risk factors. Cardiovascular, diabetes and chronic kidney disease series no. 4.* Cat. no. CDK 4. Canberra: AIHW.

16 Australian Institute of Health and Welfare (2014). *Australia's Health (2014). Australia's Health Series no. 14.* Cat. no. AUS 178. Canberra: AIHW.

17 D. R. Jacobs, Jr & L. C. Tapsell (2015). What an anticardiovascular diet should be in (2015). *Current Opinion in Lipidology*, 26(4), 270–5. doi:10.1097/mol.0000000000000184

18 R. Estruch, E. Ros, J. Salas-Salvadó, M.-I. Covas, D. Corella, F. Arós, … M. A. Martínez-González (2018). Primary prevention of cardiovascular disease with a Mediterranean diet supplemented with extra-virgin olive oil or nuts. *New England Journal of Medicine*, 378(25), e34. doi:10.1056/NEJMoa1800389

19 J. Salas-Salvadó, N. Becerra-Tomás, J. F. García-Gavilán, M. Bulló & L. Barrubés (2018). Mediterranean diet and cardiovascular disease prevention: what do we know? *Progress in Cardiovascular Diseases*, 61(6), 62–7. doi:https://doi.org/10.1016/j.pcad.2018.04.006

20 L. Chiavaroli, S. K. Nishi, T. A. Khan, C. R. Braunstein, A. J. Glenn, S. B. Mejia, … J. L. Sievenpiper (2018). Portfolio dietary pattern and cardiovascular disease: a systematic review and meta-analysis of controlled trials. *Progress in Cardiovascular Diseases*, 61(1), 43–53. doi:https://doi.org/10.1016/j.pcad.2018.05.004

21 E. Ros, M. A. Martínez-González, R. Estruch, J. Salas-Salvadó, M. Fitó, J. A. Martínez & D. Corella (2014). Mediterranean diet and cardiovascular health: teachings of the PREDIMED study. *Advances in Nutrition: An International Review Journal*, 5(3), 330S–336S. doi:10.3945/an.113.005389

22 R. Estruch, M. A. Martínez-González, D. Corella, J. Salas-Salvadó, M. Fitó, G. Chiva-Blanch, … E. Ros (2016). Effect of a high-fat Mediterranean diet on bodyweight and waist circumference: a prespecified secondary outcomes analysis of the PREDIMED randomised controlled trial. *The Lancet Diabetes & Endocrinology*, 4(8), 666–76. doi:10.1016/S2213-8587(16)30085-7

23 R. S. Rosenson, H. B. Brewer, Jr, B. J. Ansell, P. Barter, M. J. Chapman, J. W. Heinecke, … N. R. Webb (2016). Dysfunctional HDL and atherosclerotic cardiovascular disease. *Nature Reviews Cardiology*, 13(1), 48–60. doi:10.1038/nrcardio.2015.124

24 A. Trpkovic, I. Resanovic, J. Stanimirovic, D. Radak, S. A. Mousa, D. Cenic-Milosevic, … E. R. Isenovic (2015). Oxidized low-density lipoprotein as a biomarker of cardiovascular diseases. *Critical Reviews in Clinical Laboratory Sciences*, 52(2), 70–85. doi:10.3109/10408363.2014.992063

25 R. P. Heaney (2015). Making sense of the science of sodium. *Nutrition Today*, 50(2), 63–6. doi:10.1097/NT.0000000000000084

26 A. C. Guyton (1989). Dominant role of the kidneys and accessory role of whole-body autoregulation in the pathogenesis of hypertension. *American Journal of Hypertension*, 2(7), 575–85.

27 C. A. M. Anderson, R. K. Johnson, P. M. Kris-Etherton & E. A. Miller (2015). Commentary on making sense of the science of sodium. *Nutrition Today*, 50(2), 66–71. doi:10.1097/NT.0000000000000086

28 N. Esser, S. Legrand-Poels, J. Piette, A. J. Scheen & N. Paquot (2014). Inflammation as a link between obesity, metabolic syndrome and type 2 diabetes. *Diabetes Research and Clinical Practice*, 105(2), 141–50. doi:10.1016/j.diabres. 2014.04.006

29 L. Stoner, A. A. Lucero, B. R. Palmer, L. M. Jones, J. M. Young & J. Faulkner (2013). Inflammatory biomarkers for predicting cardiovascular disease. *Clinical Biochemistry*, 46(15), 1353–71. doi:http://dx.doi.org/10.1016/j.clinbiochem.2013.05.070

30 Y. Inaba, J. A. Chen & S. R. Bergmann (2010). Prediction of future cardiovascular outcomes by flow-mediated vasodilatation of brachial artery: a meta-analysis. *International Journal of Cardiovascular Imaging*, 26(6), 631–40. doi:10.1007/s10554-010-9616-1

31 D. R. Young, B. A. Waitzfelder, D. Arterburn, G. A. Nichols, A. Ferrara, C. Koebnick, ... K. H. Lewis (2016). The Patient Outcomes Research to Advance Learning (PORTAL) Network adult overweight and obesity cohort: development and description. *JMIR Research Protocols*, 5(2), e87. doi:10.2196/resprot.5589

32 G. A. Nichols, M. Horberg, C. Koebnick, D. R. Young, B. Waitzfelder, N. E. Sherwood, ... A. Ferrara (2017). Cardiometabolic risk factors among 1.3 million adults with overweight or obesity, but not diabetes, in 10 geographically diverse regions of the United States, 2012–2013. *Preventing Chronic Disease*, 14. doi:10.5888/pcd14.160438

33 J. B. Meigs (2000). Invited commentary: insulin resistance syndrome? Syndrome X? Multiple metabolic syndrome? A syndrome at all? Factor analysis reveals patterns in the fabric of correlated metabolic risk factors. *American Journal of Epidemiology*, 152(10), 908–11; discussion 912.

34 S. M. Grundy (2012). Pre-diabetes, metabolic syndrome, and cardiovascular risk. *Journal of the American College of Cardiology*, 59(7), 635–43. doi:http://dx.doi.org/10.1016/j.jacc.2011.08.080

35 K. G. Alberti, R. H. Eckel, S. M. Grundy, P. Z. Zimmet, J. I. Cleeman, K. A. Donato, ... S. C. Smith, Jr (2009). Harmonizing the metabolic syndrome: a joint interim statement of the International Diabetes Federation Task Force on Epidemiology and Prevention; National Heart, Lung, and Blood Institute; American Heart Association; World Heart Federation; International Atherosclerosis Society; and International Association for the Study of Obesity. *Circulation*, 120(16), 1640–5. doi:10.1161/circulationaha.109.192644

36 R. P. Wildman, A. P. McGinn, M. Kim, P. Muntner, D. Wang, H. W. Cohen, ... V. Fonseca (2011). Empirical derivation to improve the definition of the metabolic syndrome in the evaluation of cardiovascular disease risk. *Diabetes Care*, 34(3), 746–8. doi:10.2337/dc10-1715

37 A. Martin, E. P. Neale, M. Batterham & L. C. Tapsell (2016). Identifying metabolic syndrome in a clinical cohort: implications for prevention of chronic disease. *Preventive Medicine Reports*, 4, 502–6. doi:10.1016/j.pmedr.2016.09.007

38 D. Mozaffarian (2016). Dietary and policy priorities for cardiovascular disease, diabetes, and obesity: a comprehensive review. *Circulation*, 133(2), 187–225. doi:10.1161/circulationaha.115.018585

39 L. C. Tapsell, E. P. Neale, A. Satija & F. B. Hu (2016). Foods, nutrients, and dietary patterns: interconnections and implications for dietary guidelines. *Advances in Nutrition: An International Review Journal*, 7(3), 445–54. doi:10.3945/an.115.011718

40 National Health and Medical Research Council (2011). *A Review of the Evidence to Address Targeted Questions to Inform the Revision of the Australian Dietary Guidelines: Evidence statements.* Canberra: NHMRC. Retrieved from: www.eatforhealth.gov.au/sites/default/files/files/the_guidelines/n55d_dietary_guidelines_evidence_report.pdf.

41 D. Mozaffarian, T. Hao, E. B. Rimm, W. C. Willett & F. B. Hu (2011). Changes in diet and lifestyle and long-term weight gain in women and men. *New England Journal of Medicine*, 364(25), 2392–404. doi:10.1056/NEJMoa1014296

42 D. Aune, N. Keum, E. Giovannucci, L. T. Fadnes, P. Boffetta, D. C. Greenwood, ... T. Norat (2016). Nut consumption and risk of cardiovascular disease, total cancer, all-cause and cause-specific mortality: a systematic review and dose-response meta-analysis of prospective studies. *BMC Medicine*, 14(1), 207. doi:10.1186/s12916-016-0730-3

43 L. C. Tapsell (2015). Fermented dairy food and CVD risk. *British Journal of Nutrition*, 113(S2), S131–S135. doi:10.1017/S0007114514002359

44 A. Astrup, J. Dyerberg, P. Elwood, K. Hermansen, F. B. Hu, M. U. Jakobsen, ... W. C. Willett (2011). The role of reducing intakes of saturated fat in the prevention of cardiovascular disease: where does the evidence stand in 2010? *American Journal of Clinical Nutrition*, 93(4), 684–8. doi:10.3945/ajcn.110.004622

45 B. A. Griffin (2011). Dairy, dairy, quite contrary: further evidence to support a role for calcium in counteracting the cholesterol-raising effect of SFA in dairy foods. *British Journal of Nutrition*, 105(12), 1713–14. doi:10.1017/s0007114510005593

46 X. Tong, J. Dong, Z. Wu, W. Li & L. Qin (2011). Dairy consumption and risk of type 2 diabetes mellitus: a meta-analysis of cohort studies. *European Journal of Clinical Nutrition*, 65(9), 1027.

47 G. E. Crichton, J. Bryan, J. Buckley & K. J. Murphy (2011). Dairy consumption and metabolic syndrome: a systematic review of findings and methodological issues. *Obesity Reviews*, 12(5), e190–201. doi:10.1111/j.1467-789X.2010.00837.x

48 P. C. Elwood, J. E. Pickering, D. I. Givens & J. E. Gallacher (2010). The consumption of milk and dairy foods and the incidence of vascular disease and diabetes: an overview of the evidence. *Lipids*, 45(10), 925–39. doi:10.1007/s11745-010-3412-5

49 R. A. Gibson, M. Makrides, L. G. Smithers, M. Voevodin & A. J. Sinclair (2009). The effect of dairy foods on CHD: a systematic review of prospective cohort studies. *British Journal of Nutrition*, 102(9), 1267–75. doi:10.1017/s0007114509371664

50 J. C. Louie, V. M. Flood, D. J. Hector, A. M. Rangan & T. P. Gill (2011). Dairy consumption and overweight and obesity: a systematic review of prospective cohort studies. *Obesity Reviews*, 12(7), e582–e592. doi:10.1111/j.1467-789X.2011.00881.x

51 F. Imamura, R. Micha, S. Khatibzadeh, S. Fahimi, P. Shi, J. Powles & D. Mozaffarian (2015). Dietary quality among men and women in 187 countries in 1990 and 2010: a systematic assessment. *The Lancet Global Health*, 3(3), e132–e142. doi:10.1016/S2214-109X(14)70381-X

52 National Health and Medical Research Council (2011). *A Modelling System to Inform the Revision of the Australian Guide to Healthy Eating*. Canberra: NHMRC.

53 Y. Gan, X. Tong, L. Li, S. Cao, X. Yin, C. Gao, ... Z. Lu (2015). Consumption of fruit and vegetable and risk of coronary heart disease: a meta-analysis of prospective cohort studies. *International Journal of Cardiology*, 183, 129–37. doi:10.1016/j.ijcard.2015.01.077

54 D. Hu, J. Huang, Y. Wang, D. Zhang & Y. Qu (2014). Fruits and vegetables consumption and risk of stroke: a meta-analysis of prospective cohort studies. *Stroke*, 45(6), 1613–19. doi:10.1161/strokeaha.114.004836

55 M. Li, Y. Fan, X. Zhang, W. Hou & Z. Tang (2014). Fruit and vegetable intake and risk of type 2 diabetes mellitus: meta-analysis of prospective cohort studies. *BMJ Open*, 4(11), e005497. doi:10.1136/bmjopen-2014-005497

56 A. Afshin, R. Micha, S. Khatibzadeh & D. Mozaffarian (2014). Consumption of nuts and legumes and risk of incident ischemic heart disease, stroke, and diabetes: a systematic review and meta-analysis. *American Journal of Clinical Nutrition*, 100(1), 278–88. doi:10.3945/ajcn.113.076901

57 B. J. Rolls, J. A. Ello-Martin & B. C. Tohill (2004). What can intervention studies tell us about the relationship between fruit and vegetable consumption and weight management? *Nutrition Reviews*, 62(1), 1–17.

58 A. D. Blatt, L. S. Roe & B. J. Rolls (2011). Hidden vegetables: an effective strategy to reduce energy intake and increase vegetable intake in adults. *American Journal of Clinical Nutrition*, 93(4), 756–63. doi:10.3945/ajcn.110.009332

59 L. C. Tapsell, A. Dunning, E. Warensjo, P. Lyons-Wall & K. Dehlsen (2014). Effects of vegetable consumption on weight loss: a review of the evidence with implications for design of randomized controlled trials. *Critical Reviews in Food Science and Nutrition*, 54(12), 1529–38. doi:10.1080/10408398.2011.642029

60 A. V. Saunders, W. J. Craig, S. K. Baines & J. S. Posen (2013). Iron and vegetarian diets. *Medical Journal of Australia*, 199(suppl. 4), S11–16.

61 A. V. Saunders, B. C. Davis & M. L. Garg (2013). Omega-3 polyunsaturated fatty acids and vegetarian diets. *Medical Journal of Australia*, 199(4 Suppl.), S22–S26.

62 A. V. Saunders, W. J. Craig & S. K. Baines (2012). Zinc and vegetarian diets. *Medical Journal of Australia*, 9(1 suppl. 2), 17–21.

63 A. Saunders, K. Marsh, C. Zeuschner & M. E. Reid (2012). Is a vegetarian diet adequate? Concepts and controversies in plant-based nutrition. *Medical Journal of Australia Open*, 1(suppl. 2), 1–48.

64 H. M. Sinclair (1956). Deficiency of essential fatty acids and atherosclerosis, etcetera. *The Lancet*, 270(6919), 381–3.

65 W. C. Willett (2012). Dietary fats and coronary heart disease. *Journal of Internal Medicine*, 272(1), 13–24. doi:10.1111/j.1365-2796.2012.02553.x

66 M. C. de Oliveira Otto, D. Mozaffarian, D. Kromhout, A. G. Bertoni, C. T. Sibley, D. R. Jacobs, Jr & J. A. Nettleton (2012). Dietary intake of saturated fat by food source and incident cardiovascular disease: the Multi-Ethnic Study of Atherosclerosis. *American Journal of Clinical Nutrition*, 96(2), 397–404. doi:10.3945/ajcn.112.037770

67 J. Salas-Salvado, J. Fernandez-Ballart, E. Ros, M. A. Martínez-González, M. Fito, R. Estruch, ... M. I. Covas (2008). Effect of a Mediterranean diet supplemented with nuts on metabolic syndrome status: one-year results of the PREDIMED randomized trial. *Archives of Internal Medicine*, 168(22), 2449–58. doi:10.1001/archinte.168.22.2449

68 J. M. Geleijnse, F. J. Kok & D. E. Grobbee (2003). Blood pressure response to changes in sodium and potassium intake: a metaregression analysis of randomised trials. *Journal of Human Hypertension*, 17(7), 471–80.

69 N. R. Cook, J. Cohen, P. R. Hebert, J. O. Taylor & C. H. Hennekens (1995). Implications of small reductions in diastolic blood pressure for primary prevention. *Archives of Internal Medicine*, 155(7), 701–9.

70 N. R. Cook, E. Obarzanek, J. A. Cutler, J. E. Buring, K. M. Rexrode, S. K. Kumanyika, ... P. K. Whelton (2009). Joint effects of sodium and potassium intake on subsequent cardiovascular disease: the Trials of Hypertension Prevention follow-up study. *Archives of Internal Medicine*, 169(1), 32–40. doi:10.1001/archinternmed.2008.523

71 C. E. Huggins, S. O'Reilly, M. Brinkman, A. Hodge, G. G. Giles, D. R. English & C. A. Nowson (2011). Relationship of urinary sodium and sodium-to-potassium ratio to blood pressure in older adults in Australia. *Medical Journal of Australia*, 195(3), 128–32.

72 D. R. Jacobs, Jr & L. C. Tapsell (2007). Food, not nutrients, is the fundamental unit in nutrition. *Nutrition Reviews*, 65(10), 439–50.

CHAPTER 18

NUTRITION IN OLDER AGE

KAREN CHARLTON AND KAREN WALTON

CHAPTER OBJECTIVES

This chapter will enable the reader to:

- identify some of the nutrition-related conditions associated with old age
- discuss the implications for increased nutrient requirements in old age
- outline the risk factors associated with malnutrition in old age
- discuss possible nutritional considerations for older people living in institutions.

KEY TERMS

Cognitive and physical function
Community-dwelling

Frailty aged care
Malnutrition

KEY POINTS

- Ageing is associated with physiological, psychological and social changes, all of which may increase the risk of a diet that is inadequate for meeting the needs of an older adult.
- Nutritional requirements change in older age, reflecting changes in activity and functional capacities, including the ability to absorb nutrients.
- Malnutrition is often seen in older people who are regularly in and out of hospital. This underlines the importance of malnutrition screening in the community setting and on admission to hospital, and ensuring adequate nutritional care on return to the community.

INTRODUCTION

The nutritional status of older people (particularly those more than 80 years of age) is a major determinant of both **cognitive and physical functioning**, as well as overall independence and quality of life. Moreover, nutrition is closely involved in the aetiology and management of various chronic diseases, such as cardiovascular disease and certain cancers.

The eminent gerontologist John Rowe [1] proposed the term 'successful ageing' to characterise the process of growing older while retaining satisfactory health, function and independence (Figure 18.1). This is contrasted with two other conditions: normative ageing and frailty. Normative ageing is the experience that covers many of the advanced years when multiple chronic diseases appear, and cognitive and/or physical function may be compromised to some degree. Frailty is at the other end of the spectrum: frail older persons have severe decline in cognitive and physical function, losing independence in **activities of daily living**, often becoming wheelchair-bound or bedridden, and requiring assistance and care. Older individuals of a similar age may be at any stage on this continuum of dependency, and thus have markedly different risk factors and requirements, leading to wide heterogeneity in this age group.

A number of factors influence older people's ability to maintain good health and participate in their community, such as sufficient income, adequate and safe housing, and a physical environment that facilitates independence and mobility [2; 3]. Older people's own lifestyle behaviours regarding health risks are also an important influence on their health status. Older adults have special nutritional needs depending on their individual circumstances. Some of this is physiological, associated with the physical process of ageing and the development of chronic disease, but others can be environmental and social. Malnutrition is a common concern associated with older age, and is one of the problems associated with frailty.

> See Chapter 17 on nutrition and the prevention of chronic disease.
>
> **Cognitive and physical functioning**
> the ability to mentally process information and maintain bodily functions such as movement.
>
> **Activities of daily living (ADL)**
> activities such as walking, sitting, eating, washing and dressing.

FIGURE 18.1 CATEGORIES OF AGEING

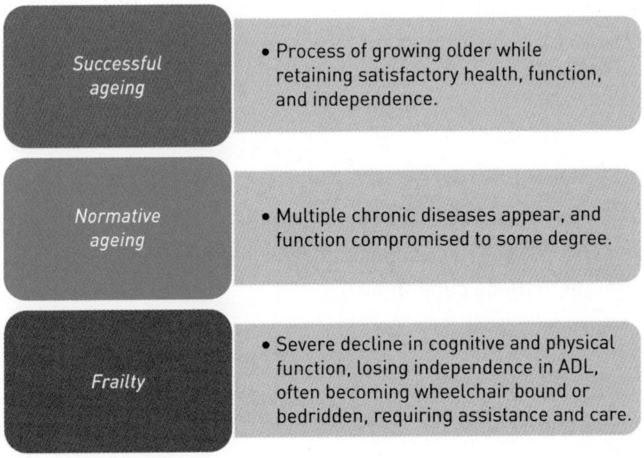

Successful ageing	• Process of growing older while retaining satisfactory health, function, and independence.
Normative ageing	• Multiple chronic diseases appear, and function compromised to some degree.
Frailty	• Severe decline in cognitive and physical function, losing independence in ADL, often becoming wheelchair bound or bedridden, requiring assistance and care.

Source: J. W. Rowe & R. L. Kahn (1987). Human aging: usual and successful. *Science*, 237(4811), 143–9

Frailty

a clinically recognisable state of increased vulnerability resulting from ageing-associated decline in function across multiple physiological systems.

Clinical syndrome

a set of signs and symptoms that tend to occur together and characterise a specific medical condition.

Phenotype

an observable set of physical characteristics of an individual resulting from the interaction between its genotype and environment.

The role of nutritional intervention in prevention and management of frailty is becoming increasingly recognised. **Frailty** is a clinically recognisable state of increased vulnerability that results from ageing-associated decline in function across multiple physiologic systems, that may be exacerbated by the presence of a disease. A frail older person is defined as one who has lost the ability to cope with everyday stressors. Fried and colleagues [4] first defined frailty as a **clinical syndrome** that meets three of five **phenotypic** criteria, namely: low grip strength; low perceived levels of energy; slowed walking speed; low physical activity; and unintentional weight loss. These criteria have been refined in subsequent studies and measures that can be used to determine presence of each of factors are shown in Table 18.1.

As well as the phenotype model, another approach to conceptualising frailty is the cumulative deficit model [5], which proposes frailty to be a non-specific multifactorial state that is better characterised by the quantity rather than quality of health/well-being disorders (called *deficits*) accumulated by individuals during their life course (e.g. signs, symptoms, impairments, abnormal lab tests, diseases). In 2012, experts reached consensus for defining frailty from a clinical perspective, as shown in Figure 18.2 [6]. A pre-frail stage is recognised as being when one or two criteria are present, and carries a high risk of progression to frailty.

The association between malnutrition and frailty, especially in older adults (over 65 years of age), has been established [4; 7–9], yet these two conditions are generally not considered together in terms of diagnosis, or strategies to address both simultaneously. Loss of body tissues, resulting in wasting, is a common phenotype for several conditions, including frailty and malnutrition [9]. The two conditions may exacerbate each other, and treatment strategies are generally similar [6; 8]. The overlapping characteristics considered in identifying frailty and malnutrition are shown in Table 18.2.

A need to focus on understanding and reversing the effects of pre-frailty is important because this is the population that may receive the most benefit from intervention. Nutritional treatment is one aspect that can be combined with other interventions including exercise (resistance and aerobic) and/or rehabilitation, given the emphasis on muscle mass and strength highlighted in the definition of frailty. Frailty and malnutrition have similar criteria for diagnosis and similar recommended treatment strategies. Whether malnutrition leads to frailty or vice versa is unknown. Prevention of overt malnutrition through early detection of risk is an important factor to consider in preventing dependency in older adults.

STOP AND THINK

- How can the distinction between 'normal ageing' and the development of frailty be made?
- What are some of the risk factors to recognise in at-risk groups?
- How does nutrition relate to these conditions?

TABLE 18.1   FRAILTY-DEFINING CRITERIA: CARDIOVASCULAR HEALTH STUDY (CHS) AND WOMEN'S HEALTH AND AGING STUDIES (WHAS)

Characteristics	CHS	WHAS
1. **Weight loss**	**Baseline:** Lost >10 pounds (4.5 kg) unintentionally in last year **Follow-up:** (weight in previous year-current weight)/(weight in previous year) ⩾0.05 and the loss was unintentional	**Baseline:** Either of: i. (weight at age 60–weight at exam)/(weight at age 60)⩾0.1 ii. BMI at exam <18.5. **Follow-up:** Either of: i. BMI at exam <18.5 ii. (weight in previous year-current weight)/ (weight in previous year) ⩾0.05 and the loss was unintentional
2. **Exhaustion**	Self report of either of: i. felt that everything I did was an effort in the last week ii. could not get going in the last week	Self report of any of: i. low usual energy level1 (<=3, range 0-10) ii. felt unusually tired in last month iii. felt unusually weak in the past month
3. **Low physical activity**	Women: Kcal <270 (1130 kJ) on activity scale (18 items) Men: Kcal <383 (1600 kJ) on activity scale (18 items)	Women: Kcal < 90 (380 kJ) on activity scale (6 items) Men: Kcal <128 (535 kJ)on activity scale (6 items)

4. **Slowness**	Walking 4.57 m at usual pace
	Women:
	   time >= 7 s for height <= 159 cm
	   time >= 6 s for height > 159 cm
	Men:
	   time >= 7 s for height <= 173 cm
	   time >= 6 s for height > 173 cm
		Walking 4m at usual pace
		Women:
		   speed <= 4.57/7 m/s for height <= 159 cm
		   speed <= 4.57/6 m/s for height > 159 cm
		Men:
		   speed <= 4.57/7 m/s for height <= 173 cm
		   speed <= 4.57/6 m/s for height > 173 cm

5. **Weakness**	Grip strength Women: <= 17 kg for BMI <= 23 <= 17.3 kg for BMI 23–26 <= 18 kg for BMI 26.1–29 <= 21 kg for BMI > 29 Men: <= 29 kg for BMI <= 24 <= 30 kg for BMI 24.1–26 <= 30 kg for BMI 26.1–28 <= 32 kg for BMI >28	Grip strength: Same as in CHS

Abbreviation: s = seconds
Rated on 0–10 scale, where 0 = 'no energy' and 10 = 'the most energy that you have ever had'.
If yes, there followed questioning 'how much of the time' the feeling persisted; responses 'most' or 'all' of the time were considered indicative of exhaustion.

Source: L. P. Fried, C. M. Tangen, J. Walston, A. B. Newman, C. Hirsch, J. Gottdiener, ... M. A. McBurnie (2001). Frailty in older adults: evidence for a phenotype. *Journals of Gerontology Series, Series A*, 56(3), M146–156

TABLE 18.2   KEY FRAILTY AND MALNUTRITION ASSESSMENT TOOLS AND THEIR OVERLAPPING CHARACTERISTICS

Identifying frailty	Identifying malnutrition	Overlapping characteristics
FRAIL: Fatigue, Resistance, Aerobic, Illness, **Loss of body weight** [10]	*ESPEN:* BMI, **weight loss**, FFMI [11]	• Weight loss/decreased body mass • Functional capacity • Weakness (grip strength) • Cognitive status
Cardiovascular Health Study Frailty Screening Measure: **Weight loss**, exhaustion, low activity, gait speed, **grip strength** [4]	*AND/ASPEN:* Insufficient energy intake, **weight loss**, loss of muscle mass, loss of subcutaneous fat/fluid accumulation, diminished **functional status** [*need 2 of 6*] [12]	
Clinical Frailty Scale: Activity, fatigue, illness, **functional status, cognitive status** [13]	*CMTF:* SGA—dietary intake, **weight**, symptoms, **functional capacity**, and metabolic requirements; physical exam for fat, muscle, oedema [14]	
Gérontopôle Frailty Screening Tool: **Functional status,** living situation, gait speed, fatigue, cognitive status [15]	*MNA:* anorexia, **weight loss**, impaired mobility, disease, **cognitive status, BMI**, living status, drug intake, meal intake, protein intake, fluid intake, fruit intake, eating dependency, perceived nutritional health status, perceived health status, arm circumference [16]	

Note: Similar characteristics are bolded. Abbreviations: AND: Academy of Nutrition and Dietetics; ASPEN: American Society of Parenteral and Enteral Nutrition; BMI: body mass index; CMTF: Canadian Malnutrition Task Force; ESPEN: European Society of Parenteral and Enteral Nutrition; FFMI: fat free mass index; MNA: Mini Nutritional Assessment; SGA: Subjective Global Assessment.

Source: C. V. Laur, T. McNicholl, R. Valaitis & H. H. Keller (2017). Malnutrition or frailty? Overlap and evidence gaps in the diagnosis and treatment of frailty and malnutrition. *Applied Physiology, Nutrition, and Metabolism*, 42(5), 449–58. doi:10.1139/apnm-2016-0652 (Table 1: Key frailty and malnutrition assessment tools and their overlapping characteristics)

WHAT ARE THE NUTRITION-RELATED HEALTH CONDITIONS ASSOCIATED WITH OLDER AGE?

Evidence is mounting that supports the need to intervene in a number of nutrition-related conditions during older age. These are discussed in detail below.

Anorexia of ageing

In the first instance, decreased appetite is common in old age, but is often the result of illness (e.g. peptic ulceration, gastric carcinoma, severe constipation and colitis, infections, liver dysfunction, renal impairment, chronic lung disease and congestive cardiac failure) or use of medication (particularly digoxin, fluoxetine, hydralazine, psychotropics, quinidine and vitamin A). Poor oral hygiene, periodontal disease, dental caries, oral mucosal problems, poorly fitting dentures and marginal zinc deficiency also contribute to a diminished sense of taste or smell, thereby adversely affecting appetite.

Anorexia of ageing
decreased appetite seen in older age.

FIGURE 18.2 DEFINITIONS OF FRAILTY

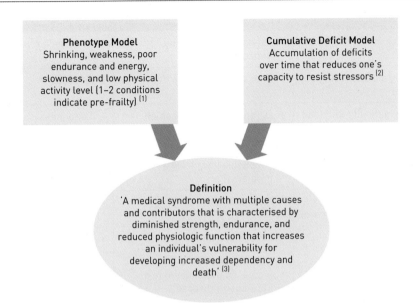

Notes: [4]; [5]; [6], p. 393.

Source: C. V. Laur, T. McNicholl, R. Valaitis & H. H. Keller. (2017). Malnutrition or frailty? Overlap and evidence gaps in the diagnosis and treatment of frailty and malnutrition. *Applied Physiology, Nutrition, and Metabolism,* 42(5), 449–58 (Figure 1. Definitions of frailty). doi:10.1139/apnm-2016-0652

Medications may induce nausea (e.g. antibiotics, aspirin and theophylline) or result in reduced salivary flow and dry mouth. A reduced thirst sensation associated with ageing increases the risk of dehydration, especially in hot weather, which may lead to confusion and forgetfulness to eat (Table 18.3).

Sarcopaenia

Sarcopaenia is defined as a skeletal muscle of <-2 SD of the mean for young persons, and is associated with loss of strength in both the upper and lower body and impairment in functional ability. Sarcopaenia has been linked to a three- to fourfold increased risk of disabilities and falls [17–19]. Measurement of body mass index (BMI) alone is unable to identify the decline in fat-free mass with ageing [20] and may mask the presence of sarcopaenic obesity, which represents an infiltration of fat into muscle. Other anthropometric measurements such as calf circumference measurement (below 31 cm) may be a more sensitive indicator of muscle-related disability and physical function in older adults [21]. The reason why **malnutrition** is related to adverse outcomes may be explained by the presence of sarcopaenia, but this has not been adequately explored.

Weight loss in older adults is common, and comprises both lean and fat mass loss, but it is likely to reflect a higher proportion of lean mass loss during periods of illness in older people. Low body weight and rapid unintentional weight loss are highly predictive of mortality and morbidity in this age group. Older people who are underweight are at greater risk of mortality than those who are overweight [22; 23]. Recent weight loss may be a more sensitive indicator of nutritional status than BMI, and the

Sarcopaenia

a condition characterised by loss of skeletal muscle mass and function, leading to loss of strength.

Malnutrition

poor nutritional intake and its consequences.

TABLE 18.3   MAJOR RISK FACTORS FOR POOR NUTRITIONAL STATUS IN OLDER PERSONS

Social factors	Physical/medical factors	Psychological/emotional factors
• Poverty	• Feeding or swallowing difficulties	• Widowed or bereaved
• Isolation (living alone or living in a remote area)	• Poor dentition	• Depression
• Poor nutrition, difficulty with food preparation, poor knowledge of food safety	• Diminished sense of smell or taste or xerostomia (dry mouth)	• Loneliness
• Elder abuse and neglect	• Dysphagia (swallowing problems)	• Dementia
• Institutional environment (hospital or residential aged care)	• Medications	• Alcoholism
	• Malabsorption	• Eating disorders or diet phobias: choking, fat, salt, etc.
	• Increased metabolism (e.g. Parkinson's disease)	• Anorexia (loss of appetite)
	• Chronic disease or chronic infection	
	• Needs assistance with feeding	
	• Needs assistance with food shopping and meal preparation	
	• Severe sight problems	
	• Physical disabilities/impaired performance of basic activities of daily living	

Source: Adapted from I. Darnton-Hill, E. T. Coyne & M. L. Wahlqvist (2001). Assessment of nutrition status. In R. Ratnaike (ed.), *A Practical Guide to Geriatric Practice*. Sydney: McGraw-Hill

TABLE 18.4   ASSESSMENT OF WEIGHT LOSS IN OLDER PERSONS OVER TIME

Time	Significant weight loss (%)	Severe weight loss (%)
One week	1–2	>2
One month	5	>5
3 months	7.5	>7.5
6 months or longer	10–20	>20

Source: I. Darnton-Hill, E. T. Coyne & M. L. Wahlqvist (2001). Assessment of nutrition status. In R. Ratnaike (ed.), *A Practical Guide to Geriatric Practice*. Sydney: McGraw-Hill

degree of weight loss over time gives an indication of whether nutrition intervention and/or further investigation is required (Table 18.4). Intentional weight loss is considered inappropriate unless excess weight is associated with functional problems. If a weight-loss program is considered necessary, referral to a dietitian is recommended as attention to adequate protein and micronutrient intake, as well as exercise, is required to preserve muscle mass.

It is well known that undernutrition is a major risk factor for a range of poor health outcomes, including mortality, in older people. What remains controversial is the risk of overweight and obesity and which BMI cut-offs indicate health risk [24]. Research on hospital mortality following cardiac surgery indicates that risk is associated mainly with BMI >40 and that having a BMI of 30–49 may carry a lower risk compared with normal weight individuals [25]. There is evidence that having a BMI less than 18.5 significantly increases risk of in-hospital mortality and post-operative outcomes [26]. It is recommended that those who are underweight or maybe even normal weight may need preoperative nutrition support for optimal outcomes. However, in determining risk, sarcopaenia may be more important than BMI. In patients admitted for abdominal surgery, those with sarcopaenia doubled their risk of in-hospital mortality within 30 days post-surgery, as well as up to one year post-surgery. For colorectal surgery, sarcopaenia resulted in a 74% risk of complications [27].

In a meta-analysis of studies in older populations, being overweight was not found to be associated with an increased risk of mortality. Mortality risk began to increase only for a BMI above 33.0 [28]. However, there was an increased risk for those at the lower end of the recommended BMI range for older adults that was evident at a BMI below 23. It is important to monitor weight status in older adults, in order to promptly address any modifiable causes of weight loss [28].

Cognitive impairment

Cognitive impairment is one of the most important issues that need to be addressed in old age. **Dementia**, a form of cognitive impairment, describes a group of irreversible neurodegenerative diseases that are currently Australia's fourth leading cause of death. Dementia is the most common manifestation of cognitive impairment and mental illness in the older population and is present in about 6.5% of Australians aged 65 years and older and 22% of people aged 85 years and over [2; 3]. This equates to around 181,000 people aged 65-plus years, including 73,500 people aged 85-plus years with dementia. Almost two-thirds of older people with dementia are female, due to women living longer than men. Several types of dementia exist, the most common type being Alzheimer's disease, which accounts for approximately two-thirds of all dementia cases. Cognitive impairment and mental illness in older persons can be a cause or an effect of malnutrition. For example, dementia can develop secondary to vitamin B12 deficiency, while dehydration can result in confusion and delirium. Conversely, dementia may be associated with forgetfulness to eat or drink, and difficulties in shopping, food preparation and self-feeding.

Cognitive impairment
reduction in memory, thinking and reasoning abilities.

Dementia
a clinically diagnosed form of cognitive impairment.

Epidemiological data on diet and cognitive decline suggest that certain macro- and micronutrients (folate, vitamins B12, C and E, flavonoids and unsaturated fatty acids) may have a protective effect, whereas a low intake of total fats has been linked to a lower risk for Alzheimer's disease or slower cognitive decline [29; 30]. Dietary patterns, such as a Mediterranean-type diet [31], may contribute to a lower incidence of dementia. Potential biological mechanisms regarding the role of diet in incidence of dementia include the protective role of antioxidants and of vitamin B12 and folate metabolism. Suboptimal status of folate and vitamin B12 at the biochemical level has been associated with significant neuropsychiatric damage, including cognitive impairment, but supplementation with vitamin B12 in those with mild deficiency [32] or healthy, well-nourished older women [33] did not improve cognitive outcomes.

>> RESEARCH AT WORK

DIET AND COGNITIVE FUNCTIONING IN OLDER AGE

Plant-based foods form an integral component of the human diet, and their consumption is consistently linked to the maintenance of health and the prevention of a vast array of diseases [34]. Non-nutritive bioactive compounds, known as phytonutrients, found in plant-based foods, contribute to the antioxidant activity of these foods [35]. Many thousands of phytonutrients exist to date, but flavonoids are a subclass showing potential in terms of beneficial effects on neurocognition [34].

Mild cognitive impairment

an intermediate stage between the expected cognitive decline of normal ageing and the more-serious decline of dementia. Mild cognitive impairment may involve problems with memory, language, thinking and judgment.

Of the six flavonoid subclasses, anthocyanins that provide the purple, red and blue pigmentation in plants are the most promising [36]. Pre-clinical evidence has shown that anthocyanin-rich food consumption can improve several cognitive functions, including long-term memory, spatial-working memory and object-recognition memory [37]. In ageing animal models, supplementation of the diet with anthocyanin-rich fruits not only maintains, but also reverses, cognitive decline [38]. A study conducted by Kent and colleagues in 2015 found that consumption of 200 mL/day of cherry juice for 12 weeks improved both short- and long-term memory and verbal fluency in older adults with mild to moderate dementia [39]. Another study in older adults with **mild cognitive impairment** showed that daily intake of concord grape juice for 16 weeks resulted in cognitive improvements, and increased activation in the posterior and anterior brain regions according to MRI [40]. Similar effects have been reported for blueberry juice [41].

While precise mechanisms of action are unclear and are likely to be multiple, neurotrophins (growth factors), particularly brain-derived neurotrophic factor (BDNF), are thought to play a role. BDNF is found in high concentrations within the hippocampus [42] and has been shown to play a critical role in neurogenesis and neuronal survival, synaptic plasticity [43] and memory formation [42]. Anthocyanins may also influence cognitive functioning through their positive impact on blood flow and peripheral vascular function that is mediated through increased bioavailability of nitric oxide due to absorbed flavonoid metabolites [34]. Increased blood flow to the brain may assist in increasing the strength and number of neuronal signals in brain regions associated with memory and learning [44]. Protection of the structure of cells in the brain, and limitation of neurodegeneration by decreased neuro-inflammation by flavonoids has also been hypothesised [44].

As more evidence emerges regarding the role of diet, including polyphenols, fibre and probiotics, on the gut microbiota, mechanisms between diet and cognition will be better understood.

Bone health

From a physical functioning perspective, bone health is also important in old age. The antithesis to bone health, osteoporosis, is a skeletal condition characterised by reduced bone strength, diminished bone density and deterioration in the microscopic architecture of bone. People achieve peak bone mass in their mid-twenties and experience decline in bone mass after about age 35 (Figure 18.3). Prevention of osteoporosis requires adequate calcium and vitamin D intake, regular weight-bearing physical activity,

FIGURE 18.3 CHANGES IN BONE MASS THROUGHOUT LIFE

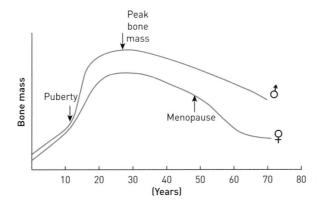

Source: R. Muir (2008). *Muir's Textbook of Pathology*, 14th edn. London: Hodder Arnold

and avoidance of smoking and excessive alcohol ingestion. Low bone density is the best predictor of fracture risk for those without prior adult fractures. Falls in older persons are common. After a first fall, about a third of patients have a drastic reduction in independence, and a third of cases result in serious injury and even death [45]. Older adults with compromised nutritional status have poorer medical outcomes after a hip fracture [46; 47]. The benefit of vitamin D supplementation in reducing the risk of fractures has been demonstrated [48; 49], but evidence for the role of vitamin D in prevention of falls is inconsistent [49].

> See Chapter 9 for more on Vitamin D.

Vitamin D deficiency has emerged as a significant public health issue in Australia. An estimated 31% of adults in Australia have inadequate vitamin D status (serum 25-hydroxyvitamin D [25-OHD] level <50 nmol/L), increasing to more than 50% in women during winter–spring and in people residing in southern states [48]. Risk factors for the prevalence of vitamin D deficiency include being housebound, **community-dwelling** disabled, those in residential care, having dark skin (particularly those modestly dressed), as well as limited sun exposure [49]. Most adults are unlikely to obtain more than 5–10% of their vitamin D requirement from dietary sources. The main source of vitamin D for people residing in Australia is exposure to sunlight. A 25-OHD level of ≥50 nmol/L at the end of winter (10–20 nmol/L higher at the end of summer, to allow for seasonal decrease) is required for optimal musculoskeletal health.

> **Community-dwelling**
> living within family and/or neighbourhood settings, not in an institution.

In order to maintain adequate vitamin D levels in the body, a walk with arms exposed for 6–7 minutes mid-morning or mid-afternoon in summer, and with as much bare skin exposed as feasible for 7–40 minutes (depending on latitude) at noon in winter, on most days, is recommended [50]. When sun exposure is minimal, vitamin D intake from dietary sources and supplementation of at least 600 IU (15 μg) per day for people aged ≤70 years and 800 IU (20 μg) per day for those aged >70 years is recommended. People in high-risk groups may require higher doses. There has been good evidence that vitamin D plus calcium supplementation may reduce fractures and falls in older men and women [47; 51–54]. However, the issue of supplementation continues to be open to debate, with new research emerging and authoritative statements being appropriately modified based on the body of evidence [52].

STOP AND THINK

• Why is it difficult to generalise about health risks of individuals, given the range of nutrition-associated problems seen in older age?

• How might some of these nutrition-related problems emerge from social and environmental or health conditions?

• What are some of the new opportunities for developing effective nutrition interventions during older age?

WHICH NUTRIENTS ARE OF PARTICULAR CONCERN IN OLD AGE?

In a general sense, adequate energy and protein intakes are key to addressing weight loss and preventing further muscle mass loss. Protein supplementation increases muscle mass, reduces complications, improves grip strength, produces weight gain [50], and also acts synergistically with resistance exercise in older persons [51; 52]. Correction of vitamin D deficiency is another nutritional strategy important for managing frailty and reducing the risk of falls, hip fractures and mortality [53–55]. There is limited evidence that vitamin D supplementation may also improve muscle function [56].

Evidence is inconsistent on the role of individual nutrients in the age disablement process, including physical and cognitive decline over time [57]; however, possible pathways linking nutrition and diet with frailty and disability are shown in Table 18.5. Nutritional epidemiology allows evaluation of the effects of overall dietary patterns and dietary quality on health outcomes. A greater adherence to a Mediterranean type of diet is significantly associated with a reduced risk of all-cause mortality [58], cardiovascular disease and cancer, as well as with a reduced incidence of Parkinson's disease and Alzheimer's disease [59], and a lower incidence of stroke [60]. Regarding mechanisms, a strong inverse association between the Mediterranean diet and oxidative stress has been demonstrated [61; 62]. The contribution of each of the individual components of the diet to the observed beneficial effects appear

TABLE 18.5   NUTRIENTS AT RISK FOR ADULTS >70 YEARS IDENTIFIED IN THE AUSTRALIAN HEALTH SURVEY 2011–12

Level of intake	Nutrient
At risk[1]	Calcium Vitamin B6 Magnesium
Marginal[2]	Fibre
Adequate[3]	Energy Protein
Above requirements	Iron Vitamin A, E Vitamin B1, B2, B12 Vitamin C

[1]Mean intakes less than 80% recommendations
[2]Around 16% below EARs
[3]Can be at risk if poor appetite/unwell

Source: Australian Bureau of Statistics (2014). *Australian Health Survey: Nutrition First results—Foods and nutrients, 2011–12.* Canberra: ABS

to be related to above median intakes of vegetables, fruits, cereals and fish, below median intakes of saturated fat, with a high ratio of unsaturated to saturated lipids being particularly important, as well as moderate alcohol consumption [58; 63–65]. Diets that contain predominantly plant-based foods (fruits, vegetables and vegetable oils) have also been linked with overall survival among older adults [66].

Along with dietary quality, dietary adequacy (amounts of nutrients and energy intake in line with recommendations) plays an important role at older ages, as nutrition deficits are found to be associated with **functional decline** [67]. Several studies have reported specific nutritional concerns in old age, including a high prevalence of vitamin D and vitamin B12 deficiency [68].

Functional decline
the reduction in ability to undertake usual activities.

Nutritional deficiencies in older persons have serious negative consequences, such as impaired immune function, poor wound healing, and loss of muscle mass, strength and function. Such outcomes result in an increased risk of infections, falls and fractures, and ultimately an increase in morbidity and mortality in frail older people.

With the exception of reduced energy requirements associated with a progressive decline in muscle mass throughout adult life, changes in body composition and digestive function increase requirements for several nutrients. A loss of skeletal muscle mass (i.e. sarcopaenia) results in a lowered metabolic rate and lowered muscle strength. With advancing age, the proportion of total body fat increases and the fat is redistributed from the extremities to the abdominal deposits. Age-related changes in body fat and muscle increase the risk of developing hypercholesterolaemia, atherosclerosis, hyperinsulinaemia, insulin resistance, type 2 diabetes and hypertension. Decreased physical activity, common in advanced age, appears to be a main contributor to age-associated changes in body fat and muscle.

>> RESEARCH AT WORK

CHANGES AFFECTING NUTRITIONAL REQUIREMENTS IN OLDER AGE

A longitudinal study of men has confirmed changes in body composition associated with ageing [20]. Fat mass increases with ageing and levels off at approximately 70 years. Fat-free mass increases slightly between age 20 and 47 years, and then steadily decreases at a non-linear rate with ageing, with approximately 40% of the loss in the eighth decade. The ageing trajectory for total body mass increases from age 20 to age 60, levels off and then decreases with ageing. The increase is primarily due to the increase in fat mass, and the decline after age 70 is due to the loss of fat-free mass. With ageing, there is a reduced capacity of the stomach to secrete hydrochloric acid, and this is probably the most significant change in gastrointestinal function in many older persons. Atrophy of the gastric mucosa (atrophic gastritis), which leads to a reduced secretion of acid, intrinsic factor and pepsin, appears to affect about a third of older persons. This leads to a lowered absorption of vitamin B12 and folate and reduced calcium and iron bioavailability.

A reduction in fat-free mass with age leads to a decrease in basal metabolic rate by about 2% per decade [69]. Physical activity usually declines and so does total energy expenditure [70]. Despite these changes, the demands for most vitamins, minerals and trace elements are not reduced or only slightly so, or in some cases increased (Table 18.6). In order to avoid deficiency in specific nutrients, older persons need to eat foods that have a high nutrient density to compensate for reduced food intakes in terms of quantity.

TABLE 18.6   AGE-RELATED PHYSIOLOGICAL CHANGES THAT AFFECT NUTRIENT REQUIREMENTS

Change in body composition or physiological function	Impact on nutrient requirement
↓ Muscle mass (sarcopaenia)	↓ Need for energy
↓ Taste and olfactory (smell) acuity	↑ Need for energy
↓ Bone density (osteopaenia)	↑ Need for calcium, vitamin D
↓ Calcium bioavailability	↑ Need for calcium, vitamin D
↓ Gastric acid (atrophic gastritis)	↑ Need for vitamin B12, folate, calcium, iron, zinc
↓ Skin capacity for cholecalciferol synthesis	↑ Need for vitamin D
↓ Hepatic uptake of retinol	↑ Need for vitamin A
↓ Efficiency in metabolic utilisation of pyridoxal	↑ Need for vitamin B6

Source: Adapted from I. Darnton-Hill, E. T. Coyne & M. L. Wahlqvist (2001). Assessment of nutrition status. In R. Ratnaike (ed.), *A Practical Guide to Geriatric Practice*. Sydney: McGraw-Hill

Recommendations for protein intake for maintenance needs remain the same over the life span, at 0.8 g of protein per kilogram of body weight. This value represents the minimum amount of protein required to avoid progressive loss of lean body mass in most individuals. However, this data was derived from short-term nitrogen balance studies in healthy young men and there has been much debate about the relevance for older age groups. Based on evidence that indicates that protein intake greater than the recommended dietary intake (RDI) can improve muscle mass, strength and function in older adults, higher protein intakes ranging from around 1 g/kg/day, up to about 1.5 g/kg/day, or 15–20% of energy have been recommended [71]. In addition, other factors, such as immune status, wound healing, blood pressure and bone health, may be improved by increasing protein intake above the RDI. Under physiological stress, older people may not be able to mobilise amino acids from the body pool to meet increased needs [72]. Protein requirements are higher still in older people who have acute or chronic illness, and/or are hospitalised [73], and are in the region of 1.2–1.5 g/kg/day in this group [71].

See Chapter 6 for more on protein.

TRY IT YOURSELF

Consider the use of these protein-rich foods as snacks for older people: cheese and biscuits; yoghurt; milk or milkshake; boiled egg; or salmon and salad sandwich. Which of the following would provide a protein-rich breakfast: toast and marmalade; omelette; muesli and milk; baked beans on toast and a glass of milk; or scrambled egg on toast?

How the protein in the diet is distributed across the day is also important. Some older adults do not consume enough protein at all, while others may consume much of their protein in a meal or two. To maximise muscle protein synthesis, it is preferred that protein is consumed in 25–30 g increments at meals across the day [74]. This further emphasises the importance of regular meals that include some protein-rich foods (e.g. eggs, dairy, fish, chicken, meat or legumes) on each occasion. This is important in the context of the position of the Society on Sarcopenia, Cachexia and Wasting Disease that exercise (both resistance and aerobic) in combination with adequate protein and energy intake is the key component for the prevention and management of sarcopaenia (www.cachexia.org).

Australia's Nutrient Reference Values (NRVs) distinguish between older adults aged 50–69 years and those aged 70-plus years. Nutrient requirement changes with advancing age are shown in Table 18.7.

TABLE 18.7 RECOMMENDED DIETARY INTAKE (RDI) AND ADEQUATE INTAKE (AI) OF NUTRIENTS FOR MEN AND WOMEN AGED 51 YEARS AND ABOVE

	Women 51–70 years	Women >70 years	Men 51–70 years	Men >70 years
Macronutrients				
Protein (RDI, g/day)	46	57	64	81
Dietary fats (AI, g/day) Linoleic acid A-linolenic acid LC n-3 (DHA/EPA/DPA)	8 0.8 90	8 0.8 90	13 1.3 160	13 1.3 160
Dietary fibre (AI, g/day)	25	25	30	30
Water (AI, L/day)	2.8 (2.1, fluid only)	2.8 (2.1, fluid only)	3.4 (2.6, fluid only)	3.4 (2.6, fluid only)
Micronutrients				
Vitamin A (retinol equivalents) (RDI, µg/day)	700	700	900	900
Thiamin (RDI, mg/day)	1.1	1.1	1.2	1.2
Riboflavin (RDI, mg/day)	1.1	1.3	1.3	1.6
Niacin (niacin equivalents) (RDI, mg/day)	14	14	16	16
Vitamin B6 (RDI, mg/day)	1.5	1.5	1.7	1.7
Vitamin B12 (RDI, µg/day)	2.4	2.4	2.4	2.4
Folate (folate equivalents) (RDI, µg/day)	400	400	400	400
Pantothenic acid (AI, mg/day)	4.0	4.0	6.0	6.0
Biotin (AI, µg/day)	25	25	30	30
Vitamin C (RDI, mg/day)	45	45	45	45
Vitamin D (RDI, mg/day)	10	15	10	15
Vitamin E (α-tocopherol equivalents) (AI, mg/day)	7	7	10	10
Calcium (RDI, mg/day)	1300	1300	1000	1300
Zinc (RDI, mg/day)	8	8	14	14
Iron (RDI, mg/day)	8	8	8	8

Source: National Health and Medical Research Council (2006). *Nutrient Reference Values for Australia and New Zealand, Including Recommended Dietary Intakes*. Canberra: NHMRC. © Commonwealth of Australia

STOP AND THINK

···

- How might nutritional requirements change for an older person, given the physical and cognitive changes that occur in the later years?
- Energy requirements may reduce with reductions in physical activity with age, but nutrient requirements do not decrease, and in some cases they may increase, particularly after 70 years of age. What does this mean for the types of foods that need to be in the diets of older people?
- Protein requirements are generally increased to avoid loss of muscle mass. What is the optimal amount of protein per kilogram body weight? How might this change if illness is present?

WHAT ARE THE RISK FACTORS ASSOCIATED WITH MALNUTRITION IN OLDER AGE?

The causes of malnutrition are multifactorial and are influenced by the metabolic effects of underlying disease, increased requirements and reduced nutritional intake. Other factors such as polypharmacy, educational level and living situation also increase the risk of nutritional deficits [75; 76]. Factors associated with malnutrition in older age are regular hospital readmission, social isolation, lack of availability of suitable foods and low muscle mass. Each of these is discussed in the following sections.

Regular hospital readmission

Tertiary care
residential facility for advanced medical and surgical treatment—that is, a hospital.

Older people are often admitted to **tertiary care** in a hospital in poor health, with multiple comorbidities such as heart and lung disease, chronic pain, dementia and depression, so the number of people with a suboptimal nutritional status, or who are 'at risk' before and on admission to hospital, is growing [77–80]. Acute illness and many chronic illnesses are characterised by hypercatabolism and hypermetabolism, which result in increased energy and protein requirements, particularly as people's reserves are often depleted. People with a lower energy intake the month before hospitalisation have been shown to have a reduced nutritional status compared with healthy people [81].

It is well known that chronically ill people, many of whom are older adults, will be in and out of hospital regularly. Adequate flagging of files on these people on admission is required, as is appropriate domiciliary follow-up on their discharge. McWhirter and Pennington [82] identified 40% of people as malnourished on admission to hospital, with three-quarters of them losing further weight when in hospital for more than one week. A mean weight loss of 5.4% during the hospital stay was reported, irrespective of the person's initial nutritional status. For many, nutritional status may continue to decline throughout their hospital stay [82–89]. Reasons for this decline may include: poor appetite and lack of interest in food, their medical condition, the variety of food options available, poor dentition, difficulty with manipulating cutlery and accessing food, lack of feeding assistance and encouragement, inaccessible food packaging, lack of recognition of malnutrition and referral for treatment, difficulties with chewing and swallowing, gastrointestinal upsets, malabsorption, depression and dementia [90–93].

Undernutrition and rapid weight loss of as little as 2–3 kg in combination with disease can increase the risk of complications, lower resistance to infection, impair physiological and mental functioning and delay recovery [94]. A patient who is consuming only 50% of their estimated daily requirements (semi-starvation) is likely to lose 15–20% of body weight in three to four weeks [95]. Undernutrition prolongs recovery and reduces quality of life [96–98]. It is suggested that functional ability is influenced with a weight loss of less than 10% [99], and nutrient deficiencies can be seen in people who have had a balanced diet withheld for as little as 10 days [100].

Risk factors for malnutrition in older people in the community include living alone, ill health, immobility, poor dentition, inability to shop and/or cook and social isolation [101]. Nutritional screening in the community, and certainly on admission to hospital, is essential to identify people who need additional nutrition support in a more time-efficient manner [102]. Innovative strategies are required to provide effective nutritional support and monitoring to the growing number of older community-dwelling adults who are at risk of malnutrition [101–105].

>> CASE 18.1

MALNUTRITION IN OLDER ADULTS IN THE COMMUNITY

Malnutrition is common among older Australians living in the community, with an estimated 10–44% of older people being at risk [103; 105; 106]. It is estimated that at least 5% of older Australians in the community are overtly malnourished, with this figure increasing to above 10% when people with one or more illnesses are included [89]. In Australia, as in many other countries, there may be problems with referral mechanisms operating between hospital and community-based medical services, perhaps with the exception of retired servicemen and servicewomen who fall under the care of the special services for the Department of Veterans' Affairs. An investigation of the home food environment of 512 older people in the United States who were transitioning from hospital to home found that, despite a variety of foods being available in their homes, a third of this group were unable to either shop or prepare food for themselves [107]. These two activities of daily living are important determinants of nutritional intake and functional ability in community-dwelling older people [108].

In 2016, the National Meal Guidelines for the Commonwealth Home Support Program were released [109]. They include recommendations regarding meals for older adults receiving home-delivered and centre-based meals [110]. As such services usually provide one meal per day, these guidelines also include much important advice about how to enrich meals and snacks and maximise nutritional intakes across the day [111; 112].

- What are the risk factors for malnutrition for community-dwelling older people?
- What recommendations can be made to further nutritionally support community-dwelling older people?
- Why might older people who are admitted to hospital in a malnourished state continue to lose weight?
- What food-based strategies can assist with intakes in hospital and on their return home?

Nutritional status tends to deteriorate in older people during a prolonged hospital stay. A study of predictors for early hospital readmission found that people with any amount of weight loss and no improvement in serum albumin during the first month after hospitalisation were at a higher risk of non-elective readmission than those who at least maintained or increased their weight and improved their serum albumin levels [113]. Hospitalised elderly people are often admitted with multiple medical problems; they may already be malnourished or may be at an increased risk of malnutrition prior to admission [114–116]. Malnourished people usually have longer lengths of stay (LOS) [117], generate increased hospital costs, and have increased rates of complications and an increased risk of adverse medical outcomes and mortality [118] than well-nourished people [115; 119–122].

>> RESEARCH AT WORK

IDENTIFYING MALNUTRITION IN HEALTHCARE SERVICES AND THE COMMUNITY

An Australian study of rehabilitation patients found that a larger proportion of malnourished patients were discharged to a higher level of residential care (32.8%, 17.0% and 4.9% for malnourished, at risk and well nourished, respectively). The risk of death at 18 months of follow-up in malnourished patients was 3.41 times those who were well nourished [118]. Adverse impacts of malnutrition have also been reported in community settings. Visvanathan and colleagues [103] studied 250 Australian elderly people living at home and receiving domiciliary care services. Initially, 38.4% of these people were nutritionally at risk, while 4.8% were malnourished. At one year follow-up, compared with those who were well nourished, those at risk or malnourished at baseline were more likely to have had two or more urgent admissions to hospital, a fall or weight loss, or to have spent more than four weeks in hospital (Figure 18.4).

FIGURE 18.4 SURVIVAL CURVE OF MORTALITY AT 18 MONTHS, ACCORDING TO CATEGORY OF NUTRITIONAL RISK

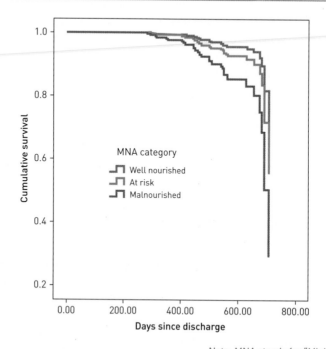

Note: MNA stands for "Mini Nutritional Assessment".

Source: K. Charlton, C. Nichols, S. Bowden, M. Milosavljevic, K. Lambert, L. Barone, et al. (2012). Poor nutritional status of older sub acute patients predicts clinical outcomes and mortality at 18 months of follow-up. *European Journal of Clinical Nutrition*, 66(11), 1224–8

Social isolation

Social isolation in the community can predispose people to malnutrition. Older community-dwelling adults may be vulnerable to malnutrition, and this may be very apparent to others in how they look (e.g. clothes look too big, belt taken in, loose rings, ill-fitting dentures), but they often do not perceive themselves to be at risk. They often reflect on how they were previously and may not see that they have lost weight and are at risk of malnutrition.

It is important that there are a number of strategies to assist in increasing nutritional intakes of older adults who are frail, have lost weight or who have a reduced appetite. Some examples include: having nourishing snacks between meals; enriching meals with additional protein; the importance of the social aspects of meals/eating with others; and receiving meal assistance or home-delivered meals, where required [123; 124]. Regular nutrition screening and assessment is a good way to monitor the nutritional status of older adults and this can be coordinated between community nurses, general practice settings and other community- and hospital-based care settings, highlighting the importance of communication.

Availability of suitable foods

It is important to consider a suitable texture; flavoursome foods (including a combination of sweet and savoury options); meal sizes that are not overwhelming; limitations from dentition issues; and the importance of snacks over the day when appetites are small or needs are increased.

Low muscle mass

Even if older people are generally well and do not suffer other chronic conditions or social isolation, the loss of muscle mass can be problematic. The Australian Longitudinal Study of Ageing found that a low corrected upper-arm muscle area (CUAMA) of <21.4 cm^2 (male) and <21.6 cm^2 (female) and weight loss of >10% body mass were independent predictors of mortality after eight years of follow-up [125]. Anthropometric measurements taken regularly provide useful information regarding changes in nutritional status over time and enable early detection of malnutrition. A number of different measurements can be taken, depending on the availability of equipment and the mobility of the older person, such as knee height, demi-span, mid-upper-arm muscle circumference (MUAC) and calf circumference (CC).

Given the significance of body weight and muscle mass in old age, being able to measure anthropometric indices is one of the first steps in addressing malnutrition in old age. A number of key measures are defined here. See also Table 18.8.

- *Weight:* may be estimated using calf circumference, knee height, MUAC, and subscapular skinfold measurements, using equations developed in the United States [126].
- *Height:* may not be able to be measured because of severe kyphosis, so estimated height can be calculated using an equation that incorporates knee height (the knee joint space-to-heel measurement (cm), measured from the sole of the foot at the heel to the anterior surface of the thigh with the foot and knee each flexed at 90°) [126]. The *arm span value*, which reflects the true length of the body frame, may be used instead of height [127].
- *BMI:* the optimal BMI range for older people is suggested to be about 23–30 kg/m^2 [28].
- *Triceps skinfold thickness (TSF):* provides a measure of subcutaneous fat.

- *Mid-upper-arm muscle circumference (MUAMC):* is derived from measurements of both the mid-upper arm circumference (MUAC) and TSF and can be used to assess protein-energy malnutrition, as the size of the muscle mass is an index of protein reserves. MUAMC measurement is most suitable for individuals who cannot be weighed, and for older persons with severe oedema in whom BMI or percentage weight loss may be misleadingly normal. At present, there are no reference values for MUAMC derived from samples of older persons.

TABLE 18.8   KEY ANTHROPOMETRIC MEASURES INDICATIVE OF BODY WEIGHT AND MUSCLE MASS IN OLD AGE

Measure	Descriptor
Weight	Men: Weight = 0.98 × calf circumference + 1.16 × knee height + 1.72 × MUAC + 0.4 × subscapular skinfold – 81.69
	Women: Weight = 1.27 × calf circumference + 0.87 × knee height + 0.89 × MUAC + 0.4 × subscapular skinfold – 62.35
Height	Men: Stature (cm) = [2.08 × knee height (cm)] + 59.01
	Women: Stature (cm) = [1.91 × knee height (cm)] – [0.17 × age (y)] + 75
Body mass index	Weight (kg) divided by height squared (m²)
Triceps skinfold thickness	Measured using calibrated callipers on the posterior surface of the arm, midway between the acromion process and the elbow (i.e. mid-upper arm) with the arm hanging loosely by the side, while the subject is in a standing position
Mid arm muscle circumference	Provides a measure of skeletal muscle mass and is calculated according to the formula:
	MUAMA (cm²) = {MUAC (cm) – [pTSF (mm)/10]}2/4p} where p = 3.14
	The corrected arm muscle area is often used since this estimates bone-free arm muscle area:
	Men: Corrected upper arm muscle area (CUAMA) = MUAMA (cm²) – 10
	Women: CUAMA = MUAMA (cm²) – 6.5

TRY IT YOURSELF

If you have access to a tape measure, try measuring the height, triceps skinfold thickness and mid-upper arm muscle circumference on a friend. Access to a floor scales and skinfold callipers (and appropriate training) would allow you to try additional measures.

STOP AND THINK

- Why is it important to screen for malnutrition in older adults undergoing regular hospital admission?
- How would social isolation contribute to malnutrition in older adults in the community?
- How could muscle mass be maintained during older age?

WHAT ARE THE PARTICULAR CONSIDERATIONS FOR OLDER PEOPLE LIVING IN INSTITUTIONAL SETTINGS?

Malnutrition is often seen among older people in institutionalised settings. Despite policies for detection and treatment of malnutrition being focused on the hospital setting, it is becoming recognised that most malnutrition is found in the community [128; 129]. For example, in the United Kingdom it has been estimated that more than three million individuals, about 93% of whom live in the community, are at risk of malnutrition, while only 2% of all malnutrition is found in hospitals [129]. In recognition of this, the National Institute for Health and Clinical Excellence [130] guidelines recommend that people should be screened not only on admission to hospitals but also on admission to aged care facilities, on their first outpatient appointment and on registration with a general practitioner.

In Australia, it is recommended that nutrition screening for older adults should occur not only in acute care, rehabilitation and **residential aged care** settings, but also regularly as part of general practice health assessments and eligibility assessments in community programs for the elderly [131]. Timely screening of older adults in general practice and community settings, and referral where required to dietitians for further nutrition assessment and support, can improve their nutritional status [132; 133]. National nutrition screening initiatives for older adults have been adopted in some countries, notably the Nutrition Screening Initiative (NSI) in the United States, which uses a self-administered 10-item checklist with the acronym DETERMINE [134; 135].

> **Residential aged care** facilities providing long-term care for older people requiring various degrees of assistance with daily living.

Malnutrition screening

There are validated instruments to assess nutritional status. The Patient Generated Subjective Global Assessment (PG-SGA) is a modified version of the SGA that is used by some researchers, which includes a score from 0 to 35, with 35 representing the highest risk of malnutrition. The validity of this tool has been determined in a number of patient groups [136; 137]. The 18-item Mini Nutritional Assessment (MNA) [138] is valid for use with community-dwelling older adults and those in care and is scored as follows: malnourished (score <17); at risk of malnutrition (17–23.9); and well nourished (≥24). The MNA comprises four domains including anthropometric assessment (recent weight loss, BMI, mid-arm circumference [MAC] and CC), global assessment (lifestyle, mobility and medications taken), dietary assessment (changes in appetite, meals per day, and daily intake of protein, fruit, vegetables and fluid) and subjective assessment (self-perception of health and nutritional status).

The usefulness of applying consistent criteria across all care settings, including the community, has been demonstrated by the British Association for Parenteral and Enteral Nutrition (BAPEN) large-scale Nutrition Screening Week surveys in the United Kingdom. Using the Malnutrition Universal Screening Tool (MUST), 28% of individuals were malnourished on admission to hospital, compared with 30–40% of those admitted to nursing care homes in the previous six months; 16–20% of outpatients were malnourished, as well as 10–14% of elderly tenants in sheltered housing accommodation. In terms of absolute numbers, there are more people at risk of malnutrition living in sheltered housing schemes than in hospitals [129]. This data highlights the need for integrated strategies to detect and treat malnutrition risk between and within care settings.

Globally, the prevalence of malnutrition in older adults has been reported to be highest in rehabilitation (51%) and acute (39%) hospital settings, but has also been detected in 50% of nursing home residents [90] and 6% of community-dwelling elderly [139]. Many countries, including Australia, have adopted clinical guidelines that recommend nutrition screening of people admitted to hospital [130; 140; 141]. But guidelines do not necessarily translate into practice. A 25-country study in Europe and Israel that included more than 21,000 patients reported wide variation in nutrition screening practices both between and within countries [142].

The combination of poor monitoring of nutritional status, inadequate nutrient intake and increased nutritional requirements during acute hospital admissions means that by the time people are discharged to rehabilitation facilities (also known as sub-acute care hospitals), they are often at higher risk of malnutrition than those in acute settings. The failure to recognise people in hospital who are at risk of malnutrition and subsequent implementation of timely nutritional intervention often results in a downward spiral whereby they are discharged back to the community or to a higher level of care, only to be readmitted later in a more compromised nutritional state. An Australian study reported that less than a quarter (23%) of older people in rehabilitation hospitals were able to consume enough energy through oral intake, including supplement prescription, despite being provided with their energy and protein requirements [143].

>> CASE 18.2

THE COSTS OF MALNUTRITION IN HOSPITALISED PATIENTS

Malnutrition is a recognised problem in older institutionalised people. How to spend the health dollar is always a controversial area. In 2006–07, one-third of all public hospital patients in New South Wales were aged over 65 years, although that group made up only 13.5% of the state's population. By 2010, those aged over 65 made up 45% of all public hospital patients [144]. Given these statistics, the high prevalence of malnutrition in older patients, coupled with the associated prolonged length of hospital stay, has significant implications for healthcare costs. Estimates from the United Kingdom indicate that malnutrition-related costs are £7.3 billion each year, more than double the projected £3.5 billion cost of obesity [129]. The bulk of these costs arise from the treatment of malnourished patients in hospital (£3.8 billion) and in long-term care facilities (£2.6 billion), followed by general practitioner visits (£0.49 billion), outpatient visits (£0.36 billion), and enteral and parenteral nutrition, tube feeding and oral nutritional supplementation in the community (£0.15 billion). The costs and average length of stay of patients receiving one of the following three interventions—high-quality nutrition support (early intervention, HPHE nutrition support and frequent review), medium-quality nutrition support (early intervention or frequent review) and low-quality nutrition support (infrequent, or late review)—were assessed. Providing high-quality care would require nutrition services to be increased by over 100%; however, a cost–benefit analysis in the United States found that for every $1 spent on quality nutrition care, $4.83 could be saved [145].

>> RESEARCH AT WORK

MALNUTRITION SCREENING TOOLS

Nutrition screening tools are used to assess the possible presence and severity of nutrition-related problems for the purposes of further assessment of nutritional status and seeking help. A number of validated nutrition screening instruments are available, including the Malnutrition Universal Screening

Tool (MUST) [146], Short Nutritional Assessment Questionnaire (SNAQ) [147], Nutritional Risk Screening 2002 (NRS) [148] and Malnutrition Screening Tool (MST) [149]. For older patients, the Mini Nutritional Assessment Short-Form (MNA-SF) [16; 150; 151] is recommended as it is the only instrument to have been validated in older people, specifically, from various settings and countries, including Australia [152]. The MNA-SF includes a measurement of BMI, or calf circumference (CC) that can be substituted for BMI if weight and height measurements are not readily available, or for those who are immobile or bedbound. The MNA-SF is quick and easy to use (takes about five minutes), is possible to administer in a wide variety of settings, requires no special training or blood sampling and targets frail older adults and the at-risk elderly population.

STOP AND THINK

- What are the particular nutritional concerns for older adults living in residential care services?
- How might nutritional support be ensured?
- What skills would be required of a healthcare team working together with older adults and their families to prevent nutritional problems from developing?

SUMMARY

- Establishing nutritional balance is a goal for nutrition throughout life.
- In older ages, the concerns vary and the special needs of older people should be considered depending on their circumstances.
- Concern for adequate nutrition is a major issue in old age, demanding an emphasis on nutritional assessment and the need to meet additional nutritional requirements.
- There are many causes for malnutrition in older people and it may be the result of underlying disease as well as inadequate nutritional intakes.
- Malnutrition in older people is associated with poor clinical outcomes, so it is important that it is taken seriously at all levels of care, and that services are developed across the community to prevent, and treat, its occurrence.

PATHWAYS TO PRACTICE

- Families, community members and healthcare workers all have a role to play in supporting the nutritional health of older Australian adults.
- Everyone associated with older adults should be able to identify risk conditions and be aware of health and community services that support adequate nutrition.
- Additional training and skills may be required for conducting nutrition assessments (including anthropometric assessments), but effective teamwork will prevail.
- Public health campaigns can promote the availability of nutritious foods for older adults and enable activity that promotes functional capacity, including the maintenance of muscle mass.

     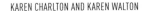KAREN CHARLTON AND KAREN WALTON

DISCUSSION QUESTIONS

1   Why are older people at greater risk of nutrition-related problems compared with younger adults in the community?
2   Which conditions that often develop with ageing require particular attention to intakes of specific nutrients?
3   Which processes in institutional settings may need attention to prevent the occurrence of malnutrition in older people?
4   What are the particular implications for nutrition when older people return to community living after being hospitalised?
5   Which are the best nutritional screening tools? Why is follow-up important?
6   How could the approaches to increasing energy and protein intakes for older people at risk be seen to be opposite to the dietary guideline recommendations?

USEFUL WEBLINKS

Ageing and Aged Care—Department of Health:
    https://agedcare.health.gov.au

Alzheimer's Australia:
    www.fightdementia.org.au

Australian and New Zealand Society of Geriatric Medicine:
    www.anzsgm.org

Australian Meals on Wheels Association (AMOWA):
    http://mealsonwheels.org.au

Global Aging Research Network, International Association of Gerontology and Geriatrics:
    www.garn-network.org

Guidelines for Food Service to Vulnerable Persons (2015):
    www.foodauthority.nsw.gov.au

Healthy Eating. A guide for older people living with diabetes:
    www.diabetesaustralia.com.au

Healthy Eating for Adults. Eat for Health and Wellbeing:
    www.eatforhealth.gov.au/sites/default/files/files/the_guidelines/n55g_adult_brochure.pdf

Nestlé Nutrition Institute—MNA Elderly:
    www.mna-elderly.com

Nutrition Standards for Adult Inpatients in NSW Hospitals:
    www.aci.health.nsw.gov.au

Society on Sarcopenia, Cachexia and Wasting Disorders:
    www.cachexia.org

Therapeutic Diet Specifications for Adult Inpatients:
    www.aci.health.nsw.gov.au

OXFORD UNIVERSITY PRESS

FURTHER READING

An, R. (2015). Association of home-delivered meals on daily energy and nutrient intakes: findings from the national health and nutrition examination surveys. *Journal of Nutrition in Gerontology and Geriatrics*, 34(2), 263–72. doi:10.1080/21551197.2015.1031604

Bowman, K., Atkins, J. L., Delgado, J., Kos, K., Kuchel, G. A., Ble, A., ... Melzer, D. (2017). Central adiposity and the overweight risk paradox in aging: follow-up of 130,473 UK Biobank participants. *American Journal of Clinical Nutrition*, 106(1), 130–5. doi:10.3945/ajcn.116.147157

Campbell, A. D., Godfryd, A., Buys, D. R. & Locher, J. L. (2015). Does participation in home-delivered meals programs improve outcomes for older adults? Results of a systematic review. *Journal of Nutrition in Gerontology and Geriatrics*, 34(2), 124–67. doi:10.1080/21551197.2015.1038463

Darnton-Hill, I., Coyne, E. T. & Wahlqvist, M. L. (2001). Assessment of nutrition status. In R. Ratnaike (ed.), *A Practical Guide to Geriatric Practice*. Sydney: McGraw-Hill

Farsijani, S., Payette, H., Morais, J. A., Shatenstein, B., Gaudreau, P. & Chevalier, S. (2017). Even mealtime distribution of protein intake is associated with greater muscle strength, but not with 3-y physical function decline, in free-living older adults: the Quebec longitudinal study on Nutrition as a Determinant of Successful Aging (NuAge study). *American Journal of Clinical Nutrition*, 106(1), 113–24. doi:10.3945/ajcn.116.146555

Fávaro-Moreira, N. C., Krausch-Hofmann, S., Matthys, C., Vereecken, C., Vanhauwaert, E., Declercq, A., ... Duyck, J. (2016). Risk factors for malnutrition in older adults: a systematic review of the literature based on longitudinal data. *Advances in Nutrition: An International Review Journal*, 7(3), 507–22. doi:10.3945/an.115.011254

Gheller, B. J. F., Riddle, E. S., Lem, M. R. & Thalacker-Mercer, A. E. (2016). Understanding age-related changes in skeletal muscle metabolism: differences between females and males. *Annual Review of Nutrition*, 36(1), 129–56. doi:10.1146/annurev-nutr-071715-050901

Hess, D. B., Norton, J. T., Park, J. & Street, D. A. (2016). Driving decisions of older adults receiving meal delivery: the influence of individual characteristics, the built environment, and neighborhood familiarity. *Transportation Research Part A: Policy and Practice*, 88, 73–85. doi:10.1016/j.tra.2016.03.011

Hozid, Z. & Fazzino, D. (2016). The sociological imagination of meals on wheels: how a home delivered meal program sheds light onto larger social issues. *Social Work and Society*, 14(2), 1–49.

Lagari, V. S. & Levis, S. (2016). Implementation of a feasible monthly vitamin D intervention in homebound older adults using a Meals-on-Wheels programme. *Evidence-Based Nursing*, 19(3), 96. doi:10.1136/eb-2016-102331

Loughrey, D. G., Lavecchia, S., Brennan, S., Lawlor, B. A. & Kelly, M. E. (2017). The impact of the Mediterranean diet on the cognitive functioning of healthy older adults: a systematic review and meta-analysis. *Advances in Nutrition: An International Review Journal*, 8(4), 571–86. doi:10.3945/an.117.015495

Ma, W., Hagan, K. A., Heianza, Y., Sun, Q., Rimm, E. B. & Qi, L. (2017). Adult height, dietary patterns, and healthy aging. *American Journal of Clinical Nutrition*, 106(2), 589–96. doi:10.3945/ajcn.116.147256

Miller, M. G., Thangthaeng, N., Poulose, S. M. & Shukitt-Hale, B. (2017). Role of fruits, nuts, and vegetables in maintaining cognitive health. *Experimental Gerontology*, 94, 24–8. doi:10.1016/j.exger.2016.12.014

Oppenheimer, M., Warburton, J. & Carey, J. (2015). The next 'new' idea: the challenges of organizational change, decline and renewal in Australian Meals on Wheels. *Voluntas*, 26(4), 1550–69. doi:10.1007/s11266-014-9488-4

Owsley, C. (2016). Vision and aging. *Annual Review of Vision Science*, 2(1), 255–71. doi:10.1146/annurev-vision-111815-114550

Petersson, S. D. & Philippou, E. (2016). Mediterranean diet, cognitive function, and dementia: a systematic review of the evidence. *Advances in Nutrition: An International Review Journal*, 7(5), 889–904. doi:10.3945/an.116.012138

Rowe, J. W., Fulmer, T. & Fried, L. (2016). Preparing for better health and health care for an aging population. *JAMA—Journal of the American Medical Association*, 316(16), 1643–4. doi:10.1001/jama.2016.12335

Shlisky, J., Bloom, D. E., Beaudreault, A. R., Tucker, K. L., Keller, H. H., Freund-Levi, Y., ... Meydani, S. N. (2017). Nutritional considerations for healthy aging and reduction in age-related chronic disease. *Advances in Nutrition: An International Review Journal*, 8(1), 17–26. doi:10.3945/an.116.013474

Soultoukis, G. A. & Partridge, L. (2016). Dietary protein, metabolism, and aging. *Annual Review of Biochemistry*, 85(1), 5–34. doi:10.1146/annurev-biochem-060815-014422

Thomas, K. S., Akobundu, U. & Dosa, D. (2016). More than a meal? A randomized control trial comparing the effects of home-delivered meals programs on participants' feelings of loneliness. *Journals of Gerontology—Series B Psychological Sciences and Social Sciences*, 71(6), 1049–58. doi:10.1093/geronb/gbv111

van de Rest, O., Berendsen, A. A., Haveman-Nies, A. & de Groot, L. C. (2015). Dietary patterns, cognitive decline, and dementia: a systematic review. *Advances in Nutrition: An International Review Journal*, 6(2), 154–68. doi:10.3945/an.114.007617

Wolfe, R. R. (2015). Update on protein intake: importance of milk proteins for health status of the elderly. *Nutrition Reviews*, 73(suppl. 1), 41–7. doi:10.1093/nutrit/nuv021

Ziylan, C., Haveman-Nies, A., Kremer, S. & de Groot, L. C. P. G. M. (2017). Protein-enriched bread and readymade meals increase community-dwelling older adults' protein intake in a double-blind randomized controlled trial. *Journal of the American Medical Directors Association*, 18(2), 145–51. doi:10.1016/j.jamda.2016.08.018

REFERENCES

1   J. W. Rowe & R. L. Kahn (1987). Human aging: usual and successful. *Science*, 237(4811), 143–9.

2   Australian Institute of Health and Welfare (2007). *Older Australia at a Glance*, 4th edn. Canberra: AIHW.

3   World Health Organization (2015). *World Report on Ageing and Health*. WHO: Geneva. Retrieved from: http://apps.who.int/iris/bitstream/handle/10665/186463/9789240694811_eng.pdf;jsessionid=8B0CB7F139AC6B82C202E41B205B26AF?sequence=1.

4   L. P. Fried, C. M. Tangen, J. Walston, A. B. Newman, C. Hirsch, J. Gottdiener, ... M. A. McBurnie (2001). Frailty in older adults: evidence for a phenotype. *Journals of Gerontology: Series A*, 56(3), M146–M157. doi:10.1093/gerona/56.3.M146

5   K. Rockwood & A. Mitnitski (2007). Frailty in relation to the accumulation of deficits. *Journals of Gerontology: Series A*, 62(7), 722–7. doi:10.1093/gerona/62.7.722

6   J. E. Morley, B. Vellas, G. A. van Kan, S. D. Anker, J. M. Bauer, R. Bernabei, ... J. Walston (2013). Frailty consensus: a call to action. *Journal of the American Medical Directors Association*, 14(6), 392–7. doi:10.1016/j.jamda.2013.03.022

7   C.V. Laur, T. McNicholl, R. Valaitis & H. H. Keller (2017). Malnutrition or frailty? Overlap and evidence gaps in the diagnosis and treatment of frailty and malnutrition. *Applied Physiology, Nutrition, and Metabolism*, 42(5), 449–58. doi:10.1139/apnm-2016-0652

8   B. Vellas, M. Cesari & J. Li (2016). *The White Book of Frailty*. France: Global Aging Research Network, International Association of Gerontology and Geriatrics..

9   K. N. Jeejeebhoy (2012). Malnutrition, fatigue, frailty, vulnerability, sarcopenia and cachexia: overlap of clinical features. *Current Opinion in Clinical Nutrition & Metabolic Care*, 15(3), 213–19. doi:10.1097/MCO.0b013e328352694f

10 G. A. Van Kan, Y. Rolland, H. Bergman, J. E. Morley, S. B. Kritchevsky & B. Vellas (2008). The IANA task force on frailty assessment of older people in clinical practice. *Journal of Nutrition Health and Aging*, 12(1), 29–37. doi:10.1007/bf02982161

11 T. Cederholm, I. Bosaeus, R. Barazzoni, J. Bauer, A. Van Gossum, S. Klek, ... P. Singer (2015). Diagnostic criteria for malnutrition—an ESPEN Consensus Statement. *Clinical Nutrition*, 34(3), 335–40. doi:https://doi.org/10.1016/j.clnu.2015.03.001

12 J.V. White, P. Guenter, G. Jensen, A. Malone & M. Schofield (2012). Consensus Statement of the Academy of Nutrition and Dietetics/American Society for Parenteral and Enteral Nutrition: characteristics recommended for the identification and documentation of adult malnutrition (undernutrition). *Journal of the Academy of Nutrition and Dietetics*, 112(5), 730–8. doi:https://doi.org/10.1016/j.jand.2012.03.012

13 K. Rockwood, X. Song, C. MacKnight, H. Bergman, D. B. Hogan, I. McDowell & A. Mitnitski (2005). A global clinical measure of fitness and frailty in elderly people. *Canadian Medical Association Journal*, 173(5), 489–95. doi:10.1503/cmaj.050051

14 A. Detsky, J. McLaughlin, J. Baker, N. Johnston, S. Whittaker, R. Mendelson & K. Jeejeebhoy (1987). What is subjective global assessment of nutritional status? *Journal of Parenteral and Enteral Nutrition*, 11(1), 8–13. doi:10.1177/014860718701100108

15 J. Subra, S. Gillette-Guyonnet, M. Cesari, S. Oustric & B. Vellas (2012). The integration of frailty into clinical practice: preliminary results from the Gérontopôle. *Journal of Nutrition, Health and Aging*, 16(8), 714–20. doi:10.1007/s12603-012-0391-7

16 B. Vellas, Y. Guigoz, P. J. Garry, F. Nourhashemi, D. Bennahum, S. Lauque & J. L. Albarede (1999). The Mini Nutritional Assessment (MNA) and its use in grading the nutritional state of elderly patients. *Nutrition*, 15(2), 116–22.

17 B. H. Goodpaster, C. L. Carlson, M. Visser, D. E. Kelley, A. Scherzinger, T. B. Harris, ... A. B. Newman (2001). Attenuation of skeletal muscle and strength in the elderly: the Health ABC Study. *Journal of Applied Physiology*, 90(6), 2157–65.

18 B. H. Goodpaster, S. W. Park, T. B. Harris, S. B. Kritchevsky, M. Nevitt, A. V. Schwartz, ... A. B. Newman (2006). The loss of skeletal muscle strength, mass, and quality in older adults: the health, aging and body composition study. *Journals of Gerontology: Series A*, 61(10), 1059–64.

19 M. Visser, B. H. Goodpaster, S. B. Kritchevsky, A. B. Newman, M. Nevitt, S. M. Rubin, ... T. B. Harris (2005). Muscle mass, muscle strength, and muscle fat infiltration as predictors of incident mobility limitations in well-functioning older persons. *Journals of Gerontology: Series A*, 60(3), 324–33.

20 A. S. Jackson, I. Janssen, X. Sui, T. S. Church & S. N. Blair (2012). Longitudinal changes in body composition associated with healthy ageing: men, aged 20–96 years. *British Journal of Nutrition*, 107(7), 1085–91. doi:10.1017/s0007114511003886

21 S. Stenholm, T. B. Harris, T. Rantanen, M. Visser, S. B. Kritchevsky & L. Ferrucci (2008). Sarcopenic obesity—definition, etiology and consequences. *Current Opinion in Clinical Nutrition and Metabolic Care*, 11(6), 693–700. doi:10.1097/MCO.0b013e328312c37d

22 D. Paddon-Jones, E. Westman, R. D. Mattes, R. R. Wolfe, A. Astrup & M. Westerterp-Plantenga (2008). Protein, weight management, and satiety. *American Journal of Clinical Nutrition*, 87(5), 1558s–1561s.

23 L. Flicker, K. A. McCaul, G. J. Hankey, K. Jamrozik, W. J. Brown, J. E. Byles & O. P. Almeida (2010). Body mass index and survival in men and women aged 70 to 75. *Journal of the American Geriatric Society*, 58(2), 234–41. doi:10.1111/j.1532-5415.2009.02677.x

24 K. N. Porter Starr & C. W. Bales (2015). Excessive body weight in older adults: concerns and recommendations. *Clinics in Geriatric Medicine*, 31(3), 311–26. doi:10.1016/j.cger.2015.04.001

25 J. Piątek, A. Kędziora, J. Konstanty-Kalandyk, G. Kiełbasa, M. Olszewska, B. H. Song, ... B. Kapelak (2016). Risk factors for in-hospital mortality after coronary artery bypass grafting in patients 80 years old or older: a retrospective case-series study. *PeerJ*, 4, e2667. doi:10.7717/peerj.2667

26 J. A. Batsis, J. M. Huddleston, L. J. Melton, P. M. Huddleston, D. R. Larson, R. E. Gullerud & M. M. McMahon (2009). Body mass index and risk of non-cardiac post-operative medical complications in elderly hip fracture patients: a population-based study. *Journal of Hospital Medicine: An Official Publication of the Society of Hospital Medicine*, 4(8), E1–E9. doi:10.1002/jhm.527

27 P. Kirchhoff, P.-A. Clavien & D. Hahnloser (2010). Complications in colorectal surgery: risk factors and preventive strategies. *Patient Safety in Surgery*, 4, 5–5. doi:10.1186/1754-9493-4-5

28 J. E. Winter, R. J. MacInnis, N. Wattanapenpaiboon & C. A. Nowson (2014). BMI and all-cause mortality in older adults: a meta-analysis. *American Journal of Clinical Nutrition*, 99(4), 875–90. doi:10.3945/ajcn.113.068122

29 S. Gillette Guyonnet, G. Abellan Van Kan, E. Alix, S. Andrieu, J. Belmin, G. Berrut, ... B. Vellas (2007). IANA (International Academy on Nutrition and Aging) Expert Group: weight loss and Alzheimer's disease. *Journal of Nutrition, Health and Aging*, 11(1), 38–48.

30 S. Gillette Guyonnet, G. Abellan Van Kan, S. Andrieu, P. Barberger Gateau, C. Berr, M. Bonnefoy, ... B. Vellas (2007). IANA task force on nutrition and cognitive decline with aging. *Journal of Nutrition, Health and Aging*, 11(2), 132–52.

31 N. Scarmeas, Y. Stern, M. X. Tang, R. Mayeux & J. A. Luchsinger (2006). Mediterranean diet and risk for Alzheimer's disease. *Annals of Neurology*, 59(6), 912–21. doi:10.1002/ana.20854

32 S. J. Eussen, L. C. de Groot, L. W. Joosten, R. J. Bloo, R. Clarke, P. M. Ueland, ... W. A. van Staveren (2006). Effect of oral vitamin B-12 with or without folic acid on cognitive function in older people with mild vitamin B-12 deficiency: a randomized, placebo-controlled trial. *American Journal of Clinical Nutrition*, 84(2), 361–70.

33 M. Wolters, M. Hickstein, A. Flintermann, U. Tewes & A. Hahn (2005). Cognitive performance in relation to vitamin status in healthy elderly German women—the effect of 6-month multivitamin supplementation. *Preventive Medicine*, 41(1), 253–9. doi:10.1016/j.ypmed.2004.11.007

34 D. Vauzour, M. Camprubi-Robles, S. Miquel-Kergoat, C. Andres-Lacueva, D. Bánáti, P. Barberger-Gateau, ... M. Ramirez (2017). Nutrition for the ageing brain: towards evidence for an optimal diet. *Ageing Research Reviews*, 35, 222–40. doi:https://doi.org/10.1016/j.arr.2016.09.010

35 J. Rodakowski, E. Saghafi, M. A. Butters & E. R. Skidmore (2015). Non-pharmacological interventions for adults with mild cognitive impairment and early stage dementia: an updated scoping review. *Molecular Aspects of Medicine*, 43–4, 38–53. doi:10.1016/j.mam.2015.06.003

36 K. Kent, K. E. Charlton, M. Netzel & K. Fanning (2017). Food-based anthocyanin intake and cognitive outcomes in human intervention trials: a systematic review. *Journal of Human Nutrition and Dietetics*, 30(3), 260–74. doi:10.1111/jhn.12431

37 K. A. Youdim & J. A. Joseph (2001). A possible emerging role of phytochemicals in improving age-related neurological dysfunctions: a multiplicity of effects. *Free Radical Biology and Medicine*, 30(6), 583–94.

38 C. Andres-Lacueva, B. Shukitt-Hale, R. L. Galli, O. Jauregui, R. M. Lamuela-Raventos & J. A. Joseph (2005). Anthocyanins in aged blueberry-fed rats are found centrally and may enhance memory. *Nutritional Neuroscience*, 8(2), 111–20. doi:10.1080/10284150500078117

39 K. Kent, K. Charlton, S. Roodenrys, M. Batterham, J. Potter, V. Traynor, ... R. Richards (2017). Consumption of anthocyanin-rich cherry juice for 12 weeks improves memory and cognition in older adults with mild-to-moderate dementia. *European Journal of Nutrition*, 56(1), 333–41. doi:10.1007/s00394-015-1083-y

40 R. Krikorian, E. L. Boespflug, D. E. Fleck, A. L. Stein, J. D. Wightman, M. D. Shidler & S. Sadat-Hossieny (2012). Concord grape juice supplementation and neurocognitive function in human aging. *Journal of Agricultural and Food Chemistry*, 60(23), 5736–42. doi:10.1021/jf300277g

41 R. Krikorian, M. D. Shidler, T. A. Nash, W. Kalt, M. R. Vinqvist-Tymchuk, B. Shukitt-Hale & J. A. Joseph (2010). Blueberry supplementation improves memory in older adults. *Journal of Agricultural and Food Chemistry*, 58(7), 3996–4000. doi:10.1021/jf9029332

42 K. I. Erickson, D. L. Miller & K. A. Roecklein (2012). The aging hippocampus: interactions between exercise, depression, and BDNF. *Neuroscientist*, 18(1), 82–97. doi:10.1177/1073858410397054

43 J. Tanaka, Y. Horiike, M. Matsuzaki, T. Miyazaki, G. C. Ellis-Davies & H. Kasai (2008). Protein synthesis and neurotrophin-dependent structural plasticity of single dendritic spines. *Science*, 319(5870), 1683–7. doi:10.1126/science.1152864

44 K. Kent, K. E. Charlton, A. Jenner & S. Roodenrys (2016). Acute reduction in blood pressure following consumption of anthocyanin-rich cherry juice may be dose-interval dependant: a pilot cross-over study. *International Journal of Food Sciences and Nutrition*, 67(1), 47–52. doi:10.3109/09637486.2015.1121472

45 T. S. Wei, C. H. Hu, S. H. Wang & K. L. Hwang (2001). Fall characteristics, functional mobility and bone mineral density as risk factors of hip fracture in the community-dwelling ambulatory elderly. *Osteoporosis International*, 12(12), 1050–5.

46 M. D. Bastow, J. Rawlings & S. P. Allison (1983). Undernutrition, hypothermia, and injury in elderly women with fractured femur: an injury response to altered metabolism? *The Lancet*, 1(8317), 143–6.

47 M. D. Bastow, J. Rawlings & S. P. Allison (1983). Benefits of supplementary tube feeding after fractured neck of femur: a randomised controlled trial. *British Medical Journal (Clinical Research Edn)*, 287(6405), 1589–92.

48 M. C. Chapuy, M. E. Arlot, F. Duboeuf, J. Brun, B. Crouzet, S. Arnaud, ... P. J. Meunier (1992). Vitamin D3 and calcium to prevent hip fractures in elderly women. *New England Journal of Medicine*, 327(23), 1637–42. doi:10.1056/nejm199212033272305

49 H. A. Bischoff-Ferrari, B. Dawson-Hughes, H. B. Staehelin, J. E. Orav, A. E. Stuck, R. Theiler, ... J. Henschkowski (2009). Fall prevention with supplemental and active forms of vitamin D: a meta-analysis of randomised controlled trials. *British Medical Journal*, 339. doi:10.1136/bmj.b3692

50 A. L. Cawood, M. Elia & R. J. Stratton (2012). Systematic review and meta-analysis of the effects of high protein oral nutritional supplements. *Ageing Research Reviews*, 11(2), 278–96. doi:10.1016/j.arr.2011.12.008

51 D. Paddon-Jones (2013). Perspective: exercise and protein supplementation in frail elders. *Journal of the American Medical Directors Association*, 14(1), 73–4. doi:10.1016/j.jamda.2012.09.028

52 V. Malafarina, F. Uriz-Otano, R. Iniesta & L. Gil-Guerrero (2013). Effectiveness of nutritional supplementation on muscle mass in treatment of sarcopenia in old age: a systematic review. *Journal of the American Medical Directors Association*, 14(1), 10–17. doi:10.1016/j.jamda.2012.08.001

53 M. H. Murad, K. B. Elamin, N. O. Abu Elnour, M. B. Elamin, A. A. Alkatib, M. M. Fatourechi, ... V. M. Montori (2011). Clinical review: the effect of vitamin D on falls: a systematic review and meta-analysis. *Journal of Clinical Endocrinology and Metabolism*, 96(10), 2997–3006. doi:10.1210/jc.2011-1193

54 H. A. Bischoff-Ferrari, W. C. Willett, E. J. Orav, P. Lips, P. J. Meunier, R. A. Lyons, ... B. Dawson-Hughes (2012). A pooled analysis of vitamin D dose requirements for fracture prevention. *New England Journal of Medicine*, 367(1), 40–9. doi:10.1056/NEJMoa1109617

55 L. Rejnmark, A. Avenell, T. Masud, F. Anderson, H. E. Meyer, K. M. Sanders, ... B. Abrahamsen (2012). Vitamin D with calcium reduces mortality: patient level pooled analysis of 70,528 patients from eight major vitamin D trials. *Journal of Clinical Endocrinology and Metabolism*, 97(8), 2670–81. doi:10.1210/jc.2011-3328

56 S. W. Muir & M. Montero-Odasso (2011). Effect of vitamin D supplementation on muscle strength, gait and balance in older adults: a systematic review and meta-analysis. *Journal of the American Geriatric Society*, 59(12), 2291–300. doi:10.1111/j.1532-5415.2011.03733.x

57 M. Inzitari, E. Doets, B. Bartali, V. Benetou, M. Di Bari, M. Visser, ... A. Salva (2011). Nutrition in the age-related disablement process. *Journal of Nutrition, Health and Aging*, 15(8), 599–604.

58 A. Trichopoulou, C. Bamia, T. Norat, K. Overvad, E. B. Schmidt, A. Tjonneland, ... D. Trichopoulos (2007). Modified Mediterranean diet and survival after myocardial infarction: the EPIC-Elderly study. *European Journal of Epidemiology*, 22(12), 871–81. doi:10.1007/s10654-007-9190-6

59 F. Sofi, F. Cesari, R. Abbate, G. F. Gensini & A. Casini (2008). Adherence to Mediterranean diet and health status: meta-analysis. *British Medical Journal*, 337. doi:10.1136/bmj.a1344

60 A. M. Euser, M. J. Finken, M. G. Keijzer-Veen, E. T. Hille, J. M. Wit, F. W. Dekker & Dutch POPS-19 Collaborative Study Group (2005). Associations between prenatal and infancy weight gain and BMI, fat mass, and fat distribution in young adulthood: a prospective cohort study in males and females born very preterm. *American Journal of Clinical Nutrition*, 81(2), 480–7.

61 T. T. Fung, K. M. Rexrode, C. S. Mantzoros, J. E. Manson, W. C. Willett & F. B. Hu (2009). Mediterranean diet and incidence of and mortality from coronary heart disease and stroke in women. *Circulation*, 119(8), 1093–100. doi:10.1161/circulationaha.108.816736

62 C. Chrysohoou, D. B. Panagiotakos, C. Pitsavos, U. N. Das & C. Stefanadis (2004). Adherence to the Mediterranean diet attenuates inflammation and coagulation process in healthy adults: the ATTICA Study. *Journal of the American College of Cardiology*, 44(1), 152–8. doi:10.1016/j.jacc.2004.03.039

63 A. Trichopoulou & V. Dilis (2007). Olive oil and longevity. *Molecular Nutrition & Food Research*, 51(10), 1275–8. doi:10.1002/mnfr.200700134

64 A. Trichopoulou, C. Bamia & D. Trichopoulos (2009). Anatomy of health effects of Mediterranean diet: Greek EPIC prospective cohort study. *British Medical Journal*, 338. doi:10.1136/bmj.b2337

65 K. T. Knoops, L. C. de Groot, F. Fidanza, A. Alberti-Fidanza, D. Kromhout & W. A. van Staveren (2006). Comparison of three different dietary scores in relation to 10-year mortality in elderly European subjects: the HALE project. *European Journal of Clinical Nutrition*, 60(6), 746–55. doi:10.1038/sj.ejcn.1602378

66 G. Masala, M. Ceroti, V. Pala, V. Krogh, P. Vineis, C. Sacerdote, ... D. Palli (2007). A dietary pattern rich in olive oil and raw vegetables is associated with lower mortality in Italian elderly subjects. *British Journal of Nutrition*, 98(2), 406–15. doi:10.1017/s0007114507704981

67 G. Abellan van Kan, G. Gambassi, L. C. de Groot, S. Andrieu, T. Cederholm, E. Andre, ... C. Latge (2008). Nutrition and aging. The Carla Workshop. *Journal of Nutrition, Health and Aging*, 12(6), 355–64.

68 R. Clarke, J. Grimley Evans, J. Schneede, E. Nexo, C. Bates, A. Fletcher, ... J. M. Scott (2004). Vitamin B12 and folate deficiency in later life. *Age Ageing*, 33(1), 34–41.

69 S. P. Tzankoff & A. H. Norris (1978). Longitudinal changes in basal metabolism in man. *Journal of Applied Physiology: Respiratory, Environmental and Exercise Physiology*, 45(4), 536–9.

70 I. Elmadfa & H. Freisling (2003). Macronutrient supply in different population groups in Austria. *Zufuhr von makronährstoffen bei verschiedenen bevölkerungsgruppen in Österreich*, 50(12), 464–8.

71 J. Bauer, G. Biolo, T. Cederholm, M. Cesari, A. J. Cruz-Jentoft, J. E. Morley, ... Y. Boirie (2013). Evidence-based recommendations for optimal dietary protein intake in older people: a position paper from the PROT-AGE Study Group. *Journal of the American Medical Directors Association*, 14(8), 542–59. doi:10.1016/j.jamda.2013.05.021

72 R. R. Wolfe, S. L. Miller & K. B. Miller (2008). Optimal protein intake in the elderly. *Clinical Nutrition*, 27(5), 675–84.

73 C. Gaillard, E. Alix, Y. Boirie, G. Berrut & P. Ritz (2008). Are elderly hospitalized patients getting enough protein? *Journal of the American Geriatric Society*, 56(6), 1045–9. doi:10.1111/j.1532-5415.2008.01721.x

74 C. Nowson & S. O'Connell (2015). Protein requirements and recommendations for older people: a review. *Nutrients*, 7(8), 6874–99. doi:10.3390/nu7085311

75 T. H. Naber, T. Schermer, A. de Bree, K. Nusteling, L. Eggink, J. W. Kruimel, ... M. B. Katan (1997). Prevalence of malnutrition in nonsurgical hospitalized patients and its association with disease complications. *American Journal of Clinical Nutrition*, 66(5), 1232–9.

76 T. H. Naber, A. de Bree, T. R. Schermer, J. Bakkeren, B. Bar, G. de Wild & M. B. Katan. (1997). Specificity of indexes of malnutrition when applied to apparently healthy people: the effect of age. *American Journal of Clinical Nutrition*, 65(6), 1721–5.

77 P. McGlone, J. Dickerson & G. J. Davies (1995). The feeding of patients in hospital: a review. *Journal of the Royal Society of Health*, 115(5), 282–8.

78 J. Edington, P. Kon & C. Martyn (1996). Prevalence of malnutrition in patients in general practice. *Clinical Nutrition*, 15(2), 60–3.

79 U. G. Kyle, M. Pirlich, T. Schuetz, H. Lochs & C. Pichard (2004). Is nutritional depletion by Nutritional Risk Index associated with increased length of hospital stay? A population-based study. *Journal of Parenteral and Enteral Nutrition*, 28(2), 99–104.

80 M. Nematy, M. Hickson, A. Brynes, C. Ruxton & G. Frost (2006). Vulnerable patients with a fractured neck of femur: nutritional status and support in hospital. *Journal of Human Nutrition and Dietetics*, 19(3), 209–18.

81 M. Mowe, T. Bohmer & E. Kindt (1994). Reduced nutritional status in an elderly population (>70 y) is probable before disease and possibly contributes to the development of disease. *American Journal of Clinical Nutrition*, 59(2), 317–24.

82 J. P. McWhirter & C. R. Pennington (1994). Incidence and recognition of malnutrition in hospital. *British Medical Journal*, 308(6934), 945–8.

83 C. S. Chima, K. Barco, M. L. A. Dewitt, M. Maeda, J. C. Teran & K. D. Mullen (1997). Relationship of nutritional status to length of stay, hospital costs, and discharge status of patients hospitalized in the medicine service. *Journal of the American Dietetic Association*, 97(9), 975–8. doi:http://dx.doi.org/10.1016/S0002-8223(97)00235-6

84 I. Kowanko (1997). The role of the nurse in food service: a literature review and recommendations. *International Journal of Nursing Practice*, 3(2), 73–8.

85 I. Kowanko (2001). Energy and nutrient intake of patients in acute care. *Journal of Clinical Nursing*, 10(1), 51–7.

86 S. Allison (2002). Institutional feeding of the elderly. *Current Opinion in Clinical Nutrition and Metabolic Care*, 5(1), 31–4.

87 J. Hallfrisch, Facn & K. M. Behall (2000). Mechanisms of the effects of grains on insulin and glucose responses. *Journal of the American College of Nutrition*, 19(suppl. 3), 320s–325s.

88 K. Hall, S. J. Whiting & B. Comfort (2000). Low nutrient intake contributes to adverse clinical outcomes in hospitalized elderly patients. *Nutrition Reviews*, 58(7), 214–17.

89 M. Banks, S. Ash, J. Bauer & D. Gaskill (2007). Prevalence of malnutrition in adults in Queensland public hospitals and residential aged care facilities. *Nutrition & Dietetics*, 64(3), 172–8. doi:10.1111/j.1747-0080.2007.00179.x

90 I. Kowanko, S. Simon & J. Wood (1999). Nutritional care of the patient: nurses' knowledge and attitudes in an acute care setting. *Journal of Clinical Nursing*, 8(2), 217–24.

91 C. Lazarus & J. Hamlyn (2005). Prevalence and documentation of malnutrition in hospitals: a case study in a large private hospital setting. *Nutrition & Dietetics*, 62(1), 41–7. doi:10.1111/j.1747-0080.2005.tb00008.x

92 M. Hickson (2006). Malnutrition and ageing. *Postgraduate Medical Journal*, 82(963), 2–8. doi:10.1136/pgmj.2005.037564

93 N. E. Adams, A. J. Bowie, N. Simmance, M. Murray & T. C. Crowe (2008). Recognition by medical and nursing professionals of malnutrition and risk of malnutrition in elderly hospitalised patients. *Nutrition & Dietetics*, 65(2), 144–50. doi:10.1111/j.1747-0080.2008.00226.x

94 Council of Europe (2002). *Food and Nutritional Care in Hospitals: How to prevent undernutrition. Report and recommendations of the Committee of Experts on Nutrition, Food Safety and Consumer Protection.* Strasbourg: Council of Europe.

95 S. P. Allison (1992). Nutritional support—who needs it and who does it? *Clinical Nutrition*, 11(4), 165–6.

96 D. B. A. Silk (1994). *Organisation of Nutritional Support in Hospitals.* Biddenden, UK: British Association for Parenteral and Enteral Nutrition.

97 J. Larsson, I. Akerlind, J. Permerth & J. O. Hornqvist (1994). The relation between nutritional state and quality of life in surgical patients. *European Journal of Surgery*, 160(6–7), 329–34.

98 L. Ovesen, J. Hannibal & E. L. Mortensen (1993). The interrelationship of weight loss, dietary intake, and quality of life in ambulatory patients with cancer of the lung, breast, and ovary. *Nutrition and Cancer*, 19(2), 159–67. doi:10.1080/01635589309514246

99 P. Mayr, S. Kalde, M. Vogt & K. S. Kuhn (2000). Safety, acceptability and efficacy of a high-energy, fibre-containing oral nutritional supplement in malnourished patients: an observational study. *Journal of Human Nutrition and Dietetics*, 13(4), 255–63. doi:10.1046/j.1365-277x.2000.00236.x

100 H. Silberman & D. Eisenberg (1982). *Parenteral and Enteral Nutrition for the Hospitalized Patient*. Norwalk, CT: Appleton-Century-Crofts.

101 D. P. S. Lipski (2003). Improving food delivery services for acute hospital geriatric inpatients: a quality assurance project. *Australasian Journal on Ageing*, 22(1), 44. doi:10.1111/j.1741-6612.2003.tb00463.x

102 S. Capra (2007). Nutrition assessment or nutrition screening—how much information is enough to make a diagnosis of malnutrition in acute care? *Nutrition*, 23(4), 356–7.

103 R. Visvanathan, C. Macintosh, M. Callary, R. Penhall, M. Horowitz & I. Chapman (2003). The nutritional status of 250 older Australian recipients of domiciliary care services and its association with outcomes at 12 months. *Journal of the American Geriatric Society*, 51(7), 1007–11.

104 M. Leggo, M. Banks, E. Isenring, L. Stewart & M. Tweeddale (2008). A quality improvement nutrition screening and intervention program available to Home and Community Care eligible clients. *Nutrition & Dietetics*, 65(2), 162–7. doi:10.1111/j.1747-0080.2008.00239.x

105 G. Sampson (2009). Weight loss and malnutrition in the elderly—the shared role of GPs and APDs. *Australian Family Physician*, 38(7), 507–10.

106 Australian and New Zealand Society of Geriatric Medicine (2007). *Under-nutrition and the Older Person*. Sydney: ANZSGM.

107 U. O. Anyanwu, J. R. Sharkey, R. T. Jackson & N. R. Sahyoun (2011). Home food environment of older adults transitioning from hospital to home. *Journal of Nutrition in Gerontology and Geriatrics*, 30(2), 105–21. doi:10.1080/21551197.2011.566525

108 H. Payette, K. Gray-Donald, R. Cyr & V. Boutier (1995). Predictors of dietary intake in a functionally dependent elderly population in the community. *American Journal of Public Health*, 85(5), 677–83.

109 Australian Meals on Wheels Association (2016). *National Meal Guidelines: A guide for service providers, caterers and health professionals providing home delivered and centre based meal programs for older Australians*. Australian Meals on Wheels Association. Retrieved from: http://mealsonwheels.org.au/wp-content/uploads/2016/10/NationalMealsGuidelines2016.pdf.

110 Department of Social Services (2014). *Key Directions for the Commonwealth Home Support Programme Discussion Paper. Best support for older people living at home*. Canberra: Commonwealth of Australia. Retrieved from: https://agedcare.health.gov.au/ageing-and-aged-care-programs-services-commonwealth-home-support-programme/discussion-paper-key-directions-for-the-commonwealth-home-support-programme.

111 C. Bunney & R. Bartl (2015). *Best Practice Food and Nutrition Manual for Aged Care Nutrition Services*, 2nd edn. Central Coast Local Health District, Gosford. Retrieved from: www.cclhd.health.nsw.gov.au/ourservices/nutrition/Documents/BestPracticeFoodandNutritionManual-Edition2.pdf.

112 C. Bunney & R. Bartl (2015). *Eating Well: A nutrition resource for older people and their carers*, 3rd edn. Nutrition Services, Central Coast Local Health District, Gosford. Retrieved from: www.cclhd.health.nsw.gov.au/ourservices/nutrition/DocumentsEatingWellResource.pdf.

113   S. E. Gariballa (2001). Malnutrition in hospitalized elderly patients: when does it matter? *Clinical Nutrition*, 20(6), 487–91. doi:10.1054/clnu.2001.0477

114   D. A. Zador & A. S. Truswell (1987). Nutritional status on admission to a general surgical ward in a Sydney hospital. *Australian and New Zealand Journal of Medicine*, 17(2), 234–40.

115   S. M. Green, H. Winterberg, P. J. Franks, C. J. Moffatt, C. Eberhardie & S. McLaren (1999). Nutritional intake in community patients with pressure ulcers. *Journal of Wound Care*, 8(7), 325–30. doi:10.12968/jowc.1999.8.7.25900

116   S. G. Dudek (2000). Malnutrition in hospitals. Who's assessing what patients eat? *American Journal of Nursing*, 100(4), 36–42.

117   K. E. Charlton, C. Nichols, S. Bowden, K. Lambert, L. Barone, M. Mason & M. Milosavljevic (2010). Older rehabilitation patients are at high risk of malnutrition: evidence from a large Australian database. *Journal of Nutrition, Health and Aging*, 14(8), 622–8.

118   K. Charlton, C. Nichols, S. Bowden, M. Milosavljevic, K. Lambert, L. Barone, ... M. Batterham (2012). Poor nutritional status of older subacute patients predicts clinical outcomes and mortality at 18 months of follow-up. *European Journal of Clinical Nutrition*, 66(11), 1224–8. doi:10.1038/ejcn.2012.130

119   A. M. Brantervik, I. E. Jacobsson, A. Grimby, T. C. Wallen & I. G. Bosaeus (2005). Older hospitalised patients at risk of malnutrition: correlation with quality of life, aid from the social welfare system and length of stay? *Age and Ageing*, 34(5), 444–9. doi:10.1093/ageing/afi125

120   N. Kagansky, Y. Berner, N. Koren-Morag, L. Perelman, H. Knobler & S. Levy (2005). Poor nutritional habits are predictors of poor outcome in very old hospitalized patients. *American Journal of Clinical Nutrition*, 82(4), 784–91.

121   M. H. Middleton, G. Nazarenko, I. Nivison-Smith & P. Smerdely (2001). Prevalence of malnutrition and 12-month incidence of mortality in two Sydney teaching hospitals. *Internal Medicine Journal*, 31(8), 455–61.

122   C. Braunschweig, S. Gomez & P. M. Sheean (2000). Impact of declines in nutritional status on outcomes in adult patients hospitalized for more than 7 days. *Journal of the American Dietetic Association*, 100(11), 1316–22. doi:10.1016/s0002-8223(00)00373-4

123   K. Walton, K. E. Charlton, F. Manning, A. T. McMahon, S. Galea & K. Evans (2015). The nutritional status and energy and protein intakes of MOW clients and the need for further targeted strategies to enhance intakes. *Appetite*, 95, 528–32. doi:10.1016/j.appet.2015.08.007

124   K. E. Charlton, K. Walton, L. Moon, K. Smith, A. T. McMahon, F. Ralph, ... J. Krassie (2013). 'It could probably help someone else but not me': a feasibility study of a snack programme offered to meals on wheels clients. *Journal of Nutrition, Health and Aging*, 17(4), 364–9. doi:10.1007%2Fs12603-012-0407-3

125   M. D. Miller, M. Crotty, L. C. Giles, E. Bannerman, C. Whitehead, L. Cobiac, ... G. Andrews (2002). Corrected arm muscle area: an independent predictor of long-term mortality in community-dwelling older adults? *Journal of the American Geriatric Society*, 50(7), 1272–7.

126   P. B. Eveleth, R. Andres, W. C. Chumlea, O. Eiben, K. Ge, T. Harris, ... B. Vellas (1998). Uses and interpretation of anthropometry in the elderly for the assessment of physical status. Report to the Nutrition Unit of the World Health Organization: the Expert Subcommittee on the Use and Interpretation of Anthropometry in the Elderly. *Journal of Nutrition, Health and Aging*, 2(1), 5–17.

127   M. L. Omran & J. E. Morley (2000). Assessment of protein energy malnutrition in older persons, part I: history, examination, body composition, and screening tools. *Nutrition*, 16(1), 50–63.

128 M. Elia (2009). The economics of malnutrition. *Nestlé Nutrition Workshop Series: Clinical & Performance Programme*, 12, 29–40. doi:10.1159/000235666

129 M. Elia, C. A. Russell & R. J. Stratton (2010). Malnutrition in the UK: policies to address the problem. *Proceedings of the Nutrition Society*, 69(4), 470–6. doi:10.1017/s0029665110001746

130 National Institute for Health and Clinical Excellence (2006). *Nutrition Support in Adults: Oral nutrition support, enteral tube feeding and parenteral nutrition*. London: NIHCE.

131 R. Visvanathan & I. Chapman (2010). Preventing sarcopaenia in older people. *Maturitas*, 66(4), 383–8. doi:10.1016/j.maturitas.2010.03.020

132 A. H. Hamirudin, K. Charlton & K. Walton (2016). Outcomes related to nutrition screening in community living older adults: a systematic literature review. *Archives of Gerontology and Geriatrics*, 62, 9–25. doi:10.1016/j.archger.2015.09.007

133 A. H. Hamirudin, K. Charlton, K. Walton, A. Bonney, G. Albert, A. Hodgkins, … A. Dalley (2016). Implementation of nutrition screening for older adults in general practice: patient perspectives indicate acceptability. *Journal of Aging Research and Clinical Practice*, 5(1), 7–13.

134 J. White (1992). Participating in the NSI (Nutrition Screening Initiative). *Food Management*, 27(8), 40.

135 J. V. White, J. T. Dwyer, B. M. Posner, R. J. Ham, D. A. Lipschitz & N. S. Wellman (1992). Nutrition screening initiative: development and implementation of the public awareness checklist and screening tools. *Journal of the American Dietetic Association*, 92(2), 163–7.

136 J. Martineau, J. D. Bauer, E. Isenring & S. Cohen (2005). Malnutrition determined by the patient-generated subjective global assessment is associated with poor outcomes in acute stroke patients. *Clinical Nutrition*, 24(6), 1073–7. doi:10.1016/j.clnu.2005.08.010

137 J. M. Thomas, E. Isenring & E. Kellett (2007). Nutritional status and length of stay in patients admitted to an acute assessment unit. *Journal of Human Nutrition and Dietetics*, 20(4), 320–8. doi:10.1111/j.1365-277X.2007.00765.x

138 Y. Guigoz & B. Vellas (1999). The Mini Nutritional Assessment (MNA) for grading the nutritional state of elderly patients: presentation of the MNA, history and validation. *Nestlé Nutrition Workshop Series: Clinical & Performance Programme*, 1, 3–11; discussion 11–12.

139 M. J. Kaiser, J. M. Bauer, C. Ramsch, W. Uter, Y. Guigoz, T. Cederholm, … C. C. Sieber (2010). Frequency of malnutrition in older adults: a multinational perspective using the mini nutritional assessment. *Journal of the American Geriatric Society*, 58(9), 1734–8. doi:10.1111/j.1532-5415.2010.03016.x

140 C. Watterson, A. Fraser, M. Banks, E. Isenring, M. Miller & C. Silvester (2009). Evidence based practice guidelines for the nutritional management of malnutrition in adult patients across the continuum of care. *Nutrition & Dietetics*, 66, S1–S34. doi:10.1111/j.1747-0080.2009.01383.x

141 J. Kondrup, S. P. Allison, M. Elia, B. Vellas & M. Plauth (2003). ESPEN guidelines for nutrition screening 2002. *Clinical Nutrition*, 22(4), 415–21.

142 K. Schindler, E. Pernicka, A. Laviano, P. Howard, T. Schutz, P. Bauer, … M. Hiesmayr (2010). How nutritional risk is assessed and managed in European hospitals: a survey of 21,007 patients findings from the 2007–2008 cross-sectional nutritionDay survey. *Clinical Nutrition*, 29(5), 552–9. doi:10.1016/j.clnu.2010.04.001

143 K. Walton, P. Williams, L. Tapsell & M. Batterham (2007). Rehabilitation inpatients are not meeting their energy and protein needs. *European e-Journal of Clinical Nutrition and Metabolism*, 2(6), e120–e126. doi:10.1016/j.eclnm.2007.09.001

144 P. Garling (2008). *Final Report of the Special Commission of Inquiry: Acute care services in NSW public hospitals.* Sydney: NSW Government.

145 P. E. Smith & A. E. Smith (1997). High-quality nutritional interventions reduce costs. *Healthcare Financial Management*, 51(8), 66–9.

146 M. Elia (2003). *Screening for Malnutrition: A multidisciplinary responsibility. Development and use of the 'Malnutrition Universal Screening Tool' (MUST) for adults.* Redditch, UK: British Association for Parenteral and Enteral Nutrition.

147 H. M. Kruizenga, J. C. Seidell, H. C. de Vet, N. J. Wierdsma & M. A. van Bokhorst-de van der Schueren (2005). Development and validation of a hospital screening tool for malnutrition: the short nutritional assessment questionnaire (SNAQ). *Clinical Nutrition*, 24(1), 75–82. doi:10.1016/j.clnu.2004.07.015

148 J. Kondrup, H. H. Rasmussen, O. Hamberg & Z. Stanga (2003). Nutritional risk screening (NRS 2002): a new method based on an analysis of controlled clinical trials. *Clinical Nutrition*, 22(3), 321–36.

149 M. Ferguson, S. Capra, J. Bauer & M. Banks (1999). Development of a valid and reliable malnutrition screening tool for adult acute hospital patients. *Nutrition*, 15(6), 458–64.

150 B. Vellas, H. Villars, G. Abellan, M. E. Soto, Y. Rolland, Y. Guigoz, … P. Garry (2006). Overview of the MNA—its history and challenges. *Journal of Nutrition, Health and Aging*, 10(6), 456–63.

151 B. Vellas, S. Lauque, S. Andrieu, F. Nourhashemi, Y. Rolland, R. Baumgartner & P. Garry (2001). Nutrition assessment in the elderly. *Current Opinion in Clinical Nutrition and Metabolic Care*, 4(1), 5–8.

152 M. J. Kaiser, J. M. Bauer, C. Ramsch, W. Uter, Y. Guigoz, T. Cederholm, … C. C. Sieber (2009). Validation of the Mini Nutritional Assessment short-form (MNA-SF): a practical tool for identification of nutritional status. *Journal of Nutrition, Health and Aging*, 13(9), 782–8.

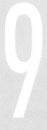

CHAPTER 19

INDIGENOUS AUSTRALIAN FOOD SECURITY: WORKING WITH AN INTERGENERATIONAL PERSPECTIVE

SCOTT WINCH

CHAPTER OBJECTIVES

This chapter will enable the reader to:

- describe the impact of colonisation on food security for Indigenous Australians
- describe the food-related health disparity between Indigenous and non-Indigenous Australians
- identify key strategies to improve food security in Indigenous communities.

KEY TERMS

Colonisation   Health disparity

Food security   Indigenous

KEY POINTS

- The diets of traditional Indigenous Australian were healthy and nutritious.
- Indigenous Australians were removed from traditional lifestyles and diets.
- Missionised communities become reliant on highly processed and unhealthy diets.
- Intergenerational dietary practices have led to food insecurity.
- Nutrition is the second-highest modifiable risk factor.
- Australian Indigenous people have higher rates of lifestyle diseases.
- Australian Indigenous people have a significantly lower life expectancy than non-Indigenous Australians.

INTRODUCTION

The context in which nutritional health is achieved must be considered beyond addressing physiological needs. Considering life stages is one way of articulating differences between groups in the population and identifying key issues in delivering adequate nutrition. Even so, the social and environmental circumstances of different age groups are clearly integrated with issues that expose specific nutritional concerns. This interrelationship is even more apparent with **Indigenous Australians**. The health of Indigenous Australians is a national public health priority, and is closely linked to nutritional issues. This chapter provides important background to this scenario and outlines ways forward linked to food security for Indigenous Australians.

Indigenous Australians
the term Indigenous is used to refer to Australian Aboriginal and Torres Strait Islander peoples.

The most widely adopted definition of Aboriginal or Torres Strait Islander (the 'Commonwealth working definition') states: 'An Aboriginal or Torres Strait Islander is a person of Aboriginal or Torres Strait Islander descent, who identifies as being of Aboriginal or Torres Strait Islander origin and who is accepted as such by the community with which the person associates'. This definition was developed during the period 1967 to 1978 and is now widely accepted by Commonwealth and other government agencies [1]. Throughout this chapter, the capitalisation of 'Indigenous' refers to the Aboriginal and Torres Strait Islander population when it is used in the Australian context [2].

Indigenous culture is rich and diverse across contemporary Australia. There are two primary cultural groups, being Aboriginal people and Torres Strait Islanders. Within the Aboriginal culture, there are six main groups, these being Murri from Queensland into central New South Wales, Koori which covers the east coast of New South Wales and Victoria, Nunga from South Australia, Noongar from Western Australia, Yolngu from the Top End of the Northern Territory, Anangu from Central Australia, and Palawa from Tasmania. Within these groups, there are about 300 language groups that form distinct social and cultural domains [3].

Traditional Aboriginal society had complex systems of law, education and health. These had been developed over thousands of years based on the Dreaming of the group. Kinship systems of family were part of lore and different camps were established for younger men and women to ensure they were segregated. Arranged marriages were part of the knowledge system where older women and men would take younger husbands and wives. They would then pass on their knowledge to their younger husbands and wives, who then would pass on their knowledge when they took younger husbands and wives later in life. This cycle of knowledge was an integral part of the knowledge system [4]. Food access (and thereby nutrition) was also an integral component.

Appreciating the impact of colonisation on food access and nutrition requires an historical perspective. Estimates of how many Aboriginal and Torres Strait Islander people lived in Australia prior to colonisation vary and range from 300,000 to 1 million, with around 250 separate languages and up to 750 associated dialect names [5]. The 1788 invasion of Australia resulted in an extreme reduction in the Aboriginal population. In 1901, it was estimated that the population had been reduced to around 93,000 [6].

These population declines and the displacement of Indigenous people from their traditional lands had a significant impact on cultural continuity, language and traditional knowledge and governance systems [7]. The British Empire had claimed its settlement of Australia was based on terra nullius, meaning there were no inhabitants of the land pre-1788, and effectively meaning that Aboriginal people were not considered human. This ideology of Western supremacy was the foundation for ensuing policies that impacted on Aboriginal and Torres Strait islander peoples, the effects of which continue today [8].

The deliberate dividing and conquering of Indigenous society and culture disrupted traditional education systems and social function. Systematic policies enacted by the colonial and later governments were aimed to destroy traditional language, knowledge and educational systems [9]. There was a deliberate segregation of older generations from the younger generations to prevent transfer of knowledge and disrupt traditional learning practices [10]. The implications of these actions were played out in many scenarios, and can be clearly seen from a nutritional perspective.

STOP AND THINK

- How have historical circumstances influenced the current health of Indigenous Australians?
- What would be the significance of traditional language and educational systems in promoting health within communities?
- What strategies might help to undo the damage of the past?

WHAT WAS A TRADITIONAL INDIGENOUS AUSTRALIAN DIET AND HOW DID THIS CHANGE WITH COLONISATION?

Based on early records, Aboriginal people were fit, strong and healthy. **Traditional Indigenous Australian diets** were typically high in protein, complex carbohydrates, fibre and micronutrients and low in saturated fat, sugar and salt. Traditional foods varied significantly based on geographical location, climate and season. There were differing types of populations, generally categorised as saltwater people, freshwater people and desert people [11].

Traditional Indigenous Australian diets
food combinations commonly consumed by Indigenous Australians before colonisation.

In the coastal areas, typical diets were rich in seafood with an abundance of fish, crustaceans and other animals such as mammals, birds and turtles. This was supplemented with land-based mammals such as kangaroos and other marsupials. There was also a large variety of plant life, which provided sustenance to coastal Aboriginal people [12]. The freshwater people typically resided in the mountainous hinterland behind the coastal fringes and inland in dense bush areas where major rivers traverse the landscape. In these regions, freshwater fish was plentiful, as was a variety of mammals similar to the coastal areas. The plant life typically varied in these locations between that of the coast and further inland [13]. In the desert area, food sources were scarcer and the types of food varied. These inland regions were the last parts of Australia to be settled. The typical diet in these areas was largely from reptiles, with also a scarcity of vegetation [14].

Where there was an abundance of fresh water and food, camps would be set up for extended periods of time lasting months. There is also evidence of more sedentary lifestyles among Aboriginal people. The role of hunting and gathering food was typically separated into males and females. Males would hunt for the larger game, while females were more responsible for gathering plants and smaller game [11].

>> RESEARCH AT WORK

EXPLORING THE INDIGENOUS DIET

Indigenous Australian author Bruce Pascoe researched journals and records made by early explorers and surveyors around Australia. From these, he was able to describe food use by Indigenous Australians in the period before colonisation. His research questions a lot of assumptions about the food use in this period—for example, agricultural practices were evident, as were other food practices such as the use of indigenous grains to bake bread. A 2016 ABC interview, 'Bruce Pascoe on the complex question of Aboriginal agriculture', is available at: www.abc.net.au/local/stories/2016/02/01/4397892.htm. His book, *Dark Emu*, won the Book of the Year in 2016 in the NSW Premier's Literary Awards [15].

TRY IT YOURSELF

Research ways to make bush bread or damper. How would the original Australian inhabitants have made this bread? How many different ingredients do you find associated with damper recipes now? What are the nutritional implications?

Colonisation

establishing control over the indigenous people of an area.

Colonisation seriously undermined people's ability to maintain these traditional practices. In essence, the profound impact of colonisation on the lifestyle and diets of much of the Indigenous population led to entirely different food practices and nutritional intake. The hunter-gatherer lifestyle suddenly became a sedentary lifestyle. The healthy, nutritional diets sustained over thousands of years suddenly became highly refined energy-dense food after Indigenous people were placed on missions and reserves. Diets became high in sugar, salt and fats. This also meant a reduction in fibre, protein and nutrients. In some instances, Aboriginal people living on reserves and not missions were still able to source traditional foods, though this was limited as traditional locations of food sources became limited due to restricted movements and the encroachment of farming [16].

Figure 19.1 outlines the many factors that have impacted on the health status of Indigenous Australians.

FIGURE 19.1 FACTORS IMPACTING ON INDIGENOUS AUSTRALIAN HEALTH STATUS

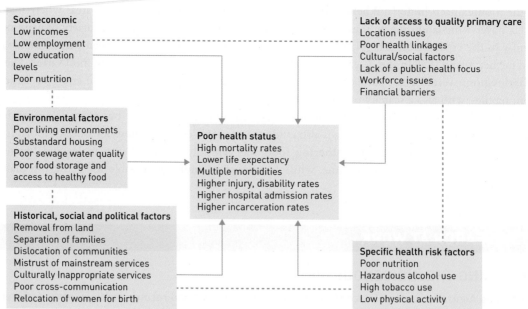

Source: Queensland Government (2012). *Queensland Health Aboriginal and Torres Strait Islander Cultural Capability Framework 2010–2033.* Brisbane: Queensland Health

>> CASE 19.1

IMPACT OF COLONISATION ON TRADITIONAL ROLES AND FUNCTIONS IN SOCIETY

With the expansion of pastoral lands, the roles of men changed and they became forced to work as labourers on farms. Their role as hunters becomes less prominent and so were the skills and knowledges that were part of the hunter lifestyle. Women, too, became more sedentary and were made to work in such roles as house servants. They also lost much of their knowledge and skills in hunting and gathering. As Aboriginal knowledge and education is oral, and language, traditional practices and ceremony were banned, much of the traditional knowledge was lost and not recorded. In addition to food practices, alcohol was also introduced and became highly used in some communities, and was even part of some payments for labourers. These drastic changes led to a much more sedentary, unhealthy and welfare-dependent existence for many Aboriginal people.

- What major rifts in understanding about land use and workforce organisation can be observed?
- What were the health implications for Indigenous Australians?
- How would this have played out in terms of access to a nutritious and sustaining diet?

STOP AND THINK

- What are the strengths of the traditional diets?
- What knowledge and skill was required to maintain these diets?
- How did colonisation impede the ongoing practice of traditional diets?

HOW HAS FOOD INSECURITY RESULTED IN NUTRITION-RELATED HEALTH DISPARITIES FOR INDIGENOUS AUSTRALIANS?

There are a number of ways in which nutrition-related problems emerge within groups in the population. In the case of Indigenous Australians, nutrition-related problems are extensive and are strongly linked to the concept of **food security**. Food security exists 'when all people at all times have access to sufficient, safe and nutritious food to maintain a healthy and active life' [17]. The Food and Agricultural Organization (FAO) of the United Nations has identified four pillars that encompass food security: availability of food; access to adequate food; utilisation of food; and stability of the food supply [18] (Figures 19.2 and 19.3).

    Food insecurity arises as a consequence of inadequate or uncertain access to appropriate quantities and quality of healthy food [19]. The prevalence of food insecurity in high-income countries ranges from 4% to 14% [20]. In Australia, the national figure is close to 4%; however, more than one in five (22%) Aboriginal and Torres Strait Islander people experience food insecurity and it is anticipated that this figure is an underestimate [21]. Rates of food insecurity are highest in remote Indigenous communities (36%). However, Indigenous people living in urban environments are still experiencing food insecurity at higher rates than non-Indigenous Australians [22].

> **Food security**
> access to safe and nutritious foods in amounts that sustain health.
>
> **Food insecurity**
> a condition of inadequate and poor-quality food supply not capable of adequately supporting health.

FIGURE 19.2 POINTS OF INTERVENTION TO IMPROVE THE FOOD SUPPLY

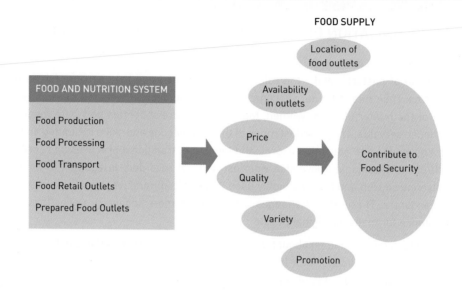

Source: L. Rychetnick, K. Webb, L. Story & T. Katz (2002). *Food Security Options Paper: A planning framework and menu of options for policy and practice interventions.* Sydney: NSW Centre for Public Health Nutrition

FIGURE 19.3 POINTS OF INTERVENTION TO IMPROVE ACCESS TO FOOD

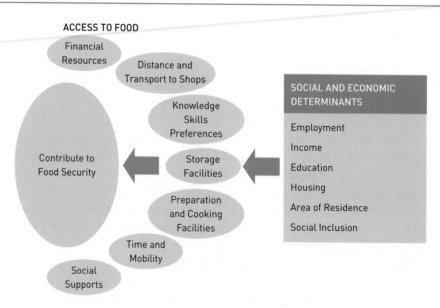

Source: L. Rychetnick, K. Webb, L. Story & T. Katz (2002). *Food Security Options Paper: A planning framework and menu of options for policy and practice interventions.* Sydney: NSW Centre for Public Health Nutrition

Food insecurity is associated with hunger, poor-quality diets, food-related health problems and psychological suffering, and is a key contributor to poor health for Australia's Indigenous communities [23; 24]. Life expectancy for Indigenous people is 17 years lower than for non-Indigenous Australians and diet-related chronic diseases such as cardiovascular disease and diabetes, and their associated risk factors, are the major causes of this health disparity [23; 25]. For Indigenous Australians, food insecurity can be attributed to low income, loss of traditional lifestyle, poor access to traditional and/or healthy foods, household infrastructure and overcrowding, limited nutrition knowledge and a lack of culturally appropriate information and education [19; 25]. Improving food security among Indigenous communities is expected to have far-reaching and long-term health and economic benefits [26]. The 2012–13 Australian Aboriginal and Torres Strait Islander Health Survey (AATSIHS) found that not only are Indigenous Australians more likely to experience food insecurity, but they are also are more likely to consume less fruit and vegetables, more saturated fat and have a higher proportion of total energy intake provided by discretionary foods than non-Indigenous Australians [21]. Reducing the burden of food insecurity by improving the affordability, quality and availability of healthy foods is likely to improve diet quality and reduce the diet-related burden of disease for Indigenous Australians [26].

Health hardware plays an important role in the environment in which food is stored and prepared. These factors include sanitation, electricity, running and hot water, storage including refrigeration and cooking facilities. These factors are disproportionately inadequate for Indigenous households and much of this is due to inadequate installation and maintenance. In addition, approximately 15% of Indigenous Australians live in overcrowded housing, three times that of the general Australian population.

> **Health hardware**
> materials and facilities that support health, such as clean water and safe food storage areas.

Geographical factors impact on the food security of Aboriginal and Torres Strait Islander peoples. A high proportion of Aboriginal people live in remote or extremely remote areas. These populations have very limited access to fresh food and vegetables and those foods available are often of low quality and sold at inflated prices. In regional areas where there may be a supply of fresh foods, these products are still at an increased cost. In urban areas, Aboriginal people are more highly concentrated in lower socioeconomic areas that are often 'food deserts' of limited supermarkets and with high levels of takeaway food as the main option.

Approximately 40% of Aboriginal and Torres Strait Islander people have incomes that lie in the bottom 20% of incomes in Australia [21]. This means that even if Aboriginal households wanted to buy healthier food, the option of cheaply priced, highly processed foods is often preferred. While it may be cheaper to purchase fresh foods and vegetables, health literacy is another factor that compromises the ability for informed food choices and preparation.

Health disparities between Indigenous and non-Indigenous Australians occur throughout the life stages. Evidence for these disparities is provided in national statistics and health surveys.

Perinatal health

Reports on Australian perinatal statistics expose the presence of nutrition-related problems in Australian communities [27]. Lower health outcomes due to poor nutrition has an impact across the life-course of Aboriginal people. This begins during the intra-uterine period, where the poor nutritional practices of many Aboriginal mothers impacts on the growth and development of the baby. Birth weight (low birth weight <2500 g), premature birth and infant mortality are critical outcomes of poor maternal nutrition (Table 19.1). This can sometimes be further exacerbated by alcohol intake during pregnancy, which is alarmingly higher for Aboriginal mothers.

TABLE 19.1   MEAN BIRTH WEIGHTS AND PERCENTAGE OF LOW BIRTH WEIGHT FOR BABIES BORN TO INDIGENOUS AND NON-INDIGENOUS MOTHERS, SELECTED JURISDICTIONS, AUSTRALIA, 2005

		NSW	Vic	Qld	WA	SA	NT	Australia
Indigenous mothers	Mean birth weight	3214	3179	3184	3080	3059	3157	3158
	% low birth weight	12.0	13.6	11.8	15.5	17.7	14.5	13.2
Non-Indigenous mothers	Mean birth weight	3382	3369	3385	3359	3361	3338	3375
	% low birth weight	5.7	6.3	6.3	6.0	6.7	6.7	6.1

Source: P. Laws, S. Abeywardana, J. Walker & E. Sullivan (2007). *Australia's Mothers and Babies 2005. Perinatal statistics series number 20.* Cat. no.: PER, 50. Sydney: AIHW National Perinatal Statistics Unit

Infant health

Breastfeeding is extremely important for Aboriginal babies in ensuring a nutrient-superior food source. There are also significant benefits for providing protective immunity through the transfer of antigens in the breast milk. Breastfeeding is also highly accessible and inexpensive, which substantially covers many of the typical food security barriers for Indigenous people. Fortunately, the rates of breastfeeding between Aboriginal and non-Aboriginal mothers is comparable at about 80% of all mothers. The rate in more remote communities is over 90% of mothers. Traditionally, breastfeeding happened for about the first four years of life, though this has been reduced in contemporary Aboriginal society. The lower level of breastfeeding in more urban Aboriginal populations could be attributed to lower levels of parental attachment due to impact of the disruption of traditional family practices through colonisation.

Child growth during the first six months of life is comparable between Aboriginal and non-Aboriginal babies. This, however, declines between six months and five years of age as Aboriginal infants become more reliant on other food sources and breastfeeding ceases at an earlier stage. This was demonstrated in a study conducted in the Northern Territory in 2007 [28] (Figure 19.4).

Overweight and obesity

The rates of overweight and obesity in the Indigenous population are higher than for non-Indigenous Australians. The proportion of Aboriginal people with a body mass index (BMI) in the overweight or obese are 28% and 29%, respectively, overall 29% of the population (Table 19.2). This is comparable to the Australian non-Indigenous population. However, there are more Aboriginal people in the obese category of 29%, compared with 17% for the non-Indigenous population. In this obese category, the risk for chronic disease or a clinical episode is significantly heightened. Of importance also is the higher rate of Aboriginal people in the underweight category [29].

FIGURE 19.4 PERCENTAGES OF REMOTE NT INDIGENOUS CHILDREN WHO WERE STUNTED, UNDERWEIGHT, WASTING OR ANAEMIC BY HEALTH DISTRICT, 2008–09

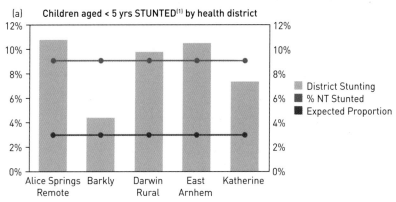

(a) Children aged < 5 yrs STUNTED[1] by health district

(1) HAZ < 2, for a child between 0 and 60 months old. HAZ is a z-score of a child's height related to averages based on growth age and gender calculated according to the US Centers for Disease Control and Prevention (CDC) rule.

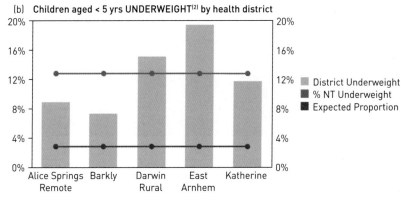

(b) Children aged < 5 yrs UNDERWEIGHT[2] by health district

(2) WAZ < 2, for a child between 0 and 60 months old. WAZ is a z-score of a child's weight related to averages based on growth age and gender calculated according to CDC rule.

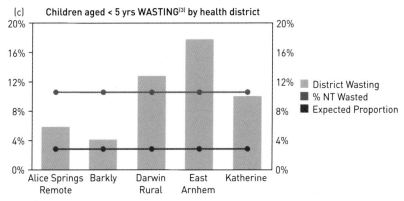

(c) Children aged < 5 yrs WASTING[3] by health district

(3) WHZ < 2, for a child between 0 and 60 months old. WHZ is a z-score of a child's weight and height combined related to averages based on height rounded and gender calculated according to CDC rule.

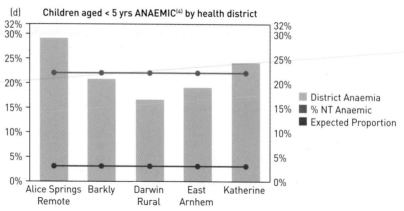

(d) Children aged < 5 yrs ANAEMIC[4] by health district

(4) Hb < 105 g/L for a child between 6–12 months old and 110 g/L for a child between 12 and 60 months old.

Source: S. Silburn, G. Robinson, F. Arney, K. Johnstone & K. McGuinness (2011). *Early Childhood Development in the NT: Issues to be addressed. Topical paper commissioned for the public consultations on the Northern Territory Early Childhood Plan.* Darwin: Northern Territory Government (Figure 1, pp. 3–4)

TABLE 19.2 BODY WEIGHT: PROPORTIONS FOR BMI CATEGORIES FOR MALES, BY INDIGENOUS STATUS AND AGE GROUP, AUSTRALIA, 2004–05

		Indigenous				Non-Indigenous			
	Age group	Underweight	Normal	Overweight	Obese	Underweight	Normal	Overweight	Obese
Males	15–24	8	52	25	15	6	64	25	6
	25–34	3	37	37	24	1	40	42	17
	35–44	1	32	31	36	1	30	47	22
	45–54	3	27	38	32	0	29	46	25
	55 and older	2	24	39	36	1	35	45	19
	All ages	4	38	32	26	2	39	42	18
Females	15–24	13	53	19	15	13	64	16	7
	25–34	5	38	22	35	5	57	25	14
	35–44	7	30	25	38	4	54	26	16
	45–54	4	29	26	41	2	48	30	20
	55 and older	3	24	30	43	3	43	33	21
	All ages	7	38	23	32	5	52	27	16

		Indigenous				Non-Indigenous			
	Age group	Underweight	Normal	Overweight	Obese	Underweight	Normal	Overweight	Obese
Persons	15–24	11	53	22	15	9	64	21	6
	25–34	4	38	29	29	3	48	34	16
	35–44	4	31	28	37	2	42	37	19
	45–54	3	28	32	37	1	38	38	22
	55 and older	2	24	34	39	2	39	39	20
	All ages	6	38	28	29	3	45	35	17

Notes:
1 Derivation of proportions excludes people for whom BMI was not known.
2 Any discrepancy in the sums of proportions results from rounding for presentation.

Source: Derived from Australian Bureau of Statistics (2006). *National Aboriginal and Torres Strait Islander Health Survey, 2004–05*. Canberra: ABS

Chronic lifestyle-related disease

General population trends for hospitalisation for chronic diseases over the past two decades reveal that there was a slight decline in the rate of hospitalisations due to cardiovascular disease (CVD), falling from 2324 in 1993–94 to 2067 per 100,000 population in 2012–13; while hospitalisations (excluding dialysis) for chronic kidney disease (CKD) increased by 17%. Indigenous people, people in the lowest socioeconomic group and those living in remote and very remote areas have the highest rates of CVD, diabetes, and CKD hospitalisations. Indigenous diabetes hospitalisation rates, for example, were four times those of non-Indigenous Australians [30].

Three chronic diseases—CVD, diabetes and CKD—acting alone or together, contribute considerably to illness, morbidity and premature mortality in the Australian Indigenous population and result in high usage of the healthcare system. All of these diseases share the end point of significant vascular pathology leading to damage of the heart, brain, lungs and kidneys.

Cardiovascular disease describes many different conditions affecting the heart, including coronary heart disease, stroke and heart failure. A number of risk factors can contribute to the risk of developing CVD, including tobacco smoking, insufficient physical activity, obesity, poor nutrition, high blood pressure, high cholesterol and diabetes, all of which are prevalent in Indigenous communities.

» RESEARCH AT WORK

MONITORING HOSPITALISATION RATES FOR CARDIOVASCULAR DISEASE IN INDIGENOUS AUSTRALIANS

Hospitalisation rates in 2012–13 for CVD among Indigenous Australians were twice as high as those for non-Indigenous Australians: 9270 compared with 4630 per 100,000 population. Indigenous males and females were hospitalised for CVD at similar rates. However, Indigenous females were hospitalised

2.3 times the rate of non-Indigenous females and Indigenous males were hospitalised at 1.7 times the rate of non-Indigenous males (Figure 19.5). A study by King and colleagues claims that CVD is a large contributor to the health gap between Indigenous and non-Indigenous Australians and was the greatest contributor to the mortality gap between Indigenous and non-Indigenous Australians [31].

One of the main problems with the data is that hospital records are for 'separations' and not individuals, and as there can be multiple admissions for the same individual, hospital separation rates do not usually reflect the incidence or prevalence of the disease or condition in question. People who receive treatment at hospital emergency departments as outpatients, but are not admitted—are not counted in hospital records. Hospital separation data are also affected by variations in admission practices, and the availability of and access to hospital and non-hospital services.

FIGURE 19.5 CORONARY HEART DISEASE HOSPITALISATION RATES, AS THE PRINCIPAL AND/OR AN ADDITIONAL DIAGNOSIS, BY INDIGENOUS STATUS AND SEX, 2012–13

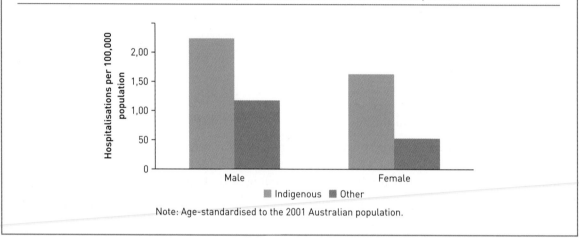

Note: Age-standardised to the 2001 Australian population.

Although length of stay (LOS) data for hospitalisation with CVD did not identify Indigenous status, the average LOS for the general population hospitalised with the principal diagnosis of CVD has decreased over the last two decades, declining from 9.6 days in 1993–94, to 7.9 days in 2007–08, and to 5.4 days in 2012–13 [30]. In 2012–13, the average LOS for a hospitalisation with CVD as an additional diagnosis was 11.2 days.

A review in 2006 by Mathur and colleagues [32] found that compared with non-Indigenous Australians, Indigenous Australians are more likely to suffer a heart attack, to die from it before being admitted to hospital, and to die from it if admitted to hospital. In hospital, they were less likely to receive key medical investigations or common procedures such as bypass surgery or angioplasty. The authors also found that Indigenous people admitted to hospital for coronary heart disease have more comorbidities than non-Indigenous Australians, but this did not appear to account for differences in procedure rates.

Diabetes is a disease that is characterised by high levels of glucose in the blood and is caused by the inability of the pancreas to produce insulin or by the body not being able to use insulin effectively. Type 2 diabetes may cause a range of complications including heart disease, CKD, loss of vision and lower limb amputation, and is the leading cause of end-stage kidney disease in Australia.

FIGURE 19.6 TYPE 2 DIABETES HOSPITALISATION RATES, AS THE PRINCIPAL AND/OR AN ADDITIONAL DIAGNOSIS, BY INDIGENOUS STATUS AND SEX, 2012–13

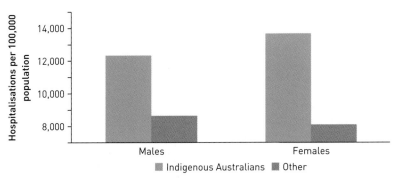

Note: Age-standardised to the 2001 Australian population.

Hospitalisation rates in 2012–13 for type 2 diabetes were four times as high among Indigenous Australians as non-Indigenous Australians. Indigenous males were three times more likely to be hospitalised for diabetes as non-Indigenous males and the rate for Indigenous females was even higher with six times more Indigenous females being hospitalised compared with non-Indigenous females (Figure 19.6) [30]. Although LOS data for hospitalisation did not identify Indigenous status, the general population data shows an average hospital stay of 8.6 days for a principal diagnosis of diabetes with a 7.4-day stay if diabetes was recorded as an additional diagnosis.

Chronic kidney disease refers to all kidney conditions where an individual has evidence of kidney damage or reduced kidney function, lasting at least three months. Many people are not aware they may have kidney disease due to considerable loss of kidney function before symptoms are evident. CKD has five stages, indicated by such markers as eGFR. End-stage kidney disease is the most severe form of kidney disease and requires either a kidney transplant or renal dialysis. Here we will examine all rates of CKD excluding regular dialysis.

In 2012–13, CKD hospitalisation rates for Indigenous Australians were nearly five times higher than for non-Indigenous Australians [30]. Indigenous males were 3.4 times more likely to be hospitalised for CKD than non-Indigenous males and the rate was even higher for Indigenous females, being 6.3 times the rate for non-Indigenous females (Figure 19.7). Although LOS data for hospitalisation did not identify Indigenous status, the general population data shows the average LOS for CKD was 4.9 days, and 9.6 days where CKD was recorded as an additional diagnosis.

Unfortunately, hospitalisation data for *respiratory diseases*, mainly asthma and chronic obstructive pulmonary disease (COPD), were only available for 2010 for all states except Tasmania; however, the trends were equally disturbing. Indigenous males and females had higher hospitalisation rates for respiratory diseases than other males and females across all age groups [30]. For both Indigenous and non-Indigenous males and females, hospitalisation rates for respiratory diseases were highest among those aged 0–4 years, and 65 years and over. The greatest ratio of Indigenous to non-Indigenous mortality from respiratory diseases occurred in the 45–54-year age group for males and females, where Indigenous males were hospitalised at about five times the rate of non-Indigenous males and Indigenous females were hospitalised at over six times the rate of non-Indigenous females. Approximately 49.4% of Indigenous Australians hospitalised for respiratory diseases were males and 50.6% were females.

FIGURE 19.7   HOSPITALISATION RATES WITH CKD, AS THE PRINCIPAL AND/OR AN ADDITIONAL DIAGNOSIS, BY INDIGENOUS STATUS AND SEX, 2012–13

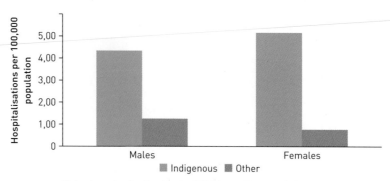

Note: Age-standardised to the 2001 Australian population.

Inequalities among populations show that Indigenous people, those in the lowest socioeconomic group and people living in remote or very remote areas have the highest rates of hospitalisation for CVD, diabetes and CKD. However, when regarding remoteness as an inequality, it should be noted that patients may be transferred from a local healthcare facility to an urban hospital for critical care, and so remote rates may be underestimated [33]. For example, 6.5% of diabetes hospitalisations in remote or very remote regions were transferred to a regional or city hospital. The higher hospitalisation rates for diabetes among the lower socioeconomic groups may reflect the higher incidence of diabetes among this population, which may be influenced by socioeconomic disadvantage limiting opportunities for lifestyle and risk modification [34].

The AIHW (2015) report shows that Indigenous Australians have higher hospitalisation rates than non-Indigenous Australians regardless of their comorbidity status and the disparity rates increase with greater comorbidity—from 1.5 times that of non-Indigenous Australians when one disease only is present to 7.3 times the rate of non-Indigenous Australians when all three diseases are present [30]. Indigenous females had the highest disparities across all comorbidity groups—2.2 times as likely as non-Indigenous females to have one disease only and 11 times more likely than non-Indigenous females to have all three diseases. Indigenous males were 1.6 times more likely than non-Indigenous males to have one disease only and five times more likely than non-Indigenous males to have all three diseases.

Australian public hospital admission records in 2007–08 show that an estimated 89% of Indigenous patients were correctly identified. In other words, 11% of Indigenous patients were not identified as Indigenous, and the true number of hospital admissions for Indigenous persons was about 12% higher than reported [35].

STOP AND THINK

- How might food insecurity issues lead to the prevalence of chronic disease and associated hospitalisations as described here?
- How might the impressively high breastfeeding rates in Indigenous Australian communities be protected and further supported?
- What are some of the challenges for health monitoring and research in accurately describing healthcare utilisation by Indigenous Australians?

OXFORD UNIVERSITY PRESS

HOW CAN INDIGENOUS HEALTH PRINCIPLES BE APPLIED FOR EFFECTIVE FOOD SECURITY AND BETTER NUTRITION FOR INDIGENOUS AUSTRALIANS?

The identification of health disparities is only the first step in developing programs that better support health for Indigenous Australians. Given the cultural discordance that has occurred from colonisation onwards, there is much to be learnt from experience in developing appropriate health-related services for Indigenous Australians. These experiences have helped to shape **Indigenous Health Principles** that can guide more culturally appropriate service development.

Indigenous Health Principles
a set of principles or guidelines for developing health services for Indigenous Australians.

» RESEARCH AT WORK

DEVELOPING INDIGENOUS HEALTH PRINCIPLES

It is not easy to determine the factors that together enable interventions to succeed. Reproducing success across services, or whole jurisdictions, is not simply a matter of identifying 'what works' and 'doing the same' elsewhere. Differences in local conditions, local personnel or community members, local histories and health status, and the dynamic, continuous interaction and evolution of all these suggest that 'one size does not fit all'. This was found in the research report commissioned by the Office of Aboriginal and Torres Strait Islander Health on the link between primary healthcare and health outcomes for Aboriginal and Torres Strait Islander Australians [36]. The report stated that these principles should include:

1 Genuine local Indigenous community engagement to maximise participation, up to and including formal structures of community control or (for non-community controlled health services) an ethic and practice of community involvement.
2 Collaborative approaches that see primary healthcare services working with (a) other service sectors—for example, housing; (b) other primary healthcare or community-based health service delivery organisations, whether government or non-government; and (c) other levels of the healthcare system, particularly hospitals/specialists.
3 Delivery of core primary healthcare programs vital to the long-term health of the community including but not restricted to (a) maternal and child health and (b) chronic disease detection and management.
4 Evidence-based approaches that are reflective of and are based on a continuous quality improvement approach and that involve the local community in adapting what is known to work elsewhere to local conditions and priorities.
5 A multidisciplinary team approach that crucially involves the employment of local Aboriginal and Torres Strait Islander community members, and that includes continuous training and support.
6 Approaches that harmonise with local Aboriginal ways of life, and in particular regionally organised service delivery and outreach services to dispersed populations.
7 Adequate and secure resourcing to allow focus on the management and delivery of non-acute care.

 SCOTT WINCH

Community kitchen
an environment centring on the concept of shared cooking space, community and culture.

Effective food security and better nutrition can be achieved by applying these principles. An example of a model approach that fits the bill is the **community kitchen**. Evidence suggests that community kitchens can play a role in improving food security through developing cooking, shopping and budgeting skills, improving nutrition education and dietary intake, and increasing social interactions [37; 38]. The community kitchens model may be particularly relevant for Indigenous communities as it is based on community development principles and supports empowerment and self-efficacy [19]. Programs that actively involve the community and consider social determinants of health have been shown to be most effective in improving health and well-being outcomes and are also the most sustainable [39].

Characteristics identified as being key to the success of other Indigenous community programs are similar to those that were adopted in the development of the community kitchen. These include undertaking substantial community consultation, developing a program to meet a community-identified need, creating relevant partnerships and transferring ownership of the program to the Aboriginal community it is targeting in order to achieve long-term sustainability [39]. While a thorough project plan and needs-based support from the community are important in ensuring the development of strong infrastructure and sustainability, participants' ability to access the program and their willingness to participate are important influential factors in determining success [40].

≫ CASE 19.2

THE COMMUNITY KITCHEN PROJECT, ILLAWARRA REGION: PLANNING, IMPLEMENTATION AND EVALUATION

The Community Kitchen Project (CKP) was developed to be strengths based, to support capacity building, to be flexible and to operate from a familiar and accessible site for the community. Its premise was supported over a period of several years to allow adequate time to achieve community ownership. Participation in the CKP initially achieved its target rate identified in planning; however, the number of attendees decreased over time. A major barrier to participation identified by the program facilitator was the intermittent nature of the program. The kitchen operated only during university semesters, with breaks during student holidays. The program facilitator identified that the community focus diminished when there was a break in the program and participant numbers decreased. Lee and colleagues [40] previously identified that for participants to be able to fully participate in community kitchens, the running of concurrent programs was useful in retaining participant interest and attendance. Plans for Stage 2 of the CKP therefore included increasing the kitchen to running weekly; however, breaks would still occur until the community took full ownership. The program facilitator also identified another barrier as not having a program champion or 'voice on the ground' to prompt community members to attend. Program champions have been shown to be vital to the success and sustainability of community-based programs in Indigenous populations [41–44]. A community member then took over the role of grocery shopping for the kitchen. While the presence of a community worker to organise and facilitate the group was also identified as important for sustainability [45], changes in people facilitating the kitchen also coincided with a decrease in participation rates. This reflected the importance of individuals being involved in the program. The community kitchen has planned support and funding until 2018, at which stage the goal is for the community to take complete ownership of the program. To achieve this, addressing barriers to participation and making improvements to the program are required to ensure the CKP can continue operation and have an impact on health and food security outcomes. The quality improvement activities modelled to enhance the nutritional composition of meals and reduce the operating costs could contribute to achieving long-term sustainability. Meals have been developed to provide substantial nutritional contributions to participants and their household's dietary intake. Decreasing the operating costs, using the strategies modelled, will ensure the available funding for the kitchen lasts longer, allowing more time for community ownership and long-term sustainability to be achieved.

• How were Indigenous Health Principles applied in the planning and implementation of the CKP?
• How did evaluation outcomes modify the direction or components of the program?
• Which key nutritional principles were embedded in the program, and how could this have an impact on health?

Poor nutrition, largely as a result of limited access to healthy food and poor nutrition knowledge, is strongly associated with high morbidity and mortality in Indigenous populations [46]. In the case of community kitchens, few programs have evaluated the nutritional contribution of the meals produced. By demonstrating low-cost, flavoursome and healthy meal ideas in a supportive environment, key issues that place Indigenous communities at risk of food security—including low income, loss of traditional lifestyle and access to traditional foods, limited nutrition knowledge and lack of culturally appropriate information—can be addressed [23; 25; 40]. Positive outcomes of community kitchens include increased nutrition, shopping and budgeting knowledge and food utilisation skills, and have also been shown to extend beyond the participants of community kitchens to their families and friends [38; 41; 47].

» RESEARCH AT WORK

COMMUNITY-DRIVEN STORE NUTRITION POLICIES

Stores for Indigenous Australians living in remote communities are typically the main source of food, so the items provided have a major impact on the health of the local community. This research showed that the implementation of a community-developed store nutrition policy changed the product lines offered, and clearly shifted trends in purchasing patterns, most notably to beverages that had a lower or zero sugar content [48]. The results reflected the work of the Mai Wiru (Good Food) Regional Stores Policy, a community-initiated, developed and implemented policy aimed at improving the health and well-being of Indigenous Australians living on the Anangu Pitjantjatjara Yankunytjatjara land through ensuring continuous access to safe, affordable and nutritious food.

Encouraging community involvement through the development of a kitchen garden to supply fresh produce for the kitchen has been shown to not only reduce costs and increase program sustainability, but also to encourage community ownership through increased responsibility, purpose and social connectedness [49]. Additional strategies to encourage community participation may include incorporating regular fishing trips by community members to supply the kitchen with fresh seafood and have more community members available to plan the meals and assist with shopping and preparation for the kitchen. Adding educational components to the kitchen sessions around budgeting and nutrition knowledge and utilising the kitchen to cater for events held within the community have also been shown to be effective [38;

41; 47]. A successful CKP in an urban Indigenous community found that encouraging the community to develop a name for the program, providing child-minding facilities, and developing connections with other programs and services within the community enhanced the sense of community and coming together, and increased participation [41]. Linking with other community and external health or welfare service providers or guest speakers to facilitate education can provide opportunities for participants to engage with services that may otherwise have barriers to access and can encourage community members to attend the CKP to utilise these [38]. It may also support the development of collaborative working relationships to support the program.

STOP AND THINK

- What are the important contributions that Indigenous Health Principles make to contemporary health service development?
- How can the concept of a community kitchen form the centre for building broader community engagement that encourages healthy dietary patterns in Indigenous Australian communities?
- What is the role of planning and evaluation in developing approaches to improving food security to support health in Indigenous Australian communities?

SUMMARY

- Before colonisation, Indigenous Australians were lean, healthy and fit, but this changed when access to traditional foods was inhibited by various factors, including type of employment.
- The traditional diet of Indigenous Australians was linked to geographical locations, but reduced food security has meant poor-quality diets and a resultant high prevalence of chronic disease.
- Programs to improve food security and nutritional health need to consider Indigenous Health Principles in planning, implementation and evaluation.

PATHWAYS TO PRACTICE

- Data on health disparities for Indigenous Australians is readily accessible to better appreciate the extent and nature of the problems that need to be addressed.
- Aboriginal Health Services and Indigenous health academics provide a starting point for consultation on their plans for research and need for collaboration.
- Community projects, including kitchens and gardens, may benefit from volunteer assistance in undertaking some of the tasks as directed by community members.

DISCUSSION QUESTIONS

1   How can the broader Australian community develop a better understanding of Indigenous Health Principles?

2   What are the implications of Indigenous Health Principles for the development of nutrition promotion programs and services?

3   What outcomes would be appropriate markers of improvements in food security for Indigenous Australians?

USEFUL WEBLINKS

Aboriginal and Torres Strait Islander Peoples—Australian Bureau of Statistics:
www.abs.gov.au/Aboriginal-and-Torres-Strait-Islander-Peoples

Australian Indigenous Health*Bulletin*:
http://healthbulletin.org.au

Australian Indigenous Health*InfoNet*:
www.healthinfonet.ecu.edu.au

Australian Institute of Aboriginal and Torres Strait Islander Studies:
https://aiatsis.gov.au

Indigenous Australians—Australian Institute of Health and Welfare:
www.aihw.gov.au/reports-statistics/population-groups/indigenous-australians/overview

FURTHER READING

Ashman, A. M., Brown, L. J., Collins, C. E., Rollo, M. E. & Rae, K. M. (2017). Factors associated with effective nutrition interventions for pregnant Indigenous women: a systematic review. *Journal of the Academy of Nutrition and Dietetics*, 117(8), 1222–53.e1222. doi:https://doi.org/10.1016/j.jand.2017.03.012

Brimblecombe, J., Bailie, R., van den Boogaard, C., Wood, B., Liberato, S. C., Ferguson, M., ... Ritchie, J. (2017). Feasibility of a novel participatory multi-sector continuous improvement approach to enhance food security in remote Indigenous Australian communities. *SSM—Population Health*, 3, 566–76. doi:10.1016/j.ssmph.2017.06.002

Browne, J., Adams, K., Atkinson, P., Gleeson, D. & Hayes, R. (2017). Food and nutrition programs for Aboriginal and Torres Strait Islander Australians: an overview of systematic reviews. *Australian Health Review*. doi:https://doi.org/10.1071/AH17082

Campbell, M. A., Hunt, J., Scrimgeour, D. J., Davey, M. & Jones, V. (2017). Contribution of Aboriginal Community-Controlled Health Services to improving Aboriginal health: an evidence review. *Australian Health Review*, 42(2), 218–26. doi:https://doi.org/10.1071/AH16149

Davy, D. (2016). Australia's efforts to improve food security for Aboriginal and Torres Strait Islander peoples. *Health and Human Rights*, 18(2), 209–18.

Genat, B., Browne, J., Thorpe, S. & MacDonald, C. (2016). Sectoral system capacity development in health promotion: evaluation of an Aboriginal nutrition program. *Health Promotion Journal of Australia*, 27(3), 236–42. doi:https://doi.org/10.1071/HE16044

Gibson, O., Lisy, K., Davy, C., Aromataris, E., Kite, E., Lockwood, C., ... Brown, A. (2015). Enablers and barriers to the implementation of primary health care interventions for Indigenous people with chronic diseases: a systematic review. *Implementation Science*, 10(1), 71. doi:10.1186/s13012-015-0261-x

Helson, C., Walker, R., Palermo, C., Rounsefell, K., Aron, Y., MacDonald, C., ... Browne, J. (2017). Is Aboriginal nutrition a priority for local government? A policy analysis. *Public Health Nutrition*, 1–10. doi:10.1017/S1368980017001902

Henryks, J. & Brimblecombe, J. (2016). Mapping point-of-purchase influencers of food choice in Australian remote Indigenous communities: a review of the literature. *SAGE Open*, 6(1). doi:10.1177/2158244016629183

Lee, A., Rainow, S., Tregenza, J., Tregenza, L., Balmer, L., Bryce, S., ... Schomburgk, D. (2016). Nutrition in remote Aboriginal communities: lessons from Mai Wiru and the Anangu Pitjantjatjara Yankunytjatjara Lands. *Australian and New Zealand Journal of Public Health*, 40, S81–S88. doi:10.1111/1753-6405.12419

MacLean, S., Ritte, R., Thorpe, A., Ewen, S. & Arabena, K. (2017). Health and wellbeing outcomes of programs for Indigenous Australians that include strategies to enable the expression of cultural identities: a systematic review. *Australian Journal of Primary Health*, 23(4), 309–18. doi:https://doi.org/10.1071/PY16061

Magnus, A., Moodie, M. L., Ferguson, M., Cobiac, L. J., Liberato, S. C. & Brimblecombe, J. (2016). The economic feasibility of price discounts to improve diet in Australian Aboriginal remote communities. *Australian and New Zealand Journal of Public Health*, 40, S36–S37. doi:10.1111/1753-6405.12391

Pettigrew, S., Jongenelis, M. I., Moore, S. & Pratt, I. S. (2015). A comparison of the effectiveness of an adult nutrition education program for Aboriginal and non-Aboriginal Australians. *Social Science & Medicine*, 145(suppl. C), 120–4. doi:https://doi.org/10.1016/j.socscimed.2015.09.025

Rogers, A. (2018). Strengthening food systems with remote Indigenous Australians: stakeholders' perspectives. *Health Promotion International*, 33(1), 38–48. doi:10.1093/heapro/daw047

Schembri, L., Curran, J., Collins, L., Pelinovskaia, M., Bell, H., Richardson, C. & Palermo, C. (2016). The effect of nutrition education on nutrition-related health outcomes of Aboriginal and Torres Strait Islander people: a systematic review. *Australian and New Zealand Journal of Public Health*, 40(S1), S42–S47. doi:10.1111/1753-6405.12392

Silburn, S., Robinson, G., Arney, F., Johnstone, K. & McGuinness, K. (2011). *Early Childhood Development in the NT: Issues to be addressed. Topical paper commissioned for the public consultations on the Northern Territory Early Childhood Plan*. Darwin: NT Government.

Stoner, L., Page, R., Matheson, A., Tarrant, M., Stoner, K., Rubin, D. & Perry, L. (2015). The Indigenous health gap: raising awareness and changing attitudes. *Perspectives in Public Health*, 135(2), 68–70. doi:10.1177/1757913915569965

REFERENCES

1 N. Thomson (1984). Aboriginal health—current status. *Internal Medicine Journal,* 14(5), 705–18.

2 NSW Department of Health (2004). *Communicating Positively: A guide to appropriate Aboriginal terminology*. Sydney: NSW Department of Health.

3 N. B. Tindale (1940). *Distribution of Australian Aboriginal Tribes: A field survey* (vol. 64). Adelaide: Royal Society of South Australia.

4 M. Langton & R. Perkins (2008). *First Australians*. Parkville: Miegunyah Press.

5 S. G. Foster & B. Attwood (2003). *Frontier Conflict: The Australian experience*: Canberra: National Museum of Australia Press.

6   D. Trewin (2002). *Population Distribution, Aboriginal and Torres Strait Islander Australians, 2001.* Canberra: Australian Bureau of Statistics.

7   R. Broome (2005). *Aboriginal Victorians: A history since 1800.* Sydney: Allen & Unwin.

8   A.-K. Eckermann, T. Dowd, E. Chong, R. Gray & L. Nixon (2010). *Binan Goonj: Bridging cultures in Aboriginal health.* Melbourne: Elsevier Australia.

9   R. McGregor (1997). *Imagined Destinies: Aboriginal Australians and the doomed race theory, 1880–1939.* Melbourne: Melbourne University Press.

10 B. F. McCoy (2008). *Holding Men: Kanyirninpa and the health of Aboriginal men.* Canberra: Aboriginal Studies Press.

11 M. Gracey (2000). Historical, cultural, political, and social influences on dietary patterns and nutrition in Australian Aboriginal children. *American Journal of Clinical Nutrition,* 72(5), 1361s–1367s.

12 K. O'Dea, N. White & A. Sinclair (1988). An investigation of nutrition-related risk factors in an isolated Aboriginal community in northern Australia: advantages of a traditionally-orientated life-style. *Medical Journal of Australia,* 148(4), 177–80.

13 K. O'Dea, P. Jewell, A. Whiten, S. Altmann, S. Strickland & O. Oftedal (1991). Traditional diet and food preferences of Australian Aboriginal hunter-gatherers [and discussion]. *Philosophical Transactions of the Royal Society of London B: Biological Sciences,* 334(1270), 233–41.

14 J. Brand & V. Cherikoff (1985). The nutritional composition of Australian Aboriginal food plants of the desert regions. In G. E. Wickens, J. R. Goodin & D. V. Field (eds), *Plants for Arid Lands* (pp. 53–68). Springer.

15 B. Pascoe (2014). *Dark Emu: Black Seeds: Agriculture or Accident?* Broome: Magabala Books. See: www.magabala.com/culture-and-history/dark-emu.html.

16 H.V. Kuhnlein & O. Receveur (1996). Dietary change and traditional food systems of indigenous peoples. *Annual Review of Nutrition,* 16(1), 417–42.

17 World Food Summit (1996). *Rome Declaration on World Food Security and World Food Summit Plan of Action.* Rome: FAO.

18 Food and Agriculture Organization (2009). *World Summit on Food Security.* Rome: FAO.

19 S. L. Godrich, C. R. Davies, J. Darby & A. Devine (2017). What are the determinants of food security among regional and remote Western Australian children? *Australian and New Zealand Journal of Public Health,* 41(2), 172–7.

20 S. Booth & A. Smith (2001). Food security and poverty in Australia: challenges for dietitians. *Australian Journal of Nutrition and Dietetics,* 58(3), 150–6.

21 Australian Bureau of Statistics (2013). *Australian Aboriginal and Torres Strait Islander Health Survey: First results, Australia, 2012–13.* Canberra: ABS.

22 J. Browne, S. Laurence & S. Thorpe (2009). Acting on food insecurity in urban Aboriginal and Torres Strait Islander communities. *Policy and Practice Interventions to Improve Local Access and Supply of Nutritious Food, 2000–2010.*

23 C. Burns (2004). *A Review of the Literature Describing the Link Between Poverty, Food Insecurity and Obesity with Specific Reference to Australia.* Melbourne: VicHealth.

24 S. L. Colles, S. Belton & J. Brimblecombe (2016). Insights into nutritionists' practices and experiences in remote Australian Aboriginal communities. *Australian and New Zealand Journal of Public Health,* 40(S1).

25 T. Vos, B. Barker, S. Begg, L. Stanley & A. D. Lopez (2009). Burden of disease and injury in Aboriginal and Torres Strait Islander peoples: the Indigenous health gap. *International Journal of Epidemiology*, 38(2), 470–7.

26 S. T. Garnett, B. Sithole, P. J. Whitehead, C. P. Burgess, F. H. Johnston & T. Lea (2009). Healthy country, healthy people: policy implications of links between Indigenous human health and environmental condition in tropical Australia. *Australian Journal of Public Administration*, 68(1), 53–66.

27 P. Laws, S. Abeywardana, J. Walker & E. Sullivan (2007). *Australia's Mothers and Babies 2005. Perinatal statistics series number 20*. Cat. no.: PER, 50. Sydney: AIHW National Perinatal Statistics Unit.

28 S. Silburn, G. Robinson, F. Arney, K. Johnstone & K. McGuinness (2011). *Early Childhood Development in the NT: Issues to be addressed. Topical paper commissioned for the public consultations on the Northern Territory Early Childhood Plan*. Darwin: NT Government.

29 Australian Bureau of Statistics (2006). *National Aboriginal and Torres Strait Islander Health Survey, 2004–05*. Canberra: ABS

30 Australian Institute of Health and Welfare (2015). *Cardiovascular Disease, Diabetes and Chronic Kidney Disease—Australian facts: Aboriginal and Torres Strait Islander people. Cardiovascular, diabetes and chronic kidney disease series no. 5*. Cat. no. CDK 5. Canberra: AIHW.

31 M. King, A. Smith & M. Gracey (2009). Indigenous health part 2: the underlying causes of the health gap. *The Lancet*, 374(9683), 76–85.

32 S. Mathur, L. Moon & S. Leigh (2006). *Aboriginal and Torres Strait Islander People with Coronary Heart Disease: Summary report: further perspectives on health status and treatment*. Sydney: AIHW.

33 R. Glazebrook & S. Harrison (2006). Obstacles and solutions to maintenance of advanced procedural skills for rural and remote medical practitioners in Australia. *Rural Remote Health*, 6(4), 502.

34 P. Azzopardi, A. D. Brown, P. Zimmet, R. E. Fahy, G. A. Dent, M. J. Kelly, ... M. Silink (2012). Type 2 diabetes in young Indigenous Australians in rural and remote areas: diagnosis, screening, management and prevention. *Medical Journal of Australia*, 197(1), 32–6.

35 Australian Institute of Health and Welfare (2010). *Indigenous Identification in Hospital Separations Data—Quality report. Health Services Series no. 35*. Cat. no. HSE 85. Canberra: AIHW.

36 R. Griew, E. Tilton, N. Cox & D. Thomas (2008). *The Link Between Primary Health Care and Health Outcomes for Aboriginal and Torres Strait Islander Australians*. Sydney: Robert Griew Consulting.

37 M. Iacovou, D. C. Pattieson, H. Truby & C. Palermo (2013). Social health and nutrition impacts of community kitchens: a systematic review. *Public Health Nutrition*, 16(3), 535–43.

38 M. Murray, E. Bonnell, S. Thorpe, J. Browne, L. Barbour, C. MacDonald & C. Palermo (2014). Sharing the tracks to good tucker: identifying the benefits and challenges of implementing community food programs for Aboriginal communities in Victoria. *Australian Journal of Primary Health*, 20(4), 373–8.

39 L. Newman, F. Baum, S. Javanparast, K. O'Rourke & L. Carlon (2015). Addressing social determinants of health inequities through settings: a rapid review. *Health Promotion International*, 30(suppl. 2), ii126–ii143.

40 J. H. Lee, J. McCartan, C. Palermo & A. Bryce (2010). Process evaluation of community kitchens: results from two Victorian local government areas. *Health Promotion Journal of Australia*, 21(3), 183–8.

41 S. Malie & L. Robertson (2011). Planting a seed and watching it blossom: Koori community kitchen making a difference. *Aboriginal and Islander Health Worker Journal*, 35(6), 4.

42 A. Viola (2006). Evaluation of the Outreach School Garden Project: building the capacity of two Indigenous remote school communities to integrate nutrition into the core school curriculum. *Health Promotion Journal of Australia*, 17(3), 233–9.

43 K. Skinner, R. Hanning, J. Metatawabin, I. Martin & L. Tsuji (2012). Impact of a school snack program on the dietary intake of grade six to ten First Nation students living in a remote community in northern Ontario, Canada. *Rural and Remote Health*, 12(2122).

44 K. Skinner, R. Hanning, J. Metatawabin & L. J. Tsuji (2014). Implementation of a community greenhouse in a remote, sub-Arctic First Nations community in Ontario, Canada: a descriptive case study. *Rural and Remote Health*, 14(2), 2545.

45 S. Crawford & L. Kalina (1997). Building food security through health promotion: community kitchens. *Journal of the Canadian Dietetic Association*.

46 Strategic Inter-Governmental Nutrition Alliance (2000). *The National Aboriginal and Torres Strait Islander Nutrition Strategy and Action Plan 2000–2010*. Canberra: National Public Health Partnership.

47 P. A. Abbott, J. E. Davison, L. F. Moore & R. Rubinstein (2012). Effective nutrition education for Aboriginal Australians: lessons from a diabetes cooking course. *Journal of Nutrition Education and Behavior*, 44(1), 55–9.

48 R. Butler, L. Tapsell & P. Lyons-Wall (2011). Trends in purchasing patterns of sugar-sweetened water-based beverages in a remote Aboriginal community store following the implementation of a community-developed store nutrition policy. *Nutrition & Dietetics*, 68(2), 115–19.

49 F. Gendron, A. Hancherow & A. Norton (2017). Exploring and revitalizing Indigenous food networks in Saskatchewan, Canada, as a way to improve food security. *Health Promotion International*, 32(5), 808–17. doi:10.1093/heapro/daw013

CHAPTER 20

SOCIAL AND BEHAVIOURAL ASPECTS OF FOOD CONSUMPTION

LAUREN WILLIAMS AND ANNE McMAHON

CHAPTER OBJECTIVES

This chapter will enable the reader to:

- outline how a social-ecological model of health underpins understanding of food choice
- identify key social and behavioural theories that are applied in nutrition interventions
- appreciate the value of social and behavioural influences on dietary change.

KEY TERMS

Agency

Foodways

Intervention

Social structure

Socio-ecological model
of health

KEY POINTS

- Food consumption is a behaviour performed by individuals in a social context.
- The influences on the foods people choose to eat operate at the level of the individual, the group and the wider society, and reflect the tension between social structure and personal agency at each of these levels.
- Strategies targeting improved food choice and nutritional status in the community need to be informed by understandings of society and human behaviour.

INTRODUCTION

The act of eating is one of the most commonly performed human behaviours. The ability to source, consume and digest a stable food supply ensures human survival. The processes of digestion and absorption are no different from those of our distant ancestors. Where we differ from our ancestors is in the complexity of the social and environmental influences around what food we choose to put in our mouths. While hunger is a biological drive and food is essential to survival, the act of food consumption is not merely based on meeting physiological needs. Food-related behaviours, including when we eat, who we eat with, how we procure and prepare our food and what foods we choose, are incredibly complex and occur in social and environmental contexts. Health science research provides evidence of the impact of diet-related illness on population health. Reversing undesirable trends in food consumption is not a simple or straightforward process. This chapter will examine the social and behavioural influences on food consumption, and explore what these influences mean for food and nutrition interventions aimed at optimising health and well-being.

> See Chapter 3 on digestion, absorption and metabolism.
>
> See Chapter 1 on the social and environmental contexts of food.

STOP AND THINK

- What is meant by the 'social and environmental' context?
- What are some of the factors in this context that influence food choice?
- Why is this relevant to practice in targeting improvements in dietary intakes?

HOW DOES A SOCIO-ECOLOGICAL MODEL OF HEALTH UNDERPIN UNDERSTANDING OF FOOD CHOICE?

Behavioural and social theories enable us to explore the links between food, behaviour and society. They are sensitive to the notion of **discourses** that can view life from a number of different perspectives. Sociology introduces concepts such as debates about **social structures** and **agency**, or people's ability to act. In considering a social behaviour like food consumption, a brief introduction to a sociological perspective is useful. Sociology is the study of how society is organised, how it influences our lives and how social change occurs. Sociologists look for patterns in social interactions where individual behaviour (agency) operates within the way in which society is organised (social structure) [1]. Structure and agency coexist in a state of tension with each other, and both influence the foods that we consume. Social structures that influence food consumption include the agricultural system, the food-processing industry, food distribution networks, the retail food industry, the food service industry, food laws and policies around the production, distribution and consumption of food, education around food and nutrition, religious practices and cultural beliefs. However, while social structure may alter the type of food available, it is important to note that humans still have agency, or free choice, over what food to eat, as well as the ability to advocate for changes to the existing food systems and laws.

> **Discourse**
> representations such as narrative forms in which a certain perspective is presented.
>
> **Social structure**
> patterns of social interaction by which people are related to each other through social institutions and social groups.
>
> **Agency**
> the ability of individuals to exercise choice in, and have influence over, their daily lives and wider society.

LAUREN WILLIAMS AND ANNE McMAHON

Socio-ecological model of health

an approach based on ecological systems theory that considers the behaviour of individuals within a social context.

The **socio-ecological model of health** is a framework that argues that individual behaviour is situated within the social and environmental context. The model notes that the individual is located within groupings, or networks, at various levels, including interpersonal, organisational structures, community, and public policy.

In terms of the influences on food choice and consumption, aspects of the socio-ecological model have been adapted to develop the model in Figure 20.1. The individual is at the centre of the model. This is the level of immediate food choice and consumption. Biology and psychology, including learning and knowledge, are major influences over people's food consumption at this level. The next circle acknowledges that individuals interact within the various groupings to which they belong, including families, peer and cultural groups. Seeking to belong to these groups means following the behaviours of the group, which includes food choice and eating behaviour. The individual level and the group level are both located within a further grouping—broader society—which includes the structure of the food supply. Policies and practices around agriculture, food processing, distribution, marketing and retail all influence food availability, affordability and accessibility, impacting on the foods individuals choose to consume.

This tension between structure and agency operates in all three sectors of Figure 20.1, resulting in patterns of food consumption in society. Each of these levels will be examined in turn below. The separation into levels does not intend to imply that the levels (individual, group and society) operate independently. The diagram illustrates their interconnectedness.

FIGURE 20.1   INFLUENCES ON FOOD BEHAVIOUR AT THE LEVEL OF THE INDIVIDUAL, GROUP AND SOCIETY (BASED ON THE SOCIO-ECOLOGICAL MODEL OF HEALTH)

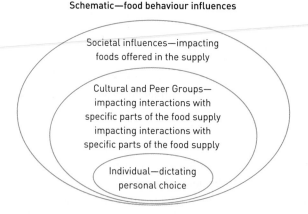

Schematic—food behaviour influences

TABLE 20.1   FACTORS INFLUENCING FOOD CHOICE

Individual-level factors	Group-level factors	Environmental factors
Behavioural	Family membership	Food system
Psychological	Gender identity	Food and health policy
Cognitive	Cultural groups	Information environment
Affective	Religion	Food consumption settings
	Social 'class'	

Individual-level influences

Eating is a type of behaviour—an act that is performed by an individual. Most people perform the act of eating several times a day, sometimes with little thought. Despite the almost taken-for-granted aspect of eating, there are complex factors underlying food consumption. For a healthy, free-living individual with a secure food supply, food consumption directly reflects food choice, which means the individual has the choice over their food behaviour, including what they eat, when and where they eat, and who they eat with. This section will explore the factors that influence food consumption (see Figure 20.2). Note: it does not explore this issue in relation to people who have little or no choice over what they eat, such as those people who live in an institution (such as an aged care home) or lack sufficient financial means to buy or prepare the foods they would like to eat (the food insecure).

See Chapter 21 on food security.

Biological and psychological influences on eating behaviour

The main influences at the level of individual consumption are *biological* (hunger and satiety, sensory perceptions) and *psychological* (taste preferences, food aversions, mood states), and these are frequently interrelated. For example, there is a difference between hunger and appetite. Hunger is a biological drive, mediated by chemical messages in the brain and gastrointestinal tract released in response to signals by the body that the proceeds of the last meal consumed have been metabolised. Hunger drives people to eat and is therefore a basic biological process aimed at keeping us alive.

Appetite, on the other hand, is a psychological drive. It is the desire to eat, in response to sensory cues such as sight, smell or taste. If we respond to appetite, we are seeking pleasure or contentment,

FIGURE 20.2 FACTORS AFFECTING FOOD CHOICE AND INTAKE

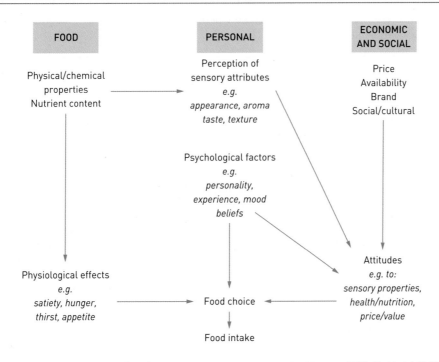

Source: D. Shepherd (1985). Dietary salt intake. *Nutrition & Food Science*, 85(5), 10–11. doi:10.1108/eb059082

LAUREN WILLIAMS AND ANNE McMAHON

rather than survival. If food consumption was driven only by hunger, people would eat anything until their physiological needs were met, and then they would stop. This is not the typical way in which people eat, which is instead more in line with appetite, responds to food preferences and aversions, and is based on past experiences and learning around food. With advances in magnetic resonance imaging (MRI) technology, neuroscientists are increasingly studying what happens in the brain when people are hungry, and what happens in response to food driven cues (appetite), as demonstrated in the Research at work feature.

» RESEARCH AT WORK

WHAT HAPPENS IN THE BRAIN IN RESPONSE TO FOOD IMAGERY?

A systematic review was conducted of 60 studies that examined the relationship between body weight and brain activity in response to food cues of 1565 adults [2]. The study participants spent time exposed to a series of images in a functional MRI machine, which measured brain activity in real time. When shown pictures of food, people had different brain responses according to whether they were healthy weight, obese or had previously lost weight.

One of the key findings was that in people who were overweight or obese, the part of the brain associated with reward was more strongly activated than in those who were healthy weight. This response was noted with respect to food cues, particular high-energy foods such as chocolate, chips and hamburgers, as compared with non-food pictures. When the observations were conducted on a full stomach, people of healthy weight responded less to food cues than those who were overweight or obese. Brain activity prior to weight-loss intervention was found to predict success in preventing weight regain. This study shows that the neural pathways in the brain activated in response to food are related to weight status. However, it was not possible to conclude whether being rewarded by thoughts of high-energy foods is a cause or effect of overweight.

Affective and cognitive influences: food experiences, learning and nutrition education

The human brain begins to learn about food and eating even before birth. There is evidence that some chemical compounds in foods are passed to the foetus through the amniotic fluid *in utero*, and through breast milk or infant formula to the newborn infant. Exposure to these food constituents has been shown to influence acceptability of foods introduced to infants [3]. Humans are conditioned to like sweet foods, as sugar helps to encourage consumption of the intended first food of babies—breast milk—which is sweet due to a high lactose content. Other taste preferences develop after birth, and there is a general aversion to foods that taste bitter or sour. Learning about taste preferences begins as conditioning, but as the brain develops, so does higher learning and the development of attitudes and beliefs about food (Figure 20.3). Learning can help to overcome the innate aversion to bitter foods, allowing humans to develop a liking for beverages such as coffee, for example.

See Chapter 14 on lactation.

Much of children's initial learning about food is from their parents and other early influencers, in providing a social context to affective (emotional) responses to foods. This may be in the form of modelling, where adults or other children provide a model for what and how to eat, and through parenting practices. Parents can have a positive or negative effect on the quality of the foods that children eat. Leann Birch, a psychologist who largely pioneered the field of the influences on childhood

FIGURE 20.3 FLAVOUR EXPERIENCES THROUGHOUT CHILDHOOD

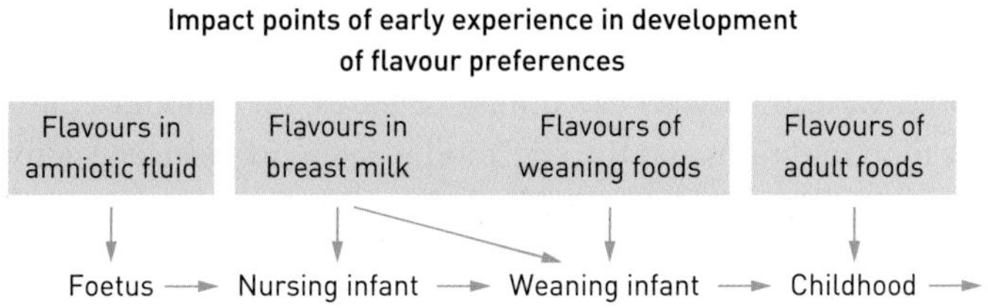

Impact points of early experience in development
of flavour preferences

| Flavours in amniotic fluid | Flavours in breast milk | Flavours of weaning foods | Flavours of adult foods |

Foetus → Nursing infant → Weaning infant → Childhood →

Source: G. K. Beauchamp & J. A. Mennella (2009). Early flavor learning and its impact on later feeding behavior. *Journal of Pediatric Gastroenterology and Nutrition*, 48, S25–S30. doi:10.1097/MPG.0b013e31819774a5

food practices, has shown that parents who use food as a reward can make health-promoting foods like vegetables less attractive, and high-fat foods more attractive, despite having the opposite intention [4]. Excessive restriction and pressuring children to eat can also have undesired consequences for food preferences.

In terms of learning about the effect that food has on the body, there is high awareness that the food people eat affects their health. The common sayings of 'an apple a day keeps the doctor away' or 'you are what you eat' are reminders of the biological effects of food. However, understanding that eating well promotes good health does not necessarily mean that healthy eating practices follow—part of food choice is a decision whether or not to eat in a healthy way. The ways in which the behavioural and social aspects of food consumption need to be considered when aiming for dietary change is addressed later in the chapter.

The development of food preferences from early childhood is a complex interplay between biology (taste perceptions, satiety), experience (liking or disliking a particular food), emotional responses to eating in a social context (food modelling, parental feeding practices) and cognitions (attitudes and beliefs). These factors provide individuals with a range of preferred foods. However, food choice is moderated to reflect the social groups and the broader society to which individuals belong. While humans all consume the same milk diet as infants, by age two to three children in different cultural groups consume diets that are composed of a variety of foods that may have no foods in common [5]. The way in which group membership influences food consumption is considered in the next section.

See Chapter 15 on nutrition during childhood.

Group-level influences

The preparation and consumption of food is an inherently social activity, one that is influenced by the groups that people belong to, or would like to belong to. Food is part of each person's identity formation and can be used to signify membership of a particular group. Food consumption becomes a marker of social identity and a way of establishing membership of some groups as distinct from others. Think about the type of takeaway coffee you buy—if you see yourself as a dedicated latte drinker, you would probably turn down the offer of an instant coffee. These choices signify more than a person's knowledge of these products; they signal the groups with which someone wants to associate themselves—for example, family, gender, cultural, religious and class-based groups. Following the distinct eating practices of the group signifies group membership, but it is important to note this is a fluid environment, and social dynamics are constantly changing.

LAUREN WILLIAMS AND ANNE McMAHON

Families

Families are the first influence on the foods that people eat and, as discussed earlier in the chapter, can have a profound effect on food choices. Food habits are largely formed in families. These habits not only include the type of foods we eat, but also the timing of meals, the amount consumed and the setting people eat in, as well as food traditions and the way food is eaten on special occasions. Ground-breaking work in the area of food sociology by Nickie Charles and Marion Kerr illustrated the way in which the social dynamics within families determined food choice in the United Kingdom in the 1980s [6]. The authors found that even though women took the main responsibility for purchasing and preparing food, they chose to serve food according to the preferences of their husband in the first instance, and then their children, and placed their own food preferences last. Charles and Kerr concluded that this reflected gender roles in society, with the men being the money earners and therefore playing the main role in setting the menu (see also the section on gender below). John Coveney [7] conducted detailed qualitative interviews with families around the meaning of food in Australia in the late 1990s. He found that family meal times were used to instruct about nutrition as a means of conveying messages about morality, particularly to children. While the findings of these studies are specific to those countries and time frames, it is noteworthy that the person within a family who has the most influence on food choice may vary. These examples illustrate that eating together in a family context is not only about food consumption, but also about the reproduction and reinforcement of family and societal values.

In Australia, the traditional concept of the evening meal includes family members sitting around the table together, sharing stories about their day. However, studies show that this traditional way of eating has diminished with broader changes in society, such as the rising number of dual-income families. This has decreased the time that women spend in the home, which means they have less time available for food preparation, resulting in an increased reliance on takeaway food and eating out. These behaviours are likely to be further influenced by the increasing number of smaller dwellings such as flats and apartments that are being built without full kitchens, which may limit opportunities to engage in food preparation activities. Given the evidence that people tend to consume more when eating in a social setting, the increased prevalence of eating out has implications for weight management and health. Again, the concept of family is also changing, as the roles people play in household units shift through the ages.

» CASE 20.1

EATING OUT OR AT HOME

In recent decades, there has been a change in the way that families eat meals, particularly the evening meal. Where the evening meal was traditionally prepared and consumed in the home, these meals are increasingly being prepared and/or consumed outside the home. A 2016 survey of 1095 consumers, commissioned by the food industry [8], found that the average Australian family eats out two to three times per week, spending $94 per week on food and alcohol in the process. In comparison, the most recent weekly household expenditure figures from the Australian Bureau of Statistics found that the average household spends $237 weekly on buying food (including eating out) and non-alcoholic beverages, and a further $32 on alcoholic beverages [9], and it is evident that a significant proportion of the family budget goes towards eating out.

The food industry study also found that the more traditional cuisines for eating out, such as Chinese and Italian, while still popular, were gradually declining in popularity, with an increase in cuisines that had a better health profile, such as Modern Australian, Japanese and vegetarian [8]. These trends aside, an analysis of data from a large survey has shown that foods prepared outside the home tend to make a significant contribution to energy and fat intake [10].

- What are the likely effects on food choice of eating outside the home?
- How has the availability of different cultural cuisines influenced food choice in Australia?
- What are the implications of these trends towards eating out for health promotion activities?

Gender

Rather than being a biological definition of sex as male or female, gender is a socially constructed classification according to whether a person considers themselves to possess characteristics and behaviours associated with being masculine or feminine [10]. Today, gender issues are at the forefront of public debate. Traditionally, being masculine or feminine required people to behave in certain ways [11], and even foods chosen can be seen as reflecting how people perform gender roles [12]. Studies have consistently found that specific types of food and drink are associated with masculine or feminine characteristics, thus making these foods 'gendered' [13]. For example, it could be argued that one of the most strongly gendered foods is red meat, which is identified with masculinity, as in the saying 'feed the man meat' [14]. Red meat is a food comprised of muscle fibres and is coloured red by blood, which could be seen as symbolising the strength and aggression needed to hunt for food. While most Western men now 'hunt' for their food in supermarket, they may still eat meat as a symbol of their strength and masculinity. Women may have avoided eating red meat because it was seen as a masculine food, opting instead for the more feminine option of 'white' flesh, such as chicken or fish, from which red blood is absent [14].

Foods such as fruit and vegetables reflect the feminine gender role of growing food and nurturing others [13]. While more men than women are overweight and obese, more women than men diet to control their body weight, making dieting a gendered behaviour [13]. Another key influence is the fact that fruits and vegetables are associated with promoting health and dieting, roles strongly associated with the female role in society. It is seen as a feminine trait to look after the health of the family through possessing food and nutrition knowledge, and women still perform the majority of food preparation [15].

Cultural groups

Culture is defined as the collective values, assumptions and beliefs shared by a group of people that influences the behaviour of the group members [16]. Around the world, culture has led people to develop different **foodways**. While these may have originally developed due to the foods and means of cooking available at the time, they continue to be reproduced as a means of signifying membership of a cultural group. One example is Chinese cuisine, which is based on foods (mostly vegetables) stir-fried in a wok and served with rice. As Chinese people migrated throughout the world, they took their foods and preparation method with them, to ensure they could still eat in a way consistent with their culture. The Australian population is largely comprised of migrant groups and its foodways have been influenced by each wave of migration. After the Second World War, migration from Italy and Greece gave Australia Mediterranean foods and ways of eating. Later migration from Asia, such as from Vietnam, followed some decades later

Foodways
the historical, cultural, social and economic practices of a group around the production and consumption of food.

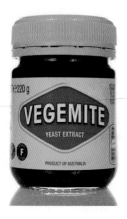

and made a strong impact on food preparation styles. By the mid-1990s, Australia's ethnically diverse society was reflected in the food-fusion style referred to as 'Modern Australian' or 'Mod Oz'. The style is characterised by fresh produce that is minimally processed, with the addition of flavours and ingredients from Asian, Mediterranean and Indigenous food cultures.

Culture also determines what is considered to be 'food'. While Australian Indigenous peoples living a traditional lifestyle might consider witchetty grubs as food, people migrating to Australia might see witchetty grubs as insects, and not consider them as food. Some individual foods are strong markers of cultural identity—for example, many Australians will have been given Vegemite™ from an early age, and may associate it with a sense of home. Australians moving overseas often describe missing Vegemite™ to symbolise homesickness, which family members seek to address by shipping Vegemite™ overseas in a 'care' package. However, the product is not loved universally. People from non-Australian countries who taste Vegemite™ often fail to see its attraction [17]. Since a liking for Vegemite™ is not genetically determined, this makes it a socially determined food preference—one that is tied to early family influences and a sense of cultural pride, even though the company that produces it has not always been Australian-owned.

It is important to note that cultural groups based on ethnicity or country of origin are not necessarily homogenous; instead, it is usually possible to distinguish certain groups within a culture, known as subcultures. Subcultures vary from the dominant culture in one or more key characteristics. As an example, young people have sufficiently different practices and behaviours to form a youth subculture, and food choice and consumption is one way they distinguish themselves from the dominant culture.

Likewise, vegetarians or vegans may be regarded as subcultural groupings based around food practices. A vegetarian eats no flesh, fish or fowl, and there are subcategories of vegetarians, such as lacto-vegetarians, who avoid eggs but consume dairy products, and ovo-vegetarians, who consume eggs but avoid dairy products. A vegan not only avoids meat, fish and poultry, but also abstains from eating (and sometimes wearing) any animal products.

≫ CASE 20.2

VEGETARIANISM: MORE THAN A DIETARY PATTERN

Some studies suggest that vegetarianism and veganism are increasing in prevalence in countries such as Australia, particularly in young adults, and they are more common among women (see the section on gender). There are many reasons people give for choosing to be vegetarian or vegan, including health reasons, concern for environmental sustainability, and animal welfare. Environmentalists argue that people should have at least two meat-free meals each week because the production of meat comes at an unsustainably high environmental cost. Health authorities promote the eating of more plant-based foods and less animal-based foods. Animal rights activists point to inhumane practices around intensive animal food production. Given these major drivers, one might imagine that vegetarians are widely recognised for taking on a social responsibility in following a healthy lifestyle and putting less burden on the food system. On the other hand, health authorities tend to take a cautious approach to vegetarianism, noting that it is possible to miss out on essential nutrients if vegetarian diets are not well balanced. These concerns are especially strong in vegan diets, given the absence of any animal-produced foods. While grounded in science, concerns for nutritional adequacy may not be the only reason that society does not embrace vegetarianism more strongly. Given that the majority of people still eat meat and that Australia is a meat-producing nation, the practice of avoiding meat also challenges the dominant culture; thus, vegetarianism is more than just a dietary pattern.

- How can the different positions presented in this case also be seen in the context of the social construction of knowledge? What information do people use to form these positions?
- What reasons besides scientific evidence might influence people's choices about meat consumption (or varieties of meat)? What is the basis for these reasons?
- Consider the reasons for meat avoidance in various contexts and discuss the role that these foodways have in religion and society.

Religions

Many religions have distinct food practices, such as the avoidance of beef by Hindus and pork by orthodox Jews and Muslims. These practices take the form of strict rules about which foods are considered acceptable to eat—that is, what is considered kosher in the Jewish religion, or halal in Islam [18] (see also Case 20.3). These rules mostly arose due to food availability and other practicalities. Following religious food rules is generally more about obeying the religion's precepts and demonstrating membership of that religion than it is about food preferences.

Hinduism and Buddhism, which originated in ancient India, have rules or aspirations for their members around meat avoidance [18]. Many Hindus follow a lacto-vegetarian diet (one that does not contain meat, poultry, fish or eggs, but does allow milk). Cows are treated as sacred animals rather than being considered as food for meat, although dairy products are highly valued. While Buddhism does not have specified food restrictions, and dietary patterns vary with religious sect or country of origin, many Buddhists avoid meat and follow a lacto-ovo vegetarian diet, which includes eggs and dairy products [18].

>> CASE 20.3

FOOD, CULTURE, RELIGION AND POLITICS

The position of food in social and cultural practices can be studied from a number of perspectives. There are many examples from disciplines outside the medical and health sciences that deal with food and society. The methods of analysis and reporting vary considerably and may require knowledge of the discipline to fully appreciate, but the ability to read across a range of discourses can provide for a fuller understanding of the role and impact of food on health.

From a medical perspective, the PREDIMED study, as discussed in previous chapters, demonstrated the preventive health value to older people in Spain returning to a traditional cuisine [19]. Food is also significant in the health and cultural history of Indigenous Australians. Analyses from other disciplines can demonstrate how food can also be implicated in the way complex political and social agendas emerge in society more broadly. For example, one analysis has presented a case of events that surrounded halal certification in Australia, which moved from social media to mainstream media in 2014 [20]. The purpose of the paper was to analyse the ramifications for Muslim

See Chapter 19 on Indigenous Australian food security.

identity of a 'stealth jihad' discourse. As such, it discussed how recent events associated with halal certification (a food-processing issue) could be associated with the social parameters of inclusion, rejection and stigmatisation (a social issue). Parallels were drawn with similar culturally identifiable food practices such as kosher certification.

- Read the papers referred to in the case. How was the reporting of food and health issues different in each of these cases?
- What was the relevance of the social context in understanding the relationship between food and health?
- What are the implications of these examples for pathways to practice in nutrition?

Social class

Class is a term used by sociologists to describe the differences in wealth, status and power among groups within society. The term 'class' is even used in travel contexts today—for example, by airlines. Sociologists use class as a category to examine the characteristics of belonging, which includes the way in which a person chooses and consumes food. Studies show that food, and the way in which it is eaten, is one of the ways in which people signify their membership of a particular social class. Even in a supposedly classless society like Australia, there are certain foods associated with the categories of working, middle or upper class—for instance, the differences between eating out at a fast-food restaurant versus a fine-dining establishment. These food choices can reflect the status and privilege associated with belonging to a particular class. Less healthy food choices can also be entrenched with negative connotations (food stigma) and might be used to judge social worth. For instance, sugar-rich foods may be spurned by the health-conscious, not because of the empty calories they represent but because they are associated with people making poor decisions leading to poor health outcomes that society has to manage.

Today, class categorisation tends to be measured as various combinations of income, occupation and education, combined to measure socioeconomic status (SES) or position (SEP). The World Health Organization (WHO) has shown that people of lower SES have a higher prevalence of diet-related diseases such as cardiovascular disease, type 2 diabetes and obesity compared with those of higher SES [21]. Some researchers have argued that this is due to inequalities inherent in the class system, rather than people merely lacking financial resources [22; 23]. It is therefore important to examine food consumption according to social class–related variables and identifiable aspects—known as the social determinants of health—to see if they may also explain differences in the prevalence these chronic diseases. A consistent finding of food-related studies is that people of higher SES/SEP tend to eat more fruit and vegetables (and therefore have a more nutrient-dense diet) than those of lower SES/SEP. However, these differences, while affecting overall diet quality, have less effect on energy density, which is reflected in overall energy and the macronutrient intake [24].

This section has considered the influence of social structures such as religious groupings and societal norms on food consumption. People can exhibit their agency in deciding which groups to belong to, or to reject. The next section considers the macro environment and the influences of broader society.

Environmental-level influences

The foods that people eat, or do not eat, are shaped by the environment in which they live. Even when a person eats alone, there are social influences on their food choice. Large structures such as the food system, policy environment, information system and lived environment all play a role in determining what foods are available to consume. Even buying petrol is no longer an activity divorced from food offerings. These additional food access points are replicated in many settings that may not have traditionally offered opportunities to eat even a decade ago, such as access to 'special health' foods in local gyms.

The food system

The food environment in developed nations such as Australia is characterised by overabundance. Technological advances following the Second World War allowed the growth of industrial food production, leading to the rise of a powerful food industry. Food is now big business, employing a large proportion of the workforce, and providing a significant source of export revenue; as such, the food industry has strong economic and political influence. To conceptualise the size and scope of food production, distribution and consumption, it is represented as a food system.

See Chapter 21 fore more on food systems.

Briefly, a food system can be considered the path that food takes from the time that it is grown in the agricultural setting, or produced/modified by the food industry, through complex distribution networks to food retailers who market and sell the products to customers, who consume a proportion of the food, and the rest becomes food waste. The system, while regulated by government (see food policy in the following paragraph), is an economic system and food is a commodity that is bought and sold. In such a system, there is a sector of the population that is food insecure. Being food insecure means they do not have regular access to available and affordable food, even in a wealthy country like Australia. Charitable agencies and governments step in to assist by providing emergency food relief to these people. This reinforces the financial basis of the food system and the government policies that support it, sometimes at the expense of humanitarian goals. The central importance of food is reflected in the fact that access to adequate food is seen as a basic human right by the United Nations (UN) in its International Covenant on Economic, Social and Cultural Rights [25]. Yet it is apparent that hunger and undernutrition are accepted as a regular way of life in some parts of the world. In 2016, 815 million people were chronically undernourished. Despite the Sustainable Development Goal of the UN to eradicate world hunger by 2030, the number of people who are undernourished increased from 777 million in 2015 [26]. It is important to recognise that this is not a failure of technology—for many years, the world has produced more than enough food to feed the entire population. The problem is one of unequal distribution, which is primarily economic, and exacerbated by extreme climate conditions, war and political unrest. Even within developed countries, where food is overly abundant, it is unavailable to some groups within society.

See Chapter 21 on food system models and food security.

Health and food policy environment

The food system is regulated by government agencies at several points, with key components enshrined in law. Economic incentives are embedded in the system for agricultural producers and for consumers; there is a consumption tax on processed food in Australia, with fresh produce being exempt in order to reduce price barriers to purchasing foods like fruit and vegetables. Governments and other agencies also develop policies that are relevant to food. A policy is a statement of intention that documents the aspirations for action of an organisation. In 1992, Australia was one of the first countries in the world to develop a national food and nutrition policy, but this was rescinded, and despite recommendations and lobbying [27], a new version was still not in place in 2018. However, large organisations, such as schools, hospitals and workplaces, might develop policies relevant to food and nutrition.

See Chapter 2 on the Australian Dietary Guidelines

Nutrition and health policies are also a potential influence on food consumption. The Australian Dietary Guidelines, as discussed throughout this book, is a set of guidelines for healthy eating based on a review of the scientific evidence for the link between food and health outcomes. The recommendations are aimed at reversing undesirable trends in food consumption in the Australian population, in particular addressing the need for people to eat more vegetables and fruit and less foods high in fat, salt and sugar [28].

>> CASE 20.4

PREVENTIVE HEALTH PARTNERSHIP

In 2017, the Australian Prevention Partnership Centre conducted a national consultation with more than 100 food and nutrition experts around Australia to evaluate policy aimed at improving population nutrition and actions to create healthier food environments [29]. The project examined the extent to which governments in Australia were implementing each of 42 policy areas shown to be important. The federal government was found to meet world best practice in some areas (including the evidence-based Australian Dietary Guidelines and the Health Star rating scheme for food labelling), and recommendations for priority actions were made for areas in which governments were not performing according to best practice. The priorities included: the need to develop a national nutrition strategy; imposing a tax on unhealthy foods (particularly sugary drinks); establishing regulations around the marketing of junk food to children; and improved monitoring of food environments to measure progress.

- To what extent do you think these strategies will address the nutrition priorities in Australia?
- What effect will they have on food consumption by individuals?

Information environment: media, food advertising and education systems

As described earlier, learning about food can impact on the food choices of individuals. The information environment relevant to food consumption comprises the food advertising and health messages distributed through mass media, social media and the formal education system. In 2009, the National Preventive Health Taskforce recommended restriction of food advertising to children in Australia due to its negative impact on their task preference and food consumption patterns [30]. Children responding to advertising may use 'pester power' in the supermarket, attempting to pressure parents to buy a desired food. Health professionals have been advocating for decades to have advertisements for unhealthy food products banned during children's television viewing time. The federal government has a voluntary code in place, but studies have shown that the number of fast-food advertisements actually increased after the introduction of the code [30]. In addition, other forms of media manipulation are being examined with respect to the effects of food messaging on children's food perceptions and intake. Food 'advergames' are another influence on children's eating behaviours that were found to impact food intake in a sustained way in a feeding study in Australia [31]. These practices are largely unregulated by government policy.

Food and nutrition form part of the school curriculum, but there is no other formal education about food and nutrition directed at the population. Health authorities, which generally have much smaller advertising budgets than large food companies, use a variety of strategies such as social marketing to educate the population on healthy eating. Social media is increasingly being used by health agencies to spread nutrition messages and conduct interventions, but it also has the potential to be used to spread misinformation and thereby create 'nutrition noise', resulting in confusion for consumers. The extent to which social media communications influence dietary intake remains to be studied.

Settings in which people live and eat

The physical environment in which people spend time, including mealtimes, is a key influence on food consumption. This includes the geographic setting—for example, people who live in remote areas of Australia pay more for food and have higher levels of food insecurity than those who live in urban areas [32]. Institutions also play a key role. Children spend 11 to 13 years of their primary and secondary level education in school settings. School canteen menus and the school's food-related policies (such as what food can be brought from home) have a significant influence over the foods that children and adolescents consume. The workplace is another setting in which people spend significant amounts of time, and large worksites may have food outlets and policies that aim to optimise the health of workers.

TRY IT YOURSELF

What influenced your food consumption the last time you ate out at a restaurant? Pick one particular eating-out occasion and consider the following questions. They are designed to illustrate the interplay between structure and agency in determining food choice at the individual, group and societal levels.

- *Deciding on the restaurant:* What was the setting? Who did you go with? How did you choose that particular place? What part did you play in the decision?
- *Ordering the food:* How much choice did you have over the food that was ordered? Did you choose a meal for yourself, or did someone else choose for you? Did you have your own meal or were the dishes shared? Did you find yourself eating foods that were different from those you would usually eat at home? Were you able to order food you really wanted or did you have to settle for something because of a limited menu? To what extent was health a factor in your food choice?

- *Eating the food:* Think about the amount of food that you ate. Did you eat more than you usually would for a similar meal at home? What influenced the amount of food you ate? To what extent was hunger an influence over how much food you ate? Did you drink alcohol with your meal?
- *Paying the bill:* How much was your share of the cost of the meal? Would you have been able to make the same meal yourself at home? How much would that have cost instead? What extra 'value' did you get from eating in the restaurant rather than at home?

These large social structures have clear effects on food availability, accessibility and affordability. Agency at this level includes the power that people have to influence these structures. The next section considers how these social and behavioural factors need to be taken into account in efforts to change the eating habits of Australians to healthier foods.

STOP AND THINK

- How strong a role should governments play in regulating the food environment?
- Should there be penalties (e.g. taxes) for food choice that is not consistent with a healthy lifestyle?
- Why is it more difficult for people who live in remote areas to eat in a healthy way?

WHICH SOCIAL AND BEHAVIOURAL THEORIES ARE COMMONLY APPLIED IN NUTRITION INTERVENTIONS?

The preceding sections have provided the background to consider why increasing nutrition knowledge alone is insufficient to change behaviour. If dietary advice, or goals for healthy eating, conflict with established or cultural foodways, or aspirational group membership, for example, permanent change in eating behaviour is unlikely to be achieved. These food attitudes and beliefs need to be appreciated, as they can form significant barriers to change. Nutrition interventions therefore need to address the structural and cultural factors influencing food choice.

Achieving a change in food consumption practices requires behaviour change, a process that is a topic of study in psychology. The study of how to change human behaviour in relation to health is an important area within this field, and the theories and models of health behaviour change are an important knowledge base for nutritionists and dietitians seeking change in dietary intake of individuals, groups and populations. Well-planned **interventions** will usually employ a behaviour-change framework to inform the strategy choice for the intervention. Some of the key models of behaviour change relevant to food consumption practices include:

Intervention

a planned program with detailed strategies aimed at achieving change.

- health belief model
- stages of change
- social cognitive theory
- theory of planned behaviour (previously theory of reasoned action).

These models vary in their framework or theoretical underpinning, and there is no one gold standard. The model chosen will depend on the aims of the intended intervention. However, all these models share recognition that changing knowledge is insufficient to achieve behaviour change (Figure 20.4).

OXFORD UNIVERSITY PRESS

FIGURE 20.4 POTENTIAL FOOD POLICIES FOR OBESITY PREVENTION BASED ON THE THEORY
OF CHANGE

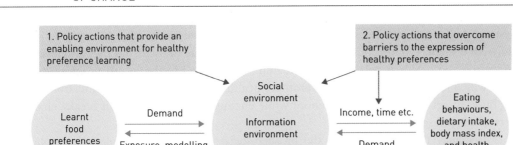

Source: C. Hawkes, T. G. Smith, J. Jewell, J. Wardle, R. A. Hammond, S. Friel, … J. Kain (2015). Smart food policies for obesity prevention. *The Lancet*, 385(9985), 2410–21. doi:10.1016/S0140-6736(14)61745-1

≫ RESEARCH AT WORK

EXPLORING INFLUENCES ON VEGETABLE CONSUMPTION: WHY NOT SPINACH?

Dietary guidelines encourage high intakes of vegetables, and health promotion activities target increased vegetable intakes, but there is a need to understand the perceptions and experiences that influence consumers' vegetable consumption [33]. This study focused on spinach, and involved semi-structured interviews with groups of different ages recruited from shopping malls located in areas of low- to middle-income earners. This was determined using the Socio Economic Indexes for Areas [34]. Participants were also recruited from non-professional staff at the local university. Bandura's social cognitive theory was considered relevant for this analysis, as it brought together concepts of self-efficacy and the influence of information sources on behaviour [35].

While participants recognised green leafy vegetables as part of a healthy diet, food selection in general was argued as being dependent on available time, convenience and food quality. Familiarity with the food, acceptability within the household, and confidence in being able to prepare the food within a culinary context formed another set of factors. Finally, nutrition knowledge and beliefs were associated with the value placed on the food, with variations present across life stages.

This qualitative research exposed the contribution that social and behavioural research plays in the translation of nutritional principles to practice, and the development of intervention programs at the population level. It shows that promoting the nutritional value of a food needs to be embedded in a social context for the benefits of consumption to be realised.

The most effective approach to interventions for complex behaviours such as dietary intake require a combination of interventions at all three of the levels in the model shown in Figure 20.1. Settings-based approaches take the local environment into account and focus on changing local food systems. As discussed earlier, schools are important environments because not only do children and adolescents spend a significant proportion of their eating time in them, but they also learn about food, nutrition and health as part of the curriculum. This has led to the health-promoting schools approach, which takes the opportunity to promote health in all aspects of school life, from creating walking buses to get children safely to school while encouraging fitness, to fruit breaks, changes in the curriculum and school policies.

Other strategies aimed at changing the broader social environment include broad policy and taxation. There is a debate in Australia about whether or not to follow the example of countries like Mexico, which introduced a tax on sugar-sweetened beverages (SSBs), a change that has achieved a 6% reduction in consumption of SSBs [36].

STOP AND THINK

- Why is behaviour change theory relevant to nutrition interventions?
- What is the relative value of the different theories?
- How does environment influence dietary behaviour?

HOW DO SOCIAL AND BEHAVIOURAL FACTORS INFLUENCE DIETARY CHANGE?

While nutrition interventions work with groups and environments in promoting dietary change, clinical healthcare services tend to work with individuals where the communication is set in the client–provider interaction of a professional consultation. Based on the early work of Carl Rogers [37], patient-centred practice is seen as fundamental in helping people manage their health conditions, particularly as it enables them to articulate meaningful personal goals [38]. In patient-centred practice, discussion on goal setting that links a person's needs with health-defined outcomes, such as weight loss, is also likely to support the behaviour change [33]. Theoretical models of behaviour change can be helpful [39], such as the stages of change model to understand key factors that influence behaviour [38; 40] (see also Table 20.2), but they need to be applied within the context of current social conditions [41–43]. Self-determination in healthcare is emerging [44], and alternative therapies are appearing in healthcare services [45–48]. In general terms, organisations such as the National Institute of Health and Clinical Excellence (NICE) acknowledge that patterns of behaviour reflect social, material and cultural contexts. From a food perspective, the emergence of 'functional' and other foods marketed on health benefits [49–51] has changed the ways people may perceive food and health [33]. While this may have positioned food more overtly with health, the relationship has not directly been used as a therapeutic tool to treat disease, but rather something that has helped to promote health and maintain functionality, in line with concepts of **wellness** and **well-being** [52].

Wellness
a sense of feeling in good health.

Well-being
a state of existence associated with a high quality of life.

TABLE 20.2 TRANSTHEORETICAL MODEL

Theory/model	Key developer	Underlying philosophy	Nutrition counselling strategies
Transtheoretical model	James O. Prochaska	Describes a sequence of cognitive (attitudes and intentions) and behavioural steps people take to change behaviour. The model offers specific strategies found effective at various points in the change process and suggests outcome measures including decision balance and self-efficacy.	Appropriate application of strategies is dependent upon the client's stage of change: • motivational interviewing • skill development training and coaching • demonstration and modelling • reinforcement • self-monitoring • goal setting and behavioural contracting • social support • stimulus control.

Source: J. M. Spahn, R. S. Reeves, K. S. Keim, I. Laquatra, M. Kellogg, B. Jortberg & N. A. Clark (2010). State of the evidence regarding behavior change theories and strategies in nutrition counseling to facilitate health and food behavior change. *Journal of the American Dietetic Association*, 110(6), 879–91. doi:https://doi.org/10.1016/j.jada.2010.03.021

» RESEARCH AT WORK

EXPLORING WOMEN'S PERCEPTIONS OF WELLNESS AND WELL-BEING IN A CLINICAL WEIGHT LOSS SETTING

Using focus group interviews, a qualitative method often used in social research, McMahon and colleagues discussed the meaning of wellness and well-being with women who had attended clinical trials at their research centre and others recruited from two community centres (a diabetes service and a fitness centre) [52]. All the women had a specific interest in food and sought some help around diet for various health-related purposes and in a range of settings.

Thematic analysis of the recorded talk showed that the terms 'wellness' and 'well-being' were significant in relation to a sense of health. The relationship with health was connected to the most sought-after result (desired outcome), strategies participants undertook themselves towards better health (taking control), personal inner factors that influenced their actions (internal influences) and external factors in the environment that also influenced their actions (external influences). The findings were consistent with other research on well-being [53; 54]. As might be expected, participants identified tension between internal and external influences in trying to achieve health outcomes, and these were expressed as both emotional and relational. In older participants, well-being was related to peace and capacity, whereas in earlier stages of life well-being was associated with energy and social acceptance. This reflected what has been termed, in other research, the 'lived experience' of well-being in a person's life [55].

Translating this to practice presents a number of challenges, although patient-centred care is stipulated in practice guidelines for dietetic professionals [56]. In social work practice, researchers have acknowledged the need to understand and work with disparate paradigms of health [57], and in dietetics there is a need to deal with multiple viewpoints and rationales in supporting behaviour change [58]. The conclusion of this focus group study of women was that assisting individuals to articulate their own notion of a satisfying life appears to be a useful starting point for working towards more detailed discussion on changing dietary behaviours.

Hence, it is likely that understanding the key motivational factors underpinning meaningful behaviour change requires more detailed exploration if individuals are to be successfully encouraged to change embedded food choice behaviour. Furthermore, practitioners need to be cognisant that what might be motivational for one person will not necessarily motivate another. Indeed, even for one individual, living in a different context or life stage may also herald different motivational needs and desires. To successfully work with individuals, groups, communities or nations, understanding these motivational imperatives requires thoughtful research to enable successful behaviour change interventions to be developed and implemented.

STOP AND THINK

- How does social science align with nutrition science in dealing with nutrition-related problems?
- What is the relative value of focusing on individuals versus society as a whole in improving nutrition in the population?
- What is the difference between researching the sociology of nutrition versus using sociology in nutrition research?

SUMMARY

- The foods people choose to consume reflect an interplay between social structure (the patterns in society) and human agency (the ability to act freely and to influence social structures).
- Influences on food consumption operate at three interrelated levels: the individual (biological and psychological factors such as hunger, sensory perception and conditioned and learnt food preferences), the group (families, gender, class groupings and foodways of the culture) and the broader society (the food system, food and health policies, the lived environment and the information system).
- The social and behavioural influences on food choice and consumption need to be considered in designing interventions. Rather than focusing on nutrition education alone, health agencies need to consider and address the attitudes and beliefs that drive food behaviours in models of behaviour change.
- The socio-ecological model of health informs interventions by going beyond behavioural change to consider the need for environmental change, including the settings in which people live and eat, the food system and the broader policy environment.

PATHWAYS TO PRACTICE

- Understanding the social and cultural factors that influence food choice is a critical element in giving effective dietary advice. For example, dietitians counselling clients on the necessary dietary changes for chronic disease management would need to understand the social and cultural contexts in which usual food consumption occurs.
- Social and cultural factors also need to be taken into account in the development of public health nutrition policies and their associated educational tools. Likewise, the development of food standards regulations may also need to consider the spectrum of cultural factors associated with foods, notwithstanding the need to assure a safe and reliable food supply.
- People working in the area of sustainable population change would also need to consider models of behaviour and environmental change where food was concerned.

DISCUSSION QUESTIONS

1　Eating is both an intensely personal and an inherently social act. Discuss.

2　Given that there are social patterns of food production, distribution and consumption, to what extent does an individual have free will over their food choice?

3　Meat, in particular red meat, is a food that can be used to convey membership of, or exclusion from, particular social groups. Discuss why red meat has meaning for different groups.

4　If people know that certain foods are detrimental to their health, why do they eat them? What would health authorities need to do to get them to change?

5　What are the advantages and disadvantages of governments establishing taxes on high-sugar or high-fat foods? To what extent does the consumer have agency in such a system?

USEFUL WEBLINKS

Australian Bureau of Statistics—Household expenditure survey:
　　http://abs.gov.au/household-expenditure

Australian Institute of Health and Welfare:
　　www.aihw.gov.au

Australian Prevention Partnership Centre:
　　http://preventioncentre.org.au

Food Standards Australia New Zealand:
　　www.foodstandards.gov.au

US Dietary Guidelines 2015–2020—The social-ecological model:
　　https://health.gov/dietaryguidelines/2015/guidelines/chapter-3/social-ecological-model

FURTHER READING

Barnes, R. D. & Ivezaj, V. (2015). A systematic review of motivational interviewing for weight loss among adults in primary care. *Obesity Reviews*, 16(4), 304–18. doi:10.1111/obr.12264

Bittner, J. V. & Kulesz, M. M. (2015). Health promotion messages: the role of social presence for food choices. *Appetite*, 87, 336–43. doi:10.1016/j.appet.2015.01.001

Bucher, T., Collins, C., Rollo, M. E., McCaffrey, T. A., De Vlieger, N., Van Der Bend, D., … Perez-Cueto, F. J. A. (2016). Nudging consumers towards healthier choices: a systematic review of positional influences on food choice. *British Journal of Nutrition*, 115(12), 2252–63. doi:10.1017/S0007114516001653

Dibb-Smith, A. & Brindal, E. (2015). Table for two: the effects of familiarity, sex and gender on food choice in imaginary dining scenarios. *Appetite*, 95, 492–9. doi:10.1016/j.appet.2015.07.032

English, L. K., Fearnbach, S. N., Wilson, S. J., Fisher, J. O., Savage, J. S., Rolls, B. J. & Keller, K. L. (2016). Food portion size and energy density evoke different patterns of brain activation in children. *American Journal of Clinical Nutrition*, 105(2), 295–305. doi:10.3945/ajcn.116.136903

Germov, J. & Williams, L. (2017). *A Sociology of Food and Nutrition: The social appetite*, 4th edn. Melbourne: Oxford University Press.

Guptill, A. E., Copelton, D. A. & Lucal, B. (2017). *Food and Society: Principles and paradoxes*, 2nd edn. Cambridge: Polity Press.

Haardörfer, R., Alcantara, I., Addison, A., Glanz, K. & Kegler, M. C. (2016). The impact of home, work, and church environments on fat intake over time among rural residents: a longitudinal observational study: health behavior, health promotion and society. *BMC Public Health*, 16(1). doi:10.1186/s12889-016-2764-z

Herman, C. P. & Higgs, S. (2015). Social influences on eating. an introduction to the special issue. *Appetite*, 86, 1–2. doi:10.1016/j.appet.2014.10.027

Higgs, S. (2015). Social norms and their influence on eating behaviours. *Appetite*, 86, 38–44. doi:10.1016/j.appet.2014.10.021

Kaisari, P. & Higgs, S. (2015). Social modelling of food intake. The role of familiarity of the dining partners and food type. *Appetite*, 86, 19–24. doi:10.1016/j.appet.2014.09.020

Kent, L. M., Morton, D. P., Rankin, P. M., Gobble, J. E. & Diehl, H. A. (2015). Gender differences in effectiveness of the complete health improvement program (CHIP). *Journal of Nutrition Education and Behavior*, 47(1), 44–59. doi:10.1016/j.jneb.2014.08.016

Loper, H. B., La Sala, M., Dotson, C. & Steinle, N. (2015). Taste perception, associated hormonal modulation, and nutrient intake. *Nutrition Reviews*, 73(2), 83–91. doi:10.1093/nutrit/nuu009

Lorenz, B. A. S., Hartmann, M. & Langen, N. (2017). What makes people leave their food? The interaction of personal and situational factors leading to plate leftovers in canteens. *Appetite*, 116, 45–56. doi:10.1016/j.appet.2017.04.014

Loth, K. A., Horning, M., Friend, S., Neumark-Sztainer, D. & Fulkerson, J. (2017). An exploration of how family dinners are served and how service style is associated with dietary and weight outcomes in children. *Journal of Nutrition Education and Behavior*, 49(6), 513–18.e511. doi:10.1016/j.jneb.2017.03.003

Marmot, M. (2004). *The Status Syndrome: How social standing affects our health and longevity*. New York: Henry Holt and Company.

Naska, A., Katsoulis, M., Orfanos, P., Lachat, C., Gedrich, K., Rodrigues, S. S. P., ... Oltarzewski, M. (2015). Eating out is different from eating at home among individuals who occasionally eat out. A cross-sectional study among middle-aged adults from eleven European countries. *British Journal of Nutrition*, 113(12), 1951–64. doi:10.1017/S0007114515000963

Patnode, C. D., Evans, C. V., Senger, C. A., Redmond, N. & Lin, J. S. (2017). Behavioral counseling to promote a healthful diet and physical activity for cardiovascular disease prevention in adults without known cardiovascular disease risk factors: updated evidence report and systematic review for the us preventive services task force. *JAMA—Journal of the American Medical Association*, 318(2), 175–93. doi:10.1001/jama.2017.3303

Peng, M., Adam, S., Hautus, M. J., Shin, M., Duizer, L. M. & Yan, H. (2017). See food diet? Cultural differences in estimating fullness and intake as a function of plate size. *Appetite*, 117, 197–202. doi:10.1016/j.appet.2017.06.032

Pfeiffer, C., Speck, M. & Strassner, C. (2017). What leads to lunch: how social practices impact (non-) sustainable food consumption/eating habits. *Sustainability (Switzerland)*, 9(8). doi:10.3390/su9081437

Polivy, J. & Herman, C. P. (2017). Restrained eating and food cues: recent findings and conclusions. *Current Obesity Reports*, 6(1), 79–85. doi:10.1007/s13679-017-0243-1

Quick, V., Martin-Biggers, J., Povis, G. A., Hongu, N., Worobey, J. & Byrd-Bredbenner, C. (2017). A socio-ecological examination of weight-related characteristics of the home environment and lifestyles of households with young children. *Nutrients*, 9(6). doi:10.3390/nu9060604

Rand, K., Vallis, M., Aston, M., Price, S., Piccinini-Vallis, H., Rehman, L. & Kirk, S. F. L. (2017). 'It is not the diet; it is the mental part we need help with.' A multilevel analysis of psychological, emotional, and social well-being in obesity. *International Journal of Qualitative Studies on Health and Well-being*, 12(1). doi:10.1080/17482631.2017.1306421

Roberts, C. & Shea, L. J. (2017). Dining behaviors: considering a foodservice theory of in-home, local community, and eating while traveling. *Journal of Hospitality and Tourism Research*, 41(4), 393–7. doi:10.1177/1096348017693053

Sleddens, E. F. C., Kroeze, W., Kohl, L. F. M., Bolten, L. M., Velema, E., Kaspers, P., ... Brug, J. (2015). Correlates of dietary behavior in adults: an umbrella review. *Nutrition Reviews*, 73(8), 477–99. doi:10.1093/nutrit/nuv007

Taillie, L. S., Ng, S. W. & Popkin, B. M. (2016). Global growth of 'big box' stores and the potential impact on human health and nutrition. *Nutrition Reviews*, 74(2), 83–97. doi:10.1093/nutrit/nuv062

Tumin, R. & Anderson, S. E. (2017). Television, home-cooked meals, and family meal frequency: associations with adult obesity. *Journal of the Academy of Nutrition and Dietetics*, 117(6), 937–45. doi:https://doi.org/10.1016/j.jand.2017.01.009

Vartanian, L. R., Reily, N. M., Spanos, S., McGuirk, L. C., Herman, C. P. & Polivy, J. (2017). Hunger, taste, and normative cues in predictions about food intake. *Appetite*, 116, 511–17. doi:10.1016/j.appet.2017.05.044

Yates, L. & Warde, A. (2017). Eating together and eating alone: meal arrangements in British households. *British Journal of Sociology*, 68(1), 97–118. doi:10.1111/1468-4446.12231

Zhou, G., Gan, Y., Hamilton, K. & Schwarzer, R. (2017). The role of social support and self-efficacy for planning fruit and vegetable intake. *Journal of Nutrition Education and Behavior*, 49(2), 100–6. doi:10.1016/j.jneb.2016.09.005

REFERENCES

1 J. Germov & L. Williams (2017). Exploring the social appetite: a sociology of food and nutrition. In J. Germov & L. Williams (eds), *A Sociology of Food and Nutrition: The social appetite*, 4th edn (pp. 3–18). Melbourne: Oxford University Press.

2 K. M. Pursey, P. Stanwell, R. J. Callister, K. Brain, C. E. Collins & T. L. Burrows (2014). Neural responses to visual food cues according to weight status: a systematic review of functional magnetic resonance imaging studies. *Frontiers in Nutrition*, 1, 7. doi:10.3389/fnut.2014.00007

3 G. K. Beauchamp & J. A. Mennella (2009). Early flavor learning and its impact on later feeding behavior. *Journal of Pediatric Gastroenterology and Nutrition*, 48, S25–S30. doi:10.1097/MPG.0b013e31819774a5

4 L. L. Birch (1998). Development of food acceptance patterns in the first years of life. *Proceedings of the Nutrition Society*, 57(4), 617–24. doi:10.1079/PNS19980090

5   L. Birch (1996). Children's food acceptance patterns. *Nutrition Today*, 31(6), 234–40.

6   N. Charles & M. Kerr (1988). *Women, Food and Families*. Manchester: Manchester University Press.

7   J. Coveney (2002). *Food, Morals and Meaning*. London: Routledge.

8   The Intermedia Group Pty Ltd (2017). Respondent summary—eating out in Australia 2017. *Hospitality Magazine*. Retrieved from: www.the-drop.com.au/wp-content/uploads/2016/11/EatingOutinAustralia_2017_Respondent-Summary.compressed.pdf.

9   Australian Bureau of Statistics (2017). *Household Expenditure Survey Australia: Summary of results, 2015–16*. Canberra: ABS. Retrieved from: http://abs.gov.au/household-expenditure.

10 L. Goffe, S. Rushton, M. White, A. Adamson & Jean Adams (2017). Relationship between mean daily energy intake and frequency of consumption of out-of-home meals in the UK National Diet and Nutrition Survey. *International Journal of Behavioral Nutrition and Physical Activity*, 14, 131. doi:10.1186/s12966-017-0589-5

11 A. Oakley (1972). *Sex, Gender and Society*. Melbourne: Sun Books.

12 C. West & D. H. Zimmerman (1987). Doing gender. *Gender & Society*, 1(2), 125–51.

13 L. F. Monaghan (2007). Body mass index, masculinities and moral worth: men's critical understandings of 'appropriate' weight-for-height. *Sociology of Health & Illness*, 29(4), 584–609. doi:10.1111/j.1467-9566.2007.01007.x

14 L. Williams & J. Germov (2017). Gender, food and the body. In J. Germov & L. Williams (eds), *A Sociology of Food and Nutrition: The social appetite*, 4th edn (pp. 232–58). Melbourne: Oxford University Press.

15 J. Sobal (2005). Men, meat, and marriage: models of masculinity. *Food and Foodways*, 13(1–2), 135–58. doi:10.1080/07409710590915409

16 J. Adams, L. Goffe, A. J. Adamson, J. Halligan, N. O'Brien, R. Purves, ... M. White (2015). Prevalence and socio-demographic correlates of cooking skills in UK adults: cross-sectional analysis of data from the UK National Diet and Nutrition Survey. *International Journal of Behavioral Nutrition and Physical Activity*, 12(1), 99. doi:10.1186/s12966-015-0261-x

17 J. Germov & M. Poole (2015). *Public Sociology: An introduction to Australian society*, 3rd edn. Sydney: Allen & Unwin.

18 A. E. Guptill, D. A. Copelton & B. Lucal (2017). Principles and paradoxes in the study of food. In *Food and Society: Principles and paradoxes*, 2nd edn (pp. 1–15). Cambridge: Polity Press.

19 J. R. Eliasi & J. T. Dwyer (2002). Kosher and halal: religious observances affecting dietary intakes. *Journal of the American Dietetic Association*, 102(7), 911–13. doi:10.1016/S0002-8223(02)90203-8

20 R. Estruch, E. Ros, J. Salas-Salvadó, M.-I. Covas, D. Corella, F. Arós, ... M. A. Martínez-González (2018). Primary prevention of cardiovascular disease with a Mediterranean diet supplemented with extra-virgin olive oil or nuts. *New England Journal of Medicine*, 378(25), e34. doi:10.1056/NEJMoa1800389

21 S. Hussein (2015). Not eating the Muslim other: halal certification, scaremongering, and the racialisation of Muslim identity. *International Journal for Crime, Justice and Social Democracy*, 4(3), 85–96. doi:10.5204/ijcjsd.v4i3.250

22 World Health Organization (2011). *Global Status Report on Noncommunicable Diseases 2010*. Geneva: WHO.

23 M. Marmot (2004). *The Status Syndrome: How social standing affects our health and longevity*. New York: Henry Holt and Company.

24 R. Wilkinson & K. Pickett (2009). *The Spirit Level: Why more equal societies almost always do better.* London: Allen Lane.

25 J. Germov & L. Williams (2017). A sociology of food and nutrition. In J. Germov & L. Williams (eds), *A Sociology of Food and Nutrition: The social appetite*, 4th edn (pp. 3–18). Melbourne: Oxford University Press.

26 United Nations (1966). *International Covenant on Economic, Social and Cultural Rights.* Retrieved from: www.ohchr.org/EN/ProfessionalInterest/Pages/CESCR.aspx.

27 Food and Agriculture Organization of the United Nations, International Fund for Agricultural Development, United Nations Children's Fund, World Food Programme & World Health Organization (2017). *The State of Food Security and Nutrition in the World 2017: Building resilience for peace and food security.* Rome: FAO.

28 Public Health Association of Australia, Dietitians Association of Australia, National Heart Foundation of Australia and Nutrition Australia (2017). *Joint Policy Statement: Towards a national nutrition policy for Australia.* Retrieved from: www.phaa.net.au/documents/item/1987.

29 National Health and Medical Research Council (2013). *Australian Dietary Guidelines.* Canberra: NHMRC.

30 G. Sacks for the Food–EPI Australia Project Team (2017). *Policies for Tackling Obesity and Creating Healthier Food Environments: Scorecard and priority recommendations for Australian governments.* Melbourne: Deakin University.

31 L. Hebden, L. King, A. Grunseit, B. Kelly & K. Chapman (2011). Advertising of fast food to children on Australian television: the impact of industry self-regulation. *Medical Journal of Australia*, 195(8), 453. doi:10.5694/mja11.11114

32 J. Norman, B. Kelly, E. Boyland & A.-T. McMahon (2016). The impact of marketing and advertising on food behaviours: evaluating the evidence for a causal relationship. *Current Nutrition Reports*, 5(3), 139–49. doi:10.1007/s13668-016-0166-6

33 National Rural Health Alliance (2015). *Food Security and Health in Rural and Remote Australia.* Canberra: Rural Industries Research and Development Corporation.

34 A.-T. McMahon, L. Tapsell, P. Williams & J. Jobling (2013). Baby leafy green vegetables: providing insight into an old problem? An exploratory qualitative study examining influences on their consumption. *Health Promotion Journal of Australia*, 24(1), 68–71. doi:https://doi.org/10.1071/HE12901

35 Australian Bureau of Statistics (2006). *Socio-Economic Indexes for Areas (SEIFA)—Technical Paper.* Canberra: ABS.

36 A. Bandura (1998). Health promotion from the perspective of social cognitive theory. *Psychology & Health*, 13(4), 623–49. doi:10.1080/08870449808407422

37 M. A. Colchero, B. M. Popkin, J. A. Rivera & S. W. Ng (2016). Beverage purchases from stores in Mexico under the excise tax on sugar sweetened beverages: observational study. *British Medical Journal*, 352. doi:10.1136/bmj.h6704

38 C. Rogers (2003). *Client Centred Therapy: Its current practice, implications and theory.* London: Constable.

39 M. C. Rosal, C. B. Ebbeling, I. Lofgren, J. K. Ockene, I. S. Ockene & J. R. Hebert (2001). Facilitating dietary change: the patient-centered counseling model. *Journal of the American Dietetic Association*, 101(3), 332–41. doi:https://doi.org/10.1016/S0002-8223(01)00086-4

40 J. M. Spahn, R. S. Reeves, K. S. Keim, I. Laquatra, M. Kellogg, B. Jortberg & N. A. Clark (2010). State of the evidence regarding behavior change theories and strategies in nutrition counseling to facilitate health and food behavior change. *Journal of the American Dietetic Association*, 110(6), 879–91. doi:https://doi.org/10.1016/j.jada.2010.03.021

41 J. O. Prochaska & W. F. Velicer (1997). The transtheoretical model of health behavior change. *American Journal of Health Promotion*, 12(1), 38–48. doi:10.4278/0890-1171-12.1.38

42 K. Ball, R. W. Jeffery, G. Abbott, S. A. McNaughton & D. Crawford (2010). Is healthy behavior contagious: associations of social norms with physical activity and healthy eating. *International Journal of Behavioral Nutrition and Physical Activity*, 7(1), 86. doi:10.1186/1479-5868-7-86

43 L. Guillaumie, G. Godin & L.-A. Vézina-Im (2010). Psychosocial determinants of fruit and vegetable intake in adult population: a systematic review. *International Journal of Behavioral Nutrition and Physical Activity*, 7, 12. doi:10.1186/1479-5868-7-12

44 G. J. Norman, J. A. Carlson, J. F. Sallis, N. Wagner, K. J. Calfas & K. Patrick (2010). Reliability and validity of brief psychosocial measures related to dietary behaviors. *International Journal of Behavioral Nutrition and Physical Activity*, 7(1), 56. doi:10.1186/1479-5868-7-56

45 E. Mattila, I. Korhonen, J. H. Salminen, A. Ahtinen, E. Koskinen, A. Särelä, ... R. Lappalainen (2010). Empowering citizens for well-being and chronic disease management with wellness diary. *IEEE Transactions on Information Technology in Biomedicine*, 14(2), 456–63. doi:10.1109/TITB.2009.2037751

46 T. L. Schuster, M. Dobson, M. Jauregui & R. H. I. Blanks (2004). Wellness lifestyles I: a theoretical framework linking wellness, health lifestyles, and complementary and alternative medicine. *Journal of Alternative and Complementary Medicine*, 10(2), 349–56.

47 E. Sointu (2006). The search for wellbeing in alternative and complementary health practices. *Sociology of Health & Illness*, 28(3), 330–49. doi:10.1111/j.1467-9566.2006.00495.x

48 R. L. Nahin, J. M. Dahlhamer & B. J. Stussman (2010). Health need and the use of alternative medicine among adults who do not use conventional medicine. *BMC Health Services Research*, 10, 220. doi:10.1186/1472-6963-10-220

49 L. M. Otto, A. Howerter, I. R. Bell & N. Jackson (2010). Exploring measures of whole person wellness: integrative well-being and psychological flourishing. *EXPLORE: The Journal of Science and Healing*, 6(6), 364–70. doi:https://doi.org/10.1016/j.explore.2010.08.001

50 D. Berry (2004). In pursuit of wellness. *Dairy Foods*, 105(5), 34–8.

51 A.-T. McMahon, P. Williams & L. Tapsell (2010). Reviewing the meanings of wellness and well-being and their implications for food choice. *Perspectives in Public Health*, 130(6), 282–6. doi:10.1177/1757913910384046

52 L. C. Tapsell, M. J. Batterham, K. E. Charlton, E. P. Neale, Y. C. Probst, J. E. O'Shea, ... J. C.Y. Louie (2013). Foods, nutrients or whole diets: effects of targeting fish and LCn3PUFA consumption in a 12mo weight loss trial. *BMC Public Health*, 13, 1231. doi:10.1186/1471-2458-13-1231

53 A. T. McMahon, J. O'Shea, L. Tapsell & P. Williams (2014). What do the terms wellness and wellbeing mean in dietary practice: an exploratory qualitative study examining women's perceptions. *Journal of Human Nutrition and Dietetics*, 27(4), 401–10. doi:10.1111/jhn.12165

54 R. A. Cummins, R. Eckersley, J. Pallant, J. van Vugt & R. Misajon (2003). Developing a national index of subjective wellbeing: the Australian Unity Wellbeing Index. *Social Indicators Research*, 64(2), 159–90. doi:10.1023/a:1024704320683

55 A. L. Duckworth, T. A. Steen & M. E. P. Seligman (2005). Positive psychology in clinical practice. *Annual Review of Clinical Psychology*, 1(1), 629–51. doi:10.1146/annurev.clinpsy.1.102803.144154

56 M. J. Healey-Ogden & W. J. Austin (2011). Uncovering the lived experience of well-being. *Qualitative Health Research*, 21(1), 85–96. doi:10.1177/1049732310379113

57 E. Hazzard, L. Barone, M. Mason, K. Lambert & A. McMahon (2017). Patient-centred dietetic care from the perspectives of older malnourished patients. *Journal of Human Nutrition and Dietetics*, 30, 574–87. doi:10:1111/jhn.12478

58 R. Ashcroft (2011). Health and wellbeing: starting with a critical pedagogical model. *Social Work Education*, 30(6), 610–22. doi:10.1080/02615479.2011.586558

59 B. B. Holli, J. A. Beto, R. J. Calabrese & J. O. S. Maillet (2009). *Communication and Education Skills for Dietetic Professionals*. Philadelphia, PA: Lippincott Williams and Wilkins.

CHAPTER 21

NUTRITION, FOOD SECURITY AND FOOD INNOVATION

LINDA TAPSELL AND JOANNA RUSSELL

CHAPTER OBJECTIVES

This chapter will enable the reader to:

- define food systems and the way in which they may influence food security
- identify ways in which nutrition can act as a driving force for food innovation
- discuss the implications for nutrition research in support of healthy foods.

KEY TERMS

Food innovation   Food systems

Food security

KEY POINTS

- The food system includes such components as primary food production, food manufacturing and processing, and food service systems (including supermarkets and restaurants). Waste streams are also part of the food system, and these can occur in production, processing and retail, and in the home.
- Food security for populations means access to safe and nutritious food in all circumstances and is affected by elements both within and outside of the food and nutrition system.
- Food innovation provides an opportunity for improving food security and the health of the population, but this requires an integrated effort among stakeholders in the food and nutrition system.
- Nutrition research provides knowledge that can underpin the development and promotion of healthy foods and the evidence base for dietary guidelines.

OXFORD UNIVERSITY PRESS

INTRODUCTION

An appreciation of the broader food environment is also necessary in applying concepts from nutrition science to practice. Rather than working with individuals, attention can be drawn to the food supply, and how exposure and access to food may influence food choices and thereby population health. This is a classic component of practice in public health nutrition. We need to know more than the nutrient value of foods to improve nutritional health. Food is a commodity and access to healthy food is subject to a range of influences within the food system, so an understanding of the food system exposes the operational nature of the food supply. Issues such as the adequacy of the food supply, innovation in food products and processes, and governance structures are all relevant. This chapter discusses these elements to set the scene for studying food, nutrition and health, and to imagine what the future food supply could look like.

WHAT ARE FOOD SYSTEMS AND HOW MIGHT THEY INFLUENCE FOOD SECURITY?

There are many ways in which food systems can be described, with a simple 'paddock to plate' concept underlying most principles. Directional descriptions may include aspects such as growing, harvesting, transporting, packaging, marketing and consuming through to waste disposal [1]. The main components of the **food system** then appear as food production, food processing, food retailing and marketing, food access, food consumption and food waste. Each part of the food system lies within a broader social, environmental and political context, so is subject to issues such as climate change, world food trade, consumer demand and scientific research. Adding human health to this scenario links the food system to nutrition [2]. The Australian Institute of Health and Welfare (AIHW) produces regular reports on these matters (see www.aihw.gov.au/reports-statistics/behaviours-risk-factors/food-nutrition/overview).

Food systems
processes and pathways that deliver food from its production (e.g. growth, processing, transport, sale) to its eventual consumption and the disposal of food waste.

Consumers' health
well-being and functionality of individuals.

Food standards
policy rules that address the management of food.

Another way of describing food systems is to refer to a 'value chain' that not only considers the direction of the pathway of food, but also the way in which value is added as the food progresses along the path (Figure 21.1). If **consumers' health** were an end point of this particular description, then a parallel value chain could be seen with the provision of healthcare. Elements of the food industry-related value chain include primary production (and use of the waste stream), ingredients and food product manufacturing, retail and regulatory inputs. Elements of the health industry value chain include health personnel education, healthcare systems and policies, and evidence-based practice guidelines. Research in nutrition (e.g. clinical trials testing the effect of foods consumed on health) provides a knowledge base for various areas of practice, including giving healthcare advice and managing regulatory aspects of health claims on food products. In this sense, the same forms of research can serve both value chains (Figure 21.1).

Food products available for purchase are governed by **food standards** that specify the type of content (what the product can and cannot contain), indicate good manufacturing practice and define the information that must be on food labels. From a legal perspective, these are managed through state/territory Public Health Acts or Food Acts, which provide for the safety and suitability of foods for human consumption. Guidelines, such as the Australian Dietary Guidelines, serve to assist the population in making food choices for which there is evidence of an association with health.

LINDA TAPSELL AND JOANNA RUSSELL

FIGURE 21.1 FOOD AND NUTRITION VALUE CHAINS

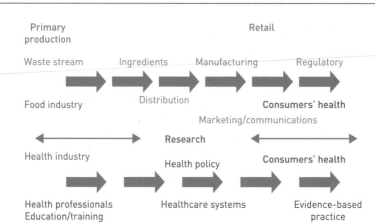

TRY IT YOURSELF

Review the supporting information available from the Australian Dietary Guidelines (www.eatforhealth.gov.au) and Foods Standards Australia New Zealand (www.foodstandards.gov.au) for guideline statements and health claims on foods. How are the evidence-based frameworks similar? Who are the end users of these guidelines and standards?

By their nature, food systems directly impact on food security. Agriculture has traditionally had a strong association with food security, with the Food and Agriculture Organization (FAO) of the United Nations defining it as 'achieved when all people at all times have physical and economic access to sufficient, safe and nutritious food to meet dietary needs and food preferences for an active and healthy life' [3]. An FAO conceptual framework for food security includes four dimensions: food availability, access and utilisation, as well as the continued stability of these [4] (see also Figure 21.2). As a general rule, consumers are unable to control the quality or availability of food offered to them, nor do they set the price.

Economic and physical access to food is the ability of a household or individual to acquire sufficient quality and quantity of food to meet all household members' nutritional requirements for productive lives. The access people have to food varies both individually and within the household situation, taking into consideration factors such as income, expenditure, employment, education and food preferences [5]. Also important is whether a household has enough resources to acquire food that is acceptable and nutritious. At this level, an individual has more control over their situation, but food access can be affected by external factors within the local environment. Even if food is available, personal physical limitations (poor mobility) or disabilities (such as arthritis) can affect a person's ability to access food, especially in an ageing population. Most measurement tools today are limited to economic access and do not address issues of physical access [6; 7]. Low income is a primary indicator for economic access to food and hence of food insecurity. Groups reported as being at higher risk of food insecurity include low-income households, particularly single-parent households with dependent children [8], Indigenous Australians, recently arrived refugees [9], people living in rented accommodation, people with disabilities, frail elderly and ethnic minorities [10–12].

FIGURE 21.2 DETERMINANTS OF FOOD SECURITY

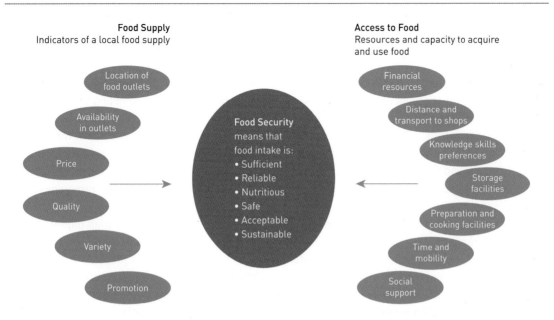

Source: L. Rychetnik, K. Webb, L. Story & T. Katz (2003). *Food Security Options Paper: A planning framework and menu of options for policy and practice interventions*. Sydney: NSW Centre for Public Health Nutrition, NSW Department of Health

In low-income households, money for food is often what is left after paying for other necessities such as housing and utility bills [13]. Food insecurity is likely to be exacerbated by rising food prices globally and in Australia [14], as well as the more rapidly escalating cost of healthier (low-energy, high-nutrient-density) foods [13; 15–17]. Research in South Australia by Wong and colleagues [17] showed that low-income families would have to spend more than 28% of their income on a 'healthy food basket' compared with 6–9% for high-income families. While the affordability of food, especially healthy food, has remained fairly constant overall for Australian households, it has declined for low-income households [18]. If additional expenses occur, such as those resulting from medical emergencies or loss of employment, the food budget is most often the first to be reduced [19]. Physical disabilities and social factors affect dietary choices. Carrying, bending and shortness of breath have been cited as physical reasons for shopping problems and difficulties in getting to and from stores, as well as in the store [20; 21]. In Australia it has been found that in households without cars, those who did not receive welfare assistance (e.g. disability support, old age or infirmity pension) had difficulties in accessing food stores. In Australia, urban planning has been developed around car use. Those that do not have a car are doubly disadvantaged by being unable to access supermarkets as well as bearing the cost of private transport to carry goods [22]. Examination of economic access to the food supply has involved collecting information on price, quality and availability of foods by auditing retail food outlets. The Healthy Food Access Basket (HFAB) has been used in Australia. It includes food items that meet 70% of nutritional and 95% of the energy requirements of a reference family of six for two weeks. The foods included are those most commonly consumed and available, but not necessarily the most nutrient-dense [23].

>> CASE 21.1

IS 'HEALTHY' FOOD MORE EXPENSIVE THAN 'UNHEALTHY' FOOD?

Until recently, monitoring of healthy food prices and affordability through healthy food access baskets in Australia has been conducted at state and territory level using a range of different methodologies such as differences in the foods included in the baskets, reference households and sampling techniques used in store [24]. For example, it has been reported that in Queensland the cost of the HFAB rose by 6.1% from 2004 to 2006, with fruit, vegetables and legumes increasing by 17.4%. This suggests that more people would be at risk of becoming food insecure due to rising food prices [25]. The price of HFAB food items has also been found to rise as distance increased from the major cities, with the highest prices reported in very remote regions [25]. The availability of healthier food options also declined as remoteness from major cities increased.

Although low-income households spend more of the weekly budget on food than higher-income households, recent research has shown that healthier diets can be cheaper than diets commonly consumed by Australian households that contain high levels of discretionary foods. This research is based on standardised tools and protocols assessing affordability of both 'healthy' and less 'healthy' diets. The **INFORMAS** framework includes three separate approaches—minimal, expanded and optimal—for monitoring food prices and affordability, both 'healthy' and 'unhealthy'. The three approaches have been designed so that they take account of differences between countries [26], as described in Table 21.1.

INFORMAS

International Network on Food and Obesity/non-communicable diseases Research, Monitoring and Action Support, a global network of organisations and researchers that aims to monitor, benchmark and support actions for the creation of healthy food environments.

In Australia, the optimal approach has been used to determine the cost of 'healthy' versus 'less healthy' diets as assessed against current dietary guidelines along with household income data [26]. Using data from the Australian Health Survey 2011–12, a 'current' (less healthy) diet basket was developed based on the quantities and proportions of foods and drinks reported to be consumed by participants. Foods for the 'healthy' basket were based on the Foundation Diet recommendations from the Australian Guide to Healthy Eating. The foods in this basket were similar to commonly consumed healthy foods [27].

The findings suggested that prices were approximately 3% higher in high socioeconomic status (SES) areas compared with low SES areas. An interesting finding was that households spent more money on buying the 'unhealthy' diet compared with a 'healthy' diet. In households without children, the healthy diet cost less than the unhealthy diet being currently being consumed by Australian households [27]. However, even though it is suggested that the current diet being consumed by Australians is more expensive than a 'healthy' diet, the cost of the unhealthy basket in high SES areas was 15.5% of median income compared with 21.5% of median income in a low SES area. Although a 'healthy' diet could be potentially cheaper than an 'unhealthy' diet currently being purchased by the Australian population, families in low SES areas were still spending more of their median income on food expenditures than those in higher SES areas.

- What factors influence the cost of food for communities?
- How is a healthy food basket decided upon?

TABLE 21.1   PROPOSED STEP-WISE FRAMEWORK TO MONITOR PRICE AND AFFORDABILITY OF 'HEALTHY' AND 'LESS HEALTHY' FOODS, MEALS AND DIETS

	Minimal approach	Expanded approach	Optimal approach
Indicator	Differential between the price of selected 'healthy' foods and 'less healthy' foods	Differential between the price of 'healthy' diets and meals, and 'less healthy' diets and meals	Affordability of 'healthy' and 'less healthy' diets and meals
Data sources	Retail prices of foods Nutrient profiling system to differentiate nutritional quality of comparable foods	Relevant country dietary guidelines and national dietary intake data (where available) Relevant country food composition tables, dietary modelling and/or food selection guides (where available)	An 'expanded' approach together with median household income data
Analysis	Comparison of the cost (and tax component) of 'healthy' and 'less healthy' equivalent foods	Diets: comparison of the cost of a 'healthy' diet for a reference (healthy weight) family over two weeks versus cost of the 'current' diet for a reference (current weight) family over two weeks Meals: cost of a reference 'healthy' meal vs the cost of a similar but less healthy meal (of equivalent weight)	As for 'expanded' but expressed as costs in relation to median household income
Stratification	No stratification	Stratification by region	Stratification by region and by household socioeconomic status
Representativeness	Country-wide	Country-wide/regional	Country-wide/regional Socioeconomic groups

Source: A. Lee, C. N. Mhurchu, G. Sacks, B. Swinburn, W. Snowdon, S. Vandevijvere, … C. Walker (2013). Monitoring the price and affordability of foods and diets globally. *Obesity Reviews*, 14(S1), 82–95. doi:10.1111/obr.12078

Food insecurity is reportedly are higher among Indigenous Australians than the general population. The 2012–13 Australian Aboriginal and Torres Strait Islander Health Survey found that 22% of Indigenous Australians reported that in the past 12 months they ran out of food and could not afford to buy more, and 7% reported that they went without food as a result. This compares with 3.7% and 1.4%, respectively, for the whole Australian population [28]. The sustainability of the food supply is also an issue for consideration with climate change. Factors such as rising sea levels, severe drought and flooding all influence local food supplies. Even though Australia exports over half of its agricultural products, climate change needs to be considered for the sustainability of the domestic food supply [29; 30]. An example of extreme environmental conditions is the flooding that damaged

See Chapter 19 for more on food security.

the Queensland banana crop in 2011. Bananas are a popular fruit for Australians and the loss in supply to the market resulted in significant price increases, with implications for food security. With a growing Australian population (estimated to be about 35 million by 2050) [31], there will be significant pressures on the food supply to remain sustainable. In addition, consideration must be given to the increasing proportion of this population who will be aged over 65 years [31]. With these issues in mind, food security needs to be considered nationally in a coordinated fashion.

In 2010, the Prime Minister's Science, Engineering and Innovation Council (PMSEIC) formed an expert working group to develop a report on food security for Australia. The FAO definition was referred to, and issues at that time were noted as vulnerability to climate change and variability; slowing primary industries productivity; declining soil fertility, land degradation and urban encroachment; increasing reliance on food imports and food production imports (e.g. fertilisers); food transport issues; nutritional intakes; and regional conflicts. Along with agricultural and technological capabilities, the report also noted Australia's expertise in human health and nutrition research among its strengths. The main messages of the report were the need for a national approach to food, investment in research and development to support agricultural productivity, meeting challenges and opportunities by building human capacity and raising awareness on the importance of food [32].

≫ RESEARCH AT WORK

SUSTAINABILITY AS A FIFTH DIMENSION OF FOOD SECURITY

It is well known that the current global food system is not sustainable, with large numbers of both undernourished and overweight and obese people. To date, aspects of food security have come under the four dimensions (availability, access, utilisation and stability), but more recently, research in this area has introduced a fifth pillar, **sustainability**. Including sustainability as a separate dimension allows for relevant issues to be discussed as all levels, including sustainable agriculture, sustainable economy,

Sustainability
the long-term maintenance and management of systems and processes.

sustainable food production and sustainable diets for all [33]. Sustainability will play a key role in monitoring and evaluating food security to ensure long-term endurance of food systems [33]. At the Rio +20 conference on Sustainable Development, the Zero Hunger Challenge was launched to highlight the importance of food and nutrition security for sustainable development. The challenge includes access to food year-round for everyone and that all food systems are sustainable [34]. These goals have also been included in the Sustainable Development Goals, specifically within goal 2 and goal 12 [35].

Australia is considered to be a food trading nation, with food exports exceeding food imports, and has a high level of food security according to the Economist Intelligence Unit [36], yet there is concern about the future of Australia's food security, perhaps due to a change in the trend for increasing food imports rather than exports. Further modelling has suggested that with the increase in Australia's population to around 35 million by 2050, there will be a need to increase the food supply, particularly imports of certain foods such as fish, fruit and vegetables. Changes in food imports and exports could have an impact on food security within Australia [37].

The distribution of food globally also has the potential to be inequitable, as climate change affects the capacity of countries to maintain a sufficient nutrient-dense food supply. The increased purchasing

TABLE 21.2   ISSUES ADDRESSED IN 2015–30 UN SUSTAINABLE DEVELOPMENT GOALS

Issues	Goals
Poverty	Ending hunger Ensuring food security, adequate nutrition Supporting sustainable agriculture
Health and well-being	Equitable quality education and lifelong learning
Gender equality and empowerment of women and girls	Water and sanitation
Affordable, reliable sustainable energy	Economic growth, productive employment, decent work
Resilient infrastructure, inclusive and sustainable industrialisation and innovation	Equality within and between countries
Inclusive, safe, resilient, sustainable cities	Sustainable production and consumption patterns
Climate change and its impacts	Conservation of oceans, seas and marine resources
Protection and sustainable use of ecosystems and protection of biodiversity	Peaceful, just and inclusive societies
Global partnerships for sustainable development	

Source: Adapted from R. Pérez-Escamilla (2017). Food security and the 2015–30 Sustainable Development Goals: from human to planetary health. *Current Developments in Nutrition*, 1(7). doi:10.3945/cdn.117.000513

power of wealthier nations will shift the flow of food away from poorer countries, increasing levels of food insecurity [38]. The effects of climate change on food supplies, an understanding of changing population dietary patterns, sources of nutrients and changing environments will have as yet unknown consequences on population health (Table 21.2).

STOP AND THINK

- Where along the food value chain can efforts be made to improve nutritional intakes in the population and promote food security?
- Which population subgroups are likely to suffer the most from food insecurity? Why?
- Why is sustainability an issue for global food systems and food security?

HOW CAN NUTRITION DRIVE FOOD INNOVATION?

From a public health perspective, nutrition is an important consideration in food product development, regardless of the degree of processing. Food delivers compounds essential for life, but the overall profile of the diet can prove beneficial or deleterious to health. The composition of food is not a trivial matter, and the degree of food processing can have an impact on the overall quality of the diet [39]. Research on the health benefits of nutrients, food ingredients and whole foods can help to drive consumer demand and influence the directions of food innovation. In recent decades, this has been reflected in the concept of **functional foods**, where the notion of health benefits is a characterising feature. There have been several drivers for this movement, including

Functional foods

foods marketed based on evidence of nutritional quality and health benefits.

Food industry

all levels of business that play a part in the food supply, including primary production (farming and grazing), ingredient and food product manufacturing, commercial food supply such as fast-food manufacturing, and food retailing.

Food innovation

the development of new product ideas and concepts arising from an open investigative framework.

advances in science (technological development and evidence-based nutrition), increasing self-care by individuals, the ageing population and rising healthcare costs, developments in food regulations and competitiveness within the **food industry** [40].

The food industry routinely undertakes **food innovation**, a process driven by new ideas. There are many business reasons for undertaking food innovation, and nutrition is not necessarily a primary consideration. The focus may originate from anywhere along the food value chain (see Figure 21.1 earlier in the chapter), but there are considerable implications for nutrition. For example, an innovative idea may be to utilise waste streams, such as developing new products using whey protein from dairy food production, or omega-3 oils from the manufacture of canned tuna. Research on protein and omega-3 fatty acids may be relevant in evaluating the nutritional value of these new products. On the other hand, nutrition may be a primary driver when there is consumer demand. For example, there may be a demand for 'healthier' white bread, so an idea may be to add novel fibres that may increase the functional value based on the effects of fibre. It is important to note that only a small percentage of new ideas make it to market, despite significant investment in product development, product testing, marketing and distribution.

Essentially, the food industry determines the types of food that are available to consumers. At most levels, particularly at the levels of primary producers and ingredient or food manufacturers, groups of researchers are involved from within an organisation or in collaboration with research providers, utilising scientific methods to answer questions and develop new ideas. The ensuing commercialisation and trade of food is influenced by a number of factors including available income, pricing competition, cuisine, social factors and taste preferences.

TRY IT YOURSELF

Visit your local supermarket and look at some products that you believe have involved significant food innovation. List areas of the possible involvement of science around the innovation, including the addition of functional ingredients or the use of health claims made on the packaging or promotions.

>> CASE 21.2

FUNCTIONAL FOODS

There are many definitions of functional foods, but underpinning this concept is the evidence that they have beneficial effects on health. It is arguable that all foods are functional, but the requirement for evidence demands a link with scientific research. This requirement is aligned with the need for scientific evidence for health claims made in food marketing on food labels [41].

The Academy of Nutrition and Dietetics has produced a number of position statements on functional foods. In 2013, functional foods were defined as foods that are potentially beneficial to health when consumed regularly as part of a varied diet at levels for which there is scientific evidence of effects [42]. They could be whole or conventional foods (vegetables, fruits, grains), or foods that have been fortified, enriched or enhanced, and which contain synthesised ingredients such as prebiotics.

In Australia, a working definition of functional foods was developed with research initiatives in that area [43]. This definition of functional foods as 'foods marketed on benefits based on scientific evidence' acknowledged the links between science, communications and the assessment of health outcomes.

The development of functional foods linked opportunities arising from analyses of the food value chain, food- and nutrition-related science and technology, consumer demand and marketing, and public health–related activity, including food standards and regulation [43].

Across the globe, a number of key organisations also developed definitions of functional foods, including food science and technology organisations (IFIC, IFT, ILSI), and governments (EU commission, Health Canada, Japanese Ministry Health, Labour and Welfare) [42]. Trends in functional foods were reported (www.ift.org) and academic conferences and journals emerged. The emergence of functional foods also created debate on the definitions of nutrients, particularly as nutrition concerns moved from prevention of deficiencies (or the inability to synthesise nutrients) to food components that could be shown to have an effect on health [44].

- Why could the term 'functional food' be seen as both something new and already in existence?
- List the various stakeholder groups that would need to work together to achieve a successful effort in functional foods.
- What are the implications of the concept of functional foods for improving the health of the population?

There are a number of sites along the food supply chain where consumers can access food (Figure 21.3). Even so, most food is purchased in grocery stores. The FOODmap 2011 published by the then Department of Agriculture Fisheries and Forestry provided a clear overview of food innovation among staple foods in the Australian food chain at that time [45] (Figure 21.4). A total turnover of $130.2 billion from food and liquor retail sales was recorded in 2010–11 in Australia. About 67% of turnover appeared in supermarkets/retail outlets (excluding alcohol) and 25% in eating out, and this latter figure could be potentially greater [45].

FIGURE 21.3 FROM FARM TO PLATE—NUTRITION AND THE FOOD INDUSTRY

Primary producers → innovation in product selection for high-yield, maximum nutrition includes genetic modification

↓

Raw ingredients → value-add through use of waste streams, concentration of bioactive components, improved delivery of bioactive components

↓

Food products → inclusion of functional ingredients, innovation in packaging and manufacture to ensure nutritional properties associated with positive health outcomes are maintained (including addition of nutrients); production of convenience products including single foods and whole meals

↓

Food distribution → systems to minimise 'food miles' of benefit for the environment but also the consumer in terms of minimising degradation of key nutrients in fresh foods, food variety provided to locations (e.g. rural/remote versus metropolitan) controlled by the food industry (limit of consumers to pay for produce)

↓

Food retail → marketing; nutrition research used in validation of nutrient content claims and health outcomes

FIGURE 21.4 LONG-TERM TRENDS AFFECTING FOOD MARKETS

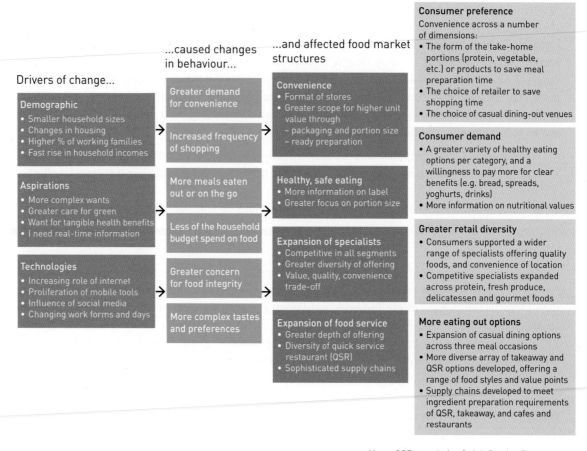

Note: QSR stands for Quick Service Restaurants.

Source: Adapted from S. Spencer & M. Kneebone (2012). *FOODmap: An analysis of the Australian food supply chain*. Canberra: DAFF

TRY IT YOURSELF

Identify the location in the food value chain for foods you have recently purchased. How much of your food was gained directly from primary producers, from a manufacturer or from a supermarket? How much of the food you eat is consumed inside the home, and how much is consumed outside the home?

STOP AND THINK

- In what locations of the food value chain do ideas for food innovation arise, and why?
- How does nutrition relate to food innovation?
- Why do different stakeholders and a range of disciplines need to work together to achieve health goals from food innovation?

HOW CAN NUTRITION RESEARCH SUPPORT THE DEVELOPMENT AND PROMOTION OF HEALTHY FOODS?

Given the 'business' side of food and agribusiness, research that aligns with the development of healthy foods will still need to consider the broader requirements for food innovation. **Value adding** tends to result from processing, whereby nutritional profile (or other features such as the shelf-life of products) is improved during food manufacture, or from differentiated production such as using organic methods or different breeding techniques [46]. On a global scale, health drivers include ageing populations, increases in chronic disease, and increasing awareness on health, well-being and food safety, but they lie alongside needs for smarter food chains, environmental issues, the global food trade and specific customer preferences [46].

> **Value adding**
> improving a quality of a food by some change in manufacturing or processing.

From a public health perspective, the need remains to position nutrition as a priority in food innovation (Figure 21.5). Research indicates, for example, that the nutritional quality of diets in the US would benefit from nutritional considerations in food processing [39], including reductions in sodium intake [47]. There are further implications for innovations in delivering foods through food service systems. This extends to restaurants and similar avenues for food provision that are also subject to innovation. The impact of the local food environment on food purchasing behaviours has been a consideration for population health, although common assumptions have been challenged by recent studies showing that purchases do not always occur in local neighbourhoods [48] and the density of fast-food or full-service restaurants may not be associated with obesity prevalence [49].

From the perspective of individual foods, nutrition research provides the evidence for the potential benefits or risks associated with foods produced with various forms of processing and formulation.

FIGURE 21.5 FOCAL POINTS FOR NUTRITION RESEARCH ON THE IMPACT OF FOOD ON HEALTH

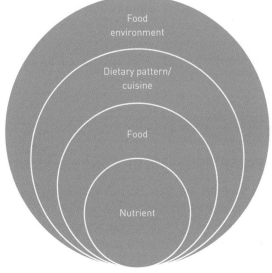

LINDA TAPSELL AND JOANNA RUSSELL

FIGURE 21.6   CONTINUUM OF NUTRIENT ESSENTIALITY

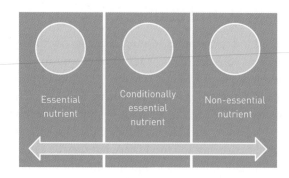

Adopted from S. Jew, J.-M. Antoine, P. Bourlioux, J. Milner, L. C. Tapsell, Y. Yang & P. J. H. Jones (2015). Nutrient essentiality revisited. *Journal of Functional Foods*, 14, 203–9.

To expose these effects, research may focus on the active ingredients in the foods, individual whole foods or dietary patterns, including key foods. Outcomes (effects) relate to disease risk factors or end points, and functional measures such as cognition, agility or well-being. Systematic reviews and meta-analyses of clinical trials and cohort studies form the basis for evidence review, but experimental approaches such as animal model studies and feeding tests can add to the plausibility of findings by exposing mechanisms by which food components have effects.

See Chapter 2 for more on evidence based review systems.

Given its close links with science, the functional food movement has challenged a number of areas of conventional nutrition, particularly in relation to biologically active food components. Historically, research on nutrients has focused on the prevention of deficiency and the inability of the body to synthesise certain nutrients. Today, alongside the ability to identify new active components in foods, nutrition researchers have been able to demonstrate effects on health that are not limited to clinical deficiency states. Dietary fibres, plant sterols and polyphenols are examples of food components for which the concept of 'deficiency' is perhaps less appropriate. Rather, a continuum of nutrient essentiality (Figure 21.6) has been proposed that would accommodate effects beyond the prevention of deficiency states [44]. It has been argued that nutrient essentiality may be considered relative to the functions that food components influence in the body under certain conditions, including state of disease and in the context of the whole diet [44].

> **» CASE 21.3**

RESEARCH ON THE HEALTH BENEFITS OF CONSUMING NUTS

Nuts are a naturally occurring food that are produced by horticultural industries and related companies involved in growing, harvesting and packaging fresh and shelled nuts for consumers. In terms of nutritional composition, this food group tends to have a high fat content alongside protein, fibre, vitamins and minerals, as well as key polyphenolic compounds found in many plant foods. As nuts also tend to be consumed as snacks they have been aligned with foods considered as 'extras' to a healthy diet, except in the case of vegetarian diets where alternative plant protein sources are required as a core part of the diet.

Over the past 20 years, a substantial amount of research has been undertaken on the health benefits of nuts. This has focused particularly on the prevention of cardio-metabolic disease, with effects relating to health outcomes such as cholesterol levels, body weight, blood pressure and cardiovascular disease events [50–52]. Much (but not all) of this research has been supported by agri-food research entities but, importantly, it has been published in independently peer-reviewed scientific literature. The full set of studies has created a body of evidence that could be systematically reviewed to determine the effects of nut consumption on health. Such reviews have been conducted for dietary guidelines in the United States [53] and Australia [54] underpinning the inclusion of nuts in guideline statements. In Australia, this has meant a recommended increase in nut consumption from a low base level.

Evidence-based review can also be undertaken for the establishment of forms of health claims. The US Department of Agriculture (USDA) website notes a qualified health claim for nuts, stating 'Eating 1.5 ounces per day of most nuts as part of a diet low in saturated fat and cholesterol may reduce the risk of heart disease' [55].

- Given earlier understandings of the relationship between diet and cardiovascular disease, why would nuts have been considered a food to avoid?
- How does the health claim on nuts address the ongoing concern for dietary saturated fat while promoting the nutritional advantages that nuts have to offer?
- What kinds of studies would have been conducted to demonstrate the health benefits of nut consumption?

» RESEARCH AT WORK

THE IMPACT OF INDIVIDUAL FOODS ON HEALTHY DIETARY PATTERNS

Dietary guidelines provide a suitable basis for advice on weight loss in the primary care setting, but how specific does this advice need to be for individuals to make sufficient and lasting changes to help them lose weight? In a study comparing general advice on dietary guidelines with individualised advice provided by a dietitian, a trial in Wollongong showed that greater weight loss was achieved with the more individualised advice. After three months of attending the same number of clinic visits, over three times as many people lost the targeted 5% body weight loss when their diets were customised. When this advice was accompanied by a sample of a healthy food (30 g walnuts/day), the difference in weight loss was still evident at six months. In addition, the group receiving the samples were consuming a higher fibre intake and their diets contained a better proportion of the right type of fats (polyunsaturated:saturated fatty acids) [56]. Secondary analyses of this study showed that the people who were given the walnuts also increased their intake of fruit and consumed less 'discretionary food' compared with those receiving general advice [57]. In addition, the diet quality scores of those receiving the individualised advice was significantly greater than for those receiving the general advice, after three months and still after 12 months [58]. This study showed that, although the total diet accounts for overall energy intake, which affects body weight, the individual foods that make up the diet are important. In this case, providing a healthy food (walnuts) appeared to influence the change in choice of other foods, increasing intakes of healthier foods and decreasing intakes of poorer-quality foods. Further research would indicate whether this influence came through changes in cuisine and/or meal patterns. Understanding how people combine individual foods in healthy dietary patterns is an important step in translating the evidence for healthy foods into dietary practices that support and promote health.

LINDA TAPSELL AND JOANNA RUSSELL

STOP AND THINK

- How do the dimensions of food systems ultimately have an impact on nutritional health?
- How does the concept of food security assist in analysing food and health-related problems for at-risk communities and populations?
- What role can the food industry play in addressing problems of nutritional health and food security?

SUMMARY

- The main components of the food system are food production, food processing, food retail and marketing, and food waste.
- The main dimensions of food security are food availability and food access, and they include the concept of nutritional quality. Indigenous Australians, refugees and people living with low incomes are all at risk of food insecurity.
- New products in the food supply remain subject to food standards requirements (including food labelling). This adds to the investment companies must make in developing, testing and marketing.
- Nutritional considerations and food innovation can occur at all stages of the food value chain, from primary production to food service.
- The connection between nutrition and food innovation is not limited to a consideration of health claims.

PATHWAYS TO PRACTICE

- Students of nutrition can drive their career paths along many pathways in the food and nutrition system, including working with the food industry in product development and nutrition messaging.
- Health professionals can also work alongside the food and nutrition system to improve nutrition and health outcomes for communities and populations.
- Supporting the recommendations for fruit and vegetable consumption as promoted in dietary guidelines also requires consideration of the production systems for fruit and vegetables.

DISCUSSION QUESTIONS

1 What are the main elements of a food and nutrition system, and how are they interrelated?
2 What does food security mean?
3 How do different personal and environmental circumstances affect food security?
4 What are the processes that food companies need to follow to address food standards?
5 What does food innovation mean?
6 What types of food innovation can occur along the food value chain?

USEFUL WEBLINKS

Australian Dietary Guidelines:
www.eatforhealth.gov.au

Australian International Food Security Research Centre:
http://aciar.gov.au/aifsc/food-security-and-why-it-matters

CSIRO:
www.csiro.au

Department of Agriculture and Water Resources:
www.agriculture.gov.au

Food Standards Australia New Zealand:
www.foodstandards.gov.au

FOODmap:
www.agriculture.gov.au/ag-farm-food/food/publications/foodmap-a-comparative-analysis

Go Nuts!—US Department of Agriculture:
www.ars.usda.gov/plains-area/gfnd/gfhnrc/docs/news-2013/go-nuts

Healthy Food Access Basket survey—Queensland Government:
www.qgso.qld.gov.au/about-us/our-services/surveys/hfab-survey.php

Institute of Food Technologists:
www.ift.org

Rural Industries Research and Development Corporation:
www.rirdc.gov.au/about-rirdc

FURTHER READING

Anand, S. S., Hawkes, C., De Souza, R. J., Mente, A., Dehghan, M., Nugent, R., ... Popkin, B. M. (2015). Food consumption and its impact on cardiovascular disease: importance of solutions focused on the globalized food system—a report from the workshop convened by the World Heart Federation. *Journal of the American College of Cardiology*, 66(14), 1590–614. doi:10.1016/j.jacc.2015.07.050

Archer, C., Gallegos, D. & McKechnie, R. (2017). Developing measures of food and nutrition security within an Australian context. *Public Health Nutrition*, 1–10. doi:10.1017/S1368980017001288

Bennett, C. J. & Palermo, C. E. (2017). Furthering food security surveillance in Australia. *Public Health Nutrition*, 20(7), 1331–2. doi:10.1017/S1368980016003438

Brimblecombe, J., van den Boogaard, C., Wood, B., Liberato, S. C., Brown, J., Barnes, A., ... Bailie, R. (2015). Development of the good food planning tool: a food system approach to food security in indigenous Australian remote communities. *Health and Place*, 34, 54–62. doi:10.1016/j.healthplace.2015.03.006

Chen, J., McCarl, B. A. & Thayer, A. (2017). Climate change and food security: threats and adaptation. *Frontiers of Economics and Globalization*, 17, 69–84.

Davis, K. F., Gephart, J. A., Emery, K. A., Leach, A. M., Galloway, J. N. & P. D'Odorico (2016). Meeting future food demand with current agricultural resources. *Global Environmental Change*, 39, 125–32. doi:10.1016/j.gloenvcha.2016.05.004

Davy, D. (2016). Australia's efforts to improve food security for Aboriginal and Torres Strait Islander peoples. *Health and Human Rights*, 18(2), 209–18.

Department of Environment Food and Rural Affairs (2009). *UK Food Security Assessment: Our approach.* Retrieved from: http://webarchive.nationalarchives.gov.uk/20130402191240/http://archive.defra.gov.uk/foodfarm/food/pdf/food-assess-approach-0908.pdf.

Ferguson, M., O'Dea, K., Chatfield, M., Moodie, M., Altman, J. & Brimblecombe, J. (2016). The comparative cost of food and beverages at remote Indigenous communities, Northern Territory, Australia. *Australian and New Zealand Journal of Public Health*, 40, S21–S26. doi:10.1111/1753-6405.12370

Godrich, S. L., Davies, C. R., Darby, J. & Devine, A. (2017). What are the determinants of food security among regional and remote Western Australian children? *Australian and New Zealand Journal of Public Health*, 41(2), 172–7. doi:10.1111/1753-6405.12636

Grundy, M. J., Bryan, B. A., Nolan, M., Battaglia, M., Hatfield-Dodds, S., Connor, J. D. & Keating, B. A. (2016). Scenarios for Australian agricultural production and land use to 2050. *Agricultural Systems*, 142, 70–83. doi:10.1016/j.agsy.2015.11.008

Hadjikakou, M. (2017). Trimming the excess: environmental impacts of discretionary food consumption in Australia. *Ecological Economics*, 131, 119–28. doi:10.1016/j.ecolecon.2016.08.006

Lindberg, R., Whelan, J., Lawrence, M., Gold, L. & Friel, S. (2015). Still serving hot soup? Two hundred years of a charitable food sector in Australia: a narrative review. *Australian and New Zealand Journal of Public Health*, 39(4), 358–65. doi:10.1111/1753-6405.12311

McCartan, J. & Palermo, C. (2017). The role of a food policy coalition in influencing a local food environment: an Australian case study. *Public Health Nutrition*, 20(5), 917–26. doi:10.1017/S1368980016003001

Myers, S. S., Smith, M. R., Guth, S., Golden, C. D., Vaitla, B., Mueller, N. D., ... Huybers, P. (2017). Climate change and global food systems: potential impacts on food security and undernutrition. *Annual Review of Public Health*, 38, 259–77.

Palermo, C., McCartan, J., Kleve, S., Sinha, K. & Shiell, A. (2016). A longitudinal study of the cost of food in Victoria influenced by geography and nutritional quality. *Australian and New Zealand Journal of Public Health*, 40(3), 270–3. doi:10.1111/1753-6405.12506

Perignon, M., Vieux, F., Soler, L.-G., Masset, G. & Darmon, N. (2017). Improving diet sustainability through evolution of food choices: review of epidemiological studies on the environmental impact of diets. *Nutrition Reviews*, 75(1), 2–17. doi:10.1093/nutrit/nuw043

Popkin, B. M. (2017). Relationship between shifts in food system dynamics and acceleration of the global nutrition transition. *Nutrition Reviews*, 75(2), 73–82. doi:10.1093/nutrit/nuw064

Reynolds, C. J., Piantadosi, J., Buckley, J. D., Weinstein, P. & Boland, J. (2015). Evaluation of the environmental impact of weekly food consumption in different socio-economic households in

Australia using environmentally extended input-output analysis. *Ecological Economics*, 111, 58–64. doi:10.1016/j.ecolecon.2015.01.007

Seto, K. C. & Ramankutty, N. (2016). Hidden linkages between urbanization and food systems. *Science*, 352(6288), 943–5. doi:10.1126/science.aaf7439

Singh-Peterson, L., Lieske, S., Underhill, S. J. R. & Keys, N. (2016). Food security, remoteness and consolidation of supermarket distribution centres: factors contributing to food pricing inequalities across Queensland, Australia. *Australian Geographer*, 47(1), 89–102. doi:10.1080/00049182.2015.1093700

Smith, K., Lawrence, G., MacMahon, A., Muller, J. & Brady, M. (2016). The resilience of long and short food chains: a case study of flooding in Queensland, Australia. *Agriculture and Human Values*, 33(1), 45–60. doi:10.1007/s10460-015-9603-1

The Lancet (2017). Addressing the vulnerability of the global food system. *The Lancet*, 390(10090), 95. doi:10.1016/S0140-6736(17)31803-2

Wycherley, T., Ferguson, M., O'Dea, K., McMahon, E., Liberato, S. & Brimblecombe, J. (2016). Store turnover as a predictor of food and beverage provider turnover and associated dietary intake estimates in very remote Indigenous communities. *Australian and New Zealand Journal of Public Health*, 40(6), 569–71. doi:10.1111/1753-6405.12571

REFERENCES

1   P. Baker & S. Friel (2016). Food systems transformations, ultra-processed food markets and the nutrition transition in Asia. *Global Health*, 12(1), 80. doi:10.1186/s12992-016-0223-3

2   United Nations Standing Committee on Nutrition (2016). *Investments for Healthy Food Systems: A framework analysis and review of evidence on food system investments for improving nutrition*. Geneva: UNSCN.

3   Food and Agriculture Organization of the United Nations (1996). *World Food Summit Declaration on World Food Security*. Rome: FAO.

4   K. Stamoulis & A. Zezza (2003). *A Conceptual Framework for National Agricultural, Rural Development, and Food Security Strategies and Policies*. Rome: FAO.

5   J. McComb, K. Webb & G. Marks (2000). What do we mean by 'food access' and 'food supply'? *Foodchain*, 1(March), 3–4.

6   Panel to Review US Department of Agriculture's Measurement of Food Insecurity Hunger National Research Council (2006). *Food Insecurity and Hunger in the United States: An assessment of the measure*. Washington, DC: National Academies Press.

7   W. S. Wolfe, E. A. Frongillo & P. Valois (2003). Understanding the experience of food insecurity by elders suggests ways to improve its measurement. *Journal of Nutrition*, 133(9), 2762–9.

8   W. Foley, P. Ward, P. Carter, J. Coveney, G. Tsourtos & A. Taylor (2009). An ecological analysis of factors associated with food insecurity in South Australia, 2002–7. *Public Health Nutrition*, 13(2), 215–21. doi:10.1017/S1368980009990747

9   D. Gallegos, P. Ellies & J. Wright (2008). Still there's no food! Food insecurity in a refugee population in Perth, Western Australia. *Nutrition & Dietetics*, 65(1), 78–83. doi:10.1111/j.1747-0080.2007.00175.x

10 M. Nord, M. Andrews & S. Carlson (2008). *Household Food Security in the United States, 2007. Economic Research Report No. (ERR-66)65.* Washington, DC: US Department of Agriculture.

11 M. Nolan, M. Williams, G. Rikard-Bell & M. Mohsin (2006). Food insecurity in three socially disadvantaged localities in Sydney, Australia. *Health Promotion Journal of Australia*, 17(3), 247–54.

12 R. Ramsey, K. Giskes, G. Turrell & D. Gallegos (2012). Food insecurity among adults residing in disadvantaged urban areas: potential health and dietary consequences. *Public Health Nutrition*, 15(2), 227–37. doi:10.1017/s1368980011001996

13 S. Lloyd, J. Lawton, M. Caraher, G. Singh, K. Horsley & F. Mussa (2011). A tale of two localities: healthy eating on a restricted income. *Health Education Journal*, 70(1), 48–56. doi:10.1177/0017896910364837

14 Food and Agriculture Organization of the United Nations, WFP & IFAD (2012). *The State of Food Insecurity in the World 2012. Economic growth is necessary but not sufficient to accelerate reduction of hunger and malnutrition.* Rome: FAO.

15 A. Drewnowski (2010). The cost of US foods as related to their nutritive value. *American Journal of Clinical Nutrition*, 92(5), 1181–8. doi:10.3945/ajcn.2010.29300

16 T. Hopgood, I. Asher, C. R. Wall, C. C. Grant, J. Stewart, S. Muimuiheata & D. Exeter (2010). Crunching the numbers: the affordability of nutritious food for New Zealand children. *Nutrition & Dietetics*, 67(4), 251–7. doi:10.1111/j.1747-0080.2010.01472.x

17 K. C. Wong, J. Coveney, P. Ward, R. Muller, P. Carter, F. Verity & G. Tsourtos (2011). Availability, affordability and quality of a healthy food basket in Adelaide, South Australia. *Nutrition & Dietetics*, 68(1), 8–14. doi:10.1111/j.1747-0080.2010.01490.x

18 C. Kettings, A. J. Sinclair & M. Voevodin (2009). A healthy diet consistent with Australian health recommendations is too expensive for welfare-dependent families. *Australian and New Zealand Journal of Public Health*, 33(6), 566–72. doi:10.1111/j.1753-6405.2009.00454.x

19 J. Wardle & M. Baranovic (2009). Is lack of retail competition in the grocery sector a public health issue? *Australian and New Zealand Journal of Public Health*, 33(5), 477–81. doi:10.1111/j.1753-6405.2009.00433.x

20 C. Wylie, J. Copeman & S. F. L. Kirk (1999). Health and social factors affecting the food choice and nutritional intake of elderly people with restricted mobility. *Journal of Human Nutrition and Dietetics*, 12(5), 375–80. doi:10.1046/j.1365-277x.1999.00177.x

21 A. Whelan, N. Wrigley, D. Warm & E. Cannings (2002). Life in a 'food desert'. *Urban Studies*, 39(11), 2083–100. doi:10.1080/0042098022000011371

22 J. Coveney (2005). A qualitative study exploring socio-economic differences in parental lay knowledge of food and health: implications for public health nutrition. *Public Health Nutrition*, 8(3), 290–7.

23 A. J. Lee, A. M. Darcy, D. Leonard, A. D. Groos, C. O. Stubbs, S. K. Lowson, ... M. D. Riley (2002). Food availability, cost disparity and improvement in relation to accessibility and remoteness in Queensland. *Australian and New Zealand Journal of Public Health*, 26(3), 266–72.

24 M. Lewis & A. Lee (2016). Costing 'healthy' food baskets in Australia: a systematic review of food price and affordability monitoring tools, protocols and methods. *Public Health Nutrition*, 19(16), 2872–86. doi:10.1017/s1368980016002160

25 M. Harrison, A. Lee, M. Findlay, R. Nicholls, D. Leonard & C. Martin (2010). The increasing cost of healthy food. *Australian and New Zealand Journal of Public Health*, 34(2), 179–86. doi:10.1111/j.1753-6405.2010.00504.x

26 A. Lee, C. N. Mhurchu, G. Sacks, B. Swinburn, W. Snowdon, S. Vandevijvere, ... C. Walker (2013). Monitoring the price and affordability of foods and diets globally. *Obesity Reviews*, 14(Suppl.1), 82–95. doi:10.1111/obr.12078

27 A.J. Lee, S. Kane, R. Ramsey, E. Good & M. Dick (2016). Testing the price and affordability of healthy and current (unhealthy) diets and the potential impacts of policy change in Australia. *BMC Public Health*, 16, 315. doi:10.1186/s12889-016-2996-y

28 Australian Bureau of Statistics (2015). *Australian Aboriginal and Torres Strait Islander Health Survey: Nutrition results—Food and nutrients, 2012–13—Food security*. Canberra: ABS.

29 L. C. Tapsell, Y. Probst, M. Lawrence, S. Friel, V. Flood, A. McMahon & R. Butler (2011). Food and nutrition security in the Australia–New Zealand region: impact of climate change. *World Review of Nutrition and Dietetics*, 102, 192–200. doi:10.1159/000327823

30 S. Friel (2010). Climate change, food insecurity and chronic diseases: sustainable and healthy policy opportunities for Australia. *NSW Public Health Bulletin*, 21(5–6), 129–33. doi:10.1071/nb10019

31 Australian Bureau of Statistics (2008). *Population Projections Australia 2006 to 2101*. Canberra: ABS.

32 The Prime Minister's Science and Engineering and Innovation Council (2010). *Australia and Food Security in a Changing World*. Canberra: PMSEIC.

33 E.M. Berry, S. Dernini, B. Burlingame, A. Meybeck & P. Conforti (2015). Food security and sustainability: can one exist without the other? *Public Health Nutrition*, 18(13), 2293–302. doi:10.1017/s136898001500021x

34 A. Meybeck & V. Gitz (2017). Sustainable diets within sustainable food systems. *Proceedings of the Nutrition Society*, 76(1), 1–11. doi:10.1017/s0029665116000653

35 R. Pérez-Escamilla (2017). Food security and the 2015–30 Sustainable Development Goals: from human to planetary health. *Current Developments in Nutrition*, 1(7). doi:10.3945/cdn.117.000513

36 The Economist Intelligence Unit (2014). *Global Food Security Index 2014: An annual measure of the state of global food security*. Retrieved from: http://foodsecurityindex.eiu.com/Resources.

37 B. Ridoutt, D. Baird, K. Bastiaans, R. Darnell, G. Hendrie, M. Riley, ... B. Keating (2017). Australia's nutritional food balance: situation, outlook and policy implications. *Food Security*, 9(2), 211–26. doi:10.1007/s12571-017-0650-x

38 S. S. Myers, M. R. Smith, S. Guth, C. D. Golden, B. Vaitla, N. D. Mueller, ... P. Huybers (2017). Climate change and global food systems: potential impacts on food security and undernutrition. *Annual Review of Public Health*, 38, 259–77. doi:10.1146/annurev-publhealth-031816-044356

39 E. Martínez Steele, B. M. Popkin, B. Swinburn & C. A. Monteiro (2017). The share of ultra-processed foods and the overall nutritional quality of diets in the US: evidence from a nationally representative cross-sectional study. *Population Health Metrics*, 15(1), 6. doi:10.1186/s12963-017-0119-3

40 American Dietetic Association (2009). Position of the American Dietetic Association: functional foods. *Journal of the American Dietetic Association*, 109(4), 735–46. doi:http://dx.doi.org/10.1016/j.jada.2009.02.023

41 Food Standards Australia New Zealand (2016). *Nutrition Content Claims and Health Claims*. Canberra: FSANZ. Retrieved from: www.foodstandards.gov.au/consumer/labelling/nutrition/Pages/default.aspx.

42 K. M. Crowe & C. Francis (2013). Position of the academy of nutrition and dietetics: functional foods. *Journal of the Academy of Nutrition and Dietetics*, 113(8), 1096–103. doi:10.1016/j.jand.2013.06.002

43 L. Tapsell (2008). Functional foods: an Australian perspective. *Nutrition & Dietetics*, 65, S23–S26. doi:10.1111/j.1747-0080.2008.00256.x

44 S. Jew, J.-M. Antoine, P. Bourlioux, J. Milner, L. C. Tapsell, Y. Yang & P. J. H. Jones (2015). Nutrient essentiality revisited. *Journal of Functional Foods*, 14, 203–9. doi:http://dx.doi.org/10.1016/j.jff.2015.01.024

45 S. Spencer & M. Kneebone (2012). *FOODmap: An analysis of the Australian food supply chain.* Canberra: Department of Agriculture, Fisheries and Forestry.

46 CSIRO Futures (2017). *Food and Agribusiness: A roadmap for unlocking value-adding growth opportunities for Australia.* CSIRO Futures. Retrieved from: www.csiro.au/en/Do-business/Futures/Reports/Food-and-Agribusiness-Roadmap.

47 M. E. Cogswell, S. M. Patel, K. Yuan, C. Gillespie, W. Juan, C. J. Curtis, … R. Merritt. (2017). Modeled changes in US sodium intake from reducing sodium concentrations of commercially processed and prepared foods to meet voluntary standards established in North America: NHANES. *American Journal of Clinical Nutrition*, 106(2), 530–40. doi:10.3945/ajcn.116.145623

48 L. E. Thornton, D. A. Crawford, K. E. Lamb & K. Ball (2017). Where do people purchase food? A novel approach to investigating food purchasing locations. *International Journal of Health Geographics*, 16(1), 9. doi:10.1186/s12942-017-0082-z

49 M. Mazidi & J. R. Speakman (2017). Higher densities of fast-food and full-service restaurants are not associated with obesity prevalence. *American Journal of Clinical Nutrition*, 106(2), 603–13. doi:10.3945/ajcn.116.151407

50 R. Micha, J. L. Peñalvo, F. Cudhea, F. Imamura, C. D. Rehm & D. Mozaffarian (2017). Association between dietary factors and mortality from heart disease, stroke, and type 2 diabetes in the united states. *JAMA—Journal of the American Medical Association*, 317(9), 912–24. doi:10.1001/jama.2017.0947

51 L. C. Del Gobbo, M. C. Falk, R. Feldman, K. Lewis & D. Mozaffarian (2015). Effects of tree nuts on blood lipids, apolipoproteins, and blood pressure: systematic review, meta-analysis, and dose-response of 61 controlled intervention trials. *American Journal of Clinical Nutrition*, 102(6), 1347–56. doi:10.3945/ajcn.115.110965

52 N. Martin, R. Germano, L. Hartley, A. J. Adler & K. Rees (2015). Nut consumption for the primary prevention of cardiovascular disease. *Cochrane Database of Systematic Reviews*, 9, Cd011583. doi:10.1002/14651858.CD011583.pub2

53 Department of Health and Human Services & US Department of Agriculture (2015). *Scientific Report of the 2015 Dietary Guidelines Advisory Committee.* Washington, DC: Department of Health and Human Services, US Department of Agriculture. Retrieved from: https://health.gov/dietaryguidelines/2015-scientific-report/pdfs/scientific-report-of-the-2015-dietary-guidelines-advisory-committee.pdf.

54 National Health and Medical Research Council (2011). *A Review of the Evidence to Address Targeted Questions to Inform the Revision of the Australian Dietary Guidelines: Evidence statements.* Canberra: NHMRC.

55 S. Raatz (2016). Go nuts! Retrieved from: www.ars.usda.gov/plains-area/gfnd/gfhnrc/docs/news-2013/go-nuts.

56 L. C. Tapsell, M. Lonergan, M. J. Batterham, E. P. Neale, A. Martin, R. Thorne, … G. Peoples (2017). Effect of interdisciplinary care on weight loss: a randomised controlled trial. *BMJ Open*, 7(7). doi:10.1136/bmjopen-2016-014533

57 E. P. Neale, L. C. Tapsell, A. Martin, M. J. Batterham, C. Wibisono & Y. C. Probst (2017). Impact of providing walnut samples in a lifestyle intervention for weight loss: a secondary analysis of the HealthTrack trial. *Food and Nutrition Research*, 61(1), article 1344522. doi:10.1080/16546628.2017.1344522

58 C. Wibisono, Y. Probst, E. Neale & L. Tapsell (2017). Changes in diet quality during a 12 month weight loss randomised controlled trial. *BMC Nutrition*, 3(1), 38. doi:10.1186/s40795-017-0157-z

CHAPTER 22

FOOD COMPOSITION AND DIETARY ASSESSMENT

YASMINE PROBST AND LINDA TAPSELL

CHAPTER OBJECTIVES

This chapter will enable the reader to:

- describe the role of food and nutrient databases and key issues surrounding their use in food and nutrition research
- critically evaluate different forms of dietary assessment methodology
- outline the function of dietary assessments for nutrition monitoring and surveillance for population health
- describe the uses of dietary modelling in nutrition practice.

KEY TERMS

Dietary assessment

Dietary modelling

Dietary surveys

Food composition

KEY POINTS

- Food composition databases provide a means for translating food information into nutrient information; food composition data may obtained from a number of sources.
- Some countries have both reference and survey food composition databases. The survey database is generally developed from population-based food surveys. INFOODS is an international program to streamline the various food composition data tables throughout the world. One of the main forms of standardisation includes the use of per 100 g nutrient values and consistent nutrient labels called TAGNAMES.
- In choosing dietary assessment methods, it is important to clarify the purpose of dietary assessment and the study population, identify the outcome measures required, and consider the number of assessments required for the purpose and the validity of the assessment for the purpose.
- Dietary modelling is used to identify the impact of public health strategies on nutrient intakes of various age and gender groups, to check that recommended dietary patterns are practically achievable and nutritionally adequate, and to develop dietary advice that addresses specific health issues and individual preferences and circumstances.

INTRODUCTION

In previous chapters, we have considered nutrition as the relationship between food intake and health. We have examined the role of food components (nutrients and other substances), and we have seen how the total diet ultimately has an impact on health. The concept of *balance* is very important in understanding nutrition. It also drives much of the application of nutrition knowledge in practice.

Se Chapter 1 on nutritional balance.

Practice generally involves the use of tools. In this chapter, we focus on core tools for nutrition practice that enable the principle of balance to be addressed. The key tools considered here are methods for assessing dietary intake, tools that enable translation of information on food intake to that of nutrients, and tools of dietary modelling, which incorporate knowledge from both food composition and dietary assessment.

STOP AND THINK

- Why do we need up-to-date information on the nutrient content of foods?
- Why do we need to measure what the population is eating?
- How important is it that these two activities are underpinned by the best available scientific methods?

WHAT IS THE ROLE OF FOOD AND NUTRIENT DATABASES?

Food database

a set of data providing the nutritional composition of different foods. The purpose of the data should be defined before a food composition database is selected.

Food and nutrient databases enable information from dietary assessment methods on food intake patterns to be converted to nutrient intake data. This is how we know that a combination of foods that makes up a person's reported diet may contain, for example, too much energy or not enough calcium. The dietary assessment tools outlined in this chapter are used to capture information about usual or actual food intakes and allow for dietary patterns and potential inadequacies of intake to be determined. To translate the food information collected in these assessments into nutrient information, another important tool needs to be used. **Food databases** assist with this process through the provision of tables of food and nutrient information.

Since the initial chemical analyses of food items to determine their composition, collections of such data have been collated in the form of nutrient databases. The first documented records appear to have arisen in 1818 as a nutrition scale for the food supply in prisons, and the first composition tables appeared in Germany in 1878 [1]. Shortly after this, Atwater and Woods (1896) published the first collection of American food composition data, including approximately 2600 food items for the key food groups and some processed foods [2]. Atwater's data is still referred to today for the conversion of food information into energy contributions from the varying macronutrients. The first Australian databases were published in 1938 and contained only seven nutrients [3].

In the present day, food composition databases have grown with the number of foods available in the food supply. The range of nutrients for analysis has increased as the techniques for analysis have been refined and further developed. For example, food composition databases prior to the 1980s included values for total energy that excluded fibre, while today's values include the contribution of dietary fibre to total energy. The global aim of food composition database experts is to have available and accessible databases for each country or region, because there are differences in nutrient yield from the varied

FIGURE 22.1 OVERVIEW OF THE HISTORY OF THE AUSTRALIAN FOOD COMPOSITION PROGRAM

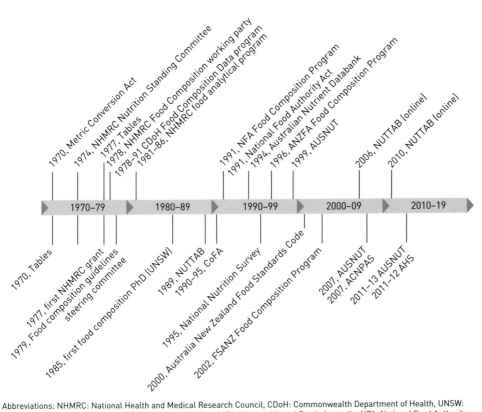

Abbreviations: NHMRC: National Health and Medical Research Council, CDoH: Commonwealth Department of Health, UNSW: University of New South Wales, NUTTAB: Nutrient Tables, CoFA: Composition of Foods Australia, NFA: National Food Authority, ANZFA: Australia New Zealand Food Authority, AUSNUT: Australian Nutrient Tables, FSANZ: Food Standards Australia New Zealand, ACNPAS: Australian Children's Nutrition and Physical Activity Survey, AHS: Australian Health Survey

Source: Y. Probst (2015). Key players of the Australian food composition program. *Procedia Food Science*, 4, 125–32. doi:http://dx.doi.org/10.1016/j.profoo.2015.06.017

climates, soil conditions and even harvest techniques used. These databases should be of a consistent format, with current practice encouraging the use of INFOODS TAGNAMES for the constituent nutrients [4]. Earlier databases attempted to report nutrient values per serving of a food item, but as serving sizes changed with time, it was decided that all food composition values be reported per 100 g of the food item to standardise the output. There are a number of key players in the Australian food composition program (Figure 22.1) [5].

In Australia, the national food composition tables were originally managed by the National Food Authority, which is today known as Food Standards Australia New Zealand (FSANZ). The first food composition data for Australia became available in 1938 with approximately 1172 [3] food items, followed by a more comprehensive collection in 1970 [6] following the development of an analytical program. From this time, food composition tables for Australia were available as the Composition of Australian Foods, which was updated almost 10 years later in 1981 and finally in seven bound volumes of 1800 foods and 28 nutrients. These were first released in 1989 and updated as required until 1995, by which time the data had been selectively updated to include 134 nutrients [7]. The 1989 database, released for the first time on a computer disc, became known the Nutrient Tables for Australian Foods (NUTTAB) [8]. The subsequent 1995 update to NUTTAB was the basis for nutritional analysis of the 1995 National Nutrition Survey (NNS) [9]. In 1991, the Nutritional Values of Australian Foods was also released, which was a collection of both NUTTAB and volumes 1–5 of the Composition of Australian Foods; it contained only 1600 foods. Two additional volumes were released at a later date. *Food for Health: A guide to good nutrition* was also published in 1991 [10]. This publication contained a limited number of foods with the focus on enabling consumers to find the foods that provide particular essential nutrients. The primary difference between this and previous publications was the presentation of the servings as common household measures rather than the traditional per 100 g measure used in other food composition tables [11]. This food serving size measure had also previously been adopted for the 1970 tables, although all other tables have followed the standard format [6; 12].

The 1995 NUTTAB database formed the basis for the development of the Australian Food and Nutrient Database (AUSNUT) 1999, and the survey database stemming from the food intake data collected in the NNS of 1995. This database contained a complete collection of nutrient data for all foods reported in the NNS, although unlike NUTTAB, which primarily contained analysed data, AUSNUT also contained some data derived from calculations and borrowed from overseas databases [13]. These two databases remained the main data of two Australian databases until the 2007 Australian National Children's Nutrition and Physical Activity Survey [14]. The year 2006 saw the release of NUTTAB 2006 [15] and, subsequently, AUSNUT 2007 [16]. It was this release of the NUTTAB database that first saw the Australian food composition database move to an online system, with a further update released in 2010. The 2007 version of AUSNUT contains 4227 foods, beverages and dietary supplements, and nutrient data for 37 nutrients [17; 18]. The 2010 version of NUTTAB contains 2668 Australian foods and up to 245 nutrients [19]. Following the completion of the 2011–13 National Nutrition and Physical Activity Survey [20; 21] component of the Australian Health Survey 2011–12 [21], a subsequent of version of the AUSNUT database was released, AUSNUT 2011–13 [22]. This database was updated with 96 foods, 307 food measures and six dietary supplements following the analysis of the National Aboriginal and Torres Strait Islander Nutrition and Physical Activity Survey [23] component of the Australian Health Survey. This is the first Australian database to include supplement information with over 5740 food items with 53 nutrients and a further 2163 supplements. In 2018 an updated version of NUTTAB was released as The Australian Food Composition Database-Release 1 (see www.foodstandards.gov.au) as on online searchable database. This became the most up to date reference nutrient database for use in Australia.

≫ RESEARCH AT WORK

DEVELOPING MATCHING FILES OF FOOD COMPOSITION DATA IN RESEARCH

Food composition data used in research projects should be carefully selected to ensure that they are suited to the region in which the data is being collected and that the database is timely in relation to the research. As food composition databases are updated over time, attempts are made to create links between the previous and the newer data available. The links are primarily via codes assigned to each food in the database, although due to changes in the food supply over time some foods from an older database may no longer be required and other foods in newer databases may need to be added. The files that demonstrate the links and changes between databases are referred to as matching files and in Australia are created by FSANZ. Further to this, changes in the eating patterns of the region may need to be considered. For this reason the AUSNUT 2011–13 food composition database contains a greater number of hot beverage/cafe options than the previous AUSNUT 1999 database and also contains additional Indigenous foods including reptiles and native fruits. A matching file was created by FSANZ to depict this [24]. Due to the substantial gap between survey databases for adults, some Australian researchers employed the AUSNUT 2007 survey database for their research, despite it relating to intakes of Australian children. Some of these projects continued to collect data following the subsequent release of AUSNUT 2011–13, but no matching file was created by FSANZ as the population target of the surveys differed. A matching file has been created by academics who were required to back-match the foods from AUSNUT 2007 to the underpinning NUTTAB data and then match it forward to the AUSNUT 2011–13 database to update the food information [25]. This now allows data analysed using AUSNUT2007 to be updated to AUSNUT 2011–13. Table 22.1 provides an outline of the number of nutrients included in the various Australian databases over eight decades.

TABLE 22.1   NUMBER OF FOOD AND NUTRIENTS INCLUDED IN AUSTRALIA FOOD COMPOSITION DATA TABLES 1938–2012 [26; 27]

Data source	Year published	Number of foods (food groups)	Number of nutrients
Report of Dr G Bourne [28]	1938	1172	7
Food Composition Tables	1941	132(6)	5
Food Composition Tables	1944	135(8)	9
Tables of the Composition of Australian Foods [29]	1946	132(13)	9
Tables of the Composition of Australian Foods [30]	1948	216(13)	11
Tables of the Composition of Australian Foods [31; 32]	1954 1961	284(16)	13
Tables of the Composition of Australian Foods [33; 34]	1979 1977	720(18)	16
NUTTAB [35]	1989	na	23
CoFA - Vol. 1 - Vol. 2 - Vol. 3 - Vol. 4 - Vol. 5 - Vol. 6 - Vol. 7	1989 1990 1990 1990 1990 1992 1995	1730 682 223 162 155 190 162 156	26
Nutritional Values of Australian Foods [36]	1991	1600(15)	23
Food for Health [36; 37]	1991	650	23
AFDB	1995	1800	108
NUTTAB	1991/92	1576(14)	27
NUTTAB [38]	1995	1805	29–34
NUTTAB [39]	1997	up to 1116	up to 50
The Nutritional Composition of Australian Aboriginal Foods [40]	1993, 1997	500	20

Data source	Year published	Number of foods (food groups)	Number of nutrients
AUSNUT	1999	4554(14)	30
NPC [41]	2001	~4000	7
NUTTAB Online [42]	2006	2600	169
AUSNUT [17]	2007	3875 (foods) 4225 (including supplements)	37
NUTTAB Online_ENREF_63 [43]	2010	2668	245
NPC [44]	2011	2520	7
AUSNUT	2013	5740 (foods) 2163 (supplements)	53
NUTTAB	2015	1542	53

Source: Adapted from Y. C. Probst & J. Cunningham (2015). An overview of the influential developments and stakeholders within the food composition program of Australia. *Trends in Food Science & Technology*, 42(2), 173–82. doi:https://doi.org/10.1016/j.tifs.2014.12.005
See also S Tompsett, R Sobolewski, A Craven, D Ballantyne, J Cunningham Updated Australian Food Composition Database (formerly NUTTAB). Proc Nutrition Society of Australia 42nd Annual Scientific Meeting. Canberra 2018. www.nsameeting.asn.au.

Food composition data has many uses, ranging from the identification of the compositional elements of a food item through to analysis of dietary intakes and dietary modelling. The purpose of the data should be defined before a database is selected—for example, the AUSNUT database is better suited to analysis of intake data due to its derivation. The food composition databases for a given country are generally managed by one central organisation, such as FSANZ in Australia. Databases are further overseen on a global level by the Food and Agriculture Organization (FAO) of the United Nations through its INFOODS program. Consideration should be given to the source of the data within the database, analysis methods used, coverage of the food items, types of values included, any coding used and modes of expression within the database [4]. It is a common assumption that all values within a food composition database have been obtained from analytical studies; however, data may also be calculated, imputed or borrowed from another country's database to fill in any missing values. Furthermore, the proportion of these missing values also requires some thought.

Within Australia and many other countries, a reference database and a survey database exist for use (NUTTAB, AUSNUT and now the new Australian Food Composition Database as described previously) [13]. In the United States, these databases are the USDA Standard Reference database and the Food and Nutrient Database for Dietary Studies (FNDDS) [45] survey database. Both of these databases are managed by the US Department of Agriculture, with regular updates occurring as new food analyses are released. Reference and survey databases have very differing purposes and should be used with care. Furthermore, some technologies draw on the values of these databases in order to provide output for the user. The age of the database and relevance to the use at hand should be noted before a database is selected. Food composition data globally moved from hardcopy tables to softcopy databases that were incorporated into software packages, and in more recent years to online formats. This allows not only the nutrient data for a food item to be displayed with ease, but also shows the background to the source of the data. This source information may include information about where the data originated, which may include whether it was based on a calculation or on analysed food items. This availability of the data has improved accessibility, allowing an increased number of uses to be developed.

Previously, a common tool that used food composition databases was the 'ready reckoner'. This tool is a summarised version of key foods or food groups to allow for a speedy analysis of information on food intake. Limits to the number of foods and the number of nutrients have meant that many nutritionists and dietitians are now using electronic forms of the data and portable technologies that can not only similarly summarise the required data but also improve the flexibility of design and application of use. The dietary assessment methods described in subsequent sections required manual calculations of the nutrients, whereas today the software available allows the data to be directly entered into it or, more efficiently, uploaded through wireless technologies; this improves not only the number of nutrients that can be assessed but also the speed with which this data can be used. Dietary modelling is another use of food composition databases that draws on the nutrient data and often, as an outcome, converts it back to food data for the development of guidelines and advice strategies.

» CASE 22.1

USES OF FOOD COMPOSITION DATA IN AUSTRALIA

One of the uses of food composition data in Australia is the provision of a nutrition information panel (NIP) on packaged foods, which is required under the Food Standards Code. Companies can either have their products analysed or match the FSANZ databases of foods for the ingredients in the product, using a 'recipe formulation'. Thus companies can contribute to the development of the food composition database and/or use the database to calculate the information for their product NIP. As costs are involved in undertaking analyses, only those with adequate resources can do the former. This also has implications for the currency of the food database.

Food researchers can also submit data from the nutrient analysis of food. They must follow analytical standards such as those outlined in AOAC International [46] and follow standards of scientific reporting, including transparency of methods used, such as sampling and techniques.

STOP AND THINK

- How do researchers decide on the number of foods to include in a food database?
- Where might the nutrient values in food composition databases be sourced from?
- If data on a food is missing from a food composition database, where might you find the data?
- When might databases need to be more specific to the country in which the dietary intake data was collected?

WHAT IS DIETARY ASSESSMENT METHODOLOGY?

Dietary assessment involves taking a measure of what people eat during a given period of time. Dietary assessment methodology is the study of the methods used, including considerations of their validity and reliability. Dietary assessment methods can be collected prospectively, at the time of consumption, or retrospectively, after the time of consumption.

Dietary assessment
the measurement of actual or usual food intakes over a specified period of time.

The main goal is to capture the types of foods and the amounts that have been consumed. Some foods are eaten every day and are easy to account for, while others are only eaten occasionally, and this makes assessment more difficult. The choice of the dietary assessment method is dependent on the purpose for which it is intended as well as the person whose intake is being recorded. The accuracy of the measurement will vary depending on the method that is used. Food records (FR) involve noting down foods consumed as they are eaten, whereas questionnaires (such as a food frequency questionnaire; FFQ) and interviews (such as the 24-hour recall or diet history) rely on memory. Commonly identified methods are outlined below, with both the traditional approach and technological advancements addressed.

The *diet history* form of dietary assessment is a retrospective interview conducted with a trained interviewer, often a dietitian, to recall the usual dietary habits of a person. Originally developed by Burke in 1947 [47; 48], the diet history follows a conversational-style approach to recalling a person's intake. Guided by the interviewer and following initial introductions [49; 50], the person is prompted to recall their intake of foods and beverages, beginning with the first meal of the day and ending with the last meal of the day. Little conversation occurs at this point, to allow the flow of the recall to be based on the order of intake; however, particular participant groups may require added direction to continue with the recall. Once the person has recalled all the meals that they usually consume, the interviewer will then prompt them to continue to provide additional information about the foods in the same order as they were recalled and using the same meal prompts as were reported.

The next stage of the diet history interview is the identification of food portion sizes and frequency of consumption. These portion sizes may already have been spoken about during the interview as the person was recalling them, although it is likely that some gaps may still exist. The frequency of consumption information needs to relate to the period of intake being address. Diet history interviews commonly range from one week to one month, although there is no specified duration. Shorter reference periods have been found to result in increased precision and validity of the data [50; 51]; However, the interview form of the recall is largely dependent on the skills of the interviewer, the recall ability of the interviewee, the use of props and utensils to assist recall, and the time and cost constraints of the setting in which it is used. Interviews can take up to an hour to complete in a research setting, but are more commonly seen in clinical settings conducted by dietitians [52]. Once the additional detail has been provided for all meals, it is common for the interviewer to ask about commonly forgotten foods. These are foods that may be affected by recall bias and, when prompted, the interviewee may recall other foods related to them [47; 52]. This recall bias is common to the diet history interview, with particular population groups known to report only the foods that may be pleasing to the interviewers or socially accepted in society [52; 53] and may vary from the types of foods to the amounts consumed. Females and overweight persons have been seen to be affected by such recall bias, tending to report less than is usual—that is, they under-report their intakes [54; 55]. This may be further impacted by the gender of the interviewer in relation to the interviewee [56]. Memory of the recall has the most impact on the results obtained and therefore groups such as the elderly or young children (below age 10 years) [57; 58] may require a carer or parent to assist the interviewer.

Diet history interviews have been conducted in an interview manner for many years, with the information recorded as handwritten notes by the interviewer, usually an accredited practicing dietitian (APD) due to the skills and food knowledge required. These handwritten notes may be entered into dietary assessment software for analysis or a ready reckoner may be applied if time or resources are limited. Few attempts to automate the diet history interview have occurred because of the conversational nature of the assessment. The DietAdvice tool attempted to follow the pedagogical process of the diet history [59–61]. This tool found a reduction in the impact of social desirability from persons who used it [62–64] as the interviewer had become the computer and not a person sitting opposite them in an interview.

USING NARRATIVE STRUCTURE TO OBTAIN A DIET HISTORY

The narrative diet history interview was developed based on an understanding that people often tell stories in a reliably structured way when accounting for events [52]. Research applying this framework to a diet history interview resulted in the following protocol:

- Explain the purpose of the interview, seek a description on usual eating patterns and suggest starting with the first meal of the day. Record the foods reported.
- If a narrative begins and clearly progresses from one meal to the next, do not interrupt but rather allow the interviewee to finish at the last eating/drinking event of the day. If the interviewee stops for any reason, use prompts to continue the narrative to the end of the day, such as 'Was that all?' or 'What comes next?' If the interviewee stops to explain food consumption patterns, respond in a non-judgmental way and keep the account of foods consumed on the narrative track.
- On reaching the end of the narrative, go back over your notes and fill in gaps based on your professional judgment (related to the purpose of the interview). If the interviewee uses hedging terms such as 'it depends', check for variations on the foods consumed at that time; if they use 'probably', in defining amounts of foods, for example, use visual aids to support estimations.
- Run through a checklist of significant foods and the frequency of their consumption (the list of foods will depend on the purpose of the interview). Summarise and check with the interviewee that this is a reasonable reflection of their usual intakes.

Food record dietary assessments collect prospective, actual intake data from a person and traditionally cover a period ranging from one to seven days. The duration of data collection is dependent on the purpose of the dietary data being collected and these assessments have been known to span longer durations in their varying forms. When completing a food record, a person is required to record all of the foods and beverages that they eat over a given period of time, documenting not only the name of the food but also the amount that was consumed. The level of detail for this portion size information is what differentiates the different forms of food records in practice. Food records may be estimated, whereby the person recording their food intake provides an estimate of the portion consumed based on their interpretation of the amount. This may equate to known, consumer-friendly measures such as 'one handful' or 'one piece'. Measures such as this may be open to interpretation and vary from person to person. If more detail is needed, a weighed food record [65] may be employed in which the person recording their intake is required to measure and weigh all food and beverage items consumed. This may be via the use of standardised measuring cups and spoons or the use of food scales. For a weighed food record, these tools need to be carried by the person to all eating occasions, a requirement which increases the burden [66] and, alongside the need to write down all foods, may result in unintentional modifications to dietary intakes by the person recording them. These modifications may include less snacking and consumption of meals that can be easily recorded [67]. Although it is preferred that the person completing a food record also includes the recipe and labels of foods consumed, in practice this occurs less often than intake modifications. Food record dietary assessments are amongst the most commonly used form of dietary assessment in the research setting, with food-based randomised controlled trails more likely to implement this form of assessment [68]. This may be due to controlled trials having been previously considered as the gold standard form of dietary assessment methodology [65], a position that has been superseded by the repeated 24-hour recall in more recent times [69]. This shift may be due to the growing consumer push for convenience, which is lessened for this method when the higher-quality data is required and weighed records are used. Food records are sometimes referred to as food diaries due to the progressive recording practice involved when they are completed correctly.

Traditionally, a food record was completed in a paper-based form and therefore required that the person completing it possessed a certain level of literacy. The growing influx of technology has seen this method undergo a degree of automation such as being placed online to improve accessibility and streamline the recording process. Completion of an online or technology-assisted food record often requires the person completing the record to type the food items and portion sizes, which reduces one of the common challenges related to this form of assessment, namely, illegible handwriting. While technology-assisted methods have improved the readability of records, the amount of detail required remains a challenge. Most users of the food record method in dietetic consultations or in research practice therefore require in-depth training for recording this intake. Without this training, information returned to the user or researcher is likely to be limited and translation of the food items into nutrients difficult if not enough food or beverage information has been provided. Attempts have been made to continue to overcome these remaining challenges to the food record method. In more recent times, food records have been completed via a web-enabled mobile phone or tablet that incorporates the use of image recognition technologies. These technologies allow the user to simply take an image of the food item they are about to consume and the technology identifies the food or beverage type. Taking a second image following consumption of the food then allows for automated calculation of the food portion size. An example of a food record is shown in Table 22.2.

The *24-hour recall* dietary assessment is a retrospective method whereby a person is required to recall the previous 24 hours of food and/or beverage intake. This method may be via a self-administered method or interviewer-assisted, and the assessment follows a validated process developed by the US National Cancer Institute. The method is referred to as the multiple pass approach [70], whereby increasing levels of detail are collected from the person whose diet is being recalled. The process initially begins with a quick list of foods or beverages consumed at each meal followed by additional detail about the foods, items consumed with the foods and at the final stage a review of all foods in the recall. When commencing the 24-hour recall dietary assessment method, the first consideration that needs to be addressed is whether the recall is the 24-hour period prior to the recall itself or the previous midnight to midnight period. Twenty-four hour recall dietary assessments are more commonly seen in large cohort studies where a larger number of persons need to report their intakes [50; 71]. The challenge is seen, however, when trying to relate the intake data to an intake that is usual or habitual to the person. For this, a repeated number of dietary recalls are required and in turn the likelihood of a person completing them is reduced due to this increased burden. A single 24-hour recall dietary assessment does not provide usual intake information; it simply provides information relevant to the period of time at which it was recalled. When completed with an interviewer present in a face-to-face or telephone-based manner, the limitations of the 24-hour recall are comparable to those of the diet history interview assessment—that is, they are impacted by memory and recall bias. However, with increasing technological applications, the 24-hour recall is more commonly seen in an online format [72], whereby an avatar or screen prompts are used to guide the person through the recall using the same multiple pass process described earlier. One example of such a tool is the Automated Self-administered Assessment, or ASA24, tool. This tool was developed by the National Cancer Institute

TABLE 22.2   EXAMPLE OF A FOOD RECORD

Date: 28 March 2019	Day of week: Monday	
Food/drink	Description and preparation	Amount
Breakfast		
Cereal with milk	Weetbix Low-fat (LF) milk	2 ½ cup
Cup of tea	1 mug made with tea bag (white with sugar)	1 tablespoon LF milk, 1 teaspoon sugar
Mid-morning		
Latte	1 medium skim latte from cafe	About 1½ cups
Lunch		
Sandwich	Wholemeal bread with margarine Cheese Ham Sliced tomato	2 slices 2 teaspoons 1 pre-packaged slice 2 deli slices Half a tomato
Fruit	Apple (red)	1
Water	Tap	2 cups
Afternoon		
Muesli bar	Yoghurt-topped apricot muesli bar	1
Dinner		
Chicken stir-fry	Chicken breast Broccoli (chopped into florets) Carrot (chopped into sticks) Capsicum (red, chopped) Soy sauce Garlic and ginger (fresh, chopped finely) Jasmine rice (steamed) Stir-fried in peanut oil	½ breast ½ cup ½ carrot ½ medium capsicum 2 teaspoon 1 clove garlic, 1 teaspoon ginger 1 cup (cooked) 2 teaspoon
After dinner		
Ice cream	Chocolate ice cream	1

[73] and has been adapted to suit other countries by modification of the types of questions asked and the underpinning food composition database from which it draws the food data. The tool has also been adapted as a children's version. The Australian ASA24 was released for adults in 2017 (see https:// epi.grants.cancer.gov/asa24/respondent/australia.html). The 24-hour recall technique has been used in national nutrition surveys [74; 75]. The steps include multiple 'passes' through a 24-hour period [76].

TRY IT YOURSELF

Starting with breakfast and working through to the last meal of the day, record all foods and beverages that you consumed yesterday. Try to follow the multiple pass format common to the 24-hour recall, starting with the general food types first and then following with the detailed information and portion sizes. Which meals were harder to recall? How did you report the portions of the foods you ate? How well did this recall represent what you would usually consume?

Now categorise the foods you have listed according to the food groups listed in the Australian Guide to Healthy Eating: vegetables, fruit, bread and cereal products, milk/cheese/yoghurt, meats/fish/eggs/ chicken/legumes, other foods. Evaluate the quality of your diet with reference to the Australian Dietary Guidelines (for types of foods) and the AGHE for amounts consumed. What can you say about your diet quality from this activity?

After introducing themselves, the interviewer explains the purpose of the interview and begins with a request to recall all foods consumed the previous day. When foods are listed, the interviewee is probed for details such as brands and type of food preparation. A second 'pass' at this detailed list then asks for portion sizes using visual aids. The third pass checks for anything missing. Today, the online ASA24Australia tool provides a new technology for conducting this interview.

The *food frequency questionnaire* (FFQ) is a retrospective dietary assessment tool often used in population surveys or epidemiological studies. The questionnaire format of the method allows for a large number of people to complete the assessment simultaneously. The FFQ is commonly found in a paper-based format but can vary in its focus. A whole-of-diet approach may be used where most food and beverages consumed are addressed, or a more targeted format can be used for a specific food group or nutrient type. FFQs generally contain a list of foods or food groups, and query how often the person has consumed each option. The number of foods or food groups depends on the purpose of the FFQ and can vary widely from 20 through to more than 100. Although the FFQ does also rely on the memory of the person completing the dietary assessment, the burden is reduced due to the food list being used as a prompt. The frequency of responses provided within the FFQ relate to the span that the FFQ is capturing. As an FFQ aims to capture usual intake information, the frequency options may span from one week to one year [67]. The responses may be categorised into never, daily, fortnightly, monthly, and so on. This frequency of consumption information may be specifically related to a standard measure of a food or food group, often from food-based dietary guidelines or national intake surveys, or the portion measures may be questioned separately or not at all. When the portion is not included, the tool is referred to as a semi-quantitative FFQ. Where food portion sizes are questioned separately, a range of text responses may be given, although more often images of graduated amounts of a sample food are provided and the person selects the closest size to what they consume. An FFQ is commonly self-administered, which means a person completes the questionnaire without any assistance; certain population groups such as children or persons with limited literacy skills may require the assistance of an interviewer, who may complete the questionnaire with them or provide assistance as needed.

For many years, analysis of FFQ dietary assessments have occurred via computer-generated answer sheets, similar to those used for exams. The person answering the FFQ selects the suitable response, and by blacking out the answer, the computer, using food composition data, can calculate the required output. This is one of the advantages of this form of assessment, as the analysis is streamlined and largely automated. More recently, the tools themselves have also been automated, with many options available in an online format. One example of an online FFQ is the Food4Me tool [77; 78]. This FFQ is a quantitative FFQ, which includes food potion images that also appear in colour (not often seen in the printed versions). The questionnaire, in addition to asking about food groups, also asks about the food habits and supplement use of the person completing the FFQ; previously, this additional information was not included in paper-based FFQs. An example of an FFQ is shown in Table 22.3.

TABLE 22.3 EXAMPLE OF A FOOD FREQUENCY QUESTIONNAIRE

PLEASE PUT A TICK (✓) ON EVERY LINE									
FOODS AND AMOUNTS	**AVERAGE USE LAST YEAR**								
FRUIT For seasonal fruits marked *, please estimate your average use when fruit is in season.									
	Never or less than once/ month	1–3 per month	Once a week	2–4 per week	5–6 per week	Once a day	2–3 per day	4–5 per day	6+ per day
Apples (1 fruit)							✓		
Pears (1 fruit)						✓			
Oranges, satsumas, mandarins (1 fruit)			✓						
Grapefruit (half)	✓								
Banana (1 fruit)						✓			
Grapes (medium serving)	✓								
Melon (1 slice)	✓								
* Peaches, plums, apricots (1 fruit)	✓								
* Strawberries, raspberries, kiwi fruit (medium serving)				✓					
Tinned fruit (medium serving)		✓							
Please check that you have a tick (✓) on EVERY line.									

TRY IT YOURSELF

Using the 24-hour recall that you created earlier, imagine you were going to analyse the food information to obtain nutrient values.

- Which food composition database would you select, and why?
- What types of variation may be apparent for the foods you have listed (e.g. seasonal, brand name)?
- Are any of the foods listed made from a recipe? How would you enter this into an analysis program?
- What would you do if a food you have written down is not available in the food composition database that you have chosen?
- Do you have accurate portion size information to include? If not, how would you figure out the portions?

Short questions, also referred to as screeners, are generally limited in number and focus on behavioural aspects of eating. These are used when dietary information is required for a large number of people but the resources are not available for a detailed assessment or the level of detail needed does not need to be precise. Short questions are generally not selected as the main form of dietary assessment, although they can provide useful additional information to complement other methods of assessment. Short questions may ask, for example, 'How many serves of fruit to you normally eat per day?' or 'Do you generally consume meat as part of your diet?' One of the most common formats for short questions is national **dietary surveys**. In Australia, these surveys are the repeated 24-hour recall form of dietary assessment and may also ask a range of short questions. In the most recent National Nutrition and Physical Activity Survey, respondents were asked about the usual number of serves of fruit and of vegetables they consume per day, with the interviewer showing them a prompt card of a usual serve size. They were also asked about the addition of and type of salt added to a meal or during cooking, the type of milk usually consumed and particular food avoidances for allergy, religious or other reasons [79].

Dietary survey
the collection of information on food and dietary intake patterns, usually via some form of questionnaire or interview.

The incorporation of *computing technologies* in dietary assessment occurred during the 1960s when computers were first introduced to assist with the analysis of food intake data [80]. Computer-assisted data collection occurred mainly with the FFQ method, followed in the next decade by the 24-hour recall method. In the 1980s and 1990s, improved computing technologies created the onset of computerised nutrient composition tables as databases and the potential for advanced and highly sophisticated statistical techniques to analyse the data obtained. The introduction and expansion of the internet saw an influx in the use of technology to support and house dietary assessment methodology, although the focus remained on the 24-hour recall and FFQ formats. These methods could include closed questioning and were seen as ideal for displaying on a computer screen. The 24-hour recall, in particular, was seen to be suited to automation because of the well-defined structure of the multiple-pass method described earlier. Involvement of a computer also added improved speed in processing the data, allowing the dietary assessment to be applied to larger groups of people without the extensive resource burden that had previously been associated with large-scale data collection. Online dietary assessment traditionally presents questions on food consumption displayed on a computer (or equivalent) screen. The method is less affected by social desirability bias [50; 81]. Greater disclosure with socially undesirable questions, in particular relating to alcohol consumption and health status, is likely [82], and there is little difference in the reliability and validity of data, especially when comparing this method with the use of pen-and-paper techniques [83]. As outlined earlier, attempts have been made to automate the diet history interview [50; 59], a resource-heavy (i.e. increased financial and personnel costs) assessment method. The complexity of its open-ended questioning and broader period of reference has created challenges for the manner in which online technologies may be used [61]. With the progression of technology, portable devices have also allowed these online technologies to be accessible via the convenience of a smartphone or tablet [84]. This is convenient for the person from whom the data is being collected and provides additional detail for the person analysing that data. The dietary assessments are now also able to include images of the actual items consumed [85], when previously food images were used mainly as an on-screen prompt to determine the portion size consumed [86]. These images no longer need to be static either. Investigations into the use of real-time recording of food intakes [87; 88] and sensors to monitor foods consumed are also being trialled [89]. As technology continues to advance, it is evident that the advantages of using technology [90] as a basis for dietary assessment outweigh the potential disadvantages. Table 22.4 summarises some forms of automated interviewing.

TABLE 22.4 FORMS OF AUTOMATED INTERVIEWING

Traditional form	Computer-assisted form	Method	Advantages	Disadvantages
Telephone interviewing	CATI (computer-assisted telephone interviewing)	Most common form of survey assessment using a computer program to display questions and information for the interviewer to read. The interviewer also enters the responses of the participant into the computer.	• First form of computer-assisted interviewing. • Decreased interviewer bias. • Standardisation of the interview. • High consumer acceptance compared with paper–pen interviews.	Interviewers sometimes complain about the rigidity of the interviews.
Telephone interviewing	TDE (Touchstone data entry)	After dialling into a computer, participants are played recorded versions of the questionnaire. Answers are indicated by pressing buttons on the telephone handset.	• Speed of processing. • User friendly for persons unable to read and/or write.	• Clarity of speech required. • Equipment needs.
Telephone interviewing	IVR (interactive voice response)/ASR (automatic speech recognition)	As above, the participant dials into the computer. Answers are given by answering aloud using voice recognition entry (VRE).		Questionnaire may be overheard by others, reducing accuracy of responses.
Face-to-face interviewing	CAPI (computer-assisted personal interviewing)	Uses very similar technology to CATI. However, the computer is generally portable and involves face-to-face interviewing.	• Only a small percentage (5%) record negative feelings. • Prevents interviewer mistakes compared with traditional paper and pen interviews (PAPI). • Diminished number of missing data such as 'don't know' or 'no answer'. • Little difference in data quality when compared with PAPI.	• Less privacy and increased bias in answering socially undesirable questions. • Not always possible to backtrack to make changes. • Typing skills and computer literacy especially with open-ended questions. • Long interview with closed questions n = 2000, 30% cost saving whereas shorter interview with few open ended questions n = 200, save 5% costs. • Approx. 1500 interviews needed to balance front-end and back-end costs when compared with PAPI.

Traditional form	Computer-assisted form	Method	Advantages	Disadvantages
Self-administered questionnaire	CASI (computer-assisted self-interviewing) or CSAQ (computer self-administered questionnaire)	The computer is used by the participant to enter in the responses to the program. Generally the questions are displayed on screen in a textual format.	• Less affected by social desirability bias. • Increased self-disclosure (yet diminishes with time as computers increase in familiarity). • Subjects find it interesting, amusing and easy to use. • >80% using computer and program. • Higher degree of privacy and anonymity. • Lower number of errors and missing responses.	• Limited populations to be studied due to computer accessibility. • Eye strain (physical problems). • No difference in reliability and validity when compared with PAPI when used in psychology.

Source: Adapted from Y. Probst (2008). *An Evaluation of Automated Dietary Assessment: A case study into self-administered computer-assisted survey interviewing for professional dietary consultation*, 1st edn. Saarbrücken: VDM Verlag Dr Müller Aktiengesellschaft and Co. KG

STOP AND THINK

Imagine you were conducting a study with 2000 primary school-aged children and needed to obtain dietary data to understand their eating patterns.

• What type of dietary assessment method do you think would be most suitable?
• Would a paper-based or a technology-assisted form of assessment be more useful?
• Does the assessment method that you chose allow you to comment on the *usual* eating patterns of the children? Is this necessary?
• Given primary schoolchildren can vary from ages 5–12 years, what additional considerations might need to be implemented when obtaining the dietary data?

≫ CASE 22.2

MEASUREMENT ERROR IN FOOD RECORDS

Measurement error
the difference between the measured, the observed and the true error of a tool.

There are many sources of **measurement error** related to the use of a food record or food diary. Many of these can be reduced by careful training and well-designed pro formas to capture the data. It is important to ensure that the food record is the best-suited form of assessment for the population with which it is being used. Further, if using a food record that incorporates the use of technology, information about the reliability and validity of the tool is also important, as it cannot be assumed that the method remains the same simply by transferring it from paper based to online, for example. Food records are more likely to be affected by random measurement error rather than systematic measurement error.

Sources of measurement error include:

- Changes to the quality of the recorded information about the food consumed based on the number of days of recording needed.
- Reported portion sizes are estimates or are missing. People completing a food record will often avoid the use of measuring cups and scales and record an observed estimate of the food portion, often in measures relevant to them (e.g. 'a small serving').
- Mixed dishes that are difficult to interpret due to variation, even when a recipe is used. A dish such as spaghetti bolognaise is likely to be made differently by different people due to taste preferences, availability of ingredients and food preparation skills. If the dish is then recorded as spaghetti bolognaise without a recipe included, analysis of the food becomes challenging.
- Food records which should aim to, at a minimum, capture the natural variation that occurs during a one-week period. For this, weekdays and weekend days are required and the recordings do not need to be consecutive, particularly if an event such as a celebration is likely to change the pattern of eating.
- Weighed food records that generally provide better quality data, although this is affected by the person recording the foods. If the person does not have adequate literacy skills or is not involved in food preparation, they may record less detail about the foods consumed. For this reason, using food records that incorporate food image technology may be advantageous, as the image can provide the detail if taken correctly.

The *validity* of a dietary assessment is a measure of how accurately it captures what it is meant to—that is, the intake of a person's diet. This accuracy will change, depending on the type of assessment being tested and the known sources of error and related bias. When considering the sources of error, there are two main forms: random error and systematic error. Random error occurs randomly and may differ depending on the context of using the tool, while systematic error is more closely related to the known bias for the tool at hand [91]. A known bias for using a diet history interview, for example, may be the known underreporting seen for persons who are overweight or obese [92]. To test how valid or accurate a tool is, it should be compared against something with a known accuracy. This known measure may be considered a **gold standard**. If the outcomes from the two measures are similar, then the tool can be considered valid. The gold standard, however, can vary substantially. Earlier it was related that the weighed food record was considered a gold standard, while more recently the repeated 24-hour recall has been the preferred standard [69; 93]. These methods are compared with the outcomes from a diet history interview or FFQ for the same person, known as relative validity [94]. The comparisons are often made using the Bland and Altman method [95]. However, both 24-hour recalls and weighed food records also contain systematic error and are not considered a 'true' measure of intake [91]. This true measure of intake is best represented by a biomarker or a biological measure of consumption that changes based on the intake of the person [96]. If this biomarker and dietary assessment agree, then it can be assumed with increasing confidence that the method is valid. A common biomarker used for energy intakes is doubly labelled water [97]. This form of validation is referred to as 'absolute validity'. The reliability or repeatability of a dietary assessment should also be considered. This is a measure of the outcomes being the same with repeated use. Reliability testing is particularly important when a new form of assessment or new format of assessment has been implemented. Table 22.5 outlines some uses and limitations of the main assessment methods.

> **Gold standard**
>
> a reference method with high precision used as a comparison to assess validity.

TABLE 22.5 USES AND LIMITATIONS OF METHODS USED TO ASSESS THE FOOD CONSUMPTION OF INDIVIDUALS

Method and procedures	Uses and limitations	Advantages/disadvantages
24-hour recall Subject or caretaker recalls food intake of previous 24 hours in an interview. Quantities estimated in household measures using food models as memory aids or to assist in quantifying portion sizes. Nutrient intakes calculated using food composition data.	Useful for assessing average *usual* intakes of a large population, provided that the sample is truly representative and the days of the week are adequately represented (i.e. repeated recalls). Used for international comparisons of relationship of nutrient intakes to health and susceptibility to chronic disease. Multiple replicate 24-hour recalls used to estimate *usual* intakes of individuals.	*Advantages:* Inexpensive, easy, quick, with low respondent burden so that compliance is high. Large coverage possible; can be used with illiterate individuals. Element of surprise so less likely to modify eating pattern. Single 24-hour recalls, likely to omit foods consumed infrequently, follows a structured multiple pass format. *Disadvantages:* Relies on memory and hence unsatisfactory for the elderly and young children.
Estimated food record Record of all food and beverages 'as eaten' (including snacks), over periods from one to seven days. Quantities estimated in household measures. Nutrient intakes calculated using food composition data.	Used to assess *actual* or *usual* intakes of individuals, depending on the number of measurement days.	*Advantages:* Data on *usual* intakes used for diet counselling and statistical analysis involving correlation and regression. *Disadvantages:* Accuracy depends on the conscientiousness of the subject and ability to estimate quantities. Longer time frames result in a higher respondent burden and lower cooperation. Subjects must be literate.
Weighed food record All food consumed over a defined period is weighed by the subject, caretaker or assistant. Food samples may be saved individually, or as a composite, for nutrient analysis. Alternatively, nutrient intakes calculated using food composition data.	Used to assess *actual* or *usual* intakes of individuals, depending on the number of measurement days.	*Advantages:* Accurate but time-consuming. Setting must permit weighing. *Disadvantages:* Subjects may change their *usual* eating pattern to simplify weighing or to impress the investigator. Requires literate, motivated and willing participants. Expensive.
Dietary history Interview method consisting of a 24-hour recall of *actual* intake, plus information on overall *usual* eating pattern, followed by a food frequency questionnaire to verify and clarify initial data. Usual portion sizes recorded in household measures. Nutrient intakes calculated using food composition data.	Used to describe *usual* food or nutrient intakes, which can be used to estimate prevalence of inadequate intakes. Used for national food policy development, for food fortification planning, and to identify food patterns associated with inadequate intakes.	*Advantages:* Narrative format can capture a relatively long period of time, allows for detailed information about foods and meals to be collated, can be used with illiterate individuals, can capture foods eaten occasionally. *Disadvantages:* Labour-intensive, time-consuming and results depend on skill of interviewer. Affected by recall bias.
Food frequency questionnaire Uses comprehensive or specific food item list to record intakes over a given period (day, week, month, year). Record is obtained by interview or self-administered questionnaire. Questionnaire can be semi-quantitative when subject asked to quantify *usual* portion sizes of food items, with or without the use of food models.	Designed to obtain qualitative, descriptive data on *usual* intakes of foods or classes of foods over a long time period. Useful in epidemiological studies for ranking subjects into broad categories of low, medium and high intakes of specific foods, food components or nutrients, for comparison with the prevalence or mortality statistics of a specific disease. Can also identify food patterns associated with inadequate intakes of specific nutrients.	*Advantages:* Method is rapid, with low respondent burden and high response rate. *Disadvantages:* Accuracy is lower than for other methods.

Source: Adapted from R. Gibson (2005). *Principles of Nutrition Assessment*, 2nd edn. New York: Oxford University Press.

STOP AND THINK

Choosing the appropriate dietary assessment methods requires an understanding of how the method is constructed, what it actually measures, how it is implemented and the limitations of the results it will generate.

- How might you evaluate the quality of dietary patterns of a group in the community?
- How would you identify the changes in food choices that might be needed for a particular person to lose weight?
- How would you assess a study participant's usual dietary intake prior to an experimental study that involved manipulating the diet?

HOW IS DIETARY ASSESSMENT CONDUCTED AT THE POPULATION LEVEL?

Australian nutrition surveys have tended to be conducted on an ad hoc basis. The 1995 National Nutrition Survey sampled 13,800 Australians aged over two years. This survey was included in the Australian Health Survey 2011–13, which collected data from about 50,000 people from across all states and territories [74]. Importantly, the survey oversampled Indigenous and Torres Strait Islander communities. Two 24-hour recalls were used: one face-to-face and the other using CATI techniques to allow for standardisation of the single 24-hour recall nutrient intake data. Table 22.6 lists dietary surveys that were conducted in Australia over 35 years. The Australian Health Survey 2011–13 was also the first national survey to include biochemical markers of health for a number of chronic diseases, as seen in Table 22.7. This has allowed new Australian research into the links between food intakes and the biochemical measures at a population level.

TABLE 22.6 DIETARY SURVEYS IN AUSTRALIA, 1980–2013

Year	Survey	Method	Population
1983	National Dietary Survey of Adults	24-hour recall	6255 adults aged 25–64 years
1985	National Dietary Survey of Schoolchildren	24-hour diary and interview	5224 children aged 10–15 years
1985	Victorian Nutrition Survey	FFQ	2862 adults aged 18+ years
1988	Australian Health and Nutrition Survey (CSIRO)	FFQ	2315 adults aged 18+ years
1989	CSIRO Survey of Elderly Australians	FFQ	1510 adults aged 55–75 years
1990	Victorian Nutrition Survey	FFQ	2687 Victorian adults
1993	Australian Food Survey (CSIRO)	FFQ	1733 adults aged 18+ years
1995	National Nutrition Survey	24-hour recall + FFQ + Ht, Wt, BP	13,800 people aged 2+ years
2007	National Children's Nutrition and Physical Activity Survey	2 × 24-hour recalls	4487 children aged 2–16 years

Year	Survey	Method	Population
2011–13	National Nutrition and Physical Activity Survey	1 × 24-hour recall 2nd 24-hour telephone recall with at least eight days after the first	12,153 people aged 2+ years 7735 people aged 5+ years
2012–13	National Aboriginal and Torres Strait Islander Nutrition and Physical Activity Survey	1 × 24-hour recall 2nd 24-hour telephone recall with at least eight days after the first (non-remote areas only)	12,947 people aged 2+ years 3753 people aged 5+ years

TABLE 22.7   BIOCHEMICAL TESTS CONDUCTED FOR THE AUSTRALIAN HEALTH SURVEY 2011–13

Biomarker	Rationale
Cardiovascular disease	
Total cholesterol	To estimate prevalence of cardiovascular disease risk factors
Fasting triglycerides	
Fasting LDL and HDL cholesterol	
Apolipoprotein B	
Type 2 diabetes	
Fasting plasma glucose	To estimate prevalence of diabetes and impaired fasting glucose
Glycated haemoglobin (HbAlc)	To monitor diabetes control
Chronic kidney disease	
Serum creatinine estimated glomerular filtration rate (eGFR)	To estimate prevalence and severity of kidney damage
Urinary albumin creatinine ratio	To estimate prevalence of albuminuria, an early indicator of kidney damage
Liver function	
Liver function tests (GGT, ALT)	To assist in assessing burden of liver disease
Nutrition status	
Erythrocyte folate	To monitor the effectiveness of folate food fortification programs and estimate prevalence of folate deficiency
Serum folate	
Serum B12	To estimate prevalence of vitamin B12 deficiency
Urinary sodium concentration	To measure sodium and potassium levels in the population
Urinary potassium concentration	

Biomarker	Rationale
Serum 25(OH)D	To estimate prevalence of vitamin D deficiency
Urinary iodine	To monitor the effectiveness of iodine food fortification programs and estimate prevalence of iodine deficiency
Serum ferritin	To estimate prevalence and severity of iron deficiency
Serum transferrin receptor	
Haemoglobin	
Inflammation marker (CRP)	To assist with iron interpretations
Other risk factors	
Serum cotinine	To estimate prevalence of active and passive smoking

Source: Department of Health and Ageing (2011). *Australian Health Survey: Rationale for expanding the National Health Survey series*. Canberra: DoHA

STOP AND THINK

* Considering the range of people about whom data is collected for the National Nutrition Survey, why do you think the 24-hour recall assessment was chosen? Could other forms of dietary assessment have been used? Why or why not?
* Why is it useful to have biomarkers collected as part of a National Health Survey that also collected information about dietary intakes? How could these biomarkers be used?
* The Australian population is now 24 million persons. Why don't we simply ask everyone what they eat for a dietary survey? How do you think dietary surveys overcome the need to ask everyone about their food intakes?

WHAT IS DIETARY MODELLING?

Data from nutrition surveys is often used in dietary modelling to assess nutritional risk. **Dietary modelling** generally involves constructing different types of diets from different combinations of foods based on what is known about the foods, including nutrient composition. The modelling can use a range of techniques that attempt to examine the potential consequences of different dietary patterns and answer theoretical questions. Key elements in dietary modelling are food groups (with standard portion sizes), food databases, patterns of usual food consumption and standard reference values. Thus, the starting points are knowing the categories of foods to 'plug into' the model, the nutrient profile of the food category, the amount and types of foods likely to be consumed by the target person or population, and the nutrient requirements of that person or population group. Exposure to (non-nutrient) chemicals in foods is assessed using dietary modelling that uses data on the chemicals in food alongside food consumption data. Toxicology is usually considered in terms of amount (such as mg) exposure from all foods per kg body weight. A custom-designed computer program, DIAMOND, was used for this purpose by FSANZ in Australia [98]. DIAMOND worked with food consumption

Dietary modelling
the use of algorithms to construct theoretical patterns of proposed dietary intake based on inputs such as the need to meet specific amounts of energy and nutrients.

YASMINE PROBST AND LINDA TAPSELL

data to identify commonly consumed foods (including mixed foods) that contained the food chemical of interest. For each person, the program could estimate the overall dietary exposure and for the population a profile exposure could be determined in terms of relative exposure. This could be used for examining the impact of, for example, fortifying bread with iodised salt. Scenarios could assume the impact of this change based on the consumption of bread at a population level.

Risk assessment considers the exposure of individuals in populations to components in the food supply and this exposure can be both detrimental (as in toxic chemicals) and desired (as in required nutrients). Nutrient Reference Values (NRVs) are an example of a reference standard used to conduct risk assessment involving nutrients. In this case exposure may be assessed in terms of adequacy or over-consumption of nutrients. Exposure to chemicals in the diet can be chronic or acute and can vary depending on whether groups within the population consume the foods delivering the chemicals or not. A model diet (also referred to as 'simulated' or 'theoretical' diets) may be constructed to represent a 'typical' diet for a given population group when no consumption data for individuals is available (e.g. when a new food category is proposed to be introduced into the food supply).

See Chapter 3 on digestion, absorption and metabolism.

The updated HARVEST system was underpinned by the same principles as DIAMOND. It was developed for the purpose of dietary modelling for dietary exposure assessment, although its main focus was to be a storage platform to house project data as well as having the analytical options for the models using the most recent food composition and food consumption data (Figure 22.2). The HARVEST

FIGURE 22.2 THE PROCESSING INVOLVED IN THE HARVEST SYSTEM

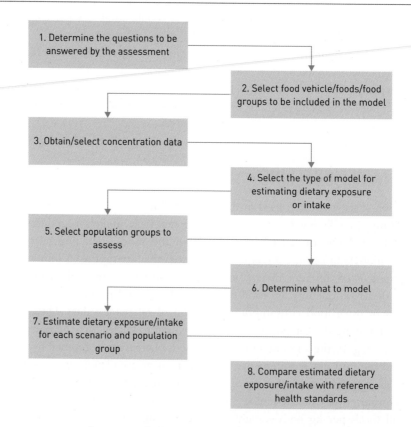

Source: www.foodstandards.gov.au/science/exposure/Pages/fsanzdietaryexposure4439.aspx

system includes nutrition survey data for Australia and New Zealand from 1995 onwards, allowing it to create timely summaries of intake data for a population, and model scenarios based on a given chemical. HARVEST also addresses the impact of one versus two days of intake from the survey data and allows users to compare data to the NRVs for Australia and New Zealand at the time.

When developing dietary advice for populations, dietary modelling is used to assess the nutritional adequacy of different dietary patterns that are being recommended. For example, the most recent review of the Australian Guide to Healthy Eating (www.eatforhealth.gov.au) used a series of systematic literature reviews to understand the links between different food groups and health risk, and combined this with extensive dietary modelling to derive dietary patterns and recommendations about the numbers of serves of different food groups that would be both nutritionally adequate and support good health for people of different ages, gender, lifestyle, body size and activity [99].

This type of dietary modelling takes into account the usual diets of populations in terms of individual food choices relative to food groups (e.g. apples compared with strawberries, or lamb compared with beef). These relative proportions were used to generate typical nutrient profiles for the food groups as a whole (e.g. fruit, meat).

>> RESEARCH AT WORK

DIETARY MODELS FOR THE DIETARY GUIDELINES

In the first stage of modelling, a range of computer-generated diets were developed that translated the NRVs into dietary patterns to describe the types, combinations and amounts of foods that deliver the nutrient requirements for each age and gender group of different physical activity level in the Australian population, while also being consistent with the patterns known to be recommended for good health (e.g. based primarily on wholegrain rather than refined cereals; using polyunsaturated margarine rather than butter) [99]. A range of models including omnivore, lacto-ovo vegetarian, pasta- and rice-based dietary patterns were developed to reflect different cuisine preferences. The second stage of the dietary modelling was to test these dietary patterns, using 100 simulated seven-day diets for each age/gender group. A computer program chose different combinations of individual foods to examine whether the models met key nutrient requirements. For example, instead of using a composite 'fruit' group, individual fruits (e.g. apples, bananas, oranges) were used in the model, and diet patterns were regarded as acceptable if all 100 diets met the estimated average requirements (EARs) for energy and a range of key nutrients: protein, thiamin, vitamin C, folate, calcium, iodine, iron, magnesium and zinc.

While food guidance and food regulation modelling is focused on the entire population, modelling in the clinical environment, whether it be for research, such as in a dietary trial, or for private consultation, is commonly focused on the needs of a particular individual. The goal of the modelling may be to achieve a particular dietary profile (e.g. 'low fat', 'high protein', 'low calorie'), and in each case a model is developed for the person, based on their estimated energy requirements and usual food intake pattern. As with the population-based models, NRVs are used to assess the overall nutritional adequacy of the diet.

Models in clinical practice are often created as the basis for developing diet or meal plans. Adequate serves of intake are therefore vital. Software used for nutrition analysis may be adapted for use during this nutrition planning stage in which a random food item is selected from each of the food groups to create a sample intake that meets the adequate number of serves suggested. The benefit of using such software allows the clinician to compare the nutrient outcomes with the NRVs quickly and easily. For the development of dietary plans, the NRVs of interest are the recommended dietary intakes (RDIs), or adequate intakes (AIs) if an RDI has not been set, and the upper levels (ULs) of intake. These values would ensure that clients who follow the dietary plan that has been created for them are at less risk of nutrient deficiency than if the EARs were used. Models can also be created using the functions and calculations of a database or spreadsheet software, although this would only form the outline for the plan [100]. Test diets would still need to be created to ensure that inadequate intake is minimised.

In clinical research, it is often necessary to work up the food groups on which modelling is to be designed to ensure the dietary targets are addressed. For example, if the type of dietary fat is to be modified it may be necessary to work with more food groups to further differentiate between foods that contain a lot of fat in terms of their fatty acid contributions [101].

TRY IT YOURSELF

Refer to the Australian Guide to Healthy Eating. Using the food patterns presented, work out the number of serves from each food group that would be suitable for someone of your age and gender. Compare this diet plan to your usual pattern of food choices. Identify the major areas of difference and discuss.

STOP AND THINK

- What are the uses of dietary models?
- What are the inputs (factors to consider) for developing a dietary model?
- Why are NRVs important in dietary modelling?

SUMMARY

- Nutrition tools represent highly developed methods and techniques for applying nutrition knowledge to protect the health of the population.
- Dietary assessment is one of the first steps in assessing how a nutritional application might be conducted.
- The choice of method and the intricate design details of that method depend on why the dietary assessment is being conducted and what needs to be known.
- At the population level, dietary assessment forms part of a much broader sphere of nutrition monitoring and surveillance.
- Converting food data to nutrients data, and then relating these to the need for nutrients to maintain health, requires comprehensive food databases with up-to-date information on the nutritional composition of foods.
- Dietary assessment data and food databases are used in dietary modelling.
- The elements that go into the modelling exercise are sets of foods, their known composition and frequency of consumption, and the dietary targets the model is trying to achieve.

PATHWAYS TO PRACTICE

- Understanding the advantages and disadvantages of dietary assessment methods allows dietitians and other health workers to choose the most appropriate method in practice. This method will differ depending on the goals of the data. A different assessment method is likely to be used for a large epidemiological cohort study that aims to verify diet–disease patterns for public health, in comparison with a dietitian in a small rural hospital who is more interested in what patients are usually eating to help them improve their health.
- Dietary surveys provide Australians with information about what they are eating. Looking at nutrition surveys over time also reveals how the food supply and eating patterns have shifted. Using this data, food manufacturers may be able to focus on particular subgroups of the population who are likely to eat a new food that they are developing. Similarly, knowing what people are eating allows the creation of more targeted public health messages to ensure eating patterns align with recommendations in the Australian Dietary Guidelines.
- Eating patterns do not remain the same over time. It is important to ensure that people who follow a particular eating pattern are still able to meet the recommendations of the NRVs and Dietary Guidelines. As we learn more about foods through food composition, researchers may also need to work out the impact of 'new' nutrients or components in foods on health. Intakes from high-quality studies can be modelled into a diet to determine the impact on eating patterns and alignment with recommendations.

DISCUSSION QUESTIONS

1   What key knowledge and skill areas are needed to utilise the tools of dietary assessment methods, food databases and dietary modelling?
2   What are the most important issues to consider at a population and individual level in choosing and developing dietary assessment methods?
3   How would you know if a dietary assessment method is providing the quality data you require?
4   What are some of the challenges in developing food databases and how are they likely to be resolved in the future?
5   What are the implications for increasing specialisation in developing practice tools in nutrition?
6   What are the nutrition practice tools of the future likely to be?

USEFUL WEBLINKS

ASA24–Australia:
> https://epi.grants.cancer.gov/asa24/respondent/australia.html

Australian Food, Supplement and Nutrient Database (AUSNUT) 2011–13:
> www.foodstandards.gov.au/science/monitoringnutrients/ausnut/pages/default.aspx

Australian Health Survey 2011–13:
> www.abs.gov.au/australianhealthsurvey

Automated Self-Administered 24-Hour (ASA24®) Dietary Assessment Tool:
https://epi.grants.cancer.gov/asa24

Dietary Assessment Primer:
https://dietassessmentprimer.cancer.gov

National Health and Nutrition Examination Survey:
www.cdc.gov/nchs/nhanes/index.htm

Nutrient tables for use in Australia (NUTTAB) 2010:
www.foodstandards.gov.au/science/monitoringnutrients/nutrientables/nuttab/Pages/default.aspx

The 'DIAMOND' (DIetAry Modelling Of Nutritional Data) computer program:
www.foodstandards.gov.au/science/exposure/Pages/fsanzdietaryexposure4439.aspx

FURTHER READING

Ahluwalia, N., Dwyer, J., Terry, A., Moshfegh, A. & Johnson, C. (2016). Update on NHANES dietary data: focus on collection, release, analytical considerations, and uses to inform public policy. *Advances in Nutrition*, 7(1), 121–34. doi:10.3945/an.115.009258

Buttriss, J. L., Briend, A., Darmon, N., Ferguson, E. L., Maillot, M. & Lluch, A. (2014). Diet modelling: how it can inform the development of dietary recommendations and public health policy. *Nutrition Bulletin*, 39(1), 115–25. doi:10.1111/nbu.12076

Cade, J. E. (2016). Measuring diet in the 21st century: use of new technologies. *Proceedings of the Nutrition Society*, 1–7. doi:10.1017/S0029665116002883

Carriquiry, A. L. (2017). Understanding and assessing nutrition. *Annual Review of Statistics and Its Application*, 4(1), 123–46. doi:10.1146/annurev-statistics-041715-033615

Church, S. M. (2015). The importance of food composition data in recipe analysis. *Nutrition Bulletin*, 40(1), 40–4. doi:10.1111/nbu.12125

Coulston, A. M., Boushey, C. J., Ferruzzi, M. & Delahanty, L. (2017). *Nutrition in the Prevention and Treatment of Disease*, 4th edn. Cambridge, MA: Academic Press.

de Keyzer, W., Bracke, T., McNaughton, S. A., Parnell, W., Moshfegh, A. J., Pereira, R. A., ... Huybrechts, I. (2015). Cross-continental comparison of national food consumption survey methods—a narrative review. *Nutrients*, 7(5), 3587–620. doi:10.3390/nu7053587

Del Gobbo, L. C., Khatibzadeh, S., Imamura, F., Micha, R., Shi, P., Smith, M., ... Mozaffarian, D. (2015). Assessing global dietary habits: a comparison of national estimates from the FAO and the global dietary database. *American Journal of Clinical Nutrition*, 101(5), 1038–46. doi:10.3945/ajcn.114.087403

Forster, H., Walsh, M. C., Gibney, M. J., Brennan, L. & Gibney, E. R. (2016). Personalised nutrition: the role of new dietary assessment methods. *Proceedings of the Nutrition Society*, 75(1), 96–105. doi:10.1017/S0029665115002086

Gemming, L. & Ni Mhurchu, C. (2016). Dietary under-reporting: what foods and which meals are typically under-reported? *European Journal of Clinical Nutrition*, 70(5), 640–1. doi:10.1038/ejcn.2015.204

Gibson, A. A., Hsu, M. S. H., Rangan, A. M., Seimon, R. V., Lee, C. M.Y., Das, A., ... Sainsbury, A. (2016). Accuracy of hands v. household measures as portion size estimation aids. *Journal of Nutritional Science*, 5, e29. doi:10.1017/jns.2016.22

Grandjean, A. C. (2012). Dietary intake data collection: challenges and limitations. *Nutrition Reviews*, 70(suppl. 2), S101–S104. doi:10.1111/j.1753-4887.2012.00545.x

Hoffman, R. & Gerber, M. (2013). Evaluating and adapting the Mediterranean diet for non-Mediterranean populations: a critical appraisal. *Nutrition Reviews*, 71(9), 573–84. doi:10.1111/nure.12040

Hooper, B., Spiro, A. & Stanner, S. (2015). 30 g of fibre a day: an achievable recommendation? *Nutrition Bulletin*, 40(2), 118–29.

Kirkpatrick, S. I., Vanderlee, L., Raffoul, A., Stapleton, J., Csizmadi, I., Boucher, B. A., ... Robson, P. J. (2017). Self-report dietary assessment tools used in Canadian research: a scoping review. *Advances in Nutrition*, 8(2), 276–89. doi:10.3945/an.116.014027

Labonté, M.-È., Kirkpatrick, S. I., Bell, R. C., Boucher, B. A., Csizmadi, I., Koushik, A., ... Lamarche, B. (2016). Dietary assessment is a critical element of health research: perspective from the partnership for advancing nutritional and dietary assessment in Canada. *Applied Physiology, Nutrition and Metabolism*, 41(10), 1096–9. doi:10.1139/apnm-2016-0146

Lamb, K. E., Olstad, D. L., Nguyen, C., Milte, C. & McNaughton, S. A. (2017). Missing data in FFQs: making assumptions about item non-response. *Public Health Nutrition*, 20(6), 965–70. doi:10.1017/S1368980016002986

Leach, H. M. (2012). Food habits. In J. Mann & A. S. Truswell (eds), *Essentials of Human Nutrition*, 4th edn. New York: Oxford University Press.

Lluch, A., Maillot, M., Gazan, R., Vieux, F., Delaere, F., Vaudaine, S. & Darmon, N. (2017). Individual diet modeling shows how to balance the diet of French adults with or without excessive free sugar intakes. *Nutrients*, 9(2). doi:10.3390/nu9020162

Lopes, T. S., Luiz, R. R., Hoffman, D. J., Ferriolli, E., Pfrimer, K., Moura, A. S., ... Pereira, R. A. (2016). Misreport of energy intake assessed with food records and 24-h recalls compared with total energy expenditure estimated with DLW. *European Journal of Clinical Nutrition*, 70(11), 1259–64. doi:10.1038/ejcn.2016.85

Maillot, M., Issa, C., Vieux, F., Lairon, D. & Darmon, N. (2011). The shortest way to reach nutritional goals is to adopt Mediterranean food choices: evidence from computer-generated personalized diets. *American Journal of Clinical Nutrition*, 94(4), 1127–37. doi:10.3945/ajcn.111.016501

Maillot, M., Vieux, F., Amiot, M. J. & Darmon, N. (2010). Individual diet modeling translates nutrient recommendations into realistic and individual-specific food choices. *American Journal of Clinical Nutrition*, 91(2), 421–30. doi:10.3945/ajcn.2009.28426

Mann, J. & Truswell, A. S. (2012). Part 5: Nutritional assessment. In J. Mann & A. S. Truswell (eds), *Essentials of Human Nutrition*, 4th edn. New York: Oxford University Press.

McClung, H. L., Champagne, C. M., Allen, H. R., McGraw, S. M., Young, A. J., Montain, S. J. & Crombie, A. P. (2017). Digital food photography technology improves efficiency and feasibility of dietary intake assessments in large populations eating ad libitum in collective dining facilities. *Appetite*, 116, 389–94. doi:10.1016/j.appet.2017.05.025

McCullough, M. L., Karanja, N. M., Lin, P.-H., Obarzanek, E. V. A., Phillips, K. M., Laws, R. L., ... Windhauser, M. M. (1999). Comparison of 4 nutrient databases with chemical composition data from the Dietary Approaches to Stop Hypertension trial. *Journal of the American Dietetic Association*, 99(8), S45–S53. doi:http://dx.doi.org/10.1016/S0002-8223(99)00416-2

McLennan, W. & Podger, A. (1995). *National Nutrition Survey Users' Guide*. Canberra: ABS and Department of Health and Family Services.

Orešković, P., Kljusurić, J. G. & Šatalić, Z. (2015). Computer-generated vegan menus: the importance of food composition database choice. *Journal of Food Composition and Analysis*, 37, 112–18. doi:http://dx.doi.org/10.1016/j.jfca.2014.07.002

Probst, Y. & Mamet, C. (2016). The evolution of food composition databases in Australia: applying data from 1944 to 2007 to current day dietary records. *Journal of Food Composition and Analysis*, 51, 24–9. doi:10.1016/j.jfca.2016.05.014

Probst, Y., Guan, V. & Kent, K. (2016). A systematic review of food composition tools used for determining dietary polyphenol intake in estimated intake studies. *Food Chemistry*. doi:10.1016/j.foodchem.2016.11.010

Rangan, A. M., Schindeler, S., Hector, D. J. & Gill, T. P. (2009). Assessment of typical food portion sizes consumed among Australian adults. *Nutrition and Dietetics*, 66(4), 227–33.

Rehm, C. D., Peñalvo, J. L., Afshin, A. & Mozaffarian, D. (2016). Dietary intake among US adults, 1999–2012. *JAMA—Journal of the American Medical Association*, 315(23), 2542–53. doi:10.1001/jama.2016.7491

Swan, G., Dodhia, S., Farron-Wilson, M., Powell, N. & Bush, M. (2015). Food composition data and public health. *Nutrition Bulletin*, 40(3), 223–6. doi:10.1111/nbu.12156

Thompson, M. E. (2015). Using longitudinal complex survey data. *Annual Review of Statistics and Its Application*, 2(1), 305–20. doi:10.1146/annurev-statistics-010814-020403

Timon, C. M., Cooper, S. E., Barker, M. E., Astell, A. J., Adlam, T., Hwang, F. & Williams, E. A. (2017). A comparison of food portion size estimation by older adults, young adults and nutritionists. *Journal of Nutrition, Health and Aging*, 1–7. doi:10.1007/s12603-017-0937-9

Woodside, J. V., Draper, J., Lloyd, A. & McKinley, M. C. (2017). Use of biomarkers to assess fruit and vegetable intake. *Proceedings of the Nutrition Society*, 1–8. doi:10.1017/S0029665117000325

Zheng, M., Wu, J. H.Y., Louie, J. C.Y., Flood, V. M., Gill, T., Thomas, B., ... Rangan, A. (2016). Typical food portion sizes consumed by Australian adults: results from the 2011–12 Australian National Nutrition and Physical Activity Survey. *Scientific Reports*, 6. doi:10.1038/srep19596

REFERENCES

1   S. M. Church (2006). The history of food composition databases. *Nutrition Bulletin*, 31(1), 15–20. doi:10.1111/j.1467-3010.2006.00538.x

2   W. Atwater & C. Woods (1896). *The Chemical Composition of American Food Materials. Experiment Station Bulletin, no. 28*. Washington, DC: US Official Experiment Stations.

3   Commonwealth of Australia (1938). *Fifth Report of the Advisory Council on Nutrition*. Canberra: Commonwealth of Australia.

4   H. Greenfield & D. Southgate (2003). *Food Composition Data: Production, management and use*, 2nd edn. Rome: FAO.

5   Y. Probst (2015). Key players of the Australian Food Composition Program. *Procedia Food Science*, 4, 125–32. doi:http://dx.doi.org/10.1016/j.profoo.2015.06.017

6   S. Thomas & M. Corden (1970). *Tables of Composition of Australian Foods*. Canberra: Commonwealth Department of Health.

7   Department of Community Services and Health National Food Authority (1989). *Composition of Foods Australia*. Canberra: AGPS.

8   Commonwealth Department of Health (1987). *Nutrient Data Tables for Use in Australia e NUTTAB87*. Canberra: Commonwealth Department of Health.

9   National Food Authority (1995). *NUTTAB95 Database*. Canberra: National Food Authority.

10 R. English & J. Lewis (1991). *Food for Health. A guide to good nutrition with nutrient values for 650 Australian foods*. Canberra: AGPS.

11 Food Standards Australia New Zealand (2012). Printed food composition tables 2012. Retrieved from: www.foodstandards.gov.au/scienceandeducation/scienceinfsanz/foodcompositionprogram/printed-foodcompositi172.cfm.

12 S. Thomas & M. Corden (1977). *Metric Tables of Composition of Australian Foods*. Canberra: Commonwealth Department of Health.

13 R. Sobolewski, J. Cunningham & D. Mackerras (2010). Which Australian food composition database should I use? *Nutrition & Dietetics*, 67(1), 37–40. doi:10.1111/j.1747-0080.2010.01393.x

14 Department of Health (2008). *2007 Australian National Children's Nutrition and Physical Activity Survey— Main findings*. Canberra: Commonwealth of Australia.

15 Food Standards Australia New Zealand (2006). *NUTTAB 2006*. Canberra: FSANZ.

16 J. Cunningham, S. Tompsett, J. Abbey, R. Sobolewski & D. Mackerras (2010). Food composition: essential data in epidemiological studies of food and health. *Australasian Epidemiologist*, 17(1), 32.

17 Food Standards Australia New Zealand (2010). *AUSNUT 2007*. 1 March. Retrieved from: www.foodstandards.gov.au/consumerinformation/ausnut2007.

18 Food Standards Australia New Zealand (2012). *AUSNUT 2007*. Canberra: FSANZ.

19 Food Standards Australia New Zealand (2012). *NUTTAB 2010*. Canberra: FSANZ.

20 Australian Bureau of Statistics (2013). *Australian Health Survey: Physical activity, 2011–12*. Canberra: ABS.

21 Australian Bureau of Statistics (2014). *Australian Health Survey: Nutrition First results—Foods and nutrients, 2011–12* Canberra: ABS.

22 Food Standards Australia New Zealand (2014). *AUSNUT 2011–13*. Canberra: FSANZ.

23 Australian Bureau of Statistics (2015). *Australian Aboriginal and Torres Strait Islander Health Survey: Nutrition results—Food and nutrients, 2012–13*. Canberra: ABS.

24 Food Standards Australia New Zealand (2014). *AUSNUT 2011–13—AUSNUT 1999 matching file*. Canberra: FSANZ.

25 E. P. Neale, Y. C. Probst & L. C. Tapsell (2016). Development of a matching file of Australian food composition databases (AUSNUT 2007 to 2011–13). *Journal of Food Composition and Analysis*, 50, 30–5. doi:http://dx.doi.org/10.1016/j.jfca.2016.05.003

26 N. Athar, J. Cunningham & W. Aalbersberg (2007). Food composition activities in the Oceania region. *Journal of Food Composition and Analysis*, 20(8), 709–12. doi:https://doi.org/10.1016/j.jfca.2007.01.003

27 B. Burlingame & J. Monro (1993). *Proceedings of the Third OCEANIAFOODS Conference, Auckland, New Zealand, 3–5 December 1991*. Palmerston North, New Zealand.

28 Commonwealth of Australia (1938). *Fifth Report of the Advisory Council on Nutrition*. Canberra: Commonwealth of Australia.

29 A. Osmond (1946). *Tables of Composition of Australian Foods*. Canberra: Commonwealth Government Printer.

30 A. Osmond (1948). *Tables of Composition of Australian Foods*. Canberra: Commonwealth Government Printer.

31 A. Osmond & W. Wilson (1961). *Tables of Composition of Australian Foods*. Canberra: Department of Health.

32 A. Osmond (1954). *Tables of Composition of Australian Foods*. Canberra: Commonwealth Government Printer.

33 S. Thomas & M. Corden (1970). *Tables of Composition of Australian Foods*. Canberra: AGPS.

34 S. Thomas & M. Corden (1977). *Metric Tables of Composition of Australian Foods*. Canberra: AGPS.

35 Commonwealth Department of Health (1987). *Nutrient Data Tables for Use in Australia—NUTTAB87*. Canberra: Commonwealth Department of Health.

36 R. English & J. Lewis (1991). *Nutritional Values of Australian Foods*. Canberra: AGPS.

37 R. English & J. Lewis (1991). *Food for Health. A guide to good nutrition with nutrient values for 650 Australian foods*. Canberra: AGPS.

38 B. Burlingame, J. Lewis, B. Aalbersberg & T. Matenga-Smith (1996). OCEANIAFOODS: national, regional and international activities. *Food Chemistry*, 57(1), 175–8. doi:http://dx.doi.org.ezproxy.uow.edu.au/10.1016/0308-8146(96)00155-0

39 Australia New Zealand Food Authority (1999). *Supplement to NUTTAB95 Database*. Canberra: ANZFA.

40 J. Brand Miller, P. Maggiore & K. James (1993). *Tables of Composition of Australian Aboriginal Foods*. Canberra: Aboriginal Studies Press.

41 J. Cunningham & L. Trevisan (2002). Nutrition panel calculator. *Food Australia*, 54(11), 494–5.

42 Food Standards Australia New Zealand (2007). *NUTTAB 2006*. Retrieved from: www.foodstandards.gov.au/monitoringandsurveillance/nuttab2006/onlineversionintroduction/onlineversion.cfm.

43 Food Standards Australia New Zealand (2013). *NUTTAB 2010*. Retrieved from: www.foodstandards.gov.au/science/monitoringnutrients/nutrientables/pages/default.aspx.

44 Food Standards Australia New Zealand (2012). *NPC Database 2011 Files*. Retrieved from: www.foodstandards.gov.au/foodstandards/nutritionpanelcalculator/npcdatabase2011files.

45 US Department of Agriculture and Agriculture Research Service (2004). *Food and Nutrient Database for Dietary Study*. Beltsville, MD: US Department of Agriculture and Agriculture Research Service.

46 W. Horwitz & G. W. Latimer (2005). *Official Methods of Analysis of AOAC International*. Gaithersburg, MD: AOAC International.

47 B. S. Burke (1947). The dietary history as a tool in research. *Journal of the American Dietetic Association*, 23, 1041–6.

48 A. M. Euser, M. J. Finken, M. G. Keijzer-Veen, E. T. Hille, J. M. Wit, F. W. Dekker & Dutch POPS-19 Collaborative Study Group (2005). Associations between prenatal and infancy weight gain and BMI, fat mass, and fat distribution in young adulthood: a prospective cohort study in males and females born very preterm. *American Journal of Clinical Nutrition*, 81(2), 480–7.

49 L. Tapsell (2000). Using applied conversation analysis to teach novice dietitians history taking skills. *Human Studies*, 23(3), 281–307.

50 H. E. d. Wardener & G. A. MacGregor. (2001). Blood pressure and the kidney. In R. W. Schrier (ed.), *Diseases of the Kidney & Urinary Tract*, 7th edn (pp. 1329–61). Philadelphia, PA: Lippincott Williams & Wilkins.

51 J. Mann & S. Bingham (2012). Dietary assessment. In J. Mann & A. S. Tuckwell (eds), *Essentials of Human Nutrition*, 4th edn. New York: Oxford University Press.

52 L. C. Tapsell, V. Brenninger & J. Barnard (2000). Applying conversation analysis to foster accurate reporting in the diet history interview. *Journal of the American Dietetic Association*, 100(7), 818–24. doi:10.1016/s0002-8223(00)00237-6

53 J. Maurer, D. L. Taren, P. J. Teixeira, C. A. Thomson, T. G. Lohman, S. B. Going & L. B. Houtkooper (2006). The psychosocial and behavioral characteristics related to energy misreporting. *Nutrition Reviews*, 64(2 Pt 1), 53–66.

54 M. Yannakoulia, D. B. Panagiotakos, C. Pitsavos, E. Bathrellou, C. Chrysohoou, Y. Skoumas & C. Stefanadis (2007). Low energy reporting related to lifestyle, clinical, and psychosocial factors in a randomly selected population sample of Greek adults: the ATTICA study. *Journal of the American College of Nutrition*, 26(4), 327–33. doi:10.1080/07315724.2007.10719619

55 F. B. Scagliusi, E. Ferriolli, K. Pfrimer, C. Laureano, C. S. F. Cunha, B. Gualano, ... A. H. Lancha, Jr (2009). Characteristics of women who frequently under report their energy intake: a doubly labelled water study. *European Journal of Clinical Nutrition*, 63, 1192. doi:10.1038/ejcn.2009.54

56 E. Stice, C. A. Palmrose & K. S. Burger (2015). Elevated BMI and male sex are associated with greater underreporting of caloric intake as assessed by doubly labeled water. *Journal of Nutrition*, 145(10), 2412–18. doi:10.3945/jn.115.216366

57 S. J. Sharman, H. Skouteris, M. B. Powell & B. Watson (2016). Factors related to the accuracy of self-reported dietary intake of children aged 6 to 12 years elicited with interviews: a systematic review. *Journal of the Academy of Nutrition and Dietetics*, 116(1), 76–114. doi:10.1016/j.jand.2015.08.024

58 D. Volkert & E. Schrader (2013). Dietary assessment methods for older persons: what is the best approach? *Current Opinion in Clinical Nutrition and Metabolic Care*, 16(5), 534–40. doi:10.1097/MCO.0b013e328363c8d1

59 Y. Probst & L. Tapsell (2007). What to ask in a self-administered dietary assessment website: the role of professional judgement. *Journal of Food Composition and Analysis*, 20(8), 696–703.

60 Y. C. Probst, C. Krnavek, L. Lockyer & L. C. Tapsell (2005). Development of a computer assisted dietary assessment tool for use in primary healthcare practice: perceptions of nutrition and computers in a sample of older adults with type 2 diabetes mellitus. *Australian Journal of Primary Health*, 11(3), 54–62.

61 S. Burden, Y. C. Probst, D. G. Steel & L. C. Tapsell (2009). Identification of food groups for use in a self-administered, computer-assisted diet history interview for use in Australia. *Journal of Food Composition and Analysis*, 22(2), 130–6.

62 Y. Probst & L. Tapsell (2007). Over- and underreporting of energy intake by patients with metabolic syndrome using an automated dietary assessment website. *Nutrition and Dietetics*, 64(4), 280–4.

63 Y. C. Probst, K. De Agnoli, M. Batterham & L. Tapsell (2009). Video-recorded participant behaviours: the association between food choices and observed behaviours from a web-based diet history interview. *Journal of Human Nutrition and Dietetics*, 22(1), 21–8.

64 Y. Probst, L. Tapsell & M. Batterham (2008). Relationships between patient age and BMI and use of a self-administered computerised dietary assessment in a primary healthcare setting. *Journal of Food Composition and Analysis*, 21, S56–S59.

65 V. Burley, J. Cade, B. Margetts, R. Thompson & D. Warm (2000). *Consensus Document on the Development, Validation and Utilisation of Food Frequency Questionnaires.* London: Ministry of Agriculture Fisheries and Food.

66 J. R. Mahalko, L. K. Johnson, S. K. Gallagher & D. B. Milne (1985). Comparison of dietary histories and seven-day food records in a nutritional assessment of older adults. *American Journal of Clinical Nutrition*, 42(3), 542–53.

67 F. E. Thompson & T. Byers (1994). Dietary assessment resource manual. *Journal of Nutrition*, 124(suppl. 11), 2245s–2317s.

68 Y. Probst & G. Zammit (2016). Predictors for reporting of dietary assessment methods in food-based randomized controlled trials over a ten-year period. *Critical Reviews in Food Science and Nutrition*, 56(12), 2069–90. doi:10.1080/10408398.2013.816653

69 A. Satija, E. Yu, W. C. Willett & F. B. Hu (2015). Understanding nutritional epidemiology and its role in policy. *Advances in Nutrition: An International Review Journal*, 6(1), 5–18. doi:10.3945/an.114.007492

70 T. P. Zimmerman, S. G. Hull, S. McNutt, B. Mittl, N. Islam, P. M. Guenther, …A. F. Subar (2009). Challenges in converting an interviewer-administered food probe database to self-administration in the National Cancer Institute Automated Self-administered 24-Hour Recall (ASA24). *Journal of Food Composition and Analysis*, 22(suppl. 1), s48–s51. doi:10.1016/j.jfca.2009.02.003

71 M. Nelson, A. E. Black, J. A. Morris & T. J. Cole (1989). Between- and within-subject variation in nutrient intake from infancy to old age: estimating the number of days required to rank dietary intakes with desired precision. *American Journal of Clinical Nutrition*, 50(1), 155–67.

72 M. Touvier, E. Kesse-Guyot, C. Mejean, C. Pollet, A. Malon, K. Castetbon & S. Hercberg (2011). Comparison between an interactive web-based self-administered 24 h dietary record and an interview by a dietitian for large-scale epidemiological studies. *British Journal of Nutrition*, 105(7), 1055–64. doi:10.1017/s0007114510004617

73 A. F. Subar, S. I. Kirkpatrick, B. Mittl, T. P. Zimmerman, F. E. Thompson, C. Bingley, … N. Potischman (2012). The Automated Self-Administered 24-Hour Dietary Recall (ASA24): a resource for researchers, clinicians and educators from the National Cancer Institute. *Journal of the Academy of Nutrition and Dietetics*, 112(8), 1134–7. doi:10.1016/j.jand.2012.04.016

74 Australian Bureau of Statistics (2014). *Australian Health Survey: Nutrition First results—Foods and nutrients, 2011–12—About the National Nutrition and Physical Activity Survey.* Canberra: ABS. Retrieved from: www.abs.gov.au/ausstats/abs@.nsf/Lookup/by%20Subject/4364.0.55.007~2011-12~Main%20Features~About%20the%20National%20Nutrition%20and%20Physical%20Activity%20Survey~731.

75 National Center for Health Statistics (2015). *National Health and Nutrition Examination Survey.* Hyattsville, MD: National Center for Health Statistics.

76 R. S. Gibson & E. L. Ferguson (1999). *An Interactive 24-Hour Recall for Assessing the Adequacy of Iron and Zinc Intakes in Developing Countries.* Washington, DC: International Life Science Institute Press.

77 R. Fallaize, H. Forster, A. L. Macready, M. C. Walsh, J. C. Mathers, L. Brennan, … J. A. Lovegrove (2014). Online dietary intake estimation: reproducibility and validity of the Food4Me food frequency questionnaire against a 4-day weighed food record. *Journal of Medical Internet Research*, 16(8), e190. doi:10.2196/jmir.3355

78 S. J. Marshall, K. M. Livingstone, C. Celis-Morales, H. Forster, R. Fallaize, C. B. O'Donovan, ... J. C. Mathers (2016). Reproducibility of the Online Food4Me Food-Frequency Questionnaire for estimating dietary intakes across Europe. *Journal of Nutrition*, 146(5), 1068–75. doi:10.3945/jn.115.225078

79 Australian Bureau of Statistics (2013). *Australian Health Survey: Users' guide, 2011–13*. Canberra: ABS.

80 C. Medlin & J. D. Skinner (1988). Individual dietary intake methodology: a 50-year review of progress. *Journal of the American Dietetic Association*, 88(10), 1250–7.

81 Y. C. Probst & L. C. Tapsell (2005). Overview of computerized dietary assessment programs for research and practice in nutrition education. *Journal of Nutrition Education and Behavior*, 37(1), 20–6. doi:http://dx.doi.org/10.1016/S1499-4046(06)60255-8

82 A. K. Illner, U. Nothlings, K. Wagner, H. Ward & H. Boeing (2010). The assessment of individual usual food intake in large-scale prospective studies. *Annals of Nutrition and Metabolism Journal*, 56(2), 99–105. doi:10.1159/000277667

83 Y. C. Probst, S. Faraji, M. Batterham, D. G. Steel & L. C. Tapsell (2008). Computerized dietary assessments compare well with interviewer administered diet histories for patients with type 2 diabetes mellitus in the primary healthcare setting. *Patient Education and Counseling*, 72(1), 49–55. doi:10.1016/j.pec.2008.01.019

84 J. D. Long, L. A. Littlefield, G. Estep, H. Martin, T. J. Rogers, C. Boswell, ... C. R. Roman-Shriver (2010). Evidence review of technology and dietary assessment. *Worldviews on Evidence-Based Nursing*, 7(4), 191–204.

85 L. Gemming, J. Utter & C. N. Mhurchu (2015). Image-assisted dietary assessment: a systematic review of the evidence. *Journal of the Academy of Nutrition and Dietetics*, 115(1), 64–77.

86 J. Ngo, A. Engelen, M. Molag, J. Roesle, P. García-Segovia & L. Serra-Majem (2009). A review of the use of information and communication technologies for dietary assessment. *British Journal of Nutrition*, 101(S2), S102–S112.

87 M. Sun, L. E. Burke, Z. H. Mao, Y. Chen, H. C. Chen, Y. Bai, ... W. Jia (2014). *eButton: A wearable computer for health monitoring and personal assistance*. Paper presented at the 2014 51st ACM/EDAC/IEEE Design Automation Conference (DAC), 1–5 June.

88 L. Gemming, A. Doherty, J. Utter, E. Shields & C. N. Mhurchu (2015). The use of a wearable camera to capture and categorise the environmental and social context of self-identified eating episodes. *Appetite*, 92, 118–25.

89 J. Shang, E. Pepin, E. Johnson, D. Hazel, A. Teredesai, A. Kristal & A. Mamishev (2012). Dietary intake assessment using integrated sensors and software. *Proceedings of the Society of Photo-Optical Instrumentation Engineers (SPIE)*, 8304. doi:10.1117/12.907769

90 Y. Probst (2006). *An Evaluation of Automated Dietary Assessment: A case study into self-administered computer-assisted survey interviewing for professional dietary consultation*. Wollongong: University of Wollongong.

91 A. F. Subar, L. S. Freedman, J. A. Tooze, S. I. Kirkpatrick, C. Boushey, M. L. Neuhouser, ... S. M. Krebs-Smith (2015). Addressing current criticism regarding the value of self-report dietary data. *Journal of Nutrition*, 145(12), 2639–45. doi:10.3945/jn.115.219634

92 G. S. Martin, L. C. Tapsell, M. J. Batterham & K. G. Russell (2002). Relative bias in diet history measurements: a quality control technique for dietary intervention trials. *Public Health Nutrition*, 5(4), 537–45. doi:10.1079/PHN2002329

93   S. A. Bingham, C. Gill, A. Welch, A. Cassidy, S. A. Runswick, S. Oakes, … N. E. Day (1997). Validation of dietary assessment methods in the UK arm of EPIC using weighed records, and 24-hour urinary nitrogen and potassium and serum vitamin C and carotenoids as biomarkers. *International Journal of Epidemiology*, 26(suppl. 1), S137–S151.

94   B. K. Armstrong, E. White & R. Saracci (1992). *Principles of Exposure Measurement in Epidemiology*. New York: Oxford University Press.

95   J. M. Bland & D. G. Altman (1986). Statistical methods for assessing agreement between two methods of clinical measurement. *The Lancet*, 1(8476), 307–10.

96   M. Jenab, N. Slimani, M. Bictash, P. Ferrari & S. A. Bingham (2009). Biomarkers in nutritional epidemiology: applications, needs and new horizons. *Human Genetics*, 125(5), 507–25. doi:10.1007/s00439-009-0662-5

97   J. Trabulsi & D. A. Schoeller (2001). Evaluation of dietary assessment instruments against doubly labeled water, a biomarker of habitual energy intake. *American Journal of Physiology-Endocrinology and Metabolism*, 281(5), E891–E899.

98   Food Standards Australia New Zealand (2009). *Principles and Practices of Dietary Exposure Assessment for Food Regulatory Purposes*. Canberra: FSANZ.

99   National Health and Medical Research Council (2011). *A Modelling System to Inform the Revision of the Australian Guide to Healthy Eating*. Canberra: NHMRC.

100 Y. Probst, E. Morrison, E. Sullivan & H. K. Dam (2016). First-stage development and validation of a web-based automated dietary modeling tool: using constraint optimization techniques to streamline food group and macronutrient focused dietary prescriptions for clinical trials. *Journal of Medical Internet Research*, 18(7), e190. doi:10.2196/jmir.5459

101 L. J. Gillen & L. C. Tapsell (2006). Development of food groupings to guide dietary advice for people with diabetes. *Nutrition and Dietetics*, 63(1), 36–47. doi:10.1111/j.1747-0080.2006.00043.x

CHAPTER 23

FOOD SCIENCE, TECHNOLOGY AND FOOD SAFETY

STUART JOHNSON, RANIL COOREY AND GARY DYKES

CHAPTER OBJECTIVES

This chapter will enable the reader to:

- describe the role of food science in food innovation
- discuss challenges addressed by food technology in delivering better foods for health
- outline the role of food microbiology and food safety systems in ensuring the quality of the food supply.

KEY TERMS

Food innovation

Food microbiology

Food safety

Food science and technology

KEY POINTS

- The provision of a safe and reliable food supply is underpinned by key disciplines within science and technology, testing and applying new methods and techniques to ensure the delivery of quality foods to consumers.
- Food innovation is an ongoing exercise involving many stakeholders and investigators along the food system, from primary producers through to processors and retailers, to produce new food products for consumers.
- Ensuring a supply of better foods for health relies on the integration of research in food science and nutrition.

INTRODUCTION

Food science is a broad topic area that incorporates aspects of many fundamental science disciplines. It is defined by the US Institute of Food Technologists as the 'study of the physical, microbiological, and chemical makeup of food'. [1]. Food scientists play a vital role in the development and provision of nutritious and safe foods, starting from when food commodities such as grain or meat leave the primary producer (e.g. the farm), and move through the food system to grading, processing, packing, distribution and retailing, and finally are delivered to the consumer.

Broadly, food science can be divided into several areas including food chemistry, food microbiology and food technology. Each of these areas links with other disciplines to deliver high-quality food to supermarkets. For example, food chemists work closely with agricultural researchers to strive for more nutritious primary produce such as grains and meat, and with nutritionists to understand the composition of the foods people eat. In turn, food technologists work side by side with engineers to develop new cost-effective and environmentally friendly food processes and packaging methods that maintain the nutritional quality, flavour and safety of food.

This chapter will provide case studies to enable you to understand the important role of different aspects of food science and technology in delivering the safe and nutritious food that consumers expect.

STOP AND THINK

What are some specific examples of where and how the following food-related scientists can assist in a safe and nutritious food supply: food microbiologist; food technologist; and food chemist?

WHAT IS THE ROLE OF FOOD SCIENCE IN FOOD INNOVATION?

Innovation is defined by the Macquarie Dictionary as 'something new or different introduced' or 'the act of innovating; introducing of new things or methods' [2]. In the current global food system, **food innovation** is crucial for solving food shortages. This is important into the future given current and predicted increases in chronic lifestyle diseases, climate variability and continued rapid population growth.

One way to study innovation is to consider the case of exemplary foods. Here we describe the renewed interest in the use of the 'ancient' cereal grain sorghum (*Sorghum bicolor*) (Figure 23.1) as a potential global staple human food [3]; this is an example of food science innovation that has helped to deliver the first-ever Australian manufactured sorghum-based staple food to consumers.

Currently, the 'pandemic' of obesity and related chronic diseases has led to a search by food and nutrition professionals for alterative food sources that might assist in their prevention and control. Approximately two in three adults and one in four children in Australia are overweight or obese. Obesity can lead to metabolic syndrome in which an increase in risk factors for chronic diseases is seen—for example, elevated blood glucose levels as a risk factor for type 2 diabetes and elevated cholesterol and blood pressure as risk factors for cardiovascular disease [4; 5].

As part of a healthy lifestyle for chronic disease prevention, the Australian Dietary Guidelines [6] recommend that every day we consume 'Grain (cereal) foods, mostly wholegrain and/or high cereal fibre varieties, such as breads, cereals, rice, pasta, noodles, polenta, couscous, oats, quinoa and barley'.

FIGURE 23.1 A. CROP OF RED AND WHITE SORGHUM READY TO HARVEST IN QUEENSLAND, AUSTRALIA

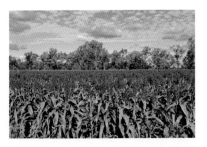

B.

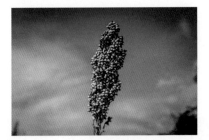

Source: Photographs courtesy of David Martin

However, there has been recent global interest in the potential of sorghum to make a major contribution to this food group due to its potential to assist in the prevention of chronic diseases [7].

Sorghum as a food exemplar

Sorghum production ranks in the top half-dozen global cereal grains and is widely grown in Central Africa, the southern United States, Mexico, Argentina, India, China and eastern Australia [8]. Like wheat and maize, sorghum is a member of the grass family (Poaceae) and thus has a grain composed of pericarp (bran) endosperm and germ. Sorghum wholegrain has a similar macronutrient composition to other cereals like wheat, with an available carbohydrates (primarily starch) content of ~70 g/100 g, a protein content of ~10 g/100 g, a lipid content of ~5 g/100 g and a total dietary fibre content of ~5 g/100 g [3]. However, like all cereal grains, these levels vary somewhat depending on the sorghum genotype, production environment and production practices. Although its macronutrient profile resembles wheat, the way in which the human body handles sorghum foods through the gastrointestinal tract is very different, as highlighted in Figure 23.2.

The food science of sorghum

As can be seen in Figure 23.2, sorghum grain storage protein, known as kafirins, is uniquely hydrophobic—that is, it does not dissolve in water and behaves more like a plastic. This makes sorghum difficult to digest; in fact, when sorghum flour is gently moist cooked such as in a simple porridge, the protein forms more cross-links and becomes even less digestible than the raw grain [9].

FIGURE 23.2   HOW THE HUMAN BODY HANDLES SORGHUM FOODS COMPARED WITH WHEAT

Protein	Starch	Polyphenolic antioxidants
Sorghum kafirins are the most hydrophobic of plant proteins	Harder to gelatinise	Level and profile vary with seed coat colour
Tightly packed in protein bodies	Harder to digest	May scavenge free radicals and inhibit oxidative enzymes in body
Harder to digest	Lower metabolisable energy	
Lower protein nutritional quality due to low digestibility		May reduce oxidative stress that is linked to chronic disease progression
Gluten free		

Source: K. G. Duodu, J. R. N. Taylor, P. S. Belton & B. R. Hamaker (2003). Factors affecting sorghum protein digestibility. *Journal of Cereal Science*, 38(2), 117–31

≫ CASE 23.1

SORGHUM USE IN DEVELOPING COUNTRIES

Traditionally, in countries such as those surrounding the Sahara Desert where sorghum is one of the few crops that will survive readily, the sorghum grain is pre-treated by methods such as alkali soaking, sprouting and fermentation to render more digestible staple foods such as porridges and flatbreads in which the protein has been partially broken down [3]. One current food technology innovation challenge is to understand the chemistry and microbiology of these traditional methods in order to translate them into commercial processes to help provide good nutrition for rapidly expanding urban African populations, many of whom have lost the traditional food skills and knowledge and now rely on energy-dense but micronutrient-poor refined maize food products.

- How can an appreciation of traditional food preparation methods provide insights for modern food science?
- What are the implications for communities living with subsistence farming losing their traditional skills in food preparation?

The 'plastic' hydrophobic nature of sorghum grain proteins also results in difficulties in incorporating sorghum into foods such as leavened bread that is traditionally made from wheat. When sorghum flour is mixed into a dough with water it does not hydrate, leading to an inability to form the cohesive, extensible and elastic dough required to make high-quality leavened bread. However, sorghum protein is gluten free and appears to have little potential to be an allergen. Due to these beneficial properties, there is great interest from food processors in developing innovative new formulations and processing strategies to manufacture sorghum-based, gluten-free foods that match mainstream consumer preferences for bread and other staple foods such as pasta and noodles.

The starch in sorghum grain is generally considered to be harder to gelatinise during cooking, and slower to digest by humans, and thus may have lower metabolisable energy than starches of other cereal foods such as wheat rice and maize. This is a negative attribute in those suffering under-energy malnutrition. On the other hand, these properties of sorghum starch may be beneficial for those at risk of obesity and related chronic diseases, given the lower level of rapidly digested starch compared with slowly digested starch, supporting the development of low glycaemic index (GI) foods [10]. These foods may also have a higher level of resistant starch, providing benefits to gut health. There is great interest in the use of sorghum as an ingredient to lower the starch digestibility of foods such as flat bread [10], pasta [11; 12] and extruded snack foods [13; 14]. While it has been reported [15] that sorghum starch *per se* is not much different from those of other common cereals, the interaction with the hydrophobic sorghum proteins and sorghum polyphenolics can reduce its starch digestibility through inhibiting hydration and gelatinisation and access to digestive enzymes.

Potential health benefits of sorghum consumption

Sorghum is unique among cereal grains for its great diversity of both the levels and types of polyphenolic phytochemicals [16; 17]. These compounds, which are widely found in cereals, fruits and vegetables, contain one or more phenolic ring structures and demonstrate antioxidant properties that are potentially beneficial to health. Sorghum grain colour can also vary widely from whitish through to red, brown and black. The colour of the grain is related to the levels and types of these polyphenolic antioxidants. For instance, red-coloured grain has high levels of the class of phenolics called anthocyanins, which also give bright colours to fruit and vegetables. However, some of the anthocyanins in sorghum are unique to this grain and are more stable to food processing, with obvious advantages as health-promoting foods through their antioxidant and associated activities [18].

Most sorghum grain used for human foods in developed countries has a whitish-coloured grain that is similar in polyphenolic antioxidant content to wholegrain wheat [19]. Traditionally, in Africa coloured sorghum grain was grown for food [20]. This is because the coloured polyphenols in red, brown and black sorghums help to protect the grain from diseases such as fungi as well as being less palatable and less digestible to insects and birds. However, these polyphenols can bind to protein in the grain, further reducing its digestibility as well as having inhibitory properties on starch and protein digestive enzymes [9]. The inhibitory effect of sorghum polyphenols in coloured grain on digestibility reduces the energy and protein bioavailability of sorghum foods for humans and feeds for domestic animals, which is a negative aspect for effective animal husbandry or for communities that are energy and protein malnourished.

» RESEARCH AT WORK

NEW PARADIGMS FOR SORGHUM-BASED FOODS

Recently, the potential of the coloured grain of sorghum to provide chronic disease protective effects for those communities with over-energy malnutrition has been highlighted [10]. To this end, sorghum can be used to manufacture palatable foods that have high antioxidant properties combined with slow starch and protein digestibility that lowers the glycaemic impact of the food and may increase it satiating effect.

This is an example of a *new paradigm* for sorghum foods, as outlined in Figure 23.3. Paradigm shifts of this nature require a high level of food science innovation in order to fill gaps in our knowledge to allow:

1   selection of best sorghum grain variety for the manufacture of the health-protective food
2   design and optimisation of the formulation of the novel sorghum food to match the target nutritional and bioactive composition and physiological handling
3   design and optimisation of a pilot scale process to manufacture the novel sorghum health food with:
    a   high consumer acceptability (sensory evaluation studies)
    b   nutritional and bioactives content (food chemical analysis)
    c   digestibility of macronutrients and bioavailability of micronutrients (*in vitro* laboratory studies)
4   assessment of health-related gastrointestinal handling of macronutrients (post-prandial human studies: glycaemic index; satiety response; lipid response)
5   chronic effect of novel sorghum foods on metabolic syndrome biomarkers—for example, blood lipids, blood pressure, oxidative stress, glucose, insulin sensitivity, and body mass index (human placebo controlled dietary intervention trials)
6   commercial scale-up of pilot scale formulation and process (food industry and test marketing trials).

FIGURE 23.3 PARADIGM SHIFT IN THE USE OF SORGHUM GRAIN FOR HUMAN FOODS

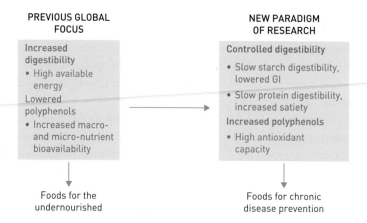

Source: A. Yousif, D. Nhepera & S. Johnson (2012). Influence of sorghum flour addition on flat bread in-vitro starch digestibility, antioxidant capacity and consumer acceptability. *Food Chemistry*, 134, 880–7

» CASE 23.2

DEVELOPMENT OF A SORGHUM-BASED BREAKFAST CEREAL

An example of the food innovation process, from initial conception to commercial launch of the first staple food in Australia made primarily of sorghum, is gluten-free Weetbix™ breakfast cereal. Figure 23.4 shows the innovation pathway leading to the commercial launch of this product by Sanitarium Health and Wellbeing, based in Cooranbong, New South Wales.

Food science and technology research and innovation were required to take sorghum grain to the new staple sorghum-based food gluten-free Weetbix™. The first stage of the study was to understand, through in-depth chemical analysis, the composition and polyphenolic levels and antioxidant properties of the main varieties of sorghum grain grown in Australia. These grains were then used for product development by Sanitarium Health and Wellbeing. Once the new process was developed, Weetbix™ flaked breakfast cereal made from wholegrains of either wheat (conventional control), white sorghum, red sorghum or brown sorghum were manufactured. The composition, polyphenolic and antioxidant properties and *in vitro* digestibility of the different flaked breakfast cereals were then measured and compared. It was found that the red and brown sorghum breakfast cereal had high levels of polyphenolics and antioxidant capacity; however, all types had similar rates of *in vitro* starch digestibility [19]. A post-prandial human study of glucose, insulin and satiety response showed that all flaked breakfast cereals give the same glycaemic response, but those made from the red and brown sorghum gave a higher insulin response and all sorghum cereals gave a higher satiety response than the wheat-base sample. In addition, the sorghum breakfast cereals influenced the level of 'appetite hormones' to match the participants' perceived higher satiety responses, in particular the red sorghum flaked breakfast cereal. Further research combining food science and nutritional physiology is now required to understand the mechanism behind the potential satiety effect in order for ongoing product development to make further enhancements. Of current interest as potential satiety enhancing components in sorghum foods are the unique 3-deoxyanthocyanidin polyphenolics found at high levels in some red and black sorghum grains. The potential role of slow protein digestibility in sorghum foods is also of interest in studying satiating effects.

- Why would sorghum emerge as a cereal of interest in food innovation?
- How can food nutritional sciences work together to produce healthier grain products?
- What further evidence would be required to make health claims on new products?

FIGURE 23.4 INNOVATION PATHWAY FROM SELECTING RAW MATERIALS TO COMMERCIAL LAUNCH OF A MAINSTREAM SORGHUM-BASED FOOD IN AUSTRALIA

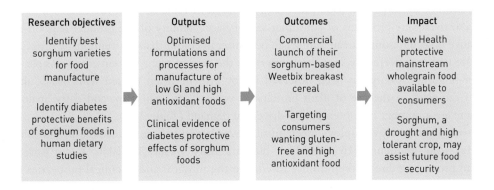

Research objectives	Outputs	Outcomes	Impact
Identify best sorghum varieties for food manufacture	Optimised formulations and processes for manufacture of low GI and high antioxidant foods	Commercial launch of their sorghum-based Weetbix breakfast cereal	New Health protective mainstream wholegrain food available to consumers
Identify diabetes protective benefits of sorghum foods in human dietary studies	Clinical evidence of diabetes protective effects of sorghum foods	Targeting consumers wanting gluten-free and high antioxidant food	Sorghum, a drought and high tolerant crop, may assist future food security

STOP AND THINK

* How does sorghum grain differ from wheat in terms of its composition, technological functionality in foods and gastrointestinal handling by humans?
* Sorghum grain comes in many different grain colours. What are the agri-food and human nutrition advantages and disadvantages of white sorghum compared with red sorghum both for consumers with (a) under-energy/protein malnutrition, and (b) over-energy/protein malnutrition?
* What were the food science innovations and the paradigm shifts in the use of sorghum for foods that led to the launch of gluten-free Weetbix™?

WHAT ARE THE CHALLENGES BEING ADDRESSED BY FOOD TECHNOLOGY IN DELIVERING BETTER FOODS FOR HEALTH?

Challenges for delivering better foods are being addressed by new food technologies such as ultrasound processing and extrusion cooking. These techniques can be considered innovative in the food industry in that they are non-traditional processes that convert raw materials to ingredients and final products for other processors to use for direct consumption by consumers (Table 23.1).

TABLE 23.1   IMPACT OF NEW FOOD TECHNOLOGIES IN THE FOOD SYSTEM

Health	Environment	Food supply
Increasing food safety	Lowering food waste	Reducing food shortages
Improving nutritional properties	Increasing cost effectiveness of processing	Increasing range and types of food products

Ultrasound processing

Ultrasound processing modifies food structure and function by using ultrasound waves that are like sound waves, but of an intensity above that detectable by human hearing [21]. Some examples of the application of ultrasound in food processing are listed in Table 23.2. In the case of milk, research continues to overcome problems of consumer sensory acceptability of the product (e.g. off-flavours). On a positive note, ultrasound-treated milk can be whiter in colour than conventionally processed milk, an attribute that is preferred by some consumers. In the case of plant proteins, for example, viscosity and water-holding capacity has been observed in soy protein when treated with ultrasound. These properties can assist in the use of plant proteins in vegetarian/vegan meat and dairy analogues, for which there are a number of contemporary drivers of demand (Table 23.3).

Ultrasound technology employs mechanical waves beyond those detectable by the human ear (>16 kHz). Low-frequency (16–100 kHz), high-intensity waves (10–1000 W/cm²) are used in ultrasound processing due to their ability to change the physical and chemical properties of foods, such as protein techno-functionality [22; 23]. During ultrasound treatment, the effect of sound wave pressure leads to the formation of gas bubbles with the phenomenon of 'cavitation'. These bubbles undergo cycles of compression and decompression, which can lead to the alteration of the structure of foods [23; 24]. As these cycles progress, the gas bubbles expand and eventually implode. This implosion releases intense energy, which creates very high temperatures of up to 5000 K and very

TABLE 23.2   USE OF ULTRASOUND PROCESSING IN FOODS

Food or ingredients	Process
Milk	One-step homogenisation (reduction of fat particle size to prevent fat separation) Pasteurisation (treatment to reduce pathogenic bacteria) of milk
Yoghurt	Used to improve its water-holding capacity to provide a more stable yoghurt with reduced syneresis (drip loss)
Cheese	Increased speed of hardening and better (increased) firmness
Whey proteins	Treated whey proteins have shown decreased viscosity and increased heat stability, conditions desirable for use of whey proteins in hot beverages
Plant proteins	Improved technological functionality

TABLE 23.3   DRIVERS OF DEMAND FOR PLANT PROTEIN FOODS AND INGREDIENTS

Dietary	Environment	Food supply
Vegetarian/vegan diets	Sustainability	Cost
High-protein foods/diets	Meat and dairy analogues	Accessibility and hunger
Healthy dietary patterns		

high pressures of up to 1000 atm in the area of the cavitation, further modifying the structure and function of the food matrix [24; 25]

In addition to the cavitation phenomenon, ultrasonic treatment of foods can result in the formation of H and ˙OH highly reactive free radicals from the division of water molecules. These free radicals can react with food molecules such as protein to form new bonds such as cross-links, which in turn can modify the food properties such as protein techno-functionality [26].

At the laboratory scale, ultrasonic baths (Figure 23.5a) are used to assist in the cleaning of difficult-to-clean parts of food processing equipment (e.g. injection valves). For small-scale batch processing, bench top ultrasonic probes can be used (Figure 23.5b). However, for large-scale continuous processing, such as that used in the dairy industry, commercial-scale in-line sonication systems are employed (Figure 23.5c). Ultrasound processing has several key advantages over other methods used to modify techno-functionality of food. For instance, it is efficient in terms of energy and time use, and is easy to scale up for in-line continuous commercial application. In addition, it does not use any chemical treatments.

FIGURE 23.5   ULTRASONIC EQUIPMENT
A. ULTRASONIC CLEANING BATH

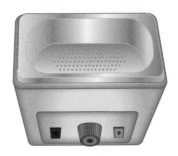

STUART JOHNSON, RANIL COOREY AND GARY DYKES

B. BATCH SMALL-SCALE ULTRASONIC PROBE SYSTEM

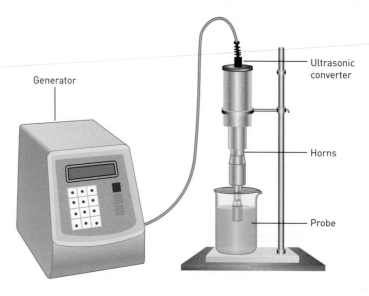

C. IN-LINE CONTINUOUS ULTRASONIC TREATMENT SYSTEM

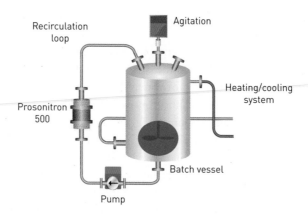

≫ RESEARCH AT WORK

USE OF ULTRASOUND FOR MODIFYING THE FUNCTIONALITY OF PLANT PROTEIN FOOD INGREDIENTS

There is increasing global demand for plant protein–based food ingredients and food products from consumers who wish to reduce animal product consumption—for example, on sustainability grounds—and for the increasing number of vegetarian and vegan consumers (Table 23.3).

Many plant proteins, however, lack the techno-functionality required for them to replace animal proteins (e.g. gelatine, egg protein, whey protein) in processed foods such as dairy and meat analogues, sauces and desserts. Required techno-functional properties include viscosity/thickening, gelling, heat stable thickening and freeze-thaw stable thickening. To this end, ultrasound treatment can be used to cause unfolding and exposure of hydrophobic groups of the globular proteins commonly found in plants [27; 28]. The free radicals produced by ultrasound processing can help form cross-linking between protein molecules such as disulphide bonds of cysteine residues [29; 30]. If carefully controlled and optimised during ultrasound processing, these changes can be used to produce new techno-functionalities in plant proteins to increase their potential applications in processed foods.

Extrusion cooking

Extrusion cooking is a versatile single process that combines mixing, shearing, heat, high pressure and chemical reactions to cook, shape and texturise foods as a continuous process [21]. Figure 23.6 shows an image of a twin screw extruder cooker.

In this process, the raw material (e.g. uncooked mixtures of wholegrain flours) are fed into the inlet in the first extruder barrel using a gravimetric feeder. Once in the barrel, water is added at a controlled flow rate and the dough is mixed, sheared, cooked and pressurised by the co-rotating twin screws combined with heating to above 100°C within the sealed barrel (note that in Figure 23.6, the barrel casing has been opened to show the screws inside). The screws convey while cooking and liquefying the material, known as the 'melt', towards the die by variation in the screw design (kneading blocks, etc.) the melt becomes even more highly sheared and thus contains super-heated water at well above 100°C. Once the 'melt' is pushed through the narrow exit and the end of the barrel (known as the die), the release of pressure causes the super-heated water to explode into steam and thus expand and texturise the material into a cooked, dried state known as the 'extrudate'. This extrudate, depending on the formulation and the configuration of the die, has many appications such as for use in snack foods, breakfast cereals, crisp breads and, when ground into a powder, as instant porridges and supplementary foods (Table 23.4).

FIGURE 23.6 PILOT-SCALE TWIN SCREW EXTRUDER COOKER

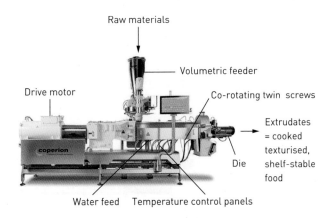

TABLE 23.4 MODIFIABLE EXTRUSION PARAMETERS TO PRODUCE THE 'IDEAL' FOOD PRODUCT

Inputs	Operation
Recipe (% of each dry ingredient)	Feed-rate (kg/h)
Moisture level in barrel (%)	Screw speed (rpm)
Barrel temperature profile (°C)	Screw configuration
	Die configuration

    STUART JOHNSON, RANIL COOREY AND GARY DYKES

Extrusion cooking is a highly controllable single-unit process and as such can be optimised to produce food products with very specific nutritional, health and textural properties, while ensuring a high level of consumer acceptability.

Many physical and chemical interactions occur during extrusion cooking. Some of the most important include:

- *Starch gelatinisation*: In the extrusion process, starch granule swelling occurs, resulting in increased starch digestibility. This may be useful for high-energy supplementary foods but tends to result in a high GI.
- *Protein denaturation and degradation*: Extrusion cooking tends to increase protein digestibility, but may lead to some loss of essential amino acid. Thus, a careful evaluation of protein digestibility corrected amino acid score for protein quality is need for extruded foods.
- *Dietary fibre modification*: Extrusion cooking can lead to chemical and structural changes in dietary fibres and cell walls of plants foods. This can lead to an increase in the ratio of soluble dietary fibre in cereal bran, for example, and thus increase the potential for the food to have beneficial effects on blood glucose and satiety.
- *Increasing bioavailability*: The breakdown of the plant food matrix during extrusion cooking can release minerals, vitamins and health-enhancing phytochemicals such as polyphenolic antioxidants from the food matrix. This can result in the increased bioavailability of these components.
- *Degradation of vitamins and phytochemicals*: Due to heat-induced reactions and chemical breakdown, vitamins and health-enhancing phytochemicals such as polyphenolic antioxidants may be destroyed during extrusion cooking, so conditions must be carefully controlled to prevent this.
- *Safety and stability of extruded products*: The high temperature and pressures used in extrusion cooking can help reduce the microbial load of the final product. Combined with the low water activity of the finished product, this provides good microbiological stability. However, dried extruded products are susceptible to oxidative rancidity and can easily absorb water from the environment, meaning air-, light- and moisture-proof packaging are required.

Figure 23.7 shows the use of extrusion cooking to increase the health functionality of high-fibre plant-food waste (e.g. cereal brans) to make new functional food ingredients.

FIGURE 23.7 POTENTIAL OF EXTRUSION COOKING TO INCREASE THE HEALTH FUNCTIONALITY OF HIGH-FIBRE PLANT-FOOD WASTE

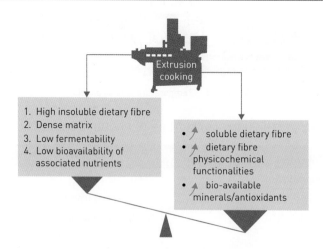

TABLE 23.5   OPPORTUNITIES AND LIMITATIONS FOR LUPIN FOODS

Opportunities	Limitations
High protein High fibre Low starch Carotenoids, phenolics Low anti-nutrient compounds Gluten-free	Difficulty integrating into leavened, baked goods (no gluten proteins, no starch, high water binding) Beany flavour Potential allergenicity

FIGURE 23.8   PROCESSING PATHWAYS ARE STILL UNDER DEVELOPMENT

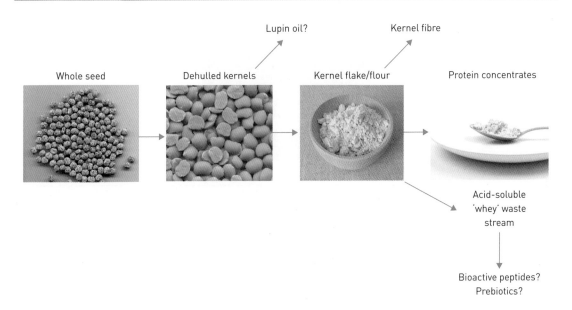

The combination of food science and technological innovation underpins a great deal of development in food in Australia. With its vast agricultural industry, there are many opportunities for food innovation across a range of domains. Lupins, for example, form part of the sustainable agricultural system in Western Australia, but there are both opportunities and limitations around their use (Table 23.5).

Figure 23.8 is a flow diagram showing the production of some lupin-based ingredients. Processing pathways are shown by the teal arrows.

» CASE 23.3

FOOD SCIENCE AND TECHNOLOGY IN PRODUCTION OF LUPIN-CONTAINING FOODS

Lupin is one of Australia's major legume seed crops. A recent review describes the potential of lupin as a sustainable crop and a health-enhancing food [31]. In rotation with cereal crops such as wheat it can help replenish the fertility of the soil through its nitrogen-fixing ability. There are several species of lupin grown around the world; however, Australia produces the majority of the world's lupin seed of the species narrow-leaved lupin (*Lupinus angustifolius*), otherwise known as the Australian sweet lupin (Figure 23.9).

STUART JOHNSON, RANIL COOREY AND GARY DYKES

FIGURE 23.9 A. AUSTRALIAN SWEET LUPIN CROP IN FLOWER

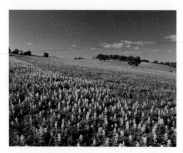

B. MATURE SEED PODS

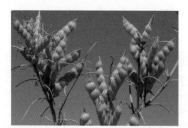

C. MATURE WHOLE SEEDS

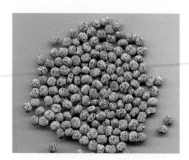

Source: Images b. and c. courtesy of Department of Primary Industries and Regional Development, WA.

Due to the very hard and inert nature of lupin seed coats (often called the hull), the seeds are commonly dehulled before milling the kernels (cotyledons) into a fine flake of flour to use as a food ingredient or for further fractionation and processing into kernel fibre and protein food ingredients. This seed coat, at ~20% of the total seed weight, is currently a low-value animal feed and even a waste-disposal problem for lupin processors and millers. There has been a recent global upsurge in the interest in using lupin as a major food ingredient in staple foods such as bread, but there are both advantages and challenges surrounding this [32] and there is mandatory labelling of lupin as an allergen on foods in Australia [33].

A wide range of lupin-derived food ingredients is available commercially around the world. Some key areas of process development for lupin seed–derived healthy ingredients include: (a) adding improved nutritional and health functionality, such as higher soluble fibre, higher fermentability and improved bioavailability of micronutrients and health-promoting phytochemicals, to the lupin seed coat [34]; and (b) developing a commercially viable isolation process and substantiation of the glucose modulating/insulin-stimulating effects of a specific lupin protein called γ-conglutin [35]. For a short video on innovation in purification and health testing of γ-conglutin, watch the clip at: www.youtube.com/watch?v=9fAuEli3tWo.

Food products containing lupin-derived ingredients still tend to be a niche market, but there are developing new markets such as gluten-free and vegan. In terms of the widespread use of lupin in staple foods such as leavened bread, product formulation and process design is still ongoing to try to overcome the lack of gluten-forming proteins in lupin and its highly water-binding kernel fibre, in order to get the nutritional benefits of lupin but in the soft and well-risen loaves that are popular with consumers [36].

One of the key drivers for the increased production and consumption of lupin foods is the developing suite of evidence from human dietary studies regarding their protective effects against metabolic syndrome [31] and their potential status as functional foods.

Short-term placebo-controlled post-meal studies on lupin kernel flour and lupin kernel fibre have generally demonstrated that lupin foods have high-satiety (appetite-suppressing) effects of potential benefit in controlling long-term food intake and maintaining healthy weight maintenance. However, long-term placebo-controlled blind interventions did not result in greater weight loss on the diet containing lupin flour foods compared with the control, leaving the efficacy of lupin flour foods for weight control under question, and requiring more research, for example, with lupin kernel fibre foods. A similar level of evidence for benefits to post-prandial blood glucose level has been found, but without significant beneficial effect on fasting glucose from the longer-term studies. One study has, however, reported lowered fasting insulin and improved HOMA (a measure on insulin sensitivity) after the lupin food diet compared with the control [37].

Beneficial effects on blood cholesterol from diets containing purified lupin kernel fibre and purified lupin protein have been reported, but similar effects were not observed in studies on lupin flour-containing foods [31]. However, consistent and important evidence from two placebo-controlled blind randomised dietary intervention studies on the effects of foods containing lupin kernel flour has indicated a potential protective role of lupin foods against hypertension.

Several placebo-controlled dietary intervention studies have investigated the effect of lupin kernel fibre on colonic function, chemistry and microbiology [31]. These studies have demonstrated beneficial changes to putative biomarkers of colonic health and a change in the balance of colonic microflora towards more beneficial types; hence, lupin kernel is considered a prebiotic food ingredient.

Based on the current level of evidence of the potential health benefits of lupin foods, further long-term blinded placebo-controlled blind dietary intervention studies are required, particularly in at-risk participants such as those with metabolic syndrome and type 2 diabetes. This increased level of evidence will be required to support any future application to Food Standards Australia New Zealand (FSANZ) to permit any high-level health claim (e.g. mention of health-related biomarkers of disease conditions) [38] to be made for lupin foods on labelling or advertising, and thus cement the status of lupin as a functional food.

In conclusion, lupin seed holds great promise as a sustainable, high-protein, high-fibre food as part of the mainstream food supply. However, continued food science research is required to improve consumer acceptability of lupin-containing foods, as well as to substantiate their health benefits in human dietary studies.

- What is the unique nutritional composition of lupin seed, highlighting how it differs from other pulses and soy beans?
- How can the lupin seed can be fractionated and processed into a wide range of food ingredients? For each type of ingredient, give an example of a commercial application in a food product.
- Based on published human dietary intervention studies in healthy participants, what would be the rationale for the types of lupin flour–based and control foods you would design for a blind placebo-controlled cross-over intervention study in people with type 2 diabetes, to investigate the effect of lupin on blood glucose control and blood pressure?

STUART JOHNSON, RANIL COOREY AND GARY DYKES

STOP AND THINK

....

- What are some of the nutrition issues that may emerge from the use of new technologies in food processing?
- What kinds of limitations emerge when considering the use of sustainable agricultural products in new food product development?
- What type of nutrition research is required to provide evidence of effects following consumption of new food products involving different plant foods?

WHAT ARE THE ROLES OF FOOD MICROBIOLOGY AND FOOD SAFETY SYSTEMS IN ENSURING THE QUALITY OF THE FOOD SUPPLY?

Food microbiology

the study of foodborne microorganisms that present major challenges for the protection of public health.

Food microbiology involves the study of foodborne microorganisms that present major challenges for the protection of public health. A foodborne disease can be defined as illness that is transmitted by the consumption of food that has been contaminated [39]. A foodborne infection is a disease that is caused by the consumption of foods containing pathogenic bacteria such as *Salmonella*. Foodborne intoxication is a disease that is caused by the ingestion of food products that contain the toxins produced by a bacterial agent such as *Bacillus cereus* [40; 41]. An increasing number of factors have been identified as contributing to the incidence of foodborne disease—for example, increasing urbanisation, prolonged storage of products under non-optimal conditions and the emergence of new bacterial strains [42].

Microbial contaminants in foodborne illness

The main microbial contaminants in foodborne illness are *Salmonella*, *Campylobacter*, *Listeria monocytogenes*, *Clostridium perfringens*, *Bacillus cereus*, *Staphylococcus aureus* and *Escherichia coli*, and these are discussed below.

Salmonella

Salmonella is a heat labile bacterium that can be easily eliminated from foods by high temperature processing [43]. Cooking a product until its core temperature reaches 75°C can eliminate *Salmonella*. However, since the organism's maximum growth temperature is 47°C, inadequate temperature control during cooking, cooling, post-processing contamination and storage are the significant contributors of *Salmonella* outbreaks [44]. The survival rate and heat resistance of the organism are mainly influenced by the effects of temperature, pH, a_w (i.e. the amount of water present in a food product that a microorganism can access for its metabolic activity) and food composition [45–49]. In low a_w food products, *Salmonella* has a slow death rate [43]. This means a food with higher salt content (lower a_w) may need to be cooked longer at the same temperature than a food that contains lower salt content (higher a_w) to eliminate *Salmonella*. Higher heat resistance of bacteria is apparent in products containing higher fat as the fat acts as a protective agent against heat [45]. This means that higher-fat products such as beef and beef lasagne may need to be heated for longer to inactivate this organism compared with lower-fat food products such as chicken breast and chicken stir-fry. The heat resistance of *Salmonella* in heterogeneous 'potentially hazardous food' (PHF) products (those with multiple ingredients such as a bolognese meal) with a variety of nutrient sources may be higher than in homogeneous food products (those with a single ingredient, such as rice). In addition to its variable heat resistance in different foods, *Salmonella* can tolerate a wide pH range, thereby increasing the risk of its growth in a variety of food products [50; 51]. PHFs are often prepared with a combination of different ingredients such as salt and spices (low a_w and pH) by marinating before the cooking and processing step (high temperature), which tends to influence *Salmonella* survival rate [48; 52–54]. Based on the above, the inactivation characteristics of *Salmonella* in different multi-ingredient foods need to be carefully determined to ensure product safety.

Campylobacter

Campylobacter is a microaerophilic bacteria that may grow under low oxygen conditions. The *Campylobacter* genus also contains thermophilic species [55–57], including *C. jejuni* and *C. coli*, that are important in foodborne diseases. Thermophilic species have the ability to grow at a high optimum temperature of around 42°C. *Salmonella* and *Campylobacter* are both prevalent in meat products, especially chicken [44; 58–61]. Several studies have shown that antibiotics added into animal feed could enhance the antimicrobial resistance of *Campylobacter* in meat products [54; 60; 62–63]. This may, in turn, impact treatment during a foodborne illness outbreak, which means proper processing of food products is important to eliminate these organisms.

As *Campylobacter* is less heat tolerant than some other foodborne pathogens such as *Salmonella* or *E. coli*, while growing outside its optimum temperature range [57], it can be relatively easily inactivated by proper temperature control. *Campylobacter* can also be easily eliminated under specific environmental conditions such as low pH or high salt concentration (a_w), conditions that reduce its survival rate [50]. For example, a bolognese meal (low pH) may have a higher lethal effect on *Campylobacter* compared with a cooked chicken product with gravy, which has a high pH and fat content. Thus, a one-size-fits-all approach may not be viable for inactivating *Campylobacter* in commercial food products.

Listeria monocytogenes

L. monocytogenes is one of the main microorganisms contaminating food after heat treatment due to its ability to survive over a wide temperature range [45; 46; 56; 64]. It possesses both psychrotrophic (can survive in extremely cold conditions) and mesophilic growth (grows best in moderate temperatures, typically 20–45°C) characteristics, which makes this organism especially problematic in cook–chill products [64–66]. *L. monocytogenes* has a long growth lag-time of up to 33 days when stored at temperatures below 5°C [40]. *L. monocytogenes*, which may survive improper initial heat processing, can multiply under refrigerated storage (<5°C), and the surviving cells can cause infection, especially if inadequate reheating is applied prior to consumption. Similarly to *Salmonella*, higher fat content has been found to favour the growth of *Listeria* and, as such, meat products need to be treated under higher lethal inactivation processes than low-fat products for both these organisms [45]. For both organisms, pH and a_w based processing has a synergistic lethal effect that can be taken into account when formulating a PHF product [52]. Although there are infrequent listeriosis outbreaks, listeriosis infection is sporadic with higher mortality and hospitalisation rates as compared with other foodborne pathogens [67–69]. It is particularly dangerous to vulnerable groups, including pregnant women, elderly people, young children and immune-suppressed groups [70].

Clostridium perfringens

C. perfringens is a spore-forming, anaerobic and widely distributed pathogen that grows in high-protein foods such as chicken- and beef-based products [71–75]. *C. perfringens* can also grow under aerobic conditions, albeit infrequently [40]. Due to this characteristic, it has the potential to cause illnesses through contaminated cook–serve (aerobic) and cook–chill products (modified atmosphere packaged; anaerobic). Although the vegetative cells can be easily killed by heat treatment, the spores remain substantially unaffected by heat, but their germination can be inhibited by the presence of salt and organic acids [75]. This means that a cooked chicken product with gravy possessing a higher salt content may have a lower probability of causing foodborne intoxication by this organism compared with boiled chicken products. Further, improper heat treatment such as using a slow heating rate during cooking will increase the heat resistance of the spores formed during processing, which could germinate during storage [75]. The undestroyed spores can germinate and multiply readily at temperatures around 43–47°C with a generation time of 10 minutes [50]. The heat-resistance properties and rate of germination of *C. perfringens* spores during storage are dependent on the strain and the food product's nutrient content [71; 75; 76]. Any surviving *C. perfringens* after processing can multiply and release enterotoxin, causing food poisoning if the temperature control during cooking and cooling is inadequate. Generally, *C. perfringens* intoxication causes only mild symptoms and medical treatment is not required in most of the cases [77]. Foodborne disease outbreaks due to *C. perfringens* can therefore easily be overlooked and misdiagnosed.

Nitrates have been used in the meat industry as preservatives against foodborne pathogens. Due to consumer trends, the decreased concentrations of nitrite (<50 ppm) used by some processes can increase the potential for *C. perfringens* growth during cooling. For this reason, additional protective measures, such as faster chilling, need to be adopted to ensure the safety of ready-to-eat meats [78]. Various predictive microbial models have been developed to estimate the survival and growth of *C. perfringens*. A Monte Carlo simulation provided an alternative method for estimating and managing the risk of cooked turkey products during cooling due to *C. perfringens* contamination [79].

Bacillus cereus

B. cereus is a spore-forming and heat-resistant bacterium [51; 56; 80; 81]. Its thermal tolerance is similar to that of other foodborne pathogens, which increase in high fat and/or low a_w products [82]. *B. cereus* synthesises an emetic toxin (cereulide) that can cause vomiting [83]. This toxin has been mainly found in high-starch foods such as rice and pasta dishes [84–87]. *B. cereus* can also synthesise enterotoxins that cause diarrhoea and these toxins are unstable in high acid and high temperatures [88; 89]. The heat- and acid-resistant spores of this organism can germinate into vegetative cells in a short time, especially at a temperature of ~28°C [89]. Such conditions may arise due to slow or improper cooling—that is, holding the product close to room temperature for an extended period of time. Previous studies have shown that lowering the pH of food products will decrease the heat resistance of *B. cereus* spores, thereby increasing the killing effect of cooking procedures [51; 81]. For instance, bolognese meals that have a lower pH compared with cooked rice would be expected to have a lower probability of spore germination during storage. In addition to the cooking procedure, rapid cooling also needs to be applied to prevent surviving spores from germinating during storage [73]. Mugadza and Buys [90] have reported both mesophilic and psychotropic characteristics in a majority of *B. cereus* strains, which indicates that this organism can grow even in refrigeration temperatures and highlights the importance of preventing spore germination [91].

Staphylococcus aureus

S. aureus is a mesophilic, non-spore-forming bacterium that grows optimally at 37°C [50]. *S. aureus* is a facultative anaerobe that is capable of growing in both aerobic and anaerobic conditions, even though it is more prevalent in aerobic environments [50]. *S. aureus* is predominantly found in challenging environments such as human skin, which is dry and has a high salt content [91]. Poor hygiene and food handling are the key factors associated with the transmission of *S. aureus* [88]. Vegetative cells of *S. aureus* formed at lower a_w have higher thermal resistance, but this is reduced in extreme pH environments [92]. Food poisoning caused by *S. aureus* is mainly due to the presence of highly heat and acid-resistant preformed enterotoxins, which triggers an emetic effect [92]. The enterotoxins' characteristics enable them to be present in foods with low pH or high heat-treated foods (such as canned foods) and cause foodborne outbreaks. The preformed enterotoxin can also cause illness when associated with well-cooked and chilled products, especially in products similar to a bolognese meal (low pH) [93; 94]. Similarly to *C. perfringens* and *B. cereus*, *S. aureus* intoxication is also likely to be underreported due to its mild symptoms [81; 88; 91].

Escherichia coli

E. coli is a member of the *Enterobacteriaceae* family and is found in the intestinal tract of mammals such as cattle, where it can easily contaminate the muscle meat (e.g. beef) that surrounds the lining of the intestinal tract [54; 95]. Most often, *E. coli* have been found in cooked ground beef rather than products such as roast beef, as grinding the beef mixes the surface bacteria from either the contaminated internal meat muscle or from the carcass surface [62; 94; 96]. These organisms are routinely used as indicators of faecal contamination and inadequate hygienic processing practices [97]. The ability of *E. coli* to survive at low temperatures is a concern in food products that are held at chilled temperatures for extended periods of time (storage and transportation) [61; 62; 94]. Shiga-toxin-producing *E. coli* (STEC) are foodborne pathogens that are closely monitored by the National Notifiable Diseases Surveillance System (NNDSS) and OzFoodNet due to their capacity to cause the fatal human disease, hemolytic-uremic syndrome (HUS) [67; 98]. The thermal-tolerance characteristic of *E. coli* is highly dependent on the physical properties of the food source it is found in (i.e. pH and a_w) [62]. A previous study reported that *E. coli* O157:H7, which is one of the strains that cause fatal disease, could survive in pasta sauce at a pH of 4.6 and at a low storage temperature of 4°C [99]. The same study concluded that the development of acid tolerance during storage could confer some cross-protection against heat, which could mean that if reheating of high-acidic food is not performed properly, *E. coli* O157:H7 could survive and cause illness. Therefore, products similar to pasta sauces, which contain minced meats, may present an increased risk due to surviving organisms from the inadequate cooking or cross-contamination, thereby causing HUS.

» RESEARCH AT WORK

MONITORING FOODBORNE ILLNESS IN POPULATIONS

Large food manufacturing organisations and their suppliers are required to implement and practise food safety standards. However, food borne diseases still occur in both developed and developing nations. In Australia, the annual cost to the economy due to foodborne illness is estimated to be around $1.2 billion [100].

Foodborne illness can result in diarrhoea and vomiting (gastroenteritis) or even illnesses such as hepatitis, similar to outbreaks in Australia in 2015 and 2017 that were attributed to frozen berries. Some of these foodborne illnesses can cause serious long-term health effects such as kidney failure and occasionally death. In Australia in 2010, there were 4.1 million reported cases of foodborne gastroenteritis and over 5000 cases of non-gastroenteritis foodborne illnesses. The most commonly implicated microorganisms were norovirus, *E. coli*, *Campylobacter* spp. and non-typhoidal *Salmonella* spp.; however, approximately 80% of illnesses were from unknown pathogens [101]. In the United States, the Centers for Disease Control and Prevention (CDC) estimates that annually 48 million people become sick due to foodborne illnesses from 9.4 million episodes. From these, there are 3000 deaths [102]. Of these illnesses, approximately 10 million are caused by 31 known pathogens and the rest—approximately 38 million—from unspecified pathogens [102]. It is important to determine incidence of foodborne illness and the implicated pathogen so that effective processes can be implemented by the food industry to prevent the spread of such illnesses. This also enables governments to develop effective food safety policies that are scientifically sound.

In the United States, the majority of foodborne illnesses are due to eight known human pathogens. Of these organisms, 58% are due to norovirus and 11% due to *Salmonella* spp. However, *Salmonella* was the leading cause of hospitalisations due to foodborne illnesses at 35% and norovirus was second at 26% of all hospitalisations due to foodborne illness [102]. This shows that much needs to be done even in developed countries to control the spread of foodborne pathogens.

Food safety systems

Food safety

activities involved in the manufacture of food products that are carried out in a manner to prevent the risk of foodborne illness.

Food safety systems operate through governments and health programs. In Australia, the food safety administration has three layers of governance and several organisations that are responsible for overseeing and implementing it. The first layer is international, the second national (or federal) and the third is at the level of the states/territories (Table 23.6). In the international arena, the two main players are the World Health Organization (WHO) and the Food and Agriculture Organization (FAO), both of which are United Nations (UN) organisations.

Food Standards Australia New Zealand was established in 1991 as a bi-national Commonwealth authority that develops food standards for composition, labelling and contaminants, including microbiological limits that apply to all foods produced or imported for sale in Australia and New Zealand. The codes and standards that FSANZ develop need to be adopted as law by the separate states and territories of Australia and New Zealand.

The other federal agency that has an interest in food safety is Biosecurity, which is an arm of the Australian Department of Agriculture and Water Resources. Biosecurity provides import, export and certification to help retain Australia's highly favourable animal, plant and human health status. The Australian food industry has been able to maintain its access to overseas export markets through this agency. It is also this agency that checks bags at airports when people arrive from overseas for food and other material that could damage Australian flora and fauna.

TABLE 23.6 LEVELS OF ADMINISTRATION OF FOOD SAFETY IN AUSTRALIA

International	Federal	State
World Health Organization	Food Standards Australia New Zealand (FSANZ)	State departments (e.g. health)
Food and Agriculture Organization (Codex Alimentarius Commission)	Biosecurity	Local governments (councils)

The next level of food safety administration at the local level is the state and territory governments. These provide input to FSANZ on the development of food standards, coordinate state-wide food recalls when necessary, and provide food monitoring, surveillance activities, and advice to industry participants.

The last level of food safety administration is local government. Local councils and shires are responsible for most of the community needs within their jurisdiction, and food safety is just one of their areas of responsibility. The authorised officers working within local government are responsible for the implementation of the food standards and codes.

The WHO, FAO and Codex Alimentarius Commission

The trade in food is a global activity, and the impact of food safety on people's health and well-being is felt worldwide, also affecting trade internationally. To manage the health impacts of this worldwide trade, different organisations have been developed, including the UN organisations, the WHO and FAO.

The WHO was established in 1948 by the UN with the objective of 'attaining the highest possible level of health for all people' [103]. WHO headquarters are based in Geneva and there and currently 192 member countries, with six regional offices, in Africa and the Americas, South East Asia, Europe, the Eastern Mediterranean and the Western Pacific. Australia is administered through the Western Pacific office, which is based in the Philippines. WHO's operations cover everything to do with health from HIV-AIDS, communicable diseases, non-communicable diseases and mental health, to pharmaceuticals, reproductive health, nutrition and food safety. Food safety comes under the portfolio of the Assistant Director-General—Non-communicable Diseases and Mental Health (see www.who.int/foodsafety/en).

The FAO was established by the UN in 1945 with the goal of leading international efforts to defeat hunger:

> Achieving food security for all is at the heart of FAO's efforts—to make sure people have regular access to enough high-quality food to lead active, healthy lives. Our three main goals are: the eradication of hunger, food insecurity and malnutrition; the elimination of poverty and the driving forward of economic and social progress for all; and, the sustainable management and utilization of natural resources, including land, water, air, climate and genetic resources for the benefit of present and future generations. [104]

The FAO serves both developed and developing countries. It provides the technical information required for countries to produce more food that is both safe and nutritious.

Currently there are 194 member nations of the FAO. There are five regional offices in addition to its headquarters in Rome. Within the FAO there are eight departments, which include the Agriculture and Consumer Protection Department, under which is the Office of Food Safety. FAO's Food Quality and Safety section is concerned with the maintenance and improvement of the quality and safety of foods at the international, regional and national levels. It promotes the establishment and operation of national regulatory frameworks compatible with international requirements, in particular those of the Codex Alimentarius Commission. Its objectives are:

> Strengthening national food control regulatory frameworks, and enhancing member country participation in Codex; Providing independent scientific advice through the JECFA and JEMRA expert bodies to support the standard setting work of Codex; Enhancing food safety management along food chains to prevent diseases and trade disruptions; Promoting food safety emergency preparedness to build resilient agri-food chains; Developing online platforms for global networking, databases for information sharing and tools to support food safety management. [105]

The Codex Alimentarius (Latin, meaning Food Law or Code) was set up in 1963 as a joint initiative of the WHO and the FAO. The organisation is 'about safe, good food for everyone—everywhere' (www.fao.org/fao-who-codexalimentarius/about-codex/en). Trading of food has existed for many thousands of years, but it is only comparatively recently that it has significantly grown in volume and value. The methods of transport and technologies to preserve perishable food for long-term travel did not exist until recently. This has made possible the growth in quantity and variety of food that can be exported. Hence, the effects of what happens to a food product in one part of the planet can be felt on the other side of the globe. The Codex Alimentarius Commission was created as a response to this need to develop food standards, guidelines and codes of practice to control and ensure the safety of the food chain. The standards are developed to protect the safety of consumers and to promote fair international trade. Other UN agencies and other organisations refer to the Codex and it is sometimes consulted as the basis for dispute resolution—there is a lot at stake for protecting consumers' health and well-being. The Codex can be accessed through its website: www.fao.org/fao-who-codexalimentarius/en.

Hazard Analysis Critical Control Point (HACCP)–based food safety programs

A food safety program is a written plan that shows how food safety and hygiene will be managed within a food manufacturing business (for example, see www.foodauthority.nsw.gov.au/ip/food-safety-programs-haccp). In many countries, the proprietors of food businesses are legally required to carry out a hazard analysis of their food manufacturing activities. In Australia, food establishments dealing with the following are required to have a HACCP-based food safety plan implemented:

- Those that provide potential hazardous food to vulnerable populations—that is, the elderly, children, pregnant women and the immunocompromised.
- Those that deal with raw oysters and other bivalves—that is, harvesting, processing and distribution of raw oysters and other bivalves.
- Catering operations that serve food for consumption.
- Those that produce manufactured and fermented meat products.

The first step in the development of a HACCP-based food safety program involves the food manufacturer looking carefully at every stage of food handling in the business and deciding at which points there could be a risk to food safety. Once these points have been identified, various measures must then be established to control the potential hazards. The control measures need to be checked and recorded to ensure that the process is working as it should and that the food safety plan is adhered to. Systems must also be in place to take prompt remedial action if a control measure fails. The food manufacturer must keep the controls under constant review to ensure that the measures are working as they should. If there are changes to the process or anything new is added, then a new analysis must be undertaken to determine whether there is a change in possible hazard that can cause a breach in the food safety plan. Something new could include the introduction of new ingredients, products or processes. The elements and advantages of a food safety plan are outlined in Table 23.7.

HACCP is a proactive system that uses a scientific approach to prevent the breakdown of food safety that could cause the outbreak of foodborne illness. The HACCP-based food safety system takes a whole-of-process approach. This means that any food safety program must encompass the following:

1 Systematically identify any potential hazards that may be reasonably expected to occur during the handling and operations during all steps of the manufacturing process. The food manufacturer

TABLE 23.7   ADVANTAGES OF A FOOD SAFETY PLAN

Element	Advantages
Contracts	A food manufacturer that can demonstrate food safety and that no foodborne illness has been attributed to their operations has a greater chance of winning contracts.
Consistency	The ability to consistently supply high-quality, safe food by following the food safety program that has been established.
Commitment	The food safety plan has to be approved, accepted and signed off by the organisation's senior manager, in most cases the chief executive officer (CEO). The CEO takes final responsibility for the implementation and running of the food safety program. The CEO has to be committed to the program to produce safe food.
Costs	The cost of product recall and the loss of market share due to the spread of foodborne illness can be huge, not to mention the cost of litigation and payment of damages. The food safety program should be designed to minimise the chance of this happening and increase an organisation's ability to consistently produce safe food, thus also increasing its profitability.
Confidence	A properly implemented food safety plan will give customers confidence that safe food products will always be manufactured consistently.
Control	With proper food safety management systems in place, the organisation will have control of its production process. It will also have good control over the safety of the products it produces, ensuring there is minimal chance of a product recall that could be costly for the organisation.
Certification	When an organisation has a food safety program in place that conforms to the principles of HACCP, it may get the system certified by a third party. Third-party certification is independent and provides confidence to the consumer that safe food is being consistently manufactured by the organisation.
Credibility	An organisation that is audited and certified by an independent body will provide credibility regarding its food safety management system to provide safe food to its consumers.

needs to look at each step of the manufacturing process, from receivable, raw material storage, through to finished goods storage and dispatch in the operation. It needs to identify what might go wrong at each point in the whole operation. *Salmonella* in a roasted chicken due to poor processing is an example of a biological hazard; detergent contamination due to improperly cleaned food preparation surface in a chicken product is a chemical hazard; or a piece of glass from a broken light bulb is a physical hazard in the product.

2   Identify where in the manufacturing process each of the identified hazards can be controlled and how it can be controlled For example, in a roasted chicken product, roasting will kill pathogens so the critical point in the process for this particular biological hazard is roasting to a core temperature that is adequate to kill all of the possible pathogens.

3   Put in place specific controls and set limits to ensure the identified hazards do not occur—for example, roasting chicken to a core temperature of 72°C for two minutes to kill any pathogen that may be present. A temperature or time below this may not kill all of the pathogens that could be present, which will then lead to a potentially hazardous food product. Limits could also be set to ensure that the product quality is not lost, in this case roasting for no less than 72°C and no more than 75°C for two minutes.

                                                      STUART JOHNSON, RANIL COOREY AND GARY DYKES

4   Be able to provide systematic monitoring of the established controls of the identified hazards. Once the controls have been set in place and their effectiveness established, it is important to monitor them to ensure they are operating properly. Records must be kept so that the organisation knows its performance—for example, the core temperature of its roast chicken has reached at least 72°C, held for two minutes and is safe for human consumption. It builds confidence within the organisation that its systems are working and can demonstrate to external stakeholders that the systems are working and the products are safe.

5   Be able to provide appropriate corrective action if and when a control measure is determined to be out of control. The food manufacturer needs to have systems in place that state what needs to be done if a control measure fails—for example, what the company should do if the core temperature of its roast chicken does not reach 72°C, only reached 65°C or was held at 72°C for one and a half minutes. These procedures are known as corrective actions. Records of corrective action taken must also be kept, as they provide not only evidence of action taken but also provide information about the effectiveness of the corrective actions. In this way, the organisation learns, can do things better next time and can demonstrate that action was taken.

6   Be reviewed regularly to ensure the adequacy of the food safety program to provide safe food consistently. The food safety system needs to be reviewed and corrected periodically, as well as when any new product or change to the process is made, to ensure that it is relevant—for example, challenge testing of the final product, in this case, roast chicken, for the presence of *Salmonella* or retention samples for shelf life verification. By doing this the organisation is verifying that its systems are still correct and effective.

7   To gain all of the benefits of a robust food safety management system, such as a HACCP system, there are a few activities that need to be carried out (see Table 23.8). The first is to bring together the HACCP team. The team must consist of committed individuals with different skills that complement each other—skills such as auditing, product knowledge, production and processing knowledge, writing and so on. The initial tasks of the team are to describe the product, understand the food product, and its intended usage. Once this is achieved, the team needs to develop a product flow diagram and then a production floor plan; both of these should be written for the specific product and production environment, and confirmed by management. The controls and their implementation could vary depending not just on the product itself, but also how the product is made, as the potential hazards could differ. Once these steps have been concluded, hazards need to be assessed, critical control points determined and the relevant controls put in place.

TABLE 23.8 REQUIREMENTS OF FOOD SAFETY SYSTEMS AND THE PRINCIPLES OF HACCP

Requirements of program	Principles
Identify hazards	Determine hazards
Identify controls	Determine critical points
Set controls	Set critical limits
Monitor	Establish monitors
Correct	Take corrective action
Review	Verify process
	Maintain records

TRY IT YOURSELF

As a food technologist, explain the steps you would take to establish a food safety management system for a company that manufactures dehydrated apple chips.

There are seven principles that need to be followed throughout the implementation of a HACCP-based food safety program:

- *Principle 1*: Determine the hazards. The food manufacturer needs to look at its entire manufacturing process and determine the potential hazards. These hazards could be: biological, such as *Salmonella* in roast chicken; chemical, such as a toxic chemical residue from a machine cleaning agent present on a work bench that the roasted chicken was left on; or physical, such as metal pieces from the roaster getting into the chicken.
- *Principle 2*: Determine the critical control points (CCPs). The food manufacturer needs to look at each processing step and determine at which point the identified hazards can be controlled and how they can be controlled. Such points could be a location in the plant (e.g. a quarantine area), a practice (e.g. trimming the surface of the product), a process (e.g. cooking or freezing) or a procedure (e.g. cleaning of the equipment). At these 'points' in the process, a preventative measure or control measure can be applied that will eliminate, prevent or minimise the identified hazard or several of the hazards. To identify and implement a step in the process as a CCP, series of questions is asked, similar to following a decision tree. Normally, if an identified hazard cannot be controlled in a processing step further down the manufacturing line, then that step becomes a CCP.
- *Principle 3*: Establish the critical limits. At this stage the food manufacturer has to put in place set limits to ensure the identified hazards do not occur. These can be measured at a given CCP. Critical limits are boundaries of safety and will be a set of factors such as temperature, time, physical product dimensions, equipment design, water activity or pH that will be able to control the given hazard. If the product is maintained within these limits, then the product will remain safe.
- *Principle 4*: Establish a monitoring system. This is the act of conducting planned observations of the control parameters that were established earlier at the CCPs to ensure that these controls are actually performing as expected. By monitoring, data can be collected and recorded for the purpose of making decisions and ensuring safe food is manufactured.
- *Principle 5*: Establish a corrective action plan. If monitoring shows a loss of control, then something needs to be done, and this is the corrective action. Corrective actions could range from stopping production, destroying products, reworking products or readjusting the process, to short-term fixes to get production back on track. The required corrective action will depend upon the severity of the problem.
- *Principle 6*: Verify the process. Verification demonstrates whether all procedures are being carried out in accordance with the HACCP plan, and its effectiveness. Verification can identify if the system is in compliance with the plan. This can be done by reviewing (looking back at) documents; by auditing (internal or external) to officially examine records, systems and procedures to see if they are still current; or by random sampling and testing to verify control records.
- *Principle 7*: Establish and maintain records. Records need to be kept so that it is known how well the HACCP system is working. The records need to be working documents that are completed and maintained by the person carrying out the specific task. A record must be made by the person who completed the task, as they need to take responsibility for carrying out the job as it should be done. Records demonstrate the effectiveness of the controls, which is evidence of product safety. These documents can be used for analysis performance and even in a court of law as evidence.

STUART JOHNSON, RANIL COOREY AND GARY DYKES

STOP AND THINK

- Given the growth characteristics of the different pathogenic microorganisms, which type of organisms you would expect to be transmitted (a) in cooked rice and (b) in a roast beef in gravy dish?
- What implications do the Australian food regulations and international food law have for Australian food exports?
- How do federal and state authorities work together to ensure the quality of the domestic food supply?

SUMMARY

- Food science represents a number of capacities that can work with the physical properties of food as they occur in nature and via processing and various forms of preparation.
- New technologies in agriculture and food processing can help to address some of the challenges of providing a safe and reliable food supply to the population.
- Food safety is critical to public health and is managed through all levels of government and at national and international levels.
- Food safety programs have characteristic steps aligned with the principles of hazard identification, control and monitoring.

PATHWAYS TO PRACTICE

- Food safety programs need to be implemented in a range of settings. Knowledge and skills in these areas can relate to work-related responsibilities in food service and food production systems.
- Food innovation, particularly where food processing is involved, requires teamwork from a range of food-related disciplines, including chemists, engineers and nutritionists.
- Understanding food law is an advantage in many areas involving food product development and commercialisation.

DISCUSSION QUESTIONS

1 How can a food scientist work with a nutritionist to improve the nutritional quality of a food product?
2 How can a food scientist work alongside an agricultural scientist to improve the quality of food?
3 What is the role of government and agricultural organisations in supporting research underpinning food innovation?

USEFUL WEBLINKS

Australian Government—Science and research priorities—Food capability statement:
www.science.gov.au/scienceGov/ScienceAndResearchPriorities/Pages/Food.aspx

Australian Institute of Food Safety:
www.foodsafety.com.au

Australian Institute of Food Science & Technology:
www.aifst.asn.au

CSIRO—Agriculture and food:
www.csiro.au/en/Research/AF/Areas/Food

Department of Agriculture and Water Resources—Research and innovation:
www.agriculture.gov.au/ag-farm-food/innovation

Food and Agriculture Organization:
www.fao.org/about/en

Food Standards Australia New Zealand:
www.foodstandards.gov.au

NSW Food Authority—Science, survey and evaluations:
www.foodauthority.nsw.gov.au/aboutus/science

The Codex Alimentarius—International food standards:
www.fao.org/fao-who-codexalimentarius/en

US Department of Agriculture:
www.usda.gov

US Food and Drug Administration:
www.fda.gov

World Health Organization—Food safety:
www.who.int/foodsafety/en

FURTHER READING

Awika, J. (2017). Sorghum: its unique nutritional and health-promoting attributes. In J. Taylor & J. Awika (eds), *Gluten-Free Ancient Grains: Cereals, pseudocereals, and legumes—sustainable, nutritious, and health-promoting foods for the 21st century* (pp. 21–54). Amsterdam: Elsevier.

Baugreet, S., Hamill, R. M., Kerry, J. P. & McCarthy, S. N. (2017). Mitigating nutrition and health deficiencies in older adults: a role for food innovation? *Journal of Food Science*, 82(4), 848–55. doi:10.1111/1750-3841.13674

Botelho, R., Araújo, W. & Pineli, L. (2017). Food formulation and not processing level: conceptual divergences between public health and food science and technology sectors. *Critical Reviews in Food Science and Nutrition*, 1–12. doi:10.1080/10408398.2016.1209159

Brennan, C. S. (2015). The importance of food science and technology in modern society. *International Journal of Food Science and Technology*, 50(1), 1–2. doi:10.1111/ijfs.12747

Bustamante, M. Á., Fernández-Gil, M. P., Churruca, I., Miranda, J., Lasa, A., Navarro, V. & Simón, E. (2017). Evolution of gluten content in cereal-based gluten-free products: an overview from 1998 to 2016. *Nutrients*, 9(1). doi:10.3390/nu9010021

Cepanec, K., Vugrinec, S., Cvetković, T. & Ranilović, J. (2017). Potassium chloride-based salt substitutes: a critical review with a focus on the patent literature. *Comprehensive Reviews in Food Science and Food Safety*, 16(5), 881–94. doi:10.1111/1541-4337.12291

Fang, Z., Zhao, Y., Warner, R. D. & Johnson, S. K. (2017). Active and intelligent packaging in meat industry. *Trends in Food Science and Technology*, 61, 60–71. doi:10.1016/j.tifs.2017.01.002

Fellows, P. J. (2017). *Food Processing Technology Principles and Practice*, 4th edn. Duxford, UK: Woodhead Publishing.

Foegeding, E. A. (2015). Building on the first 75 years of food science. *Journal of Food Science*, 80(12), iv. doi:10.1111/1750-3841.12610

Gobbetti, M., Pontonio, E., Filannino, P., Rizzello, C. G., De Angelis, M. & Di Cagno, R. (2017). How to improve the gluten-free diet: the state of the art from a food science perspective. *Food Research International*, 110, 22–32. doi:10.1016/j.foodres.2017.04.010

Goldfein, K. R. & Slavin, J. L. (2015). Why sugar is added to food: food science 101. *Comprehensive Reviews in Food Science and Food Safety*, 14(5), 644–56. doi:10.1111/1541-4337.12151

Johnson, S., Clements, J., Villarino, C. & Coorey, R. (2017). Lupins: their unique nutritional and health-promoting attributes. In J. Taylor & J. Awika (eds), *The Gluten-free Ancient Grains: cereals, pseudocereals and legumes—sustainable, nutritious and health-promoting foods for the 21st century*. Amsterdam: Elsevier.

Kentish, S. & Feng, H. (2014). Applications of power ultrasound in food processing. *Annual Review of Food Science and Technology*, 5(1), 263–84. doi:10.1146/annurev-food-030212-182537

Lund, D. B. (2017). Who would have thought? The story of a food engineer. *Annual Review of Food Science and Technology*, 8, 1–20. doi:10.1146/annurev-food-030216-030225

Melini, F., Melini, V., Luziatelli, F. & Ruzzi, M. (2017). Current and forward-looking approaches to technological and nutritional improvements of gluten-free bread with legume flours: a critical review. *Comprehensive Reviews in Food Science and Food Safety*, 16(5), 1101–22. doi:10.1111/1541-4337.12279

Misra, N. N., Koubaa, M., Roohinejad, S., Juliano, P., Alpas, H., Inácio, R. S., ... Barba, F. J. (2017). Landmarks in the historical development of twenty first century food processing technologies. *Food Research International*, 97, 318–39. doi:10.1016/j.foodres.2017.05.001

Peng, X. & Yao, Y. (2017). Carbohydrates as fat replacers. *Annual Review of Food Science and Technology*, 8, 331–51. doi:10.1146/annurev-food-030216-030034

Rostami, K., Bold, J., Parr, A. & Johnson, M. W. (2017). Gluten-free diet indications, safety, quality, labels, and challenges. *Nutrients*, 9(8). doi:10.3390/nu9080846

Sadeghi, R., Rodriguez, R. J., Yao, Y. & Kokini, J. L. (2017). Advances in nanotechnology as they pertain to food and agriculture: benefits and risks. *Annual Review of Food Science and Technology*, 8, 467–92. doi:10.1146/annurev-food-041715-033338

Schaffer-Lequart, C., Lehmann, U., Ross, A. B., Roger, O., Eldridge, A. L., Ananta, E., ... Robin, F. (2017). Whole grain in manufactured foods: current use, challenges and the way forward. *Critical Reviews in Food Science and Nutrition*, 57(8), 1562–8. doi:10.1080/10408398.2013.781012

Valdramidis, V. P. & Koutsoumanis, K. P. (2016). Challenges and perspectives of advanced technologies in processing, distribution and storage for improving food safety. *Current Opinion in Food Science*, 12, 63–9. doi:10.1016/j.cofs.2016.08.008

van Buren, L., Dötsch-Klerk, M., Seewi, G. & Newson, R. S. (2016). Dietary impact of adding potassium chloride to foods as a sodium reduction technique. *Nutrients*, 8(4). doi:10.3390/nu8040235

van der Linden, E. & Foegeding, E. A. (2015). Food science needs for 2050. *Journal of Food Science*, 80(4), iii–iv. doi:10.1111/1750-3841.12619

Werner, B. G., Koontz, J. L. & Goddard, J. M. (2017). Hurdles to commercial translation of next generation active food packaging technologies. *Current Opinion in Food Science*, 16, 40–8. doi:10.1016/j.cofs.2017.07.007

Wickramarachchi, K. S., Sissons, M. J. & Cauvain, S. P. (2015). Puff pastry and trends in fat reduction: an update. *International Journal of Food Science and Technology*, 50(5), 1065–75. doi:10.1111/ijfs.12754

Wyrwa, J. & Barska, A. (2017). Innovations in the food packaging market: active packaging. *European Food Research and Technology*, 243(10), 1681–92. doi:10.1007/s00217-017-2878-2

Yu, H., Gibson, K. E., Wright, K. G., Neal, J. A. & Sirsat, S. A. (2017). Food safety and food quality perceptions of farmers' market consumers in the United States. *Food Control*, 79, 266–71. doi:10.1016/j.foodcont.2017.04.010

Zganiacz, F., Wills, R. B. H., Mukhopadhyay, S. P., Arcot, J. & Greenfield, H. (2017). Changes in the sodium content of Australian processed foods between 1980 and 2013 using analytical data. *Nutrients*, 9(5). doi:10.3390/nu9050501

REFERENCES

1. Institute of Food Technologists (2017). *IFT Feeding the Minds that Feed the World*. Retrieved from: www.ift.org.

2. *Macquarie Dictionary* (2017). Macmillan Publishers Australia. Retrieved from: www.macquariedictionary.com.au.

3. J. Awika (2017). Sorghum: its unique nutritional and health-promoting attributes. In J. Taylor & J. Awika (eds), *Gluten-Free Ancient Grains: Cereals, pseudocereals, and legumes—sustainable, nutritious, and health-promoting foods for the 21st century* (pp. 21–54). Amsterdam: Elsevier.

4. World Health Organization (2013). *Nutrition, Physical Activity and Obesity: United Kingdom of Great Britain and Northern Ireland*. Retrieved from: www.euro.who.int/__data/assets/pdf_file/0020/243335/United-Kingdom-WHO-Country-Profile.pdf?ua=1.

5. Australian Government Australian Institute of Health and Welfare (2017). *Australia's Health: Glossary*. Retrieved from: www.aihw.gov.au/reports-statistics/health-welfare-overview/australias-health/glossary.

6. Australian Government Department of Health and Ageing (2013). *Australian Dietary Guidelines*. Canberra: NHMRC.

7. A. Stefoska-Needham, E. J. Beck, S. K. Johnson & L. C. Tapsell (2015). Sorghum: an underutilized cereal whole grain with the potential to assist in the prevention of chronic disease. *Food Reviews International*, 31, 401–37.

8. Food and Agriculture Organization of the United Nations (2017). *Production: Sorghum*. Retrieved from: http://faostat.fao.org/site/339/default.aspx.

9. K. G. Duodu, J. R. N. Taylor, P. S. Belton & B. R. Hamaker (2003). Factors affecting sorghum protein digestibility. *Journal of Cereal Science*, 38(2), 117–31.

10. A. Yousif, D. Nhepera & S. Johnson (2012). Influence of sorghum flour addition on flat bread in-vitro starch digestibility, antioxidant capacity and consumer acceptability. *Food Chemistry*, 134, 880–7.

11 I. Khan, A. Yousif, S. K. Johnson & S. Gamlath (2013). Effect of sorghum flour addition on resistant starch content, phenolic profile and antioxidant capacity of durum wheat pasta. *Food Research International*, 54(1), 578–86. doi:http://dx.doi.org/10.1016/j.foodres.2013.07.059

12 I. Khan, A. M. Yousif, S. K. Johnson & S. Gamlath (2014). Effect of sorghum flour addition on in vitro starch digestibility, cooking quality, and consumer acceptability of durum wheat pasta. *Journal of Food Science*, 79(8), S1560–S1567. doi:10.1111/1750-3841.12542

13 R. Licata, J. Chu, S. Wang, R. Coorey, A. James, Y. Zhao & S. Johnson (2014). Determination of formulation and processing factors affecting slowly digestible starch, protein digestibility and antioxidant capacity of extruded sorghum–maize composite flour. *International Journal of Food Science & Technology*, 49(5), 1408–19. doi:10.1111/ijfs.12444

14 R. Licata, R. Coorey, Y. Zhao, J. Chu & S. Johnson (2015). Maximizing slowly digested starch in an expanded sorghum-maize extruded food using response surface methodology. *Starch—Stärke*, 67(3–4), 285–93. doi:10.1002/star.201400191

15 J. R. N. Taylor & M. N. Emmambux (2010). Developments in our understanding of sorghum polysaccharides and their health benefits. *Cereal Chemistry*, 87(4), 263–71. doi:10.1094/cchem-87-4-0263

16 J. M. Awika & L. W. Rooney (2004). Sorghum phytochemicals and their potential impact on human health. *Phytochemistry*, 65, 1199–221.

17 G. Wu, S. K. Johnson, J. F. Bornman, S. J. Bennett & Z. Fang (2017). Changes in whole grain polyphenols and antioxidant activity of six sorghum genotypes under different irrigation treatments. *Food Chemistry*, 214, 199–207. doi:10.1016/j.foodchem.2016.07.089

18 J. M. Awika, L. W. Rooney & R. D. Waniska (2004). Properties of 3-deoxyanthocyanins from sorghum. *Journal of Agricultural and Food Chemistry*, 52, 4388–94.

19 A. Stefoska-Needham, E. J. Beck, S. K. Johnson, J. Chu & L. C. Tapsell (2016). Flaked sorghum biscuits increase postprandial GLP-1 and GIP levels and extend subjective satiety in healthy subjects. *Molecular Nutrition and Food Research*, 60(5), 1118–28. doi:10.1002/mnfr.201500672

20 P. S. Belton & R. H. Taylor (2004). Sorghum and millets: protein sources for Africa. *Trends in Food Science & Technology*, 15, 94–8.

21 P. J. Fellows (2017). *Food Processing Technology Principles and Practice*, 4th edn. Duxford, UK: Woodhead Publishing.

22 A. C. Soria & M. Villamiel (2010). Effect of ultrasound on the technological properties and bioactivity of food: a review. *Trends in Food Science & Technology*, 21(7), 323–31. doi:https://doi.org/10.1016/j.tifs.2010.04.003

23 T. S. Awad, H. A. Moharram, O. E. Shaltout, D. Asker & M. M. Youssef (2012). Applications of ultrasound in analysis, processing and quality control of food: a review. *Food Research International*, 48(2), 410–27. doi:https://doi.org/10.1016/j.foodres.2012.05.004

24 M. J. W. Povey & T. J. Mason (1998). *Ultrasound in Food Processing*. London; New York: Blackie Academic & Professional.

25 J. O'Sullivan, B. Murray, C. Flynn & I. Norton (2016). The effect of ultrasound treatment on the structural, physical and emulsifying properties of animal and vegetable proteins. *Food Hydrocolloids*, 53, 141–54. doi:https://doi.org/10.1016/j.foodhyd.2015.02.009

26 C. Ozuna, I. Paniagua-Martínez, E. Castaño-Tostado, L. Ozimek & S. L. Amaya-Llano (2015). Innovative applications of high-intensity ultrasound in the development of functional food ingredients: production of protein hydrolysates and bioactive peptides. *Food Research International*, 77, 685–96. doi:https://doi.org/10.1016/j.foodres.2015.10.015

27 A. R. Jambrak, T. J. Mason, V. Lelas, Z. Herceg & I. L. Herceg (2008). Effect of ultrasound treatment on solubility and foaming properties of whey protein suspensions. *Journal of Food Engineering*, 86(2), 281–7. doi:https://doi.org/10.1016/j.jfoodeng.2007.10.004

28 A. R. Jambrak, V. Lelas, T. J. Mason, G. Krešić & M. Badanjak (2009). Physical properties of ultrasound treated soy proteins. *Journal of Food Engineering*, 93(4), 386–93. doi:https://doi.org/10.1016/j.jfoodeng.2009.02.001

29 İ. Gülseren, D. Güzey, B. D. Bruce & J. Weiss (2007). Structural and functional changes in ultrasonicated bovine serum albumin solutions. *Ultrasonics Sonochemistry*, 14(2), 173–83. doi:https://doi.org/10.1016/j.ultsonch.2005.07.006

30 C. Arzeni, O. E. Pérez & A. M. R. Pilosof (2012). Functionality of egg white proteins as affected by high intensity ultrasound. *Food Hydrocolloids*, 29(2), 308–16. doi:https://doi.org/10.1016/j.foodhyd.2012.03.009

31 S. Johnson, J. Clements, C. Villarino & R. Coorey (2017). Lupins: their unique nutritional and health-promoting attributes. In J. Taylor & J. Awika (eds), *The Gluten-free Ancient Grains: Cereals, pseudocereals and legumes—sustainable, nutritious and health-promoting foods for the 21st century*. Amsterdam: Elsevier.

32 C. Villarino, V. Jayasena, R. Coorey, S. Chakrabarti-Bell & S. Johnson (2016). Nutritional, health and technological functionality of lupin flour addition to baked products: benefits and challenges. *Critical Reviews in Food Science and Nutrition*, 56, 835–57. doi:10.1080/10408398.2013.814044

33 Food Standards Australia New Zealand (2017). Standard 1.2.3 Information requirements—warning statements, advisory statements and declarations. Retrieved from: www.legislation.gov.au/Details/F2017C00418.

34 L. Zhong, Z. Fang, M. Wahlqvist, G. Wu, J. Hodgson & S. Johnson (Under review). Seed coats of pulses as a food ingredient: characterization, processing, and applications. *Trends in Food Science & Technology*.

35 S. Mane, S. Johnson, M. Duranti, V. Pareek & R. Utikar (Under review). Lupin seed γ-conglutin: extraction and purification methods: a review. *Trends in Food Science & Technology*.

36 C. Villarino, V. Jayasena, R. Coorey, S. Chakrabarti-Bell & S. Johnson (2015). Optimization of formulation and process of Australian sweet lupin (ASL)-wheat bread. *LWT—Food Science and Technology*, 61(2), 359–67. doi:http://dx.doi.org/10.1016/j.lwt.2014.11.029

37 R. Belski, T. Mori, I. Puddey, S. Sipsas, R. Woodman, T. Ackland, … J. Hodgson (2011). Effects of lupin-enriched foods on body composition and cardiovascular disease risk factors: a 12-month randomized controlled weight loss trial. *International Journal of Obesity*, 35, 810–19.

38 Food Standards Australia New Zealand (2017). Australia New Zealand Food Standards Code—Schedule 4—Nutrition, health and related claims. Retrieved from: www.legislation.gov.au/Details/F2017C00711.

39 Food Standards Australia and New Zealand (2014). *Standard 3.2.2 Food Safety Practices and General Requirements*. Canberra: FSANZ.

40 M. Adams & M. Moss (2008). *Food Microbiology*. Cambridge, UK: The Royal Society of Chemistry.

41 Food Standards Australia and New Zealand (2017). *Essential Food Safety Practices. Cool and reheat food safely to the right temperatures*. Retrieved from: www.foodstandards.gov.au/consumer/safety/faqsafety/Pages/default.aspx.

42 J. Christian, M. Cole & T. Luba (2003). Food safety and testing in perspective. In A. Hocking (ed.), *Foodborne Microorganisms of Public Health Significance*, 6th edn (pp. 1–20). Waterloo Dc, NSW: AIFST Incorporated.

43 S. Jay, D. Davos, M. Dundas, E. Frankish & D. Lightfoot (2003). Salmonella. In H. AD (ed.), *Food Microorganisms of Public Health Significance* (pp. 207–66). Waterloo Dc, NSW: AIFST Incorporated.

44 The OzFoodNet Working Group (2012). *Monitoring the Incidence and Causes of Diseases Potentially Transmitted by Food in Australia: Annual Report of the OzFoodNet, 2010.* Canberra: Communicable Disease Intelligence.

45 R. Y. Murphy, L. K. Duncan, B. L. Beard & K. H. Driscoll (2003). D and z values of *Salmonella*, *Listeria innocua*, and *Listeria monocytogenes* in fully cooked poultry products. *Journal of Food Science*, 68(4), 1443–7. doi:10.1111/j.1365-2621.2003.tb09664.x

46 R. Y. Murphy, T. Osaili, L. K. Duncan & J. A. Marcy (2004). Thermal inactivation of *Salmonella* and *Listeria monocytogenes* in ground chicken thigh/leg meat and skin. *Poultry Science*, 83(7), 1218–25. doi:10.1093/ps/83.7.1218

47 V. K. Junej (2007). Thermal inactivation of *Salmonella* spp. in ground chicken breast or thigh meat. *International Journal of Food Science & Technology*, 42(12), 1443–8. doi:10.1111/j.1365-2621.2006.01362.x

48 E. Mani-López, H. S. García & A. López-Malo (2012). Organic acids as antimicrobials to control *Salmonella* in meat and poultry products. *Food Research International*, 45(2), 713–21. doi:https://doi.org/10.1016/j.foodres.2011.04.043

49 K. Karuppasamy, A. S. Yadav & G. K. Saxena (2015). Thermal inactivation of *Salmonella enteritidis* on chicken skin previously exposed to acidified sodium chlorite or tri-sodium phosphate. *Journal of Food Science and Technology*, 52(12), 8236–43. doi:10.1007/s13197-015-1922-0

50 International Commission on Microbiological Specifications for Foods (ICMSF) (1996). *Microorganisms in Foods 5: Microbiological specifications of food pathogens*, 1st edn. London: Blackie Academic and Professional.

51 M. A. Casadei, R. Ingram, E. Hitchings, J. Archer & J. E. Gaze (2001). Heat resistance of *Bacillus cereus*, *Salmonella typhimurium* and *Lactobacillus delbrueckii* in relation to pH and ethanol. *International Journal of Food Microbiology*, 63(1), 125–34. doi:https://doi.org/10.1016/S0168-1605(00)00465-7

52 M. R. Rodríguez, J. S. Aguirre, A. Lianou, J. Parra-Flores & G. D. García de Fernando (2016). Analysis of the variability in microbial inactivation by acid treatments. *LWT—Food Science and Technology*, 66, 369–77. doi:http://dx.doi.org/10.1016/j.lwt.2015.10.056

53 K. Karuppasamy, A. Yadav & G. Saxena (2015). Thermal inactivation of *Salmonella enteritidis* on chicken skin previously exposed to acidified sodium chlorite or tri-sodium phosphate. *Journal of Food Science and Technology*, 52(12), 8236–43. doi:10.1007/s13197-015-1922-0

54 A. Cook, R. Reid-Smith, R. Irwin, S. A. McEwen, V. Young & C. Ribble (2011). Antimicrobial resistance in *Campylobacter*, *Salmonella*, and *Escherichia coli* isolated from retail grain-fed veal meat from southern Ontario, Canada. *Journal of Food Protection*, 74(8), 1245–51. doi:10.4315/0362-028X.JFP-10-483

55 R. Wallace (2003). Campylobacter. In A. Hocking (ed.), *Food Microorganisms of Public Health Significance* (pp. 311–32). Waterloo Dc, NSW: AIFST Incorporated.

56 J. Jay, M. Loessner & D. Golden (2005). *Modern Food Microbiology*, 7th edn. New York: Springer Science Business Media Inc.

57 H. T. T. Nguyen, J. E. L. Corry & C. A. Miles (2006). Heat resistance and mechanism of heat inactivation in thermophilic *Campylobacters*. *Applied and Environmental Microbiology*, 72(1), 908–13. doi:10.1128/aem.72.1.908-913.2006

58 R. J. Stafford, P. J. Schluter, A. J. Wilson, M. D. Kirk, G. Hall, L. Unicomb, … I. McKay (2008). Population-attributable risk estimates for risk factors associated with *Campylobacter* infection, Australia. *Emerging Infectious Diseases*, 14(6), 895–901. doi:10.3201/eid1406.071008

59 L. E. Unicomb, K. E. Fullerton, M. D. Kirk & R. J. Stafford (2009). Outbreaks of *Campylobacteriosis* in Australia, 2001 to 2006. *Foodborne Pathogens and Disease*, 6(10), 1241–50. doi:10.1089/fpd.2009.0300

60 M. A. McCrackin, K. L. Helke, A. M. Galloway, A. Z. Poole, C. D. Salgado & B. P. Marriott (2016). Effect of antimicrobial use in agricultural animals on drug-resistant foodborne *Campylobacteriosis* in humans: a systematic literature review. *Critical Reviews in Food Science and Nutrition*, 56(13), 2115–32. doi:10.1080/10408398.2015.1119798

61 C.V. Asiegbu, S. L. Lebelo & F. T.Tabit (2016).The food safety knowledge and microbial hazards awareness of consumers of ready-to-eat street-vended food. *Food Control*, 60, 422–9. doi:10.1016/j.foodcont.2015.08.021

62 J. N. Sofos (2008). Challenges to meat safety in the 21st century. *Meat Science*, 78(1), 3–13. doi:https://doi.org/10.1016/j.meatsci.2007.07.027

63 T. Luangtongkum, B. Jeon, J. Han, P. Plummer, C. Logue & Q. Zhang (2009). *Antibiotic Resistance in Campylobacter: Emergence, transmission and persistence*. London: Future Medicine Ltd.

64 S. G. Goh, A.-H. Leili, C. H. Kuan, Y. Y. Loo, Y. L. Lye, W. S. Chang, ... R. Son. (2014). Transmission of *Listeria monocytogenes* from raw chicken meat to cooked chicken meat through cutting boards. *Food Control*, 37, 51–5. doi:https://doi.org/10.1016/j.foodcont.2013.08.030

65 A. Pal, T. P. Labuza & F. Diez-Gonzalez (2008). Shelf life evaluation for ready-to-eat sliced uncured turkey breast and cured ham under probable storage conditions based on *Listeria monocytogenes* and psychrotroph growth. *International Journal of Food Microbiology*, 126(1), 49–56. doi:https://doi.org/10.1016/j.ijfoodmicro.2008.04.028

66 E. M. Fox, P. G.Wall & S. Fanning (2015). Control of *Listeria* species food safety at a poultry food production facility. *Food Microbiology*, 51, 81–6. doi:https://doi.org/10.1016/j.fm.2015.05.002

67 Department of Health (2014). OzFoodNet Reports. Retrieved from: www.ozfoodnet.gov.au/internet/ozfoodnet/publishing.nsf/content/reports-1.

68 M. Elmali, H. Y. Can & H. Yaman (2015). Prevalence of *Listeria monocytogenes* in poultry meat. *Food Science and Technology*, 35(4), 672–5. doi:10.1590/1678-457X.6808

69 Y. Gu, X. Liang, Z. Huang & Y. Yang (2015). Outbreak of *Listeria monocytogenes* in pheasants. *Poultry Science*, 94(12), 2905–8. doi:10.3382/ps/pev264

70 P. S. Sutherland, D. W. Miles & D. A. Laboyrie (2003). Listeria monocytogenes. In: A. D. Hocking (ed.), *Food Microorganisms of Public Health Significance* (pp. 381–443).Waterloo Dc, NSW: AIFST Incorporated.

71 F. M. Steele & K. H.Wright (2001). Cooling rate effect on outgrowth of *Clostridium perfringens* in cooked, ready-to-eat turkey breast roasts. *Poultry Science*, 80(6), 813–16. doi:10.1093/ps/80.6.813

72 D. Olds, J. Sneed, A. Mendonca & B. Bisha (2006). Influence of four retail foodservice cooling methods on the behavior of *Clostridium perfringens* ATCC 10388 in turkey roasts following heating to an internal temperature of 74°C. Food Protection 69; 112-117.

73 M. Márquez- González, E. Cabrera- Díaz, M. D. Hardin, K. B. Harris, L. M. Lucia & A. Castillo (2012). Survival and germination of *Clostridium perfringens* spores during heating and cooling of ground pork. *Journal of Food Protection*, 75(4), 682–9. doi:10.4315/0362-028X.JFP-11-409

74 V. K. Juneja, D. A. Baker, H. Thippareddi, O. P. Snyder & T. B. Mohr (2013). Growth potential of *Clostridium perfringens* from spores in acidified beef, pork, and poultry products during chilling. *Journal of Food Protection*, 76(1), 65–71. doi:10.4315/0362-028X.JFP-12-289

75 Y. Xiao, A. Wagendorp, T. Abee & M. H. J. Wells-Bennik (2015). Differential outgrowth potential of *Clostridium perfringens* food-borne isolates with various cpe-genotypes in vacuum-packed ground beef during storage at 12°C. *International Journal of Food Microbiology*, 194, 40–5. doi:10.1016/j.ijfoodmicro.2014.11.008

76 A. M. Fazil, T. Ross, G. Paoli, P. Vanderlinde, P. Desmarchelier & A. M. Lammerding (2002). A probabilistic analysis of *Clostridium perfringens* growth during food service operations. *International Journal of Food Microbiology*, 73(2–3), 315–29. doi:10.1016/S0168-1605(01)00667-5

77 J. Bates & P. Bodnaruk (2003). *Clostridium perfringens*. In A. Hocking (ed.), *Food Microorganisms of Public Health Significance*, 6th edn (pp. 479–504). Waterloo Dc, NSW: AIFST Incorporated.

78 M. I. Myers, J. G. Sebranek, J. S. Dickson, A. M. Shaw, R. Tarté, K. R. Adams & S. Neibuhr (2016). Implications of decreased nitrite concentrations on *Clostridium perfringens* outgrowth during cooling of ready-to-eat meats. *Journal of Food Protection*, 79(1), 153–6. doi:10.4315/0362-028X.JFP-15-301

79 L. Huang & B. T. Vinyard (2016). Direct dynamic kinetic analysis and computer simulation of growth of *Clostridium perfringens* in cooked turkey during cooling. *Journal of Food Science*, 81(3), M692–M701. doi:10.1111/1750-3841.13202

80 I. Leguerinel & P. Mafart (2001). Modelling the influence of pH and organic acid types on thermal inactivation of *Bacillus cereus* spores. *International Journal of Food Microbiology*, 63(1–2), 29–34. doi:10.1016/S0168-1605(00)00394-9

81 C. B. Dalton, J. Gregory, M. D. Kirk, R. J. Stafford, R. Givney, E. Kraa & D. Gould (2004). Foodborne disease outbreaks in Australia, 1995 to 2000. *Communicable Diseases Intelligence Quarterly Report*, 28(2), 211–24.

82 I. Jenson & C. Moir (2003). *Bacillus cereus* and other *Bacillus* species. In A. Hocking (ed.), *Food Microorganisms of Public Health Significance*, 6th edn (pp. 455–78). Waterloo Dc, NSW: AIFST Incorporated.

83 D. M. McElroy, L. A. Jaykus & P. M. Foegeding (1999). A quantitative risk assessment for *Bacillus cereus* emetic disease associated with the consumption of Chinese-style rice. *Journal of Food Safety*, 19(3), 209–29. doi:10.1111/j.1745-4565.1999.tb00246.x

84 T. I. Pirhonen, M. A. Andersson, E. L. Jääskeläinen, M. S. Salkinoja-Salonen, T. Honkanen-Buzalski & T. M. L. Johansson (2005). Biochemical and toxic diversity of *Bacillus cereus* in a pasta and meat dish associated with a food-poisoning case. *Food Microbiology*, 22(1), 87–91. doi:https://doi.org/10.1016/j.fm.2004.04.002

85 H. Rosenquist, L. Smidt, S. R. Andersen, G. B. Jensen & A. Wilcks (2005). Occurrence and significance of *Bacillus cereus* and *Bacillus thuringiensis* in ready-to-eat food. *FEMS Microbiology Letters*, 250(1), 129–36. doi:10.1016/j.femsle.2005.06.054

86 C. Ankolekar & R. G. Labbé (2009). Survival during cooking and growth from spores of diarrheal and emetic types of *Bacillus cereus* in rice. *Journal of Food Protection*, 72(11), 2386–9. doi:10.4315/0362-028X-72.11.2386

87 J. Wang, T. Ding & D. H. Oh (2014). Effect of temperatures on the growth, toxin production, and heat resistance of *Bacillus cereus* in cooked rice. *Foodborne Pathogens and Disease*, 11(2), 133–7. doi:10.1089/fpd.2013.1609

88 S. D. Bennett, K. A. Walsh & L. H. Gould. (2013). Foodborne disease outbreaks caused by *Bacillus cereus*, *Clostridium perfringens*, and *Staphylococcus aureus*—United States, 1998–2008. *Clinical Infectious Diseases*, 57(3), 425–33. doi:10.1093/cid/cit244

89 A. Rajkovic, M. Kljajic, N. Smigic, F. Devlieghere & M. Uyttendaele (2013). Toxin producing *Bacillus cereus* persist in ready-to-reheat spaghetti Bolognese mainly in vegetative state. *International Journal of Food Microbiology*, 167(2), 236–43. doi:https://doi.org/10.1016/j.ijfoodmicro.2013.09.001

90 D. T. Mugadza & E. Buys (2018). *Bacillus* and *Paenibacillus* species associated with extended shelf life milk during processing and storage. *International Journal of Dairy Technology*, 71(2), 301–8. doi:10.1111/1471-0307.12474

91 J. Kadariya, T. C. Smith & D. Thapaliya (2014). *Staphylococcus aureus* and *Staphylococcal* food-borne disease: an ongoing challenge in public health. *BioMed Research International*, 2014. doi:10.1155/2014/827965

92 C. Stewart (2003). *Staphylococcus aureus* and *Staphylococcal* enterotoxins. In A. Hocking (ed.), *Foodborne Microorganisms of Public Health Significance*, 6th edn (pp. 359–79). Waterloo Dc, NSW: AIFST Incorporated.

93 L. Valik & F. Görner (1993). Growth of *Staphylococcus aureus* in pasta in relation to its water activity. *International Journal of Food Microbiology*, 20(1), 45–8. doi:https://doi.org/10.1016/0168-1605(93)90059-P

94 E. Durack, M. Alonso-Gomez & M. G. Wilkinson (2011). Growth of *Escherichia coli* and *Staphylococcus aureus* in individual lasagne layers and evidence for migration of *E. coli* throughout the product. *Food Control*, 22(12), 2000–5. doi:10.1016/j.foodcont.2011.05.019

95 E. A. Dlusskaya, L. M. McMullen & M. G. Gänzle (2011). Characterization of an extremely heat-resistant *Escherichia coli* obtained from a beef processing facility. *Journal of Applied Microbiology*, 110(3), 840–9. doi:10.1111/j.1365-2672.2011.04943.x

96 W. E. Hill, R. Suhalim, H. C. Richter, C. R. Smith, A. W. Buschow & M. Samadpour (2011). Polymerase chain reaction screening for *Salmonella* and enterohemorrhagic *Escherichia coli* on beef products in processing establishments. *Foodborne Pathogens and Disease*, 8(9), 1045–53. doi:10.1089/fpd.2010.0825

97 Food Standards Australia and New Zealand (2001). *Guidelines for the Microbiological Examination of Ready to Eat Foods*. Canberra: FSANZ.

98 National Notifiable Diseases Surveillance System (NNDSS) (2015). *Notifications for All Diseases by State & Territory and Year*. Canberra: Department of Health.

99 B. Eribo & M. Ashenafi (2003). Behavior of *Escherichia coli* O157:H7 in tomato and processed tomato products. *Food Research International*, 36(8), 823–30. doi:10.1016/S0963-9969(03)00077-2

100 OzFoodNet (2011). *Monitoring the Incidence and Causes of Diseases Potentially Transmitted by Food in Australia: Annual report of the OzFoodNet network, 2011*. Retrieved from: www.health.gov.au/internet/main/publishing.nsf/content/cda-cdi3902g.htm.

101 M. Kirk, K. Glass, L. Ford, K. Brown & G. Hall (2014). *Foodborne Illness in Australia: Annual incidence circa 2010*. Canberra: Department of Health.

102 Centers for Disease Control and Prevention (CDC) (2016). *Burden of Foodborne Illness: Findings*. Retrieved from: www.cdc.gov/foodborneburden/2011-foodborne-estimates.html.

103 World Health Organization (1946). *Constitution of the World Health Organization. New York, 22 July 1946*. Retrieved from: https://treaties.un.org/doc/Treaties/1948/04/19480407%2010-51%20PM/Ch_IX_01p.pdf.

104 Food and Agriculture Organisation of the United Nations. 2019. Sustainable Development Goals. Available at http://www.fao.org/sustainable-development-goals/en/.

105 Food and Agriculture Organisation of the United Nations. 2019. Food Safety and Quality. Available at http://www.fao.org/food/food-safety-quality/about-us/en/.

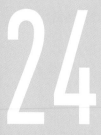

CHAPTER 24

FOOD, NUTRITION AND HEALTH: MOVING FORWARD

LINDA TAPSELL

CHAPTER OBJECTIVES

This chapter will enable the reader to:

- debate why food is fundamental to nutrition science and practice
- discuss new areas of knowledge emerging for practice
- examine global and regional challenges to dealing with food, nutrition and health.

KEY TERMS

Dietary intervention	Food environment
Food	Nutrition research

KEY POINTS

- Understanding and valuing food is fundamental to nutrition science and related practices.
- Nutrition research is becoming more integrative, enabling a better understanding of the actions of nutrients, and the effects of foods and dietary patterns on health.
- The double burden of malnutrition and obesity presents the global community with difficult challenges. These require integrating research on the health effects of foods, nutrients and dietary patterns with social, cultural and environmental factors.

OXFORD UNIVERSITY PRESS

INTRODUCTION

The study of food, nutrition and health is one of the most intriguing areas of science. It brings together an incredible range of disciplines and methodologies, but translates to something as everyday as eating a meal. It is not surprising then that 'nutrition experts' are aplenty and we encounter unintended consequences from simple messages such as 'eat less fat'. To quote one of Einstein's most famous sayings, 'everything should be made as simple as possible, but not simpler'. This is one of the greatest challenges for nutrition researchers and health practitioners alike.

Contemporary nutrition science developed alongside Western science, but it extends back to the ancient Greek philosophers, when Aristotle founded a scientific approach to the study of biology and Hippocrates made the significant proclamation: 'let food be thy medicine and medicine be thy food'. The delivery of essential compounds from food has long been recognised. The empirical tradition underlying the Hippocratic approach can be seen in major developments in eighteenth-century chemistry, which led to the identification of chemical compounds and the study of chemical reactions. These disciplined observational and experimental traditions carried through to what is often considered the origins of modern nutritional science. Thus the study of chemistry is one of the platforms for understanding nutrition.

See Chapter 1 on the origins of nutritional science.

Advances in many disciplines of science, including biochemistry, molecular biology, genetics and quantum physics, have ensured ongoing intrigue for today's scientists. For nutrition, this knowledge consolidates the view that molecules from food are powerful in terms of an individual's health, but at the same time the individual needs to be placed in perspective in terms of their unique genetic profile and their place in the ecology of the planet. To this end, we must see the spectrum of science that serves nutrition practice, from molecules to environments, and develop knowledge systems that enable this spectrum to hold together and deliver effectively.

Each of the chapters of this book has considered this integration of knowledge in terms of pathways to practice, with an emphasis on human health. Just as there are many locations in which nutrition knowledge can be employed, nutrition research utilises scientific methods from many disciplines. However, for research to have relevance to practice, studies should address questions that concern the population health needs, and research designs need to address these questions adequately.

Nutrition concerns the effect of food on health, so related health problems can be seen from the extremes of not enough quality food to too much food altogether. Both of these problems tend to be social in nature, relating to availability and access to food and an individual's ability to manage food consumption. Whether the knowledge concerns social or biological issues, it will reflect the **methodology** that has been applied to generate it. Ensuring transparency in research is critical to rigorous scientific endeavour. It involves clearly stating the inherent assumptions and limitations of the study design and methods applied, plus outlining the steps undertaken so that other researchers can repeat them and confirm the results. **Peer review** in science results in debates on methodology as much as results.

Methodology
the study of methods ensuring transparent use of methods in research; exposes assumptions about the type of knowledge generated, and the limitations of study designs.

Peer review
critical assessment of science by others with knowledge and experience in the stated field.

Developing conceptual positions on the biological effect of food on health is problematic, because it relies on different forms of knowledge arising from different study designs. For example, the discovery of a nutrient-driven pathway of action through carefully controlled animal model studies does not immediately translate to benefits to humans, but it does generate hypotheses that could be tested in trials involving humans. This process of **research translation** has many dimensions. It enables discrimination between effects of diet on

Research translation
the paths taken whereby new knowledge from research moves towards practice.

See Chapter 2 on dietary guidelines.

See Chapter 3 on the NRVs.

individuals under clinical care and the likely benefits to populations. The development of dietary guidelines and Nutrient Reference Values (NRVs) exemplifies the translation of research to create statements to inform the public and practitioners. In turn, these materials are referred to in various health promotion strategies, including the development of school canteen policies, food standards and regulations, and food service systems in aged care facilities. In a number of areas of nutrition, it is possible to see the path between basic concepts in science translated to practice domains and actions at a societal level (Table 24.1).

TABLE 24.1   INTERDEPENDENCE OF KNOWLEDGE IN NUTRITION-RELATED RESEARCH

Knowledge generation level	Category of research	Exemplars
Does it work in practice?	Implementation research	Evaluation of interventions Social research Health economics research
What are the effects in humans?	Randomised controlled trials	Epidemiology—clinical trials
Is there evidence of associations between factors in populations?	Observational studies	Epidemiology—cohort studies
Can the mechanisms be seen in humans?	Laboratory experiments	Human experimental studies
What are the likely mechanisms of action?	Laboratory experiments	Animal model studies
What are the molecular pathways?	Basic science laboratory studies	Research at molecular and cellular level

Integrative approach
piecing together knowledge in a defined and sequential manner to arrive at a position.

Integrative approaches are required to piece together the different forms of knowledge and establish evidence-based statements for practice at a particular point in time. Recall from previous chapters that clinical trials provide definitive evidence but are limited by design for testing effects of foods and diets. Cohort studies provide strong evidence of associations that may better serve the nature of food consumption and how health outcomes emerge. Research at the molecular level provides an understanding of the mechanisms at play and this knowledge can contribute to arguments of plausibility of the clinical and epidemiological observations.

Authoritative references such as dietary guidelines and food standards represent the best available knowledge at a particular point in time. They are revised at regular intervals because new knowledge is published in the scientific literature and needs to be incorporated. While this could be interpreted simply as 'changing our minds', it is the nature of science that inquiry is ongoing and positions are tested and re-tested. Some accepted hypotheses or parts thereof may fail to remain valid, so guidelines need to be updated with new or modified positions. Usually the changes to recommendations are subtle or nuanced because only certain aspects of the original position change, not the whole position. In addition, policy-related positions need to be implemented—for example, through healthcare services, guidelines for individual behaviour change and improvements in the food environment to better support health. Implementation calls for different types of research again, but it is all part of the integration of knowledge that occurs between nutrition science and practice.

STOP AND THINK

....

- Why does food lie at the heart of understanding nutrition?
- How will the challenges for nutrition science and practice develop in the future?
- What are the opportunities for working in different areas of food and nutrition science?

WHY WILL FOOD REMAIN FUNDAMENTAL TO NUTRITION SCIENCE AND PRACTICE?

Now, as always, consuming food is the first step in obtaining the combinations of nutrients and other food components required to build and maintain the functionality of the human system. Thus, for populations food will clearly remain fundamental to health. Associated research will extend from broad environmental issues to population health, food components and their actions or the development of nutrition interventions.

From an environmental perspective, the interdependence between humans and their food is not only reflected in their relative nutritional compositions but also in the environment in which they survive. Concerns for the future are adequate water to grow food, the micronutrient status of soils in which plant foods are grown, the chemicals that are added in the production and processing of food, and the impact of food waste (including water and nutrients) on ecological systems. Understanding the increasingly complex systems of food production and distribution is an important start (Table 24.2). Dietary guidelines, which distil the scientific evidence of the relationships between health outcomes and the consumption of foods, may soon be evaluated for environmental impacts [1; 2], and new methodologies for doing so will expand the capabilities of the nutrition scientist. From a preventive health perspective, the move from a nutrient to a food focus for populations is likely to continue, as a greater appreciation of the food matrix evolves [3; 4]. Nevertheless, while this is a simple message, the implementation is not simple.

TABLE 24.2   EXAMPLES OF EMERGING FOOD ISSUES FOR NUTRITION SCIENCE

Food issue	Research issue
Food versus supplements	Safe consumption levels
	Evidence of effects of dietary patterns versus supplements
	Clinical trials versus observational studies
Food composition	Changing nature of food
	Processed versus unprocessed foods
	Protective food components (e.g. flavonoids)
	Deleterious food components (e.g. advanced glycation end-products)
Food fortification	Monitoring effects and levels of dietary insufficiency
Food allergy	Establishing evidence for policies and guidelines

Food versus supplements

The value of foods rather than supplements in delivering nutrients to the population remains a significant issue. For example, unlike in healthy dietary patterns, a recent meta-analysis of 49 trials pooling together nearly 300,000 participants found insufficient evidence to support the use of nutrient supplements (including vitamins, minerals and fatty acids) in the primary prevention of incidence of cardiovascular disease (CVD) and cancer, and cause-specific death [5]. This also comes with expressions of concern for the use of supplements, particularly in children and in consideration of potential health risks [6]. On the other hand, a meta-analysis of 19 prospective studies and optimal consumption of 12 food groups demonstrated reduced risk of all-cause mortality with the consumption of wholegrains, vegetables, fruit, nuts and fish [7], showing clear health benefits from food consumption. The relationships in this study were non-linear (for vegetables, fruits, nuts and dairy), but this may reflect the limitations of food categorisation in observational research. Nevertheless, reliance on observational studies for food–health relationships are likely to remain, and are arguably more relevant given the nature of food consumption and the time required to see effects.

≫ RESEARCH AT WORK

HERBS AND SPICES: CULINARY FOODS OR SUPPLEMENTS?

Herbs and spices tend to lie somewhere between a food and a supplement. Although they originate from plant foods, their culinary use implies they tend not to be eaten as single foods, and some aspects of their cultural use suggests they may be taken as supplements. The latter is not surprising given that many pharmaceutical agents have been developed from plants, while the former acknowledges their role in healthy cuisines. However, their consumption may be overlooked in reductionist studies that focus on foods groups consumed in large quantities, rather than the cuisines characterised by the use of herbs and spices.

Given the connection with pharmacology, research on the molecular effects of chemicals delivered by herbs and spices can be found in quality scientific literature, including cutting-edge areas such as the isolation and analysis of microbial function of spice extracts [8]. A recent systematic analysis involving the integration of spice-phytochemical–disease data identified bioactive spice phytochemicals and their potential relationships with health [9]. Cinnamon, for example, has been investigated for its glucose-lowering properties, and alongside this is research examining its safety of use [10]. The distinction needs to be made between controlled doses of spices as supplements (e.g. saffron as a novel treatment for depression [11]) versus the culinary use of spices in dietary interventions. An example of the latter is the use of herbs and spices to reduce salt intake as an intervention for lowering blood pressure. In one study, for example, where mechanisms were also considered, the flavour of spices was seen to influence salt sensitivity and preference, suggesting it may be a particularly effective approach to influencing salt reduction behavioural strategies [12].

Research on herbs and spices occupies an interesting space for nutrition research, extending from molecular understandings of chemical components to supplemental, food, dietary pattern and behavioural studies. The evidence base for practice will vary depending on the questions asked, but the demands on the quality of science remain the same as for other foods (and supplements).

Food composition

While food may remain at the centre of health debates, the composition of food is constantly changing. The nature of food processing continues to emerge as an important consideration in nutritional epidemiology [13], which is dependent on accurate food composition databases. Staple foods can be modified with added ingredients during manufacturing, making them dissimilar to the original food category referred to in dietary guidelines. Indeed, preventive health research has shown that cooking at home may be associated with greater compliance with dietary guidelines [14].

New food composition analyses on unprocessed staple foods (such as flavonoids in fruit) is highly informative. For example, one study of around 45,000 men showed that higher intakes of fruit-based flavonoids (anthocyanins and flavanones) were associated with lower risk of non-fatal heart attack and ischaemic stroke [15]. This analysis based on data from a primary food component added support for the health benefits of fruit consumption. Rather than dichotomise the argument around foods versus nutrients, this type of analysis shows how research on food components can be applied to better understand the effects of food. Given the increasing evidence to support plant-based diets, research on the phytochemical composition [16] and the actions of phytochemicals [17] are increasingly supporting research on both the production and consumption of plant-based foods.

» RESEARCH AT WORK

THE RISE OF DIETARY FLAVONOIDS IN STUDIES OF AGEING

Flavonoids are important components of plant-based (carbohydrate-rich) foods. They have emerged in research as important dietary components in slowing a number of degenerative pathways associated with ageing, including age-related cognitive decline, macular degeneration and type 2 diabetes. The literature in this area is rapidly expanding as we better understand how flavonoids work, how they are delivered into the gut and then modified by the body, and their relationships with functional health outcomes.

New research on dementia and age-related cognitive decline suggests that the mechanisms for effects of flavonoids are associated with the function of neurones in the brain. These include modulating signalling pathways associated with synaptic activity, reducing neuro-inflammation and promoting vascular effects that help stimulate new nerve cell growth in parts of the brain associated with memory. There are also suggestions of interactions with the gut microbiota and controlling effects on proteins implicated in brain degeneration [18]. This knowledge appears to be translating across to animal model studies and it now needs to be adequately translated into human studies [19]. More clinical studies on flavonoid-rich diets and cognitive decline are anticipated.

Epidemiological research supports the growing body of evidence. In Australia, researchers from the Blue Mountains Eye study (using a cohort of 2856 adults residing west of Sydney) found that dietary intake of flavonoids had an independent and protective association with the likelihood of having age-related macular degeneration. Interestingly, a reduced risk was found after 15 years in those reporting consumption of at least one orange a day compared with those who never consumed oranges at baseline [20]. On a much broader scale, a meta-analysis and systematic review of prospected cohort studies published the same year (2018) showed that diets rich in polyphenols (in particular flavonoids) were inversely associated with the risk of type 2 diabetes. This research also examined the dose–response relationship, which helps to derive recommendations for a protective level of intake. As most of the associations were non-linear, further research was suggested in this area [21].

See Chapter 4 for a discussion on flavonoids.

The study of flavonoids demonstrates the relative contribution and interrelationship between mechanistic, animal model, clinical and epidemiological research in exposing the effects of food components, and ultimately foods and dietary patterns that support healthy ageing. The shift towards prevention of disease and maintaining functionality is also apparent, highlighting the position of nutrition in health and demonstrating the significance of rigorous nutrition science practices.

Not all the components of foods are naturally occurring or protect health, and some, such as dietary advanced glycation end-products (AGEs), are deleterious and require toxicological studies. AGEs are pathogenic glycotoxins formed in foods that are heat processed in combination with fat and sugar, a feature of Western dietary patterns known to be deleterious to health [22]. It is well to remember that just as food delivers components for health, there will always be negative elements that need to be understood, researched and monitored.

Food fortification

Food fortification remains integral to public health interventions given evidence of nutrient insufficiency in the population. For example, introducing greater access to folate in the Australian population occurred through the fortification of a staple food (bread) and involved many stakeholders in the food system [23]. It has been a great success, reducing the incidence of neural tubal defects by 30%, and more in the Indigenous population [24].

Food allergy

Food allergy continues to emerge as an issue of public health significance. The rising incidence of food allergy has implications for institutional food availability, such as in child care centres, and action relies on sound scientific research. For example, recently it has been shown that, contrary to the common practice of avoiding allergenic foods (namely, eggs and peanuts) in the first year of life, earlier exposure to these foods is associated with reduced risk of allergy [25]. The research has supported evidence-based statements for introducing solid foods to infants when they are ready (but not before four months), when they should also be offered allergenic foods including peanut butter, cooked egg, dairy and wheat products (see https://foodallergyresearch.org.au). The area of food allergy research is constantly developing, particularly alongside research in immunology. This means position papers will need to be consistently updated as new research informs the area, and practitioners will need to keep up with current knowledge.

>> **CASE 24.1**

SALT IN FOOD

There is a need to reduce sodium intakes in the diet, but the realities of reducing population sodium consumption demands close monitoring of food composition, in particular of manufactured foods. Just before the 2017 festive season, a collaboration of the George Institute for Global Health, the Heart Foundation and Victoria Health launched a report on the salt content of 849 chilled dip products and 1285 cracker product lines found in major food stores in Australia [26] within their Unpack the Salt campaign (www.unpackthesalt.com.au). The report noted that while the salt content of chips had reduced by 16% during that time, it had increased by 14% in dips. Olive, seafood and aioli dips had the highest levels, whereas dips based on vegetables, such as hummus, guacamole, eggplant and spinach, contained the least. A serve of the most salty dip (2.4 g/serve) and most salty cracker (0.5 g/serve) would take up half the targeted minimum intake of salt, leaving little for natural healthy foods.

> See Chapter 11 on reducing sodium intake.

- What does this case study expose about single foods when trying to achieve target levels of nutrients that are in oversupply?
- What is the significance of these foods in everyday meal planning and in festive seasons?
- How does research on food composition and the diet–disease relationship translate to practice in this case study?

STOP AND THINK

- What different aspects of food need to be understood in working effectively in nutrition promotion?
- How is food technology implicated in the development of a nutritious food supply?
- What are the challenges for governments and food and health agencies in protecting the health of populations through food and dietary intervention?

WHAT ARE SOME OF THE NEW AREAS OF KNOWLEDGE INFORMING PRACTICE?

The nutrition knowledge base is founded on ongoing research, regardless of whether the research questions arise from the laboratory or practice contexts. A better understanding of the diet–disease relationship continues to unfold. From a biological perspective, new dimensions to this understanding come from such areas as genetics, metabolomics, immunology (including the role of the gut) and further exploration in food composition. New areas of knowledge that may inform practice are multiple, and may in time create more formal nutrition specialisations. Drawing on the contents of the previous chapters, some of the emerging areas are discussed below (see also Table 24.3).

TABLE 24.3   EXAMPLES OF EMERGING KNOWLEDGE FOR PRACTICE

Topic	Research issues
Dietary patterns	Management and analysis of large data sets Food patterns versus cuisines in varying populations and settings
Energy, macronutrients	Understanding the mechanics of energy balance Clarifying the pathways of fuel utilisation Impact of macronutrients on body composition across the lifecycle
Food sources of macronutrients	Relative impact of macronutrients versus food sources of macronutrients
Nutrigenomics	Individual requirements for and responses to nutrients New research technologies in 'omics'
Gut microbiome	Effects of food intake on microbiome and the consequences New research technologies for the study the diet-gut-brain interrelationship

Dietary patterns and health

Epidemiological research

studies of the relationship between environmental factors (such as diet) and health or disease in populations.

Epidemiological research and experimental research have made significant contributions to understanding the diet–health relationship and will continue to do so, but the challenge is to integrate this knowledge. This is particularly relevant to developing health-related policies and guidelines for practice, as well as priorities for further research. The term 'big data' is often referred to, and managing this requires not only more sophisticated computational technology but also advances in biostatistics.

A shift in focus from nutrients to foods can also be seen. For example, a recent complex analysis of dietary surveys conducted in large samples from Western populations showed that consumption of both specific foods (such as nuts, fish and vegetables) and specific nutrients (such as sodium and fatty acids) are implicated in deaths from heart disease, stroke and type 2 diabetes [27]. The ability to detect these associations may also reflect the range of consumption levels of these foods and nutrients (high to low) across populations. As nutrients are consumed in foods and foods are consumed in dietary patterns, these analyses still reduce dietary behaviour to individual food choices. How these foods and nutrients combine in reality to meals consumed still needs to be understood.

Studies of food combinations in established cuisine patterns of known nutritional quality demonstrate favourable associations with biomarkers of cardiometabolic and endocrine-related risk [28]. However, very large samples are required and confounding can still limit the ability to expose the relationship. For example, in one meta-analysis, after adjustments for body mass index (BMI), the DASH diet pattern and a Mediterranean diet score were only associated with lower triglyceride concentrations rather than a full set of risk factors [28]. Studies need to be replicated in a number of different contexts, but as food combinations are influenced by cuisine factors in different regions, much more work may be required in translating dietary principles across to different settings. For example, translating the effects of the Mediterranean diet tested in Spain for the PREDIMED study may require a different set of changes to food choice in the United States than were required for the PREDIMED study sample [29].

≫ RESEARCH AT WORK

EVIDENCE-BASED LIBRARIES

Despite consistency in the evidence defining healthy dietary patterns, there are gaps in the understanding of dietary effects. Ongoing research is still required, for example, on nuances of the diet–heart disease relationship. To assist practitioners, professional groups publish regular reviews summarising the evidence to date and providing continuing professional development— for example, the Academy of Nutrition and Dietetics produces regular publications from the Evidence Analysis Laboratory [30–32]. The American College of Cardiology (ACC) review on diet and cardiovascular disease highlights the differences in the type of research available and the translation to clinical recommendations [33]. Presenting the uneven platform of research also helps to identify emerging areas for investigation (see Table 24.4). These topics will keep this area open for science for some time.

TABLE 24.4 FOODS INCLUDED IN ACC CLINICAL RECOMMENDATIONS

Recommended use of food	Nature of research reviewed
FREQUENT	
Antioxidant-rich fruits and vegetables	RCTs/observational studies
Green leafy vegetables	Meta-analyses, observational studies
Protein from plant sources	Observational /prospective studies
IN MODERATION	
Nuts	RCTs, meta-analyses, observational studies
Olive oil	RCTs
Canola oil	RCTs, meta-analyses
Sunflower oil	No RC, observational studies for CVD
AVOID	
Dietary pattern combining fried food, eggs, processed meats, and sugar-sweetened beverages (Southern diet pattern)	Prospective studies
Palm oil	RCTs and observational studies

Abbreviations: CVD: cardiovascular disease; RCT: randomised controlled trial.

Source: A. M. Freeman, P. B. Morris, N. Barnard, C. B. Esselstyn, E. Ros, A. Agatston, P. Kris-Etherton (2017). Trending cardiovascular nutrition controversies. *Journal of the American College of Cardiology*, 69(9), 1172–87. doi:10.1016/j.jacc.2016.10.086

Energy and macronutrient requirements

With obesity remaining a major public health issue, research on energy balance and fuel utilisation remains fundamental. At the centre of this lies debate about mechanistic models of obesity. One such debate is the 'calories in, calories out' principle versus the 'carbohydrate-insulin model' of obesity [34; 35]. Research on energy balance and fuel utilisation is ongoing, so arguments about the complexities of neuroendocrine mechanisms that regulate energy homeostasis versus the relative significance of carbohydrate intake and insulin action can be expected. There remain no quick fixes or magic diets. The translation to practice lies in how both the calorie value of the diet and the type and amount of carbohydrate-rich foods consumed might best be managed. In addition, while research from both these areas has been informative for adjusting energy intakes during weight loss and choosing more appropriate plant foods, dietary advice still has to address other issues related to the individual's weight-loss environment, including social and psychological factors.

See Chapters 4 and 7 on energy balance and fuel utilisation.

As with carbohydrate metabolism, the issue of dietary fat also remains fundamental, including the positioning of fat-rich foods in the diet. The mechanisms by which fatty acids act in the body, particularly in relation to effects on cholesterol levels, insulin action, fat oxidation and inflammatory pathways, have been well researched to date. While fatty acids are required by the body, high intakes of saturated fat appear deleterious, and these negative associations are supported by human studies in Western populations. It is not saturated fat *per se*, however, that is potentially deleterious, but the relative amount. A point that is often missed is that guidance on the level of saturated fat relates to

See Chapter 5 on fats and lipids.

Total dietary fat
the percentage of energy contributed by fat from all foods consumed in the diet.

total dietary fat. Arguments have rightly been made for the inclusion of individual foods, such as nuts, that contain some saturated fats, but higher amounts of the desired and less available unsaturated fats, or full-fat dairy foods that contain higher amounts of saturated fat but in the company of multiple essential nutrients. The limitation of focusing on individual foods and nutrients is clearly problematic, but again the issue should not be reduced to a dualistic argument. The level of single nutrients in foods, and the overall nutrient value of single foods and of total diets must be considered together.

Likewise, research on dietary protein remains fundamental in nutrition science, particularly given the significance of delivering nitrogen to the body. There are numerous examples of cutting-edge areas in research in this area. For example, with the ageing population significant interest is now emerging in how dietary protein is supporting healthy ageing; in particular, in preventing the loss of muscle mass and strength. Research on the type of amino acids delivered in protein-rich foods spread across the day will throw light on the mechanisms of satiety and of muscle repair that will have significant implications for dietary strategies.

Food sources of macronutrients

As research has shifted to studies at the food level, questions have been asked whether nutrients have the same effects if delivered from different foods. The interdependence between nutrients, foods and whole diets is well demonstrated in the case of saturated fat. If enough energy is available it may be possible, for example, to include high-fat dairy foods and keep the percentage of energy from saturated fat low with judicious choices of other foods. The research in this area continues to contribute to this understanding. For example, an analysis of the PREDIMED study found that while baseline intakes of saturated fatty acids were not associated with type 2 diabetes, the yearly uptake of saturated fat was associated with higher risk, particularly from butter and cheese (but not yoghurt) [36]. Because total diet is central to this question, the differences may also reflect the relative amount of these foods consumed and the combinations of foods consumed. The detection of a relationship should be considered seriously, however, because blunting influences of the total diet make it difficult to expose any association. Studies such as these continue to support current recommendations to choose low-fat dairy products and limit intakes of butter. This advice, however, is formulated bearing in mind the other foods concurrently consumed in the diet. High dietary saturated fat appears to remain a problem where cardiovascular disease is prevalent.

The monitoring of dietary interventions is part of the ongoing research in this area. Margarines have been introduced to replace butter, providing more omega-6 fatty acids in the food supply. This has presented further questions, particularly as omega-6 and omega-3 fatty acids share similar pathways. Again, mechanistic studies remain important in clarifying this position, but they need to be considered together with observational studies. For example, given mechanistic understandings of dietary fat and insulin action [37], a recent international cohort study of biomarkers of omega-6 fatty acids in almost 40,000 adults found circulating linoleic acid may be protective against type 2 diabetes [38]. A further study showed that dietary fat may modulate a gene variant influencing glucose tolerance in type 2 diabetes [39]. From the study of dietary fat, this research is indicative of the move to focus on individual variations in responses to dietary composition and thereby the need for nutrigenomic dietary counselling.

Nutrigenomics
the study of how the supply of nutrients influences genetic expression.

Nutritional Genomics

Nutrigenomics is a cutting-edge area of science and is providing significant opportunity for better health through 'precision nutrition', or by targeting of diets based on an understanding of individual variation. The concept of nutrigenomics acknowledges that nutrients, foods and dietary patterns influence disease risk by direct effects on metabolic processes. In the first instance, nutrients can alter the expression of genes and influence pathways involving genetic products that emerge further down the cascade of genetic expression (e.g. **proteome** and **metabolome**). Diet can influence the extent to which genetic polymorphisms are expressed. In other words, nutrigenomics acknowledges that health and disease are states in which diet acts as a powerful agent in the gene–environment interaction [40]. This is particularly the case in **epigenetic** stages of life, which can have profound influences on future health. Having said that, depending on their genetic profile, one person may have greater requirements for a specific nutrient than another (**nutrigenetics**).

TRY IT YOURSELF

Search quality medical and nutrition science journals for studies of diet and gene interactions. Identify nutrients, foods and dietary patterns that appear to be implicated. Discuss the extent of research that may be required before this knowledge can reasonably contribute to integrated reviews of the evidence for practice.

Proteome
the profile of proteins produced from genetic expression.

Metabolome
the profile of compounds produced from the action of a metabolic process or pathway.

Epigenetic events
stages when gene functions are established.

Nutrigenetics
the study of how genetic profile influences requirements for nutrients.

Developments in the 'omics' have provided opportunities for better assessment of dietary intakes and dietary requirements. Applying nutritional metabolomics has introduced new potential biomarkers of dietary intake [41; 42]. In addition to measures associated with transport and storage of nutrients in the body, metabolomics enables a more dynamic view of nutrients in action. This new technology is already adding another dimension to reviews of science required in determining nutrient reference standards [43].

Importantly, 'omics' research technology can assist with greater integration of knowledge when assessing nutritional status. This new way of thinking takes us from reductionist views based on single nutrients to a more complex systems-based approach that is more reflective of the human body and the dynamic interrelationships that exist between nutrients alongside basic functions such as growth and host defence. For example, using proteomics in a study of undernourished children in Nepal, researchers were able to identify proteins associated with lean mass and the assessment of growth in these children. They were also able to put into perspective the status of treatment with associated micronutrients [44]. In another piece of research, this group was able to identify a plasma proteome comprising functional biomarkers that reflected defensive measures (homeostatic and induced inflammatory responses) as well as the metabolism of nutrients and tissue repair. This set of proteins gave an integrated view of the state of inflammation at a point in time that involved a wide range of nutrients, their transport through the body and their actions [45]. This research has the potential to take nutritional diagnostics and treatment to a new level.

The principles behind this more dynamic and integrative understanding of human nutrition can be seen in other areas of health, such as bone health. Bone is a living tissue with multiple nutrients coming in and going out as the human organism lives through each day. There is a focus in research and healthcare on certain nutrients such as calcium and vitamin D, possibly because intakes of these nutrients may be at risk due to inadequate dietary sources. Moving to the study of dietary patterns ensures that the 'bigger picture' of multiple nutrients in combination is not missed.

See Chapter 9 on research into vitamin D.

See Chapter 11 on research into calcium.

Gut microbiome

The profile of microbes present in the gut (gut microbiome) and their metabolic products (metabolome) is pushing the boundaries of knowledge in human health. A significant area moving forward in nutrition science is the appreciation of the gut as the 'engine room' in metabolic health (Table 24.5). Vast numbers of microbes coexist in the human body—the statistic often cited is that bacterial genes outnumber human genes by over 200 to 1. This sets the stage for a great deal of scientific investigation and increased demands for interdisciplinary research in nutrition, particularly with microbiology and immunology.

TABLE 24.5   EXAMPLES OF BACTERIA IN THE HUMAN GUT

Genus	Phylum	Comment
Lactobacillus	*Firmicutes*	Used in fermented milk
Ruminococcus	*Firmicutes*	Digest resistant starches
Escherichia	*Proteobacteria*	*E. coli is* pathogenic
	Bacteroides	Very abundant in human gut

Biological classification systems need to be understood; for the domain of bacteria, categorisation is phylum, class, order, family and genus, much of which is reflected in the name. A genus, such as *Lactobacillus* (belonging to the *Firmicutes* phylum category) can have many different species with diverse actions. As the name indicates, these bacteria produce lactic acid from glucose. *Lactobacillus* strains are used in yoghurts and fermented milk products. As these products deliver bacteria they are often referred to as *probiotics*.

Omics technology is also used in the study of the gut microbiome. It enables identification of the molecules produced by the actions of bacteria and their action on gene expression (hence the interest in bacterial genes alongside human genes). Of specific interest to nutrition is the study of which fuel sources are used by gut microbes. The microbiome interacts with all macronutrients and has particular relevance to a number of micronutrients. The nutrition of the microbiome is itself an area of interest, with nitrogen also being a limiting nutrient, and dietary energy accessibility shared between host and bacteria. Nutrition lies at the heart of this symbiotic relationship.

The effects of dietary fibre are studied intensely because it escapes to the large bowel, providing a fuel source for gut bacteria, which then produce short chain fatty acids (e.g. acetate, butyrate and propionate). The study of dietary fibre is very sophisticated, with major global efforts in determining categories based on structure and function. Many different types of dietary fibre exist, but given the utilisation of some by bacteria that may produce health benefits, they can be referred to as *prebiotics*. Examples are in fructo oligosaccharides (FOS), galacto oligosaccharides (GOS) and inulin. There are commercial opportunities in the development of new fibres targeting the modulation of the gut microbiome to better support health.

Metabolomics is of particular value in understanding the role of the gut microbiome in mechanisms associated with obesity. For example, new research has shown that dietary patterns may influence the production of the metabolite known as CD14, which is produced by macrophages on exposure to endotoxins [46]. This biomarker is indicative of gut hyper-permeability, which is now considered to be part of the pathophysiology of entrenched obesity [47]. This research adds a novel dimension to the evidence associated with dietary patterns

See Chapter 4 on dietary fibre.

See Chapter 7 on entrenched obesity.

and health. As gastric surgery takes hold as a procedure for obesity treatment, 'omics' technology is also throwing light on implications for the gut microbiome. For example, in one study using multi-omic approaches, significant differences were found in the microbiomes of morbidly obese patients who had undergone different forms of gastric surgery, and these differences were mirrored in their metabolomes [48]. Understanding the interrelationships between individual genetic profiles, the gut environment and dietary patterns will extend the knowledge underpinning nutrition-related practice in the future (Table 24.6).

TABLE 24.6 GUT MICROBIOME: FUNCTIONS AND HEALTH CONSIDERATIONS

Functions	Health considerations
Fermenting non-digested food	Cognition and brain health
Vitamin, secondary bile acid, neurotransmitter synthesis	Obesity and insulin resistance
Pathogen displacement	Intestinal health/disease

» RESEARCH AT WORK

FAECAL SAMPLING AND THE GUT MICROBIOME

New technologies are constantly under development for studying effects associated with the gut microbiome [49]. Given the huge numbers of microbes, the dynamic nature of the environment under study and genetic potential of both host (human) and bacteria, it represents a real scientific challenge. A collaborative team led by scientists in the Twin Research and Genetic Epidemiology Department in the United Kingdom has shown that faecal metabolic profiling is a novel tool that can be used to examine links between the composition of the microbiome, the (genetically expressed) phenotypes of humans and heritable complex traits. The researchers examined 1116 products of metabolism (metabolites) delivered in the faeces from 786 individuals from the TwinsUK study. They found the profile of these metabolites (the metabolome) largely reflected the composition of the gut microbe community, explaining about two-thirds of the variance in this population. A strong association was found with visceral fat mass, confirming the emerging knowledge on the impact of the gut environment on abdominal obesity. This is a good example of how new technologies provide breakthroughs for advancing nutrition research. We can expect to see many more studies of the diet–disease relationship that include faecal sampling to better understand the complexities of a science that is anything but simple. The outcomes will contribute to more precise implementation of dietary strategies that support health.

STOP AND THINK

- How have recent developments in scientific technologies pushed the boundaries for understanding the roles of food in health and disease?
- What will be required for evidence-based reviews of effects of food on health, given the broader scientific landscape addressing this topic?
- What are the implications for education in the discipline of nutrition science?

WHAT ARE THE CURRENT GLOBAL CHALLENGES FOR FOOD AND NUTRITION SCIENCE?

At the most basic level, the main issue for nutrition is access to food, and this still varies across the globe. The quality and quantity of available food has also changed, bringing its own challenges. In the 1950s, observations were made between dietary fat intake, cholesterol levels and coronary heart diseases [50]. This led to dietary guidance for reducing saturated fat intake and replacing it with food sources of unsaturated fats. Food innovation followed, representing a shift towards developing foods for a specific preventive health purpose. The concept of 'functional foods' emerged, with rising consumer recognition that food formulation could have significant impacts on health. Table margarine (or spreads) appeared as one of the first of these foods targeting the dietary ratio of polyunsaturated fats to saturated fats by serving as a replacement food for butter. This was also commercially feasible because sandwiches formed a key component of the Australian cuisine. These new foods required marketing based on health claims that were predicated on scientific evidence and regulated by governments. One of the problems in focusing on individual foods with strong marketing support, however, is the loss of a sense of the total diet, and thereby total energy intake. The lack of attention to total dietary energy has been implicated in the rising prevalence of obesity in the population. Paradoxically, this health problem has occurred alongside a greater recognition of the value of food to human health. There is a better appreciation now that foods deliver more than just energy—they deliver a multitude of compounds with specific actions that influence the ability to live well for longer.

There is an increasing need for integrative research and practice, where information from a range of scientific disciplines is connected to solve nutrition-related problems at the individual, population and environmental levels. The study of dietary patterns across different regions and in various populations is a first step. Another is the application of nutrigenomics and metabolomics to develop more precise dietary interventions at the clinical level. Meanwhile, global expansion in the production and trade in food and the evolution of health services demand a focus on key priorities for action.

See Chapter 21 on the UN Sustainable Development Goals.

In 2017, an independent collaboration of poverty management and global development stakeholders produced the peer-reviewed Global Nutrition Report, providing an account of the world's nutrition [51]. This comprehensive report links the United Nations' global Sustainable Development Goals with an analysis of nutrition strategies and targets, including information about country expenditure on nutrition. It confirms that the double burden of obesity and undernutrition relates to nearly every country, and that greater attention to nutrition is needed to address both poverty and chronic disease. Importantly, the report goes further to put nutrition in the context of educational standards and the need to confront climate change.

The UN Decade of Action on Nutrition [52] called for coordinated action on the double burden of malnutrition throughout the globe, namely the coexistence of undernutrition with overweight and obesity or nutrition-related non-communicable disease throughout the life course. Given the need for adequate nutrition in supporting growth, development and cognitive function, optimal nutrition is crucial to achieving the Sustainable Development Goals. Action relates to a number of contexts, including those related to the environment, population health and the home.

Decadal plans are also available at the Australian Academy of Science, with the 2017–26 plan for Agriculture currently available (see www.science.org.au/support/analysis/decadal-plans-science). In 2017, a discussion paper for Nutrition was developed and consultation undertaken (Table 24.7). Education and training was also addressed, recognising the interdisciplinary nature of nutrition science and the need for clearly defined scopes of practice (Figure 24.1).

TABLE 24.7 TOWARDS A DECADAL PLAN FOR AUSTRALIAN NUTRITION SCIENCE

Location of benefits	Nutrition science	New connections	Workshop topics
Informed preventive health approaches	Cause–effect mechanisms	Genomics, IT, big data analytics, environmental/ agricultural sciences	Solutions to nutrition science challenges
High-quality nutritious foods with economic benefits	Diet–health relationships	Nutrients–foods–dietary patterns	Context—environmental factors
Innovation in healthcare	Innovations in policy, products and services	Education, context and communications	Personalised nutrition

Source: Adapted from: Australian Academy of Science National Committee for Nutrition (2018). *Towards a Decadal Plan for Australian Nutrition Science*. Retrieved from: www.science.org.au/files/userfiles/support/national-committees/nutrition-decadal-plan-consultation-paper.pdf

FIGURE 24.1 SCOPE OF PRACTICE FRAMEWORK FOR NUTRITION

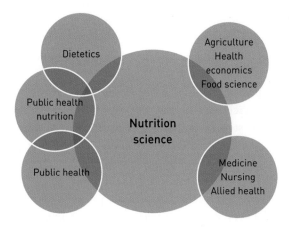

Source: Adapted from: www.science.org.au/nutrition

With an array of stakeholders in food, nutrition and health, clarity in terms of governance is critical to deal with issues such as concern about conflicts of interest [53–55]. This occurs in an environment dependent on cooperation and knowledge sharing to address the dual burdens of obesity and malnutrition.

Training in nutrition is central to these efforts. As with all areas of health, there are many dimensions, from basic understandings for personal use through to accredited professional practice and high-level research and policy development. Ongoing developments across the globe are being undertaken by authoritative and scientific bodies, including those associated with the Sustainable Development Goals [56] and collaborative nutrition education research centres (for example, www.nnedpro.org.uk).

The determinants of the spread of obesity across the globe are multiple and reflect conditions of the day. One analysis has shown 'globesity' may reflect more on social rather than economic factors, and more specifically the flow of information and social proximity. The analysis showed that one standard deviation in social globalisation was associated with a 13.7% increase in obesity [57]. This emphasises the role of social context in nutrition.

See Chapter 1 on research and policy development.

See Chapter 20 on social and behavioural aspects of food consumption.

LINDA TAPSELL

Population-based interventions should not only consider behaviour change but also the environments in which people live. Research should continue to question assumptions. For example, a recent Mediterranean diet intervention in rural North Carolina found, contrary to hypotheses, that participants living in less favourable environments (based on factors such as food outlet quality and exercise support) showed greater improvements in diet, physical activity and weight [58]. More research in this area will provide evidence for understanding and addressing the impact of social context on behaviour.

Interventions may achieve weight loss, but it is now well known and accepted that weight loss is usually not maintained [59]. Whether this is due to the pathophysiology of obesity, whereby mechanisms acting at the cellular and systems level defend the obese state, or recidivism in lifestyle behaviours remains open to debate, but the realities of prevalence have seen a move to view obesity as a chronic condition requiring long-term and possibly intermittent preventive health action. Monitoring weight-loss maintenance and weight regain has become a component of evaluating interventions, modifying the shape of ongoing research—for example, success is being redefined in realistic conditions, but there needs to be agreement on standards. A follow-up study on one of the largest preventive health trials involving nearly 1800 US participants, the Look AHEAD (Action for Health in Diabetes) trial found that different criteria were being used in the literature to classify people in terms of weight-loss maintenance or regain. The authors found a definition of regaining <25% of initial weight loss during maintenance was realistic [60]. This standard can now be used in clinical and population research on weight change.

Translating research to practice means more research needs to be conducted within the real-life context of health services. Examining the feasibility of routinely weighing patients in primary care services is a first step in building this platform [61]. From a nutrition perspective, evidence is being established on the effectiveness of individualised dietary counselling provided by accredited practising dietitians [62; 63]. As in any discipline, ensuring professional assessment and translation of evidence-based reviews to the individual context is now being shown for nutrition and health. Understanding how food delivers nutrients provides some in principle parallels with pharmacotherapy, but the delivery context is very different. Some aspects of pharmacodynamics may apply under more controlled conditions, but from a biological point of view, what food and nutrition delivers aligns more with multi-pharmacy. Most importantly, the consumption of food is set in a context that addresses social, cuisine and quality-of-life issues, including pleasure and enjoyment.

Thus, an appreciation of the interdisciplinary nature of nutrition and the inextricable link between food, nutrition and health provides the basic platform for launching the study of nutrition. While the applications are many, the origins and strengths of nutrition as a discipline lie in sound science. Translational pathways are critical for practices in healthcare, public policy and food innovation. Nutrition advice will evolve with science and so it will be modified with time, but transparency in evidence-based methodologies will enable this to occur effectively. New foods will continue to appear on the market and there is great opportunity for public good when this is aligned to nutrition principles—and it must be seen as an imperative. The study of food, nutrition and health has enormous potential to build a sustainable and healthy environment supporting productive populations sensitive to the ecosystem of which they are a part. There are many pathways to practice and vast opportunities for research. These all need to be built on a solid foundation of basic principles, and a willingness to challenge, question and continue learning along the way.

STOP AND THINK

- Why are we seeing a dual burden of disease across the globe?
- What are the differences between strategies targeting population health versus individuals?
- What elements of the food industry could play a significant role in addressing the double burden of disease, and how might this happen?

SUMMARY

- Nutrition science has gone through a number of stages of development, moving towards a greater emphasis on food and the need to integrate knowledge from an expanding scientific platform.
- Opportunities continue to emerge for improving health and quality of life through optimising food and applications of 'precision nutrition'.
- New methodologies, in which evidence is reviewed for effects of food on health, enable transparency and an ability to keep up with advancements in science.
- Nutrition-related disease can now be described at a global level, with a focus on the double burden of malnutrition and obesity.
- Strategies for dealing with global nutrition problems have been developed by international and national agencies and relate to all levels of society and governance.
- Future directions in food, nutrition and health reflect developments in science and technology, with global challenges that require multidisciplinary research teams and strong foundations in nutrition principles.

PATHWAYS TO PRACTICE

- There are many career paths associated with food, nutrition and health, where the focus may vary from working with food itself, to healthcare contexts, environment and policy.

- As food is fundamental to health, all registered healthcare providers should have an appreciation of basic nutrition principles and the ability to discern between core and discretionary foods. In addition to a basic education in nutrition science, accredited practising dietitians have health professional skills training and must meet requirements for continuing professional development. They are recognised by Australian health authorities to treat and manage nutrition-related conditions.

- Nutrition research can be undertaken in a range of contexts—for example, from molecular biology to animal model studies, clinical trials, epidemiology and social/behavioural research. The line of inquiry may need a range of research capacities, even within the nutrition discipline, making integrated teams better able to deliver across the translational spectrum.

- Linking food scientists to nutritionists is an important step in building a healthier food supply.

- Evidence-based statements, standards and guidelines are regularly provided by authoritative agencies (e.g. World Health Organization, US Department of Agriculture and National Health and Medical Research Council) and should be a first reference point in dealing with food, nutrition and health issues.

DISCUSSION QUESTIONS

1 What are some of the big questions that research in food and nutrition should address today?

2 How can the discipline of nutrition maintain an identity in an ever-expanding field?

3 What is the role of standards—for example, in research, publishing, media reporting, professional education, healthcare practice and collaborative work? Who is responsible for them?

4 How can the complex science of nutrition be communicated so that it is 'made as simple as possible, but not simpler'?

USEFUL WEBLINKS

Academy of Nutrition and Dietetics:
www.eatright.org

Academy of Nutrition and Dietetics—Evidence Analysis Library:
www.andeal.org

American College of Cardiology:
www.acc.org

Australian Academy of Science—Decadal plans for science:
www.science.org.au/support/analysis/decadal-plans-science

Centre for Food & Allergy Research:
http://foodallergyresearch.org.au

Dietitians Association of Australia:
https://daa.asn.au

Food Standards Australia New Zealand:
www.foodstandards.gov.au/Pages/default.aspx

National Health and Medical Research Council—Health topics:
www.nhmrc.gov.au/health-topics

NNEdPro Global Centre for Nutrition and Health:
www.nnedpro.org.uk

Nutrition Society of Australia:
www.nsa.asn.au

Unpack the Salt:
www.unpackthesalt.com.au

US Department of Agriculture—Food and nutrition:
www.usda.gov/topics/food-and-nutrition

World Health Organization—Nutrition:
www.who.int/nutrition/en

FURTHER READING

Binks, M. & Chin, S. H. (2017). What are the challenges in developing effective health policies for obesity? *International Journal of Obesity*, 41, 849. doi:10.1038/ijo.2017.1

FOOD, NUTRITION AND HEALTH

FOOD, NUTRITION AND HEALTH

SECOND EDITION

EDITED BY LINDA TAPSELL

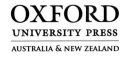

OXFORD

UNIVERSITY PRESS

AUSTRALIA & NEW ZEALAND

Oxford University Press is a department of the University of Oxford.
It furthers the University's objective of excellence in research,
scholarship, and education by publishing worldwide. Oxford is a registered
trademark of Oxford University Press in the UK and in certain other
countries.

Published in Australia by
Oxford University Press
Level 8, 737 Bourke Street, Docklands, Victoria 3008, Australia.

© Linda Tapsell 2019

The moral rights of the author/s have been asserted

First published 2013
Second Edition

A catalogue record for this
book is available from the
National Library of Australia

ISBN 9780190304867

Edited by Anne Mulvaney
Cover design by OUPANZ
Cover Image: Shutterstock
Text design by Sardine Design
Typeset by Newgen KnowledgeWorks Pvt. Ltd., Chennai, India
Proofread by Pete Cruttenden
Indexed by Jenny Browne
Printed in China by Golden Cup Printing Co. Ltd.

CONTENTS

EXTENDED CONTENTS

CHAPTER 8: WATER, ALCOHOL AND BEVERAGES
Vinodkumar Gopaldasani and Rebecca Thorne

CHAPTER 9: FAT-SOLUBLE VITAMINS: A, D, E AND K
Olivia Wright, Vicki Flood and Linda Tapsell

CHAPTER 10: WATER-SOLUBLE VITAMINS: B AND C
Linda Tapsell

CHAPTER 11: MAJOR MINERALS: SODIUM, POTASSIUM, CALCIUM, MAGNESIUM AND PHOSPHORUS
Linda Tapsell

OXFORD UNIVERSITY PRESS

LIST OF FIGURES AND TABLES

FIGURES

TABLES

OXFORD UNIVERSITY PRESS

OXFORD UNIVERSITY PRESS

LIST OF CASE STUDIES

OXFORD UNIVERSITY PRESS

OXFORD UNIVERSITY PRESS

LIST OF ABBREVIATIONS

AA	arachidonic acid
ABS	Australian Bureau of Statistics
ADH	anti-diuretic hormone
AEE	activity energy expenditure
AGHE	Australian Guide to Healthy Eating
AI	adequate intake
AIHW	Australian Institute of Health and Welfare
AMD	age-related macular degeneration
AMDR	acceptable macronutrient distribution range
AOAC	Association of Official Analytical Chemists
APD	accredited practising dietitian
AUSNUT	Australian Food and Nutrient Database
BGL	blood glucose level
BMI	body mass index
BMR	basal metabolic rate
CDC	Centers for Disease Control and Prevention
CHO	carbohydrate
CHS	Cardiovascular Health Study
CKD	chronic kidney disease
CMRF	cardiometabolic risk factors
CSIRO	Commonwealth Scientific and Industrial Research Organisation
CVD	cardiovascular disease
DASH	Dietary Approaches to Stop Hypertension
DIT	diet-induced thermogenesis
DNA	deoxyribonucleic acid
DPA	docosahexaenoic acid
EAR	estimated average requirement
EER	estimated energy requirement
EPA	eicosapentaenoic acid
FAO	Food and Agriculture Organization (United Nations)

FDA	Food and Drug Administration (USA)
FFQ	food frequency questionnaire
FOS	fructo oligosaccharides
FSANZ	Food Standards Australia New Zealand
GDM	gestational diabetes mellitus
GI	glycaemic index
GOS	galacto oligosaccharides
GRAS	generally recognised as safe
HACCP	Hazard Analysis Critical Control Point
HDL	high-density lipoprotein
HFAB	Healthy Food Access Basket
IDA	iron deficiency anaemia
IDD	iodine deficiency disorders
IDL	intermediate-density lipoprotein
LA	linoleic acid
LBM	lean body mass
LCN	low-calorie sweetener
LCPUFA	long chain polyunsaturated fatty acids
LDL	low-density lipoprotein
LOAEL	lowest observed adverse effect level
LOS	length of stay
MAMP	microbe associated molecular patterns
MCT	medium chain triglyceride
ME	metabolisable energy
MET	metabolic equivalent
MNA	Mini Nutritional Assessment
MUFA	monounsaturated fatty acid
NHMRC	National Health and Medical Research Council
NIP	nutrition information panel
NOAEL	no adverse effect level
NRV	Nutrient Reference Values
NUTTAB	Nutrient Tables for Australian Foods
PAL	physical activity level
PCA	principal component analysis

OXFORD UNIVERSITY PRESS

PHF	potentially hazardous food
PMSEIC	Prime Minister's Science, Engineering and Innovation Council
PTN	protein
PUFA	polyunsaturated fatty acids
RCT	randomised controlled trial
RDI	recommended dietary intake
REE	resting energy expenditure
ROS	reactive oxygen species
SCFA	short chain fatty acids
SDT	suggested dietary target
SES	socioeconomic status
SFA	saturated fatty acids
SSB	sugar-sweetened beverage
TEF	thermic effect of food
TFA	trans fatty acids
UIC	urinary iodine concentration
UL	upper level of intake
UPF	ultra-processed food
USI	universal salt iodisation
VDR	vitamin D receptor
VLDL	very-low-density lipoprotein
WHAS	Women's Health and Aging Studies
WHO	World Health Organization

ABOUT THE EDITOR

LINDA TAPSELL AM PHD FDAA

Linda Tapsell is a Senior Professor, Nutrition and Dietetics in the School of Medicine at the University of Wollongong, and the Illawarra Health and Medical Research Institute, New South Wales. She holds a Bachelor of Science (Biochemistry and Pharmacology) and Post Graduate Diploma in Nutrition and Dietetics from the University of Sydney, a Masters of Health Personnel Education from the University of New South Wales and a PhD in Nutrition and Public Health from the University of Wollongong. Professor Tapsell began her career in healthcare working in large teaching hospitals and community health. She has been an academic for 28 years, teaching multitudes of nutrition and dietetic students and supervising more than 20 PhD graduates. She has had a stellar research career, having led two major food research centres and been the chief investigator of dietary trials conducted over a 25-year period examining the effects of food consumption on health. Professor Tapsell has had over 200 articles published in scientific journals and has served on a number of national and international nutrition science advisory committees, including those relating to grant reviews, dietary guidelines and nutrient reference values. She is a Fellow of both the Dietitians Association of Australia (DAA) and the Nutrition Society of Australia, and a long-standing member of the American Society of Nutrition. In 2015, Professor Tapsell was named a member of the Order of Australia (AM) for 'significant service to health science as an academic and clinician specialising in diet and nutrition'.

OXFORD UNIVERSITY PRESS

CONTRIBUTORS

ANNE MCMAHON

Dr Anne-Therese McMahon is a Senior Lecturer at the University of Wollongong whose research focuses on understanding food behaviour and health outcomes. Her work primarily draws upon qualitative health research methodologies to understand complex human behaviour from the perspectives of the participants themselves. Dr McMahon is now also broadening her work to include planetary health imperatives and intersections with human health, focusing her attention on food sustainability practices. This includes identifying, implementing and evaluating local and international food initiatives involving students, community partners and researchers in public health and nutrition disciplines with a view to supporting healthy communities overall.

ANNETTE MURPHY

Annette Murphy is a Senior Clinical Dietitian working at the John Hunter Hospital in Newcastle. She has nearly 20 years of experience working in research fields and as a clinical dietitian. She has held positions as a Lecturer at the University of Newcastle in the areas of Paediatric Dietetics and Community and Clinical Dietetics. She has co-authored numerous book chapters and assisted in the writing of a number of academic papers.

CLARE COLLINS

Professor Clare Collins is a National Health and Medical Research Council (NHMRC) Senior Research Fellow, Professor of Nutrition and Dietetics and Director of Research for the School of Health Sciences, Faculty of Health and Medicine, and Deputy Director, Priority Research Centre in Physical Activity and Nutrition at the University of Newcastle. In 2017, Professor Collins was awarded the Hunter Medical Research Institute's Researcher of the Year. Her research areas include dietary intake assessment and evaluating the impact of food and nutrition across key life stages and chronic disease conditions. Professor Collins is a Fellow of the DAA, has published over 300 manuscripts, supervised 25 higher degree research candidates, has been a DAA media spokesperson for 18 years and is a sought-after nutrition media commentator.

ELIZABETH NEALE

Dr Elizabeth Neale is an Accredited Practising Dietitian whose current role is as a Career Development Fellow (Lecturer) in the School of Medicine at the University of Wollongong. Dr Neale's research focuses on the evidence-based framework in nutrition, with a particular focus on the methodologies of systematic reviews and meta-analyses in nutrition. She also has research expertise in exploring the impact of whole foods and dietary patterns on risk factors for chronic diseases.

GARY DYKES

Professor Gary Dykes is currently the Acting Head, School of Public Health at Curtin University. He holds a PhD in microbiology from the University of the Witwatersrand in South Africa.

Professor Dykes is an experienced researcher who has pursued a diverse international career spanning a number of research organisations and universities in South Africa, New Zealand, Canada and Malaysia, as well as in Australia. He is an active researcher in the area of public health microbiology with a focus on enteric bacterial foodborne pathogens and has published widely in this area.

JOANNA RUSSELL

Dr Joanna Russell is a public health nutritionist, lecturer and early career researcher based in the Faculty of Social Sciences at the University of Wollongong. She was awarded her PhD in 2014 and her research focuses on the methodological challenges of measuring population level food security and diet quality. Building on her PhD research, Dr Russell is involved in developing appropriate measurement tools to assess food security in Australian older adults.

KANITA KUNARATNAM

Kanita Kunaratnam is currently pursuing her PhD at the University of Sydney, looking into child and maternal dietary patterns. She has a background in nutrition and dietetics and has over 10 years of experience working as a dietitian in many different settings including hospitals, public health and community health. Her research interests are in child and maternal nutrition, nutrition policy and public health, and childhood obesity. As a mother of three young children, she thoroughly enjoys combining the experience of motherhood and parenting with evidence-based research to positively influence the growth and development of children.

KAREN CHARLTON

Dr Karen Charlton, PhD AdvAPD RPHNutr, is an Associate Professor who teaches public health nutrition at the University of Wollongong. She researches the role of diet in the prevention and management of chronic diseases, particularly hypertension and cognitive decline. She advocates for improved models of nutritional care across the lifespan, from pregnancy to nutrition in old age. Her work has been translated into policy, in the context of salt reduction strategies and iodine deficiency.

KAREN WALTON

Dr Karen Walton is an Advanced Accredited Practising Dietitian and an Associate Professor at the University of Wollongong. Her research interests include nutrition support for older adults in the community, hospitals and residential aged care; particularly regarding access to food and beverage packaging and food service interventions to enhance dietary intakes among older adults.

KRISTINE PEZDIRC

Dr Kristine Pezdirc works as a clinical trial project officer in the School of Medicine and Public Health at the University of Newcastle. She was awarded her PhD from the University of Newcastle in February 2016. She also completed a Bachelor of Nutrition and Dietetics (Hons I) at the University of Newcastle in 2010. Dr Pezdirc's research areas of interest include young adults, fruit and vegetable intake, biomarkers (carotenoids) and skin colour.

LAUREN WILLIAMS

Professor Lauren Williams is Head of Discipline of Nutrition and Dietetics at Griffith University, and has honorary professorial appointments at the University of Newcastle and the University of Canberra.

Her undergraduate degree was in science (Honours) and she also holds tertiary qualifications in social science, health promotion and dietetics, and a PhD in public health nutrition. Professor Williams has been an academic for over 25 years, primarily in dietetic education, and previously worked as a public health nutritionist. Lauren has published books, book chapters and journal articles in her research areas of weight control, gendered dieting, the rural and allied health workforce, and the sociological aspects of food and eating. She has co-edited four editions of the OUP academic text and reader *A Sociology of Food and Nutrition: The Social Appetite* with John Germov. She is a Fellow of the DAA.

LEE ASHTON

Dr Lee Ashton is a Postdoctoral researcher in the Priority Research Centre for Physical Activity and Nutrition at the University of Newcastle. He was awarded his PhD from the University of Newcastle in March 2017. He also completed a Master of Science in Nutrition, Obesity & Health at the University of Leeds in 2011 and a Bachelor of Science (Hons) in Sport and Exercise Science at Leeds Beckett University in 2010, both in the United Kingdom. His research investigates physical activity and nutrition for population health, with particular emphasis on health promotion strategies for chronic disease prevention and well-being.

MICHAEL LEVERITT

Dr Michael Leveritt is a Senior Lecturer in Nutrition and Dietetics at the University of Queensland. His research and teaching activities focus on developing a better understanding of how nutrition can positively enhance athlete participation, well-being and performance in a variety of sport and exercise contexts. He is a passionate educator, practitioner and researcher with over 100 peer-reviewed research publications and his career to date has included positions with the Australian Institute of Sport as well as academic positions in New Zealand and the United Kingdom.

OLIVIA WRIGHT

Dr Olivia Wright is a Lecturer in Nutrition and Dietetics at the University of Queensland. She is passionate about helping people to remain healthy as they age, enjoys assisting the food and nutraceutical industry to design and trial innovative products to assist people's well-being, and is driven to provide high-quality education through novel teaching and assessment strategies. She has published over 30 research papers and has mentored numerous postgraduate students to achieve their nutrition practice and/or research goals. Dr Wright has a strong focus on research collaboration across disciplines and has achieved continued success in multidisciplinary research.

RANIL COOREY

Dr Ranil Coorey he is a Senior Lecturer at Curtin University. He has developed commercial food safety management systems and worked in the food industry in research and development and product innovation. His research includes a variety of industry-funded projects on chicken and red meat safety. These projects have included active packaging for microbial inactivation, modelling storage temperature and spoilage-related changes to the microbial flora and biochemistry of meat. Dr Coorey also holds an international collaborative research project on safe chicken processing. He teachers food safety and food processing and has published in these areas.